Current Trends in Immunity and Respiratory Infections

Current Trends in Immunity and Respiratory Infections

Editor: Nikolas Stephen

AMERICAN
MEDICAL PUBLISHERS
www.americanmedicalpublishers.com

American Medical Publishers
www.americanmedicalpublishers.com

Cataloging-in-Publication Data

Current trends in immunity and respiratory infections / edited by Nikolas Stephen.
p. cm.
Includes bibliographical references and index.
ISBN 979-8-88740-039-6
1. Respiratory infections. 2. Respiratory infections--Immunological aspects.
3. Respiratory infections--Immunodiagnosis. 4. Infection. 5. Respiratory organs--Diseases.
6. Immune system. 7. Immunology. I. Stephen, Nikolas.
RC740 .C87 2023
616.2--dc23

American Medical Publishers,
41 Flatbush Avenue,
1st Floor, New York,
NY 11217, USA

ISBN 979-8-88740-039-6 (Hardback)

Contents

Preface

Respiratory infections or respiratory tract infections (RTIs) are infections that lead to diseases that affect the respiratory tract. Infections of the respiratory tract may be caused due to microbes like virus, bacteria, and fungi. The common respiratory tract infections include common cold, pneumonia, bronchitis and tonsillitis. All beings have an innate ability to resist and fight with infection causing agents and this ability is known as immunity. In case of RTIs, immunity acts as the protective line of defense. Researchers have been working to understand respiratory immunopathology by understanding the mechanisms involved in human body fighting different types of RTIs. Such knowledge would be important for developing effective therapies for treatment and prevention of RTIs. The aim of this book is to present breakthrough researches that have been conducted on respiratory tract infections. It also discusses the role of immunity with respect to respiratory infections. This book will help the readers in keeping pace with the rapid changes in this area of study.

This book is the end result of constructive efforts and intensive research done by experts in this field. The aim of this book is to enlighten the readers with recent information in this area of research. The information provided in this profound book would serve as a valuable reference to students and researchers in this field.

At the end, I would like to thank all the authors for devoting their precious time and providing their valuable contribution to this book. I would also like to express my gratitude to my fellow colleagues who encouraged me throughout the process.

Editor

1

Necrosis Driven Triglyceride Synthesis Primes Macrophages for Inflammation During *Mycobacterium tuberculosis* Infection

Neetika Jaisinghani[1,2], Stanzin Dawa[1,2†], Kaurab Singh[1,2†], Ananya Nandy[1,2†], Dilip Menon[1,2†], Purva Deepak Bhandari[1,2†], Garima Khare[3], Anil Tyagi[3,4] and Sheetal Gandotra[1,2†]*

[1] Chemical and Systems Biology Group, CSIR-Institute of Genomics and Integrative Biology, New Delhi, India, [2] Academy of Scientific and Innovative Research (AcSIR), New Delhi, India, [3] Department of Biochemistry, University of Delhi South Campus, New Delhi, India, [4] Guru Gobind Singh Indraprastha University, New Delhi, India

***Correspondence:**
Sheetal Gandotra
sheetal.gandotra@igib.res.in

Pulmonary tuberculosis (TB) exhibits granulomatous inflammation, a site of controlling bacterial dissemination at the cost of host tissue damage. Intrigued by the granuloma type-dependent expression of inflammatory markers in TB, we sought to investigate underlying metabolic changes that drive amplification of inflammation in TB. Here, we show an association of higher inflammation in necrotic granulomas with the presence of triglyceride (TG)-rich foamy macrophages. The conspicuous absence of these macrophages in solid granulomas identified a link between the ensuing pathology and the metabolic programming of foamy macrophages. Consistent with *in vivo* findings, *in vitro* infection of macrophages with *Mycobacterium tuberculosis* (Mtb) led to increase in TG synthesis only under conditions of ~60% necrosis. Genetic and pharmacologic intervention that reduced necrosis prevented this bystander response. We further demonstrate that necrosis independent of Mtb also elicits the same bystander response in human macrophages. We identified a role for the human enzyme involved in TG synthesis, diacylglycerol *O*-acyltransferase (DGAT1), in this phenomenon. The increased TG levels in necrosis-associated foamy macrophages promoted the pro-inflammatory state of macrophages to infection while silencing expression of diacylglycerol *O*-acyltransferase (DGAT1) suppressed expression of pro-inflammatory genes. Our data thus invoke a role for storage lipids in the heightened host inflammatory response during infection-associated necrosis. Our data provide a functional role to macrophage lipid droplets in host defense and open new avenues for developing host-directed therapies against TB.

Keywords: necrosis, tuberculosis, macrophage, triglyceride, inflammation

INTRODUCTION

Tuberculosis (TB) is the major cause of worldwide mortality due to any single infectious agent (1). Inflammation in TB plays a dual role—onset of the innate inflammatory response is crucial for the recruitment and activation of macrophages while dysregulation of this response leads to disease exacerbation (2). The inflammatory response in TB also contributes to tissue necrosis and

Abbreviations: Mtb, *Mycobacterium tuberculosis*; TB, tuberculosis; MOI, multiplicity of infection; NcS, necrotic cell supplement; NAFMs, necrosis-associated foamy macrophages.

cavitation which is the characteristic end-stage tissue damage (3, 4) leading to chronic impairment of pulmonary function (5, 6). Moreover, the heterogeneity of the inflammatory response in human TB granulomas within the same tissue suggests that local alterations in macrophage function might lead to gradation of responses (7, 8). Understanding the trajectory of macrophage fate during infection holds key to targeting immunopathogenesis of an active TB infection.

We sought to investigate if local metabolic alterations can alter the inflammatory response of human macrophages to the bacilli. The importance of lipid metabolism in infection induced inflammatory response has emerged from benefits of treatments that target lipid metabolism in preclinical models of TB (9). These models have revealed that nuclear receptors responsive to lipids, such as peroxisome proliferator-activated receptor-γ and liver X receptors (LXRα and LXRβ), protect against TB by regulating both pro- and anti-inflammatory pathways (9, 10). In addition, targeting the synthesis of lipid mediators of inflammation derived from arachidonic acid, by the non-steroidal anti-inflammatory drug Ibuprofen, has shown promise toward limiting pathology in the mouse model of infection (11). Given that triglyceride (TG) is a major lipid in human TB granulomas (12) and acts as a sink of fatty acids and signaling mediators such as diacylglycerides, phosphatidic acid, and phospholipids, its role in TB infection needs to be addressed. Understanding the mechanistic basis for differentiation of macrophages to TG-rich foamy macrophages during infection would be the first step in addressing whether TGs are important in control of inflammation and essential for bacterial survival.

In an attempt to understand the relationship of local inflammatory responses and TG accumulation in foamy macrophages, we established an association between high TNFα expression and appearance of TG-rich foamy macrophages in guinea pig granulomas. Both were conspicuously present in regions surrounding necrosis. Using a combination of biochemical and genetic tools we demonstrate that, during *Mycobacterium tuberculosis* (Mtb) infection of macrophages, necrosis is key to the increase in TG synthesis and accumulation in bystander cells. Importantly, we describe an *ex vivo* model of necrosis-associated foamy macrophages (NAFMs). These lipid-laden foamy macrophages mount a heightened inflammatory response to infection which can be suppressed by targeting diacylglycerol *O*-acyltransferase (DGAT1). Together, our data demonstrate that necrosis-associated inflammatory responses in TB may be mediated through bystander TG accumulation.

MATERIALS AND METHODS

Cell Culture and Reagents

THP1 monocytes obtained from ECACC were cultured in RPMI 1640 (with glutamax, high glucose, HEPES, and sodium pyruvate) from Himedia with 10% FBS from Himedia. Phorbol 12-myristate 13-acetate (PMA), orlistat, T863 (2-((1,4-trans)-4-(4-(4-Amino-7,7-dimethyl-7H-pyrimido[4,5-b][1,4]oxazin-6-yl)- phenyl) cyclohexyl)acetic acid), chlorpromazine (CPZ) (C8138), and C75 (4-Methylene-2-octyl-5-oxotetrahydrofuran-3-carboxylic acid) were obtained from Sigma, IM54 (ALX-430-137-M001) was obtained from Enzo life sciences. THP1 monocyte culture media were analyzed for *Mycoplasma* contamination using a luminescence based kit (*Lonza*, LT07-118). THP1 cell line authentication was performed at Lifecode technologies Private Limited using 10 genetic loci *viz*: TH01, D21S11, D5S818, D13S317, D7S820, D16S539, CSF1PO, AMEL, vWA, and TPOX. The sample genotypes were queried against reference genotypes available in ATCC and DSMZ® reference cell line STR databases to authenticate sample identity. Mtb H37Rv and *Mycobacterium bovis* BCG Tokyo were kind gifts from Dr. Vivek Rao, ΔRD1, and its wild-type control were kind gifts of Dr. David Sherman and Dr. Krishnamohan Atmakuri. Mycobacterial strains were transformed with the plasmids expressing fluorescent reporter proteins. pCherry3 was a kind gift from Dr. Tanya Parish (addgene#24659), pMV261-emGFP was a kind gift from Dr. Vivek Rao, and pTEC18 was kind gift from Dr. Lalita Ramakrishnan (addgene#30177).

Guinea Pig Lung Histology Analysis

Guinea pigs were infected with Mtb H37Rv *via* the respiratory route in an aerosol chamber (Inhalation exposure system, Glas-Col, IN, USA) at ~30 cfu per animal. At week 4 and week 10 post infection, three guinea pigs per time point were euthanized by using CO_2 asphyxiation. After dissecting the animals, three lobes (right caudal, middle, and cranial) of each lung were fixed in 10% buffered formalin. The left caudal portion of the lung was used for the enumeration of the bacillary load. For this, the left caudal portion was weighed and homogenized in 5 ml saline in a polytron PT2100 homogenizer followed by plating on 7H11(OADC) media. Colony counts were extrapolated for the whole lung based on weight of the left caudal lobe and the entire lung for each animal. Macroscopic granulomatous tissues were cut from the lung and kept in 20% sucrose solution overnight at 4°C followed by cryosectioning at section depth of 5 μm using *Leica Cryostat CM 1850*.

Hematoxylin and Eosin Staining

Sections on the slides were rehydrated using water for 5 min. The slides were then dipped in hematoxylin solution (1:10 Delafield's Hematoxylin solution) for 5 min and then rinsed in water. The slides were then stain intensified by placing in ammonia solution (0.08%) for 1 min, followed by rinsing in water for 5 min. The sections were then equilibrated in 95% ethanol solution followed by dipping them in eosin stain (1%) for 15 s. The sections were then dehydrated in 95% and 100% ethanol for 2 min in each solution, and finally rinsed in water for 5 min. The slides were then cleaned and mounted using 20% glycerol.

Hematoxylin and Oil Red O Staining

The sections were first dipped in a prewarmed Oil Red O solution (0.18% in 60% isopropanol) for 1 h at 60°C, then rinsed twice with water for 5 min each. The slides were then dipped in hematoxylin solution for 5 min, rinsed, and mounted in 20% glycerol. Images were acquired using Leedz Microimaging 5 MP camera attached to a Nikon Ti-U microscope. Analysis was performed by four individuals independently including a trained pathologist.

Immunofluorescence of Guinea Pig Lung Sections

Serial sections to those used for oil red O staining were used for TNFα and MAC1 immunostaining. TNFα immunostaining: sections were blocked with 5% bovine serum albumin (BSA) for 1 h, followed by overnight incubation with anti-TNFα antibodies (1:50, ab1793). Alexa-633 tagged secondary antibody was used for detecting the primary antibody reactivity, followed by DAPI counterstaining. Images were acquired using a laser scanning microscope in the widefield mode. MAC1 immunostaining: cryosections were incubated with 0.25% Tween-20 in 1× PBS for 10 min for permeabilization, sections were rinsed thrice with 1× PBS for 10 min each. Sections were incubated with primary antibody, 1:50 dilutions, Anti-MAC [MAC387] (ab22506) for 2 h at room temperature after blocking with 1% BSA for 1 h. Sections were then incubated with Alexa 633 conjugated secondary antibody (1:200 dilutions, Life Technologies, A21052) for 30 min at room temperature, sections were washed well with 1× PBS thrice for 10 min each. Sections were counterstained with BODIPY 493/505 for 1 h at room temperature. Coverslips were mounted on the sections using Prolong Diamond Antifade mountant with DAPI. Images were acquired using Leica SP8 Confocal microscope.

Extraction of Lipids From Granulomatous Lesions of Guinea Pig Lungs

Visible lesions from infected lungs and anatomically comparable regions from uninfected lungs were dissected out at indicated time points and then weighed. These tissues were then sonicated in 600 μl of chloroform:methanol (2:1) at 60°C in a water bath sonicator. Lipids were extracted using the modified Bligh and Dyer method by first making the sonicated extract to 1,200 μl of chloroform:methanol (1:2) by adding 600 μl of methanol. One-fourth volume of 50 mM citric acid, half volume of water, and one-fourth volume of chloroform were added and vortexed. This was then centrifuged at 9,600 *g* for 10 min and then the lower phase taken and dried. The dried lipid extracts were weighed and then resuspended in chloroform:methanol (2:1) such that the concentration of the extract was 0.1 mg/μl and extracts corresponding to 0.5 mg were loaded on TLC. TLCs were developed in 4°C in the solvent system hexane:diethyl ether:acetic acid (70:30:1) for neutral lipids.

DGAT1 Knockdown

Lentiviral particles for *DGAT1* knockdown were obtained from Transomic technologies (shRNA sequences used DGAT1 pZIP-hEF1 alpha zsgreen: TGCTGTTGACAGTGAGCGCCCTAC CGGGATGTCAACCTGATAGTGAAGCCACAGATG TATCAGGTTGACATCCCGGTAGGATGCCTACTGCCTC GGA).

50,000 THP1 monocytes were transduced with lentiviral particles at multiplicity of infection (MOI) 10 for 24 h. Transduced cell lines were maintained for stable cell line generation in puromycin at 0.6 μg/ml for about 3–4 weeks. Knockdown efficiency was checked using qRT-PCR and also validated using TG analysis from TLC.

RNA Isolation and qRT-PCR Analysis

1.2 million cells were used for isolation of RNA from a single replicate of a condition, with three replicate wells per experiment. Cells were infected at MOI 50 for 3 h. The monolayers were washed three times with media and replaced with RPMI media supplemented with 10% FBS. At 24 h post infection, cells were scraped in TRIzol (Ambion) or RNAzolRT (Sigma). RNA was extracted into the aqueous phase, precipitated, and further purified using the Qiagen RNeasy kit or by organic precipitation. The purified RNA was DNase treated using Turbo DNAse (*Ambion, AM2238*) for 1 h at 37°C. 1 μg of purified RNA was used for cDNA synthesis (*Invitrogen, 18080-093*). cDNA was diluted 10 times and 2 μl of the diluted cDNA was used for expression analysis of selected genes by qRT-PCR (*Roche, LightCycler Sybr green master mix, 04707516001*). Primer sequences used for qRT-PCR were as follows:

Gene name	Primer	Sequence
PPIA	Forward	ATGCTGGACCCAACACAAAT
	Reverse	TCTTTCACTTTGCCAAACACC
DGAT1	Forward	GCCTGCAGGATTCTTTCTTC
	Reverse	AGACATTGGCCGCAATAACC
TNFA	Forward	CCCCAGGGACCTCTCTCTAATC
	Reverse	GGTTTGCTACAACATGGGCTACA
IL1B	Forward	CTCGCCAGTGAAATGATGGCT
	Reverse	GTCGGAGATTCGTAGCTGGAT

Lipid Extraction From Macrophages (Modified Bligh and Dyer Method)

For making a total lipid extract from THP1 monocyte-derived macrophage and human MDMs, the cells were first washed with PBS twice and then lysed in 1% Triton X100. After lysis, four volumes of methanol:chloroform (2:1) was added, and the lysate was vortexed. One volume of 50 mM citric acid, one volume of water, and one volume of chloroform were added and vortexed. This was then centrifuged at 10,000 *g* for 10 min, and then the lower phase isolated and dried. The dried lipid extract was then resuspended in chloroform:methanol (2:1) and loaded on TLC. TLCs were developed in 4°C in the solvent system hexanes:diethyl ether:acetic acid (70:30:1) for neutral lipids. For cholesterol estimation, the TLCs were pre-run in chloroform:methanol (90:10) followed by baking them at 110°C for 30 min. After spotting the samples and standards, the TLCs were developed sequentially in solvent system 1: chloroform:methanol:water (65:25:4) and solvent system 2: hexane:diethyl ether:acetic acid (70:30:2).

For visualization of unlabeled lipids on TLC, the TLCs were stained either using 10% copper sulfate (w/v) in 8% phosphoric acid (v/v) solution or phosphomolybdic acid (10% in ethanol) solution followed by charring at 150°C. Quantification of unlabeled lipid spots was done using ImageJ.

Measurement of Cellular TG Synthesis

THP-1 monocytes were differentiated into macrophages using 100 μM PMA at a density of 0.6 million cells/ml for 24 h, followed by 2 days in media without PMA. Subsequently, cells were infected with Mtb H37Rv at respective MOI for 24 h, in the presence of general lipase inhibitor orlistat (13) and 1 μCi/ml C^{14} oleic acid (*ARC0297*) or 1 μM BODIPY558/568C12 as described previously (14). This duration of treatment and concentration of orlistat was not found to affect mycobacterial viability. Total cellular lipids were extracted at 24 h post addition of pulse using the modified Bligh and Dyer method, dried, and then analyzed using thin layer chromatography. TLCs were scanned using the Typhoon Scanner and densitometry analysis performed using Image Quant 5.2. Fatty acid incorporation into TG during necrotic cell supplement (NcS) stimulation was measured in the same manner as explained above.

Cell Death Assays

Annexin V and Propidium Iodide (PI) Staining

THP1 macrophages seeded at a density of 0.6 million cells/ml were infected with Mtb, MtbΔRD1, or *M. bovis* BCG at indicated MOI. Cell death by apoptosis or necrosis in macrophages infected with different strains was quantified by Alexa Flour® 488 Annexin V/Dead cell Apoptosis kit from Invitrogen. This was done at 8 h post infection rather than 24 h as in all other experiments so as to reduce likelihood of secondary necrosis being measured along with primary necrosis. This also allowed sufficient number of cells to be left for accurate quantification of % annexin and PI positivity in case of wild-type H37Rv without analysis being skewed by the decrease in total number of cells. Monoloyers were washed with 1× Annexin binding buffer twice, and then stained with 10 μl Alexa Flour 488 Annexin V and 1 μl of 10 mg/ml PI in 100 μl of 1× Annexin binding buffer for 15 min at room temperature. Monolayers were again washed with buffer twice and fixed with 4% formaldehyde for 30 min at room temperature. The coverslips were washed with PBS and mounted using ProLong Antifade with DAPI. Wide field z-stacks were acquired using Leica TCS SP8 (40× objective) followed by counting annexin V or PI positive cells manually from five images for each group.

Lactate Dehydrogenase Release Assay

Culture supernatants from uninfected and infected THP1 macrophages were used for LDH activity assays using Cytotoxicity detection kit from Roche. Cell death was enumerated as a percentage of cells dying in treatment groups as compared to cell death in cells treated with Triton X100 (lysis buffer in kit).

Cell Death Estimation by Cell Counts

THP1 macrophage monolayer was fixed with 4% formaldehyde for 15 min at room temperature followed by washing with PBS three times for 5 min each. Cells were then stained with 2% DAPI solution for 30 min at room temperature followed by washing with PBS three times for 5 min each. 10 images for each well were acquired in EVOS Floid cell imaging system using the UV lamp. Images from different groups were subjected to cell counts using Volocity software from Perkin Elmer.

Supernatant Transfer Experiments

Donor Cell Preparation

THP1 macrophages were seeded in 12-well plates at a density of 0.6 million cells per well, and their lipids were labeled using BODIPY 558/568 C12 overnight. Post 16 h of labeling, they were washed with PBS to remove the extracellular label and then infected at MOI 50 for 24 h in the presence or absence of IM54 (20 μM). After 24 h, the supernatant was collected and transferred to recipient cells thought a 0.45 μm transwell filter (Milipore). *Recipient cells*: THP1 macrophages were seeded on coverslips in 12-well plates. Third day after differentiation with as above, medium was changed to supernatant from infected macrophages (for each well supernatant for three wells were combined) through the filter. CPZ (10 μM) was added to recipient cells during treatment. After 48 h of treatment, coverslips were fixed and stained with BODIPY493/503, followed by confocal microscopy.

Immunofluorescence

Cells were fixed using neutral buffered, methanol-free 4% formaldehyde, permeabilized using 0.5% Saponin, blocked with 3% BSA, and incubated overnight with primary antibodies. Primary antibodies used for immunostaining: CD44 (BD Pharmingen 550392) and Adipophilin (ADRP) (Progen 610102). Secondary antibodies used for detection were highly cross adsorbed antibodies conjugated to Alexa fluor dyes (Invitrogen).

Lipid Droplet (LD) Imaging and Analysis

Lipid droplet size distribution in THP1 cells expressing either non-targeting shRNA or shRNA against *DGAT1* was performed using InCell6000 (GE) in the confocal mode. Two days post PMA removal, they were treated with 1 μM BODIPY665/676 or LipidTox Deep Red to visualize LDs. 10 min post staining, cells were imaged. LDs were identified using built-in vesicle identification tools with additional segmentation restrictions to allow object separation. Analysis was done by compartmentalization of LDs per cell using built-in scripts. For all other experiments, THP-1 monocytes were seeded with 100 μM PMA on glass coverslips of 0.17 mm thickness for 24 h, followed by 2 days in media without PMA. In all experiments, macrophages were fixed using 4% methanol-free formaldehyde for 30 min. Fixed coverslips were washed with PBS and then stained using BODIPY493/503 (Invitrogen, D3922) solution at 10 μM for 1 h at room temperature, followed by three washes in 1× PBS. After staining, the coverslips were mounted on slides and sealed. Confocal z-stacks of 0.30 mm thickness were taken using Leica TCS SP8. LD volume measurements were done based on BODIPY493/503 fluorescence using VOLOCITY (Perkin Elmer) image analysis software. Statistical significance was calculated from non-parametric Kruskal–Wallis test with a *post hoc* Dunn's test for comparison of groups. Mean LD volume from multiple experiments was tested for significance using Student's *t*-test. Mean cellular fluorescence (for either BODIPY493/503 or BODIPY558/568) was calculated using the Leica LAX 3.1.1 software; cell boundaries were made using a free hand selection tool and total fluorescence in the selected region of interest reported. Total fluorescence/cell from each experiment was taken and data from three to four such experiments were pooled.

Measurement of Mean Bacterial Fluorescence Per Cell in Infected Macrophages

THP1 macrophages seeded at a density of 0.3 million cells/ml were infected with Mtb strains expressing mCherry-H37Rv and

H37RvΔRD1, at indicated MOI for 24 h. After fixation using 4% methanol-free formaldehyde, macrophages were stained with BODIPY493/503 at 10 μM, Cell Mask (Invitrogen, C10046) at 1 μg/ml and DAPI at 1 μg/ml concentration for half an hour at room temperature. The wells were then washed with PBS three times for 5 min each and proceeded with imaging. Nine confocal z-stacks were acquired randomly for each well at 63× objective in IN CELL 6000 High content imager (GE Health care). Images were analyzed for estimation of mean fluorescence intensity of bacteria per cell was analyzed using IN CELL Developer toolbox. Cell boundaries and nuclei were marked using Cell mask and DAPI fluorescence. Mean fluorescence density of bacteria overlapping with the fluorescence in the Cell mask channel was quantified. This arbitrary fluorescence measure was background corrected and thereafter plotted as a surrogate measure for bacterial uptake per cell.

THPM Necrosis and Media Preparation

Cells were scraped in media and then frozen at −20°C temperature followed by thawing at room temperature. This was repeated five times to make the NcS. NcS was then added on THP1 monocyte-derived macrophages at a density of 1.2 million necrosed cells/ml media for 8 days, changing media every 2 days with PMA addition at day 1 and day 5 post additions of NcS. The "normal media" control group was cultured in the same manner except necrotic cells were not added as supplement.

Biochemical Estimations

Quantification of cholesterol, TG, and protein concentration in necrotic supplement and normal media was performed by specific colorimetric reactions for each of the analytes using COBAS INTEGRA 400 plus (Roche Diagnostics). Glucose estimation was performed using the anthrone method.

Glucose Uptake Assays

14C-2-deoxyglucose (ARC 0112A) (1 μCi/ml) was added to differentiated THP1 macrophages in media or NcS for 5, 24, and 48 h. At these time points, cells were washed four times with media, and cell lysates were prepared. Cell lysates at each time point were added to 100 μl of scintillation cocktail (*Microscint PS, Perkin Elmer, 6013631*) in a white 96-well flat bottom plate and then read in the Perkin Elmer TopNXT Scintillation counter. Glucose uptake was plotted as ratio of radioactivity present in the cell lysate to the total radioactivity added.

Cytokine Analysis

THP1 macrophages were cultured as described above for 8 days, followed by infection with Mtb at MOI 50 for 3 h at which point extracellular bacilli were removed. The monolayers were washed three times with media and replaced with RPMI media supplemented with 10% FBS. Cell culture supernatants were harvested at 24 h post infection and assayed for TNFα using an ELISA kit (eBioscience) or Milliplex human cytokine/chemokine bead panel (HCYTOMAG-60K).

Isolation and Culture of Human PBMCs

Blood (9 ml) was drawn from five individuals with their consent in K3EDTA containing vacutainers. Blood was first diluted in RPMI to 30 ml which was then layered on top of 10 ml Histopaque (Sigma, 10771) and centrifuged at 500 *g* for 30 min at 20°C with acceleration 9 and deceleration 1. After centrifugation, the buffy coat was collected in a separate tube and washed with PBS once. To remove platelets from the pellet, the pellet was resuspended in RPMI and then layered on top of 5 ml FBS followed by centrifugation. For removal of RBCs, the pellet was resuspended in 9 ml of water for 10 s followed by addition of 1 ml of 10× PBS. Cells were collected by centrifugation and then allowed to differentiate into macrophages in RPMI media containing FBS or human pooled serum, with or without human M-CSF or GMCSF for 6 days. In between, at day 4, the monolayer was washed to remove non-adherent cells with PBS. Infections were done at day 8 post isolation. For TNFα release measurements, PBMCs were differentiated in 50 ng/ml GMCSF for 6 days, followed by 8 days in media or NcS in the presence of 10 ng/ml GMCSF.

Intracellular Mycobacterial Growth Assay

Macrophages were seeded in 48-well plates at a density of 0.6 million/ml and infected at MOI of 0.1 for 4 h, followed by removal of extracellular bacilli by 3 washed with PBS and addition of complete growth media. Cells were lysed in 100 μl of 1% Triton-X100 and serial dilutions plated on 7H10 OADC plates. Media was changed after every 48 h.

Statistics

All statistics were computed using Prism. ANOVA and *t*-test were used for all parametric data wherein data from three to four independent experiments were combined. For testing statistical significance of change in median of the LD size (**Figure 2C**) and per cell signal of BODIPY558/568 (**Figure 4C**), Kruskal–Wallis test was used.

Ethics Statement

The animals were housed and handled at the Department of Biochemistry, University of Delhi South Campus according to directives and guidelines of the Committee for the Purpose of Control and Supervision of Experiments on Animals (CPCSEA). Use of Mtb infected guinea pig lung tissue for this work was approved by the CPCSEA as per ethics proposal #IGIB/IAEC/14/15. Blood was drawn from healthy human volunteers with informed written consent as per approval #11dtd. March30th2015 of the Institutional Human Ethics Committee.

RESULTS

Necrotic TB Granulomas Exhibit Heightened Inflammation Associated With Increased TG Accumulation

The guinea pig model of pulmonary TB presents with the array of granulomas observed in human TB, including solid and necrotic granulomas which may be caseous, fibrocaseous, or cavitary lesions (12, 15, 16). To study how lesion types differ in their inflammatory nature and abundance of lipid-loaded foamy macrophages, we investigated lesions from infected guinea pigs at week 4 and 10 post aerosol infection with virulent Mtb strain H37Rv with ~30 bacilli/lung. By 4 weeks post infection, the bacterial burden per lung was found to be $4.1 \times 10^5 \pm 1.7 \times 10^5$ (**Figure 1A**). Bacterial burden increased further 4-folds by 10 weeks post infection (**Figure 1A**). At 4 weeks post infection 92.8% of the granulomas were non-necrotic (referred to as solid) while at week 10 approximately half of the granulomas were found to be necrotic, with amorphous eosin staining (**Figure 1B**) interspersed with pyknotic and karyorrhectic nuclei at the core (Figure S1A in Supplementary Material). These findings were consistent with bacterial burden associated necrosis in TB (17). Consistent with previous reports in humans (18), we observed distinctive staining for TNFα at the cellular cuff of the necrotic core (**Figure 1C**). By contrast, TNFα immunostaining in solid granulomas seemed to be more diffuse and in general lower compared to necrotic granulomas (**Figures 1C,D**). This suggested that perhaps exposure to necrosis would lead to the higher expression of TNFα.

Further histological analysis using oil red O staining revealed that necrotic granulomas also exhibited a cellular cuff of oil red O positive cells (**Figure 1E**). While 100% of necrotic granulomas were oil red O positive, this staining was conspicuously absent from solid granulomas (**Figures 1E,F**). These cells with higher abundance of neutral lipid content were confirmed to be macrophages using immunostaining for mac-1, a macrophage marker, and staining for BODIPY493/503, a neutral lipid fluorescent dye (Figures S1B,C in Supplementary Material). Lipid analysis from macroscopic granulomas verified the neutral lipid to be mainly TG (Figure S1D in Supplementary Material). TG content from macroscopic granulomas likely to be necrotic (week 10) was higher as compared to anatomically similar regions of lungs from animals that were infected for 4 weeks or

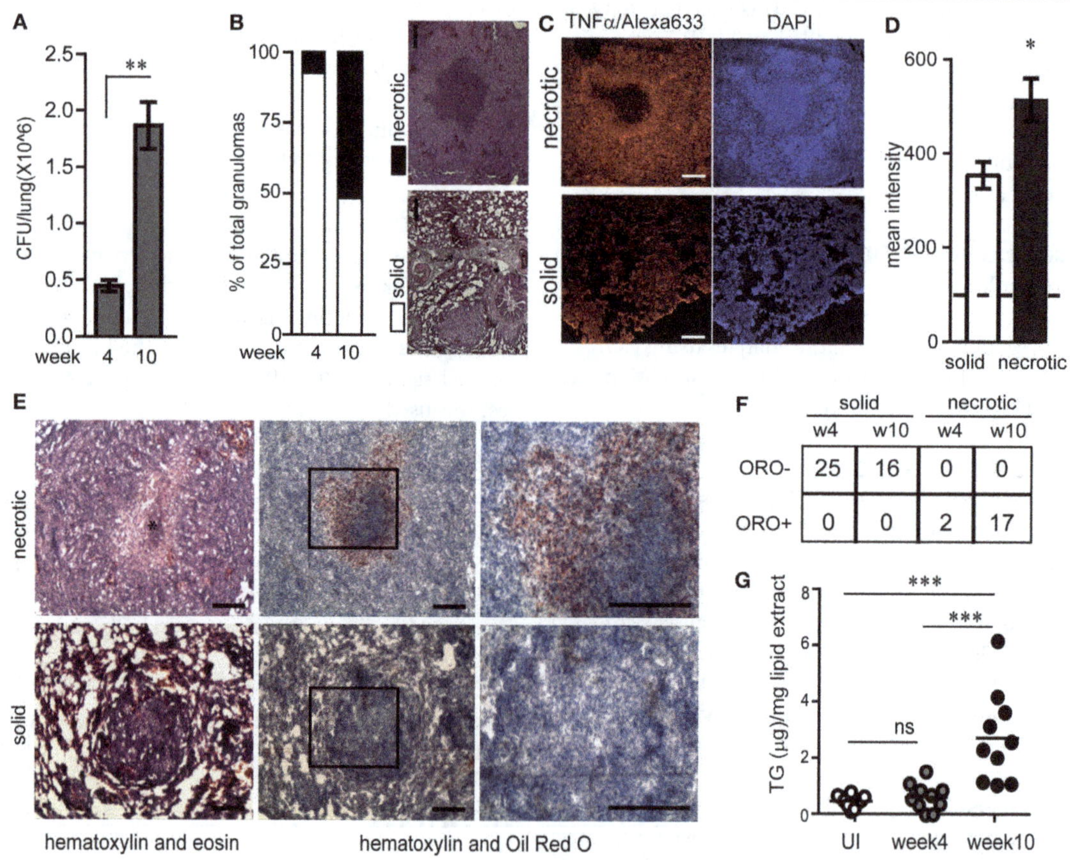

FIGURE 1 | Necrotic tuberculosis granulomas exhibit increased TNFα production and spatial polarization of triglyceride-rich foamy macrophages. **(A)** CFU/lung per guinea pig ($N = 3$ per time point) at week 4 and 10 post aerosol infection with ~30 cfu/lung. **(B)** Percentage of solid and necrotic granulomas of total granulomas in tissue sections analyzed from three animals at each time point. Images are examples of a typical solid and necrotic granuloma stained with haematoxylin + eosin. Scale bar = 100 µm. **(C)** TNFα immunofluorescence in solid and necrotic guinea pig granulomas. Right panel shows nuclear staining with DAPI (scale bar = 250 µm). **(D)** Quantification of TNFα immunofluorescence as mean intensity/granuloma from four solid and three necrotic granulomas. Dashed horizontal line is the mean value from controls without primary antibody. **(E)** Sequential cryosections stained with haematoxylin + eosin (left panels) and haematoxylin + Oil red O (center and right panels) from a necrotic and solid granuloma. * indicates necrotic center filled with pyknotic nuclei. Scale bar = 100 µm. **(F)** Table showing number of oil red O negative (ORO⁻) and positive (ORO⁺) solid and necrotic granulomas at week 4 and week 10 post infection. **(G)** TG quantification from 10 individual macroscopic granulomas from a single animal at each time point, calculated using densitometry of thin layer chromatographs. Each circle represents TG from a single macroscopic granuloma or anatomically similar section from control animals. Line indicates mean TG of each group (*$p < 0.05$, **$p < 0.01$, ***$p \leq 0.001$, ns, not significant). Also see Figure S1 in Supplementary Material.

were uninfected (**Figure 1G**). These data demonstrated that as granulomas evolved to develop necrosis, they exhibited presence of TG rich foamy macrophages proximal to the necrotic core. In addition, the presence of TG rich foamy macrophages correlated with higher local TNFα in the cellular cuff of the necrotic core.

TG Levels and LD Abundance in THP1 Macrophages Is Dependent on *DGAT1* Expression

To further understand the possible relationship between TG metabolism and inflammation in TB infection, we sought to investigate whether TGs constitute the major neutral lipid in human macrophages. We used THP1 monocyte-derived macrophages for this purpose. TG storage can occur from either the MGAT pathway or the Kennedy pathway. Both pathways converge to generate diacylglycerol, which is then converted to TG by a diacylglycerol *O*-acyl transferase (19). Using lentivirus transduced THP1 cells expressing shRNA against the enzyme DGAT1, we achieved an 80–90% knockdown in *DGAT1* expression (**Figure 2A**) and 60% decrease in TG levels (Figure S1E in Supplementary Material). TG and other neutral lipids are bound by a monolayer of phospholipid membrane within cytosolic LDs (20). Neutral lipid staining using LipidTox also showed a decrease in abundance and size of LDs upon DGAT1 knockdown (**Figures 2B–D**). This demonstrated that in THP1 cells, majority of the neutral lipid is TG and its levels can be regulated efficiently using a *DGAT1* knockdown.

Mtb Infection Increases Macrophage TG Synthesis During Necrosis

We investigated if Mtb infection itself increases TG synthesis during macrophage infection. To understand how acute Mtb infection alters host total lipid content, we measured the size of LDs in PMA differentiated THP1 macrophages upon Mtb infection using BODIPY493/503. Mtb infection of THP1 macrophages for 24 h at a MOI of one (MOI 1^{24h}) or five (MOI 5^{24h}) led to infection of approximately 80% cells with at least one bacterium per cell. However, neither of these conditions led to an increase in size or content of LDs (**Figures 3A,B**). Human peripheral blood monocyte-derived macrophages, similar to THP1 macrophages, also did not show an increase in LD size or lipid content under the same infection conditions (Figures S2A–C in Supplementary Material). However, an increase in MOI to 50 led to a shift in the proportion of LDs of larger size (**Figures 3A,B**). Consistent with an increase in LD size, we observed an increase in TG synthesis (**Figure 3C**) and absolute levels of TG (**Figure 3D**) under MOI 50^{24h} condition of infection while no increase was observed at MOI 1^{24h} and MOI 5^{24h}.

Incident to the increase in TG synthesis at MOI 50^{24} was an increase in cell death from 40% to over 60% (**Figure 3E**; Figure S2D in Supplementary Material). Therefore, the increase in TG levels could be a bystander response of remaining viable cells to necrosis. TG content in the remaining adherent cells revealed a linear correlation with the relative necrosis in that well ($R^2 = 0.59, p = 0.0002$) (Figure S2E in Supplementary Material).

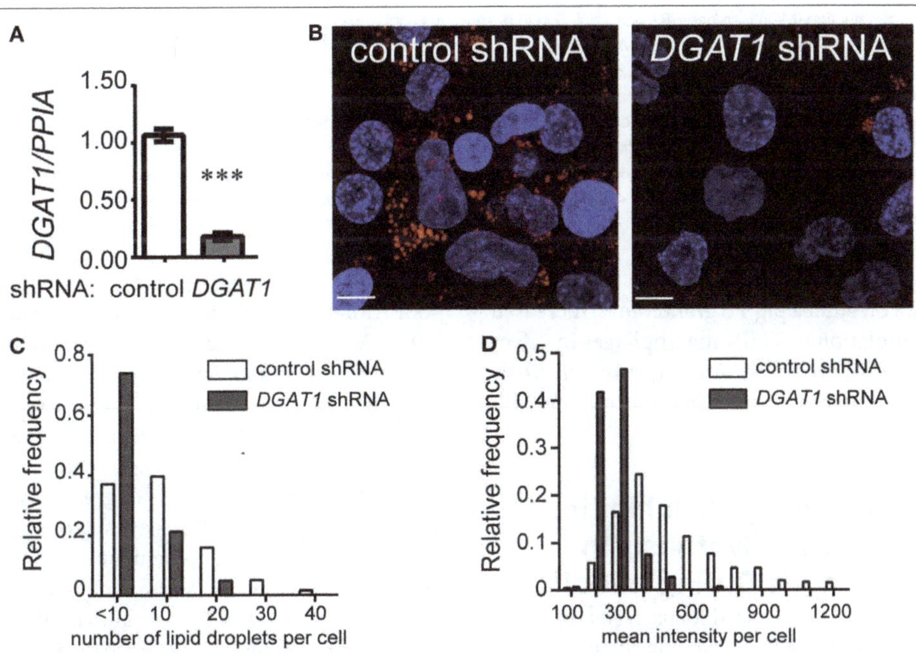

FIGURE 2 | Triglycerides are the major neutral lipids in human THP1 macrophages. **(A)** *DGAT1* expression in stable THP1 cell lines derived upon transduction with lentiviruses expressing non-targeting (control) and *DGAT1*-targeting shRNA. Data are mean ± SEM from three independent experiments. **(B)** LipidTox (red) and DAPI (blue) stained control (non-targeting) and *DGAT1* shRNA expressing stable THP1 macrophages. Graphs representing distribution of lipid droplet size **(C)** and content (mean fluorescence intensity per cell) **(D)** from LipidTox stained images. Data are representative of 2 independent experiments. See also Figure S1 in Supplementary Material.

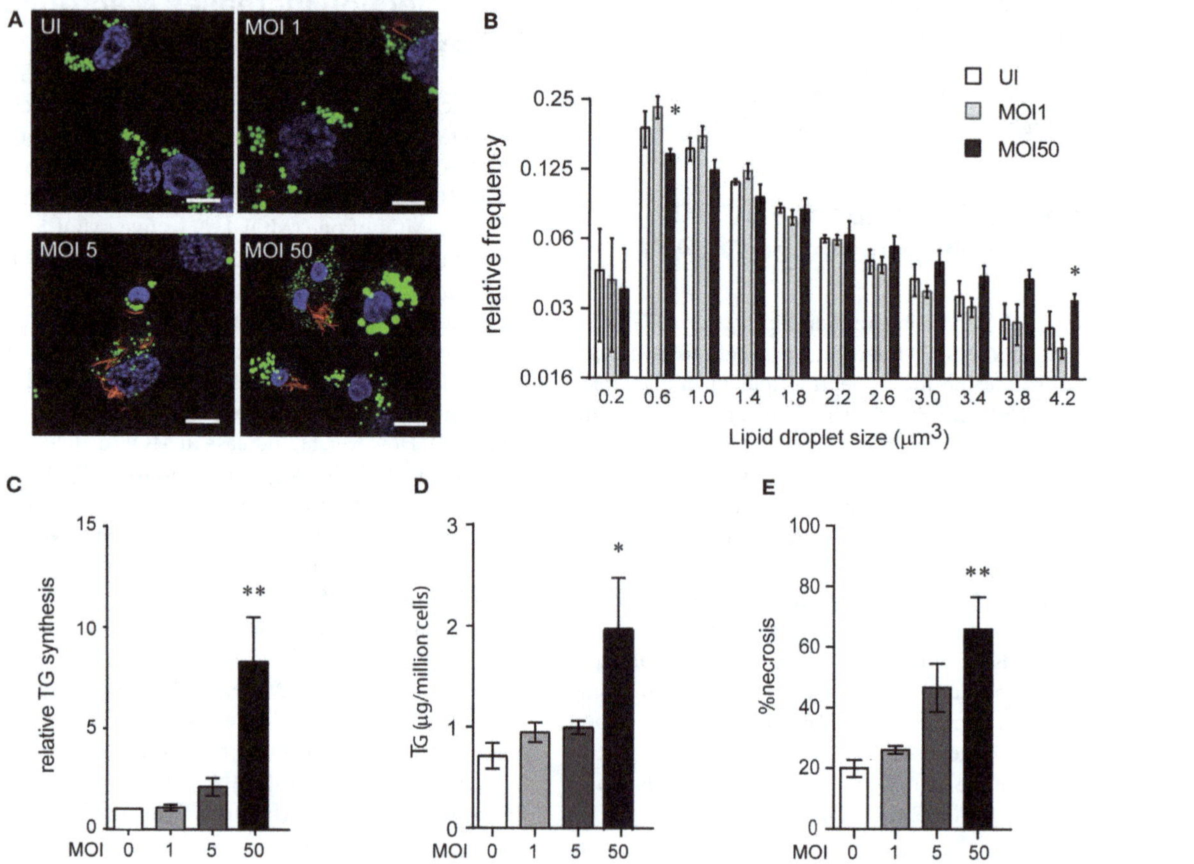

FIGURE 3 | High multiplicity of infection (MOI) increases TG accumulation in human macrophages concomitant to necrosis. **(A)** BODIPY 493/503 (green) and DAPI (blue) stained THP1 macrophages at 24 h post infection with MOI 1. mCherry+ *Mycobacterium tuberculosis* can be seen in red. Scale bar = 10 μm. **(B)** Assessment of mean LD size estimated from five confocal z-stacks of each condition per experiment. Data are mean ± SEM from two to three independent experiments. **(C)** TG synthesis relative to uninfected cells, estimated in macrophages infected with indicated MOI at 24 h post infection and normalized to number of cells at the end of 24 h infection. Data are mean ± SEM from three independent experiments. **(D)** TG estimation in adherent cells at 24 h post infection with indicated MOI. Data are mean ± SEM from three independent experiments. **(E)** Quantification of cell death measured by LDH activity and represented as % of necrosis relative to detergent lysed cells. Data are mean ± SEM from three experiments. One-way ANOVA followed by Dunnett's test derived *p*-values are indicated only for the significantly different groups relative to uninfected cells (**$p < 0.01$, and *$p < 0.05$). Also see Figure S2 in Supplementary Material.

Consistent with our data on guinea pig TB granulomas, increased TG synthesis and accumulation in THP1 macrophages in infection conditions with increased cell death suggested necrosis as a key player in foamy macrophage formation during Mtb infection.

Genetic and Pharmacological Inhibition of Necrosis Prevents TG Synthesis in Bystander Macrophages During Infection

The mycobacterial pathogenicity associated locus, *region of difference 1* (RD1), has been shown to be involved in inducing atypical cellular necrosis (21–23) *via* a bacterial contact-dependent membrane deformation (24). The vaccine strain *M. bovis* BCG harbors a deletion of the RD1 locus (25) and is known to induce apoptosis rather than necrosis in macrophages (26, 27). Consistent with literature, we also observed Mtb infection to cause necrosis instead of apoptosis of THP1 macrophages with poor Annexin V staining (1–15%, $N = 3$) and efficient PI staining (20–85%, $N = 3$) within 8 h of infection at MOI 50 (**Figure 4A**; Figures S3A,B in Supplementary Material). In comparison, infection with ΔRD1 strain and *M. bovis* BCG led to 10–20% annexin V positivity and 10% or lower PI positivity (Figures S3A,B in Supplementary Material). Infection with ΔRD1 strain or *M. bovis* BCG led to retention of greater number of adherent cells at MOI 50 (**Figures 4B,D**) as a result of significantly lower necrosis (Figures S3C,D in Supplementary Material). We found fewer number of adherent cells remaining at MOI 1 in case of ΔRD1 compared to the wild-type strain (**Figure 4B**), probably due to higher apoptosis, as LDH release assays indicated no difference in necrosis at this MOI (Figure S3C in Supplementary Material). High MOI-dependent increase in TG synthesis did not occur during infection with ΔRD1 strain or BCG to the extent it did in H37Rv infection (**Figures 4C,E**). Increased TG synthesis was consistent with increase in incidence of larger LDs and higher total cellular BODIPY493/503 fluorescence in macrophages infected

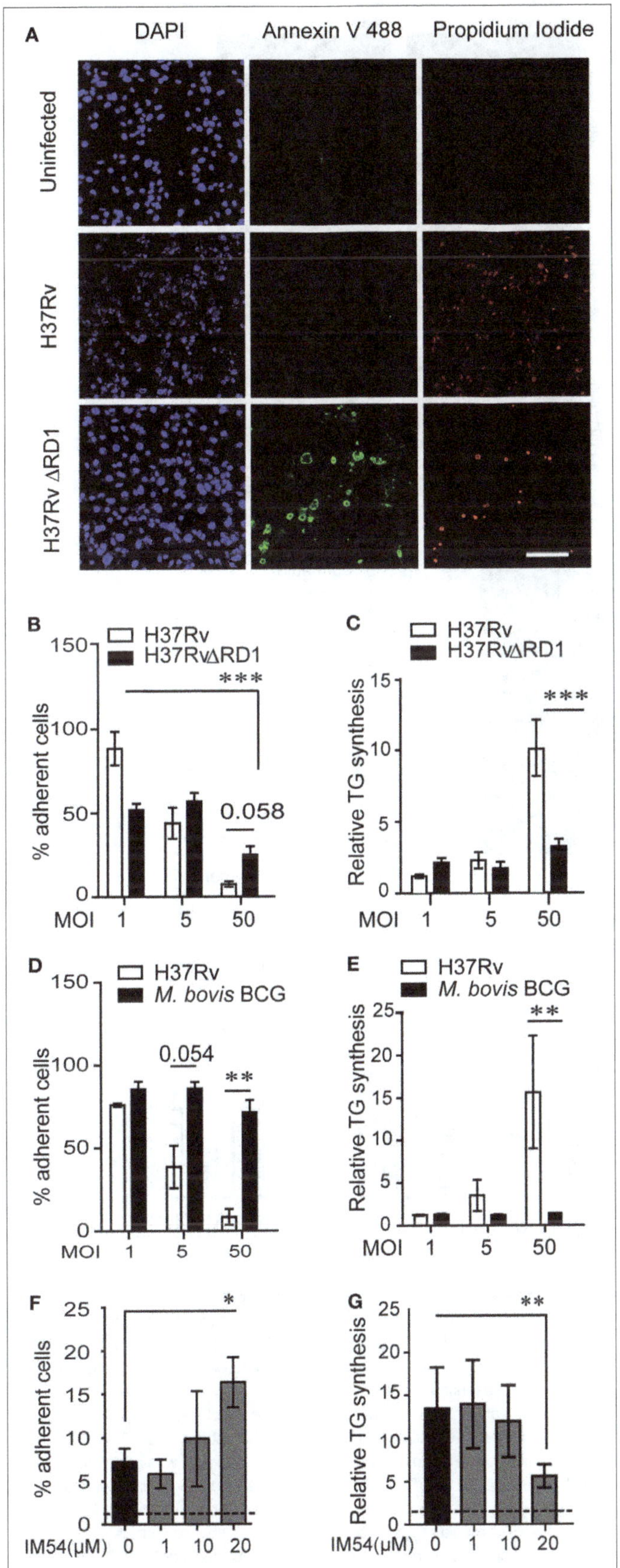

FIGURE 4 | Continued

FIGURE 4 | Inhibition of necrosis during *Mycobacterium tuberculosis* infection prevents TG accumulation in bystander macrophages. **(A)** Representative images of Annexin V and propidium iodide staining of uninfected and infected THP1 macrophages at 8 h post infection with the indicated strains at multiplicity of infection (MOI) 50. Scale bar = 100 µm. Graphs in **(B,D)** represent percentage of THP1 macrophages remaining adherent at 24 h post infection with H37Rv, H37RvΔRD1 **(B)**, or *Mycobacterium bovis* BCG **(D)** at indicated MOI as a percentage of uninfected control. Data are mean ± SEM from three independent experiments. Quantification of TG synthesis relative to uninfected cells at 24 h post infection with H37Rv, H37RvΔRD1 **(C)**, or M. *bovis* BCG **(E)** at indicated MOI. Data are mean ± SEM from three independent experiments. **(F)** Graph represents percentage of THP1 macrophages remaining adherent at 24 h post infection with H37Rv at MOI 50 in the presence of increasing concentration of IM54 as a percentage of uninfected control. Data are mean ± SEM from three independent experiments. **(G)** Quantification of relative TG synthesis in THP1 macrophages at 24 h post infection with H37Rv at MOI 50 in the presence of increasing dosage of IM54. Data are mean ± SEM from three independent experiments. *t*-test derived *p*-values are indicated (***$p < 0.001$, **$p < 0.01$, and *$p < 0.05$). Also see Figure S3 in Supplementary Material.

with H37Rv compared to H37RvΔRD1 at MOI 50 (Figures S3E–G in Supplementary Material). To rule out the possibility of these differences arising out of differential uptake of H37Rv and H37RvΔRD1, we quantified mean bacterial fluorescence intensity per cell in both conditions at all MOIs. While the mean bacterial fluorescence intensity per cell increased with increasing MOI, it was not different between macrophages infected with H37Rv and H37RvΔRD1 infections at the same MOI (Figure S3H in Supplementary Material). This further validates the role of RD1-mediated necrosis in increasing TG accumulation as a bystander response to necrosis.

To rule out the possibility that RD1 regulates fatty acid uptake by macrophages independent of necrosis, we used IM54, an inhibitor of H_2O_2 induced necrosis (28), to inhibit necrosis in Mtb infected THP1 macrophages at MOI 50. IM54 at 20 µM increased number of adherent cells by 2.5-folds when compared with the vehicle control (**Figure 4F**). This was consistent with a dose-dependent inhibition of necrosis by IM54, where 20 µM concentration reduced cell death from 70 to 40% at MOI 50^{24h} (Figure S3I in Supplementary Material). This concentration of IM54 led to 2.5-fold reduction in TG synthesis (**Figure 4G**), confirming a role for infection induced necrosis to be a player in stimulating TG synthesis in bystander macrophages.

Development of an *Ex Vivo* Model of NAFMs

To further understand if lipids released from necrotic cells were contributing to the TG pool of uninfected or bystander macrophages, we employed a transwell assay in which uninfected THP1 macrophages were seeded in the lower chamber and supernatant from MOI 50^{24h} infected cells was added to the upper chamber (**Figure 5A**). The transwell prevented effects due to bacterial infection of recipient (bystander) cells (Figure S4A in Supplementary Material). To chase the lipids from the donor cells, they were labeled with BODIPY558/568-C12 FA prior to infection. BODIPY558/568-C12 FA labeled lipids from MOI 50^{24h}

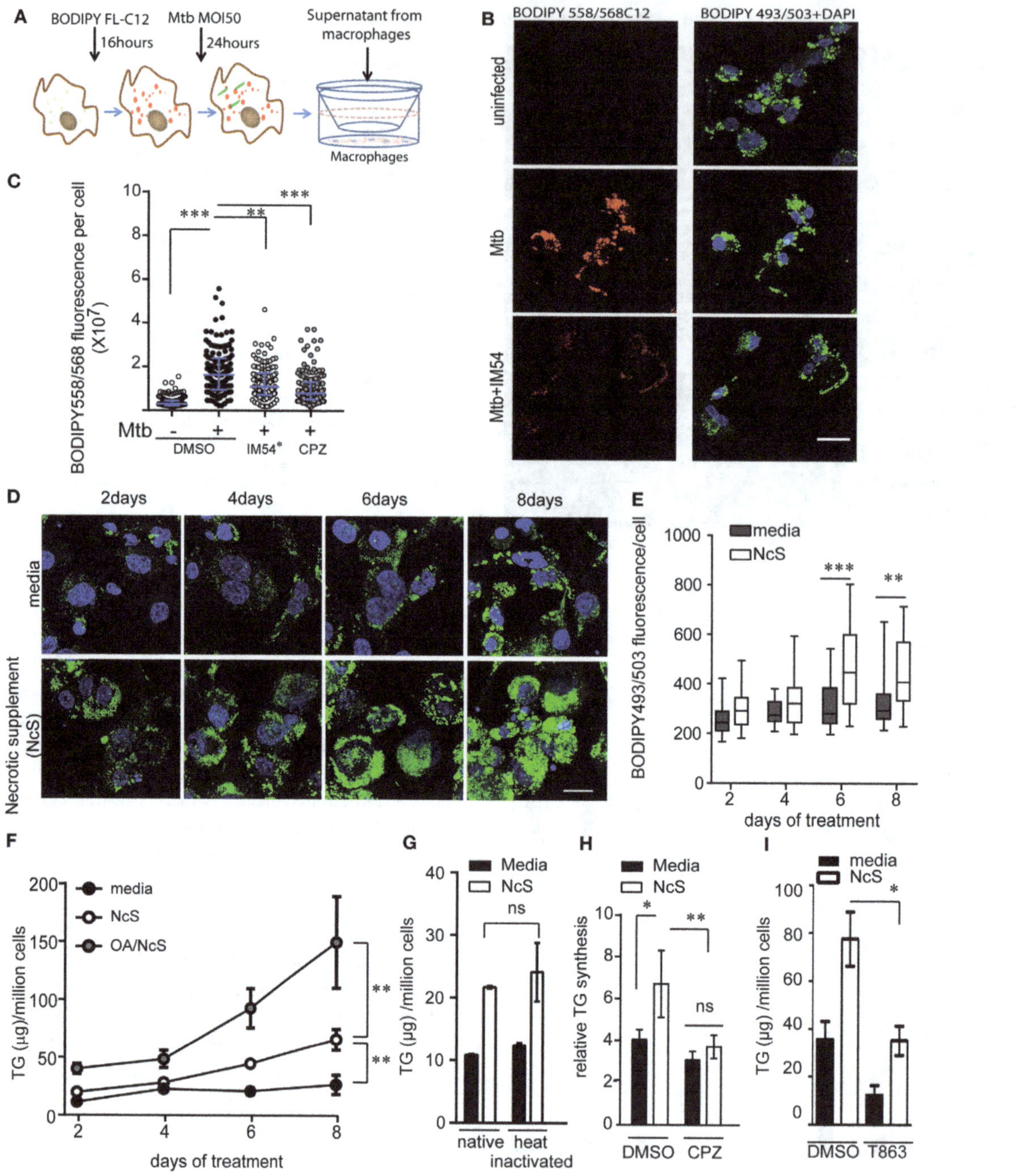

FIGURE 5 | *Ex vivo* model of necrosis-associated foamy macrophages. **(A)** Schematic representing experimental setup for supernatant transfer from BODIPY558/568C12 labeled infected THP1 macrophages. **(B)** BODIPY 493/503 and DAPI staining in THP1 macrophages treated with supernatant from uninfected or *Mycobacterium tuberculosis*-infected THP1 macrophages labeled with BODIPY558/568C12 prior to infection. Scale bar = 25 µm. **(C)** Quantification of BODIPY558/568 fluorescence per recipient cell from experiment shown in **(A)**. IM54* indicates treatment of donor cells with IM54 during infection while chlorpromazine (CPZ) was added to recipient cells. DMSO was used as a vehicle control at 0.1% vol/vol. Data are from three independent experiments, with approximately 100 cells per group. **(D)** BODIPY493/503 (green) and DAPI (blue) stained THP1 macrophages at days 2, 4, 6, and 8 post treatment with media or necrotic cell supplement (NcS). Scale bar = 25 µm. **(E)** Quantification of total cellular BODIPY493/503 signal from a representative experiment. **(F)** TG estimation from THP1 macrophages post 2, 4, 6, and 8 days of differentiation. Gray circles represent NcS prepared from oleic acid pre-treated cells. 150 µM bovine serum albumin-conjugated oleic acid was added to cells 48 h prior to NcS preparation. Data are mean ± SEM from three independent experiments. **(G)** TG estimation from THP1 macrophages at 8 days post differentiation with normal media, NcS, or heat-inactivated normal media or heat inactivated NcS. Data are mean ± SD from triplicate wells. Data are representative of two independent experiments. **(H)** TG synthesis over 2 days in THP1 macrophages in response to heat inactivated NcS or media in the presence of DMSO or chlorpromazine (CPZ). Data are mean from three independent experiments, normalized to 5 h time point for normal media. **(I)** TG estimation in macrophages exposed to media or NcS after 8 days of treatment in the presence of DMSO (vehicle control) or T863 (10 µM). Data are mean ± SEM from three independent experiments. Kruskal–Wallis test derived *p*-values are shown in **(C,E)**. Linear regression analysis for slopes was done in **(F)**. *T*-test derived *p*-values are indicated in **(E,G–I)** (***$p < 0.001$, **$p < 0.01$, *$p < 0.05$, ns, not significant).

infected cells could be assimilated into the neutral lipid pool of uninfected cells across the transwell (**Figures 5A,B**). The transwell allowed transfer of lipids with a lower tendency for most neutral lipids such as TGs to pass through while more polar lipids such as diacylglycerides, phospholipids, and fatty acids passed through more readily (Figure S4B in Supplementary Material). While free fatty acids could traverse the filter, they were the least abundant species and did not increase during the course of the transwell experiment, suggesting lipid esterified BODIPY558/568-C12 to be the major source of the label in this experiment. Prevention of necrosis with IM54 prevented transfer of labeled lipids to the LDs of recipient cells, confirming that lipids of cells undergoing necrosis can provide a source of fatty acids for TG synthesis in bystander cells (**Figures 5B,C**). For recipient macrophages to acquire fatty acids from lipids for new synthesis, these lipids must first undergo lysosomal degradation (29). CPZ, an inhibitor of lysosomal lipases (30), could significantly inhibit label transfer, confirming a role for new TG synthesis from incoming lipids that included diacylglyceride and TG (**Figure 5C**).

The above experiments suggested that lipids released from necrotic cells may be sufficient to develop "necrosis-associated foamy macrophages" *ex vivo*. To further test if exposure to necrotic cells was sufficient to stimulate TG accumulation in bystander macrophages, we stimulated healthy THP1 macrophages with mechanically necrotized macrophages (NcS). NcS generated by mechanical disruption of healthy macrophages contained 1.4-fold higher TG than media, while protein and glucose concentration of both media and NcS was similar (Figure S4C in Supplementary Material). We evaluated the ability of NcS to enable TG storage in recipient macrophages at a donor cell to recipient ratio of 2:1. This ratio simulated the scenario of Mtb infection at MOI 50, wherein at least two-thirds of the cells were lost for a lipogenic response to be observed in the remaining one-third bystander macrophages. NcS was able to stimulate accumulation of LDs in healthy macrophages in a time-dependent manner (**Figures 5D,E**), corresponding to a temporal increase in total cellular TG (**Figure 5F**). NcS-stimulated cells increased their TG levels in a time-dependent manner with a 3- to 5-fold increase by day 8 compared with day 0 while normal media treated cells exhibited only 1.2-fold increase in TG content during the same time (**Figure 5F**). Dilutions of the NcS led to decreased LD abundance in recipient cells (Figure S4D in Supplementary Material) while increasing the lipid load of donor cells by prior treatment with oleic acid (31) further increased the TG content of recipient cells by twofolds in a time-dependent manner (**Figure 5F**), validating a role for exogenous lipid in increasing TG content of recipient macrophages. Heat inactivation of the NcS failed to abrogate TG accumulation in recipient cells, suggesting active process from the donor not likely to contribute to the phenomenon (**Figure 5G**). Fatty acids could be mediating this response if they are first degraded by the cellular machinery as majority of cellular fatty acids are present in esterified form. Inhibition of lysosomal lipases by CPZ led to impairment in NcS stimulated TG synthesis (**Figure 5H**), consistent with the mode of lipid uptake during high MOI Mtb infection. While exogenous lipids were assimilated in the presence of NcS, exogenous glucose uptake was in fact decreased in response to NcS (Figure S4E in Supplementary Material). Because glucose feeds into *de novo* fatty acid synthesis, we speculated that *de novo* FA synthesis might not be required for NAFMs formation. Inhibition of FA synthase with C75 did not lead to any change in total TG levels upon stimulation with NcS (Figure S4F in Supplementary Material) even though it led to 80% inhibition of *de novo* FA synthesis (Figure S4G). NcS-dependent TG synthesis was abrogated by T863, an inhibitor of DGAT1 (32), verifying the role of endogenous esterification of incoming lipid-derived FA rather than *en masse* storage of the excess exogenous TG (**Figure 5I**). TG-rich macrophages generated by exposure to NcS are hereafter referred to as NAFMs.

TG Storage in Human Macrophages Upregulates Infection Induced Pro-Inflammatory Response

During infection, necrosis is a progressive phenomenon arising due to increased bacterial burden in infected macrophages, wherein NAFMs would form as a bystander response and then subsequently get infected. Our *in vivo* data suggested possibility of increased inflammatory response in oil red O positive foamy macrophages. To investigate the role of TG content in altering the inflammatory response, we questioned whether infection of *ex vivo* generated NAFMs, exhibit differences in immune response to Mtb infection. We found that Mtb infected NAFMs (THP1 derived) released 1.5- to 3-fold higher TNFα compared with infected THP1 NMs (**Figure 6A**) while neither did NAFMs exhibit a heightened basal secretion of TNFα (**Figure 6A**) nor did the NcS media itself contain detectable levels of TNFα (data not shown). We questioned if this increase was due to increased bacterial uptake in foamy macrophages. We found no difference between NM and NAFM in the uptake of Mtb, suggesting inherent potential of NAFMs to mount a higher pro-inflammatory response independent of bacterial burden (Figure S5A in Supplementary Material). These infection conditions led to approximately 40% necrotic cell death (Figure S5B in Supplementary Material), which we previously found to be insufficient for necrosis-triggered TG synthesis (**Figures 4C–E**; Figure S3C in Supplementary Material), suggesting priming of cells during NAFM differentiation for the heightened responses rather than necrosis induced TG synthesis during infection. Primary human MDMs also exhibited increased staining with BODIPY493/503 and 1.2- to 2-fold increase in cellular TG in response to NcS over a period of 8 days (Figures S5C,D in Supplementary Material). Three out of four donors also exhibited increase in infection induced TNFα release upon differentiation to NAFMs (Figure S5E in Supplementary Material).

To further test if cytokine production in response to infection was proportional to intracellular TG levels, we differentiated DGAT1 shRNA and control shRNA expressing THP1 cells with NcS and then sought to measure release and expression of TNFα in response to Mtb infection. *DGAT1* knockdown cells exhibited approximately 50% decrease in TG levels in case of NMs and 30–40% decrease in case of NAFMs (**Figure 6B**).

DGAT1 knockdown led to approximately 50% decrease in infection induced TNFα in the supernatant in case of NM (**Figure 6C**). To check a broader range of cytokines, chemokines,

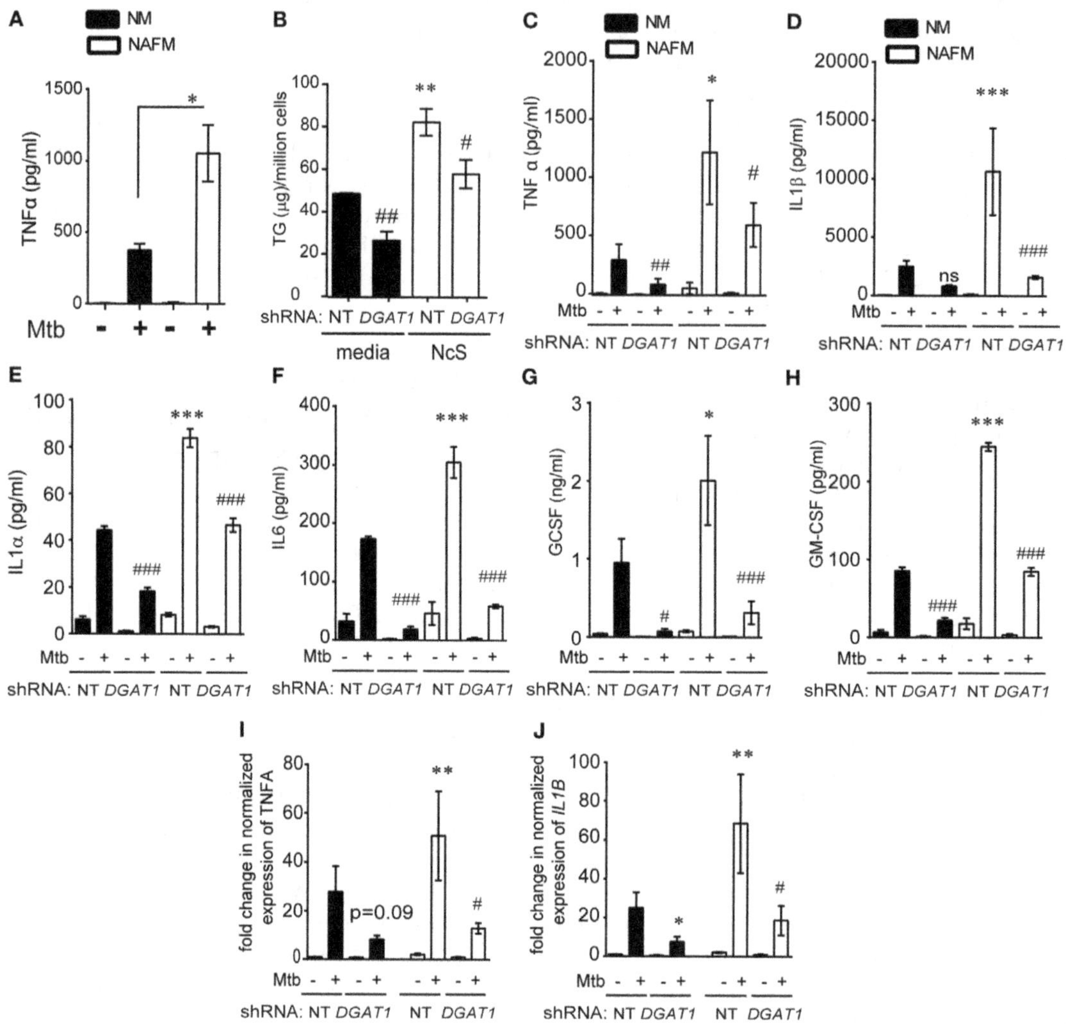

FIGURE 6 | DGAT1-mediated TG synthesis is responsible for the heightened inflammatory response to *Mycobacterium tuberculosis* (Mtb) infection in foamy macrophages. **(A)** TNFα release measured by ELISA in supernatants from THP1 cells that were normal media treated (termed as normal macrophages or NM) or treated with necrotic cell supplement (NcS) for 8 days [termed as necrosis-associated foamy macrophages (NAFMs)] at 24 h after infection with Mtb at multiplicity of infection (MOI) 50 for 3 h. Data are mean ± SEM from three independent experiments (*$p < 0.05$). **(B)** TG estimation from NT and *DGAT1* knockdown THP1 macrophages at 8 days post differentiation with media or NcS. Data are mean ± SEM from triplicate experiments. **(C)** TNFα release measured by ELISA in supernatants from NM and NAFM of NT and *DGAT1* knockdown THP1 macrophages at 24 h post infection with Mtb at MOI 50 for 3 h. Data are mean ± SEM from three independent experiments. **(D–H)** Luminex-based detection of indicated cytokines in supernatants from Mtb-infected NM and NAFM of *DGAT1* and non-targeting shRNA expressing macrophages. Data are mean ± SEM from five to six wells from two independent experiments. Transcript abundance of *TNFα* **(I)** and *IL1B* **(J)** normalized to that of PPIA in NMs and NAFMs of NT and DGAT1 shRNA expressing THP1 macrophages. Data are mean ± SEM from three experiments (*** or $^{\#\#\#}p \leq 0.01$, ** or $^{\#\#}p \leq 0.01$, * or $^{\#}p \leq 0.05$, ns, not significant). * represents comparison between NAFM and NM and # represents comparison between *DGAT1* knockdown and non-targeting control (NT) expressing macrophages for each group. See also Figure S5 in Supplementary Material.

and growth factors that are expressed by macrophages in response to Mtb infection, we performed a luminex multiplex assay. We observed that besides TNFα, IL-1β, IL-1α, IL-6, GCSF, and GMCSF release upon Mtb infection was 2- to 2.5-fold higher from NAFMs compared to NMs (**Figures 6D–H**). Infection induced release of all of these cytokines decreased upon depletion of *DGAT1* transcripts (**Figures 6D–H**) in macrophages despite their prior stimulation with NcS, confirming the role of TGs in the inflammatory response to infection. To further verify whether *DGAT1* regulated levels of these key cytokines and growth factors at the level of secretion or transcription, we quantified transcript abundance for *TNFα* and *IL1β*. Infection-induced *TNFα* transcript abundance was reduced by approximately 60–80% upon *DGAT1* knockdown (**Figure 6I**). *IL1β* transcript abundance was also found to be 40–80% lower in NMs and 60–80% lower in NAFMs upon depletion of *DGAT1* expression (**Figure 6J**). Cholesterol is also known to regulate inflammation (33) but estimations from NMs and NAFMs showed that neither NcS stimulation nor DGAT1 silencing altered total cellular cholesterol levels (Figure S5F in Supplementary Material), delinking the possibility of cholesterol mediated control of inflammation in this model. Therefore, the pro-inflammatory response of human macrophages to Mtb was indeed dependent on their intracellular TG abundance. Surprisingly, we found no significant differences in the uptake or growth of Mtb in NM and NAFM, whether in the wild-type or *DGAT1* knockdown background (Figures S5G–I in Supplementary Material). Therefore, intracellular TG levels regulate specific innate immune responses during Mtb infection without affecting growth of the intracellular bacilli.

DISCUSSION

This study, for the very first time, illustrates the role of macrophage TG levels in the pro-inflammatory response of foamy macrophages during Mtb infection. Here, we demonstrate that Mtb-induced necrosis stimulates TG accumulation in foamy macrophages is a bystander response. Once TG loaded cells encounter bacilli, they mount a higher pro-inflammatory response than cells with lower TG levels. We demonstrate that lysosomal degradation of incoming lipids is important for neosynthesis of TGs in a DGAT1-dependent manner in the bystander cells. In this process, the bystander foamy cells reduce their uptake of glucose and do not rely on *de novo* fatty acid synthesis for synthesis of the new TG. This model is able to explain the *in vivo* tripartite association of increased inflammatory response, presence of TG-rich foamy macrophages, and necrotic granulomas and is able to provide insights into the relevant carbon sources that polarize macrophages into a metabolically altered state in TB (**Figure 7**). We demonstrate that RD1 dependent necrosis in the context of TB infection is crucial for this, but can be generalized to necrosis independent of infection also. This suggests that TG accumulation in macrophages in the context of other necrotic pathologies might also be important for sustaining inflammation to infectious insult. These findings could be relevant in the case of necrotic atherosclerotic plaques and necrotic infections.

Triglycerides have been considered inert storage lipids; our data reveals that TG levels are important in titrating the inflammatory response to infection with Mtb. There are several possible mechanisms whereby this could happen. First, metabolites of TGs, namely fatty acids and glycerides, could regulate inflammation (34–37). Eicosanoids derived from fatty acid precursors such as prostaglandin E2, lipoxins LXA4, and LTB4 are known mediators of the inflammatory response in TB infection (38, 39). PGE2 in particular is important for IL1β expression in monocytes and macrophages (2, 40). Antagonistic to PGE2, which prevents

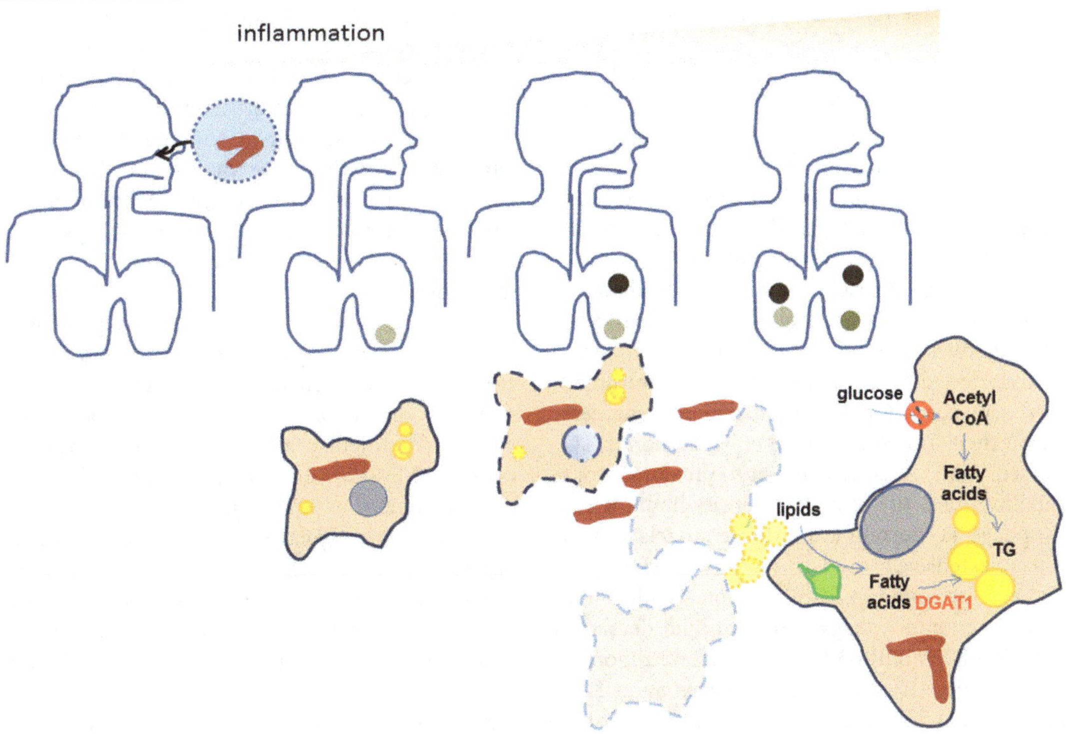

FIGURE 7 | Proposed scheme for the amplification of inflammation as a result of neosynthesis of triglycerides (TGs) in bystander foamy macrophages in TB. Bacteria are indicated as red rods while lipid droplets are indicates as yellow spheres. Darkened regions in the lung indicate granulomas. During initial infection of macrophages with *Mycobacterium tuberculosis* (Mtb), low levels of TGs are present in infected macrophages. The inflammatory response of macrophages recruits immune cells that help in granuloma formation. As bacteria multiply, both host and bacterial factors may synergize to bring about necrosis of infected cells, leading to formation of necrotic granulomas. Macrophages surrounding the necrotic center differentiate to TG-rich (yellow) foamy macrophages using lipids available from the necrotic cells, by first degrading them using lysosomal lipases (green). In doing so, they downregulate their glucose uptake and do not rely on *de novo* fatty acid synthesis for the increase in TG levels. Upon infection with Mtb, these necrosis-associated foamy macrophages release higher levels of pro-inflammatory mediators. The pro-inflammatory response of macrophages is dependent on the increased TG levels. The evolution of granulomas to necrotic granulomas, thereby amplifies the inflammatory response.

necrosis (41), H37Rv induced LXA4 production promotes necrosis (38). By contrast, the avirulent strain H37Ra induces PGE2 production which inhibits LXA4 production, thereby preventing necrosis (38). PGE2 is also a negative regulator of type I IFN induction (2) and early Type I IFN response during murine infection promotes cell death (42). Our investigations thus far have revealed that infection induced production of prostaglandin E2 or of infection-induced necrosis are not, however, regulated by TG levels (data not shown) even though IL1β expression in our model is dependent on TGs. This suggests that lipids other than TGs may be more important sources of PGE2 production during infection. A further investigation into all possible eicosanoid classes generated by macrophages upon Mtb infection is warranted to understand the role of TGs in inflammation. Besides eicosanoids, sphingolipids and phospholipids also share common metabolites of TG degradation. These lipid classes are also known activators of pro-inflammatory signal transduction within cells (43, 44). While these pathways involve the classical outside-to-inside signaling, signal transduction within the cell could also be regulated by specific proteins that interact with LDs. ER and mitochondrial membranes act as signaling hubs that modulate NOD2 and inflammasome, respectively (45, 46). Recently, viperin was demonstrated to mediate recruitment of TLR adaptors to LDs in plasmacytoid dendritic cells (47). It remains to be understood whether and how LD surface regulates signal transduction in infected macrophages.

Previous studies have suggested a role for mycobacterial lipids in stimulating macrophage neutral lipid accumulation (48, 49); while the carbon source for these lipids itself is not mycobacterial lipids, we suspect that in addition to necrosis, these lipids could additionally stimulate lipogenic signaling in infected cells. Human macrophages cultured *in vitro* tend to store TGs; therefore, evaluating modulation of the TG content upon infection requires the use of pulse chase-based assays while steady-state level metabolite analysis without flux analysis may prove to be misleading. Thus, this study provides evidence for unaltered rate of TG synthesis under conditions where cell death is minimal. Furthermore, our data suggest that cells that are bystanders of necrosis increase their TG content further if the donor TG content is increased. This is consistent with previous work describing the ability of TG-rich very low-density lipoproteins to increase macrophage TG content (50). Mouse models of Mtb infection have been extensively used to identify mechanisms of foamy macrophage formation in Mtb infection. While some studies report inhibition of autophagy-mediated lipid degradation regulated by microRNA miR-33 (51), others have reported a TLR2-dependent increase in lipid synthesis genes upon Mtb infection to be responsible for this process (52). A recent study suggested that IFNγ and Mtb synergize for foamy macrophage formation using mouse bone marrow-derived macrophages (53). However, the human TB and guinea pig models of TB suggest a possible role for incident pathology in driving foamy macrophage formation. While Mtb induced necrosis is operative in C57BL6 model of infection (54), it is not evident as "necrotic lesions" unless probed with specific markers. Therefore, ascertaining inherent variability in granuloma types and the role of necrosis has probably not been addressed in the resistant mouse models used in the above described studies. Moreover, building a causal role for necrosis-mediated foamy macrophage formation *in vivo* is challenging as strains such as RD1 deletion mutant induce largely lymphocytic granulomas (55) and inhibitors of Mtb induced cell death during *in vitro* experiments have shown limited potency *in vivo* (56). Based on our data, and studies summarized above, we suggest that any primary trigger that leads to increase in cellular TG may be further amplified to increase the abundance of TG-rich foamy macrophages once necrosis takes place. Our study here recapitulates the strong correlation between necrosis and foamy macrophage formation found in human TB (48) and helps explain the coincidence of spatially polarized expression of TNFα (18). Importantly, our work provides a new *ex vivo* model of foamy macrophages which can be used in future for studies pertaining to host response and antibiotic sensitivity.

Mycobacterium tuberculosis evades host immunity and adapts to the host's lipid rich environment (57, 58). Therefore, the importance of lipids for mycobacterial growth in macrophages has been a major area of investigation (59). Cholesterol utilization pathways of Mtb and host fatty acids are essential for bacterial survival in macrophages (60, 61). An important paradigm shift that appears from our work, consistent with that recently reported by the Stanley group using mouse macrophages (53), is that Mtb growth is not dependent on host TG accumulation by DGAT1. Phospholipids, sphingolipids, and free fatty acids could be the other carbon sources utilized by Mtb within macrophages. Alternatively, TG synthesis by DGAT2 could also contribute to enough TGs such that bacterial growth can be sustained. It remains to be ascertained whether TG accumulation *in vivo* alters Mtb growth. These findings can help us understand the contribution of foamy macrophages to disease and could possibly be coupled with antimicrobial drugs as a host-directed therapy to decrease host damage and synergistically help clear infection.

Lipid metabolism in macrophages plays a critical role in inflammation during metabolic disorders (62), atherosclerosis (63), and neurodegeneration (64). Increased TG accumulation in metabolic disorders has been reported to be majorly diet induced, where excess dietary fatty acids are stored into TG in the form of cytosolic LDs (20). Increased inflammation in a murine model of diet-induced obesity can be reversed by overexpression of DGAT1 in macrophages (65). Similarly, increasing fatty acid degradation by overexpressing CPT1, the rate-limiting enzyme in fatty acid oxidation, also plays a protective role against lipid-induced inflammation (66). While it is tempting to speculate that there may be species-specific regulation of lipid metabolism, as suggested earlier (67, 68), presentation of cellular lipids in the context of necrosis versus circulating free fatty acids and lipids as under condition of dietary excess might underlie the distinction between our model and these studies. An in-depth understanding of the mechanism involved in uptake of lipids from necrotic cells would be important in regulating functions of the foamy macrophage. Processes such as efferocytosis, phagocytosis, or receptor-mediated endocytosis could be involved. Our preliminary investigations ruled out efferocytosis or phagocytosis to be involved (data not shown). Finally, culmination of uptake into TG synthesis is important for attainment of a state primed for pro-inflammatory responses. Future work is required to assess the role of lipid uptake and synthesis machinery in regulating inflammation in animal models of TB.

AUTHOR CONTRIBUTIONS

Conceptualization, supervision, funding acquisition: SG. Methodology: SG and NJ. Investigation: NJ and SD. Microscopy: NJ, SD, KS, AN, DM, and SG. Validation: DM, KS, AN, and PB. Analysis: NJ, DM, and SG. Resources: GK, AT, and SG. Writing: NJ and SG.

ACKNOWLEDGMENTS

The authors thank Dr. Vivek Rao and Dr. Rajesh S. Gokhale for constructive comments and suggestions during the course of the research work. The authors thank Mr. Manish Kumar for maintenance of the imaging facility. A pre-print version of this manuscript is available on BioRxiv (69).

REFERENCES

1. WHO Report. (2015). Available from: http://www.who.int/mediacentre/factsheets/fs310/en/
2. Mayer-Barber KD, Andrade BB, Oland SD, Amaral EP, Barber DL, Gonzales J, et al. Host-directed therapy of tuberculosis based on interleukin-1 and type I interferon crosstalk. *Nature* (2014) 511(7507):99–103. doi:10.1038/nature13489
3. Cooper AM. Cell-mediated immune responses in tuberculosis. *Annu Rev Immunol* (2009) 27:393–422. doi:10.1146/annurev.immunol.021908.132703
4. O'Garra A, Redford PS, McNab FW, Bloom CI, Wilkinson RJ, Berry MP. The immune response in tuberculosis. *Annu Rev Immunol* (2013) 31:475–527. doi:10.1146/annurev-immunol-032712-095939
5. Hnizdo E, Singh T, Churchyard G. Chronic pulmonary function impairment caused by initial and recurrent pulmonary tuberculosis following treatment. *Thorax* (2000) 55(1):32–8. doi:10.1136/thorax.55.1.32
6. Menezes AM, Hallal PC, Perez-Padilla R, Jardim JR, Muino A, Lopez MV, et al. Tuberculosis and airflow obstruction: evidence from the PLATINO study in Latin America. *Eur Respir J* (2007) 30(6):1180–5. doi:10.1183/09031936.00083507
7. Orme IM, Robinson RT, Cooper AM. The balance between protective and pathogenic immune responses in the TB-infected lung. *Nat Immunol* (2015) 16(1):57–63. doi:10.1038/ni.3048
8. Cadena AM, Fortune SM, Flynn JL. Heterogeneity in tuberculosis. *Nat Rev Immunol* (2017) 17(11):691–702. doi:10.1038/nri.2017.69
9. Wallis RS, Hafner R. Advancing host-directed therapy for tuberculosis. *Nat Rev Immunol* (2015) 15(4):255–63. doi:10.1038/nri3813
10. Korf H, Vander Beken S, Romano M, Steffensen KR, Stijlemans B, Gustafsson JA, et al. Liver X receptors contribute to the protective immune response against *Mycobacterium tuberculosis* in mice. *J Clin Invest* (2009) 119(6):1626–37. doi:10.1172/JCI35288
11. Vilaplana C, Marzo E, Tapia G, Diaz J, Garcia V, Cardona PJ. Ibuprofen therapy resulted in significantly decreased tissue bacillary loads and increased survival in a new murine experimental model of active tuberculosis. *J Infect Dis* (2013) 208(2):199–202. doi:10.1093/infdis/jit152
12. Kim MJ, Wainwright HC, Locketz M, Bekker LG, Walther GB, Dittrich C, et al. Caseation of human tuberculosis granulomas correlates with elevated host lipid metabolism. *EMBO Mol Med* (2010) 2(7):258–74. doi:10.1002/emmm.201000079
13. Brasaemle DL, Rubin B, Harten IA, Gruia-Gray J, Kimmel AR, Londos C. Perilipin A increases triacylglycerol storage by decreasing the rate of triacylglycerol hydrolysis. *J Biol Chem* (2000) 275(49):38486–93. doi:10.1074/jbc.M007322200
14. Palmer AM, Nova E, Anil E, Jackson K, Bateman P, Wolstencroft E, et al. Differential uptake of subfractions of triglyceride-rich lipoproteins by THP-1 macrophages. *Atherosclerosis* (2005) 180(2):233–44. doi:10.1016/j.atherosclerosis.2004.12.038
15. McMurray DN. Guinea pig model of tuberculosis. In: Bloom B, editor. *Tuberculosis*. Washington, DC: ASM Press (1994).
16. Turner OC, Basaraba RJ, Orme IM. Immunopathogenesis of pulmonary granulomas in the guinea pig after infection with *Mycobacterium tuberculosis*. *Infect Immun* (2003) 71(2):864–71. doi:10.1128/IAI.71.2.864-871.2003
17. Hoff DR, Ryan GJ, Driver ER, Ssemakulu CC, De Groote MA, Basaraba RJ, et al. Location of intra- and extracellular *M. tuberculosis* populations in lungs of mice and guinea pigs during disease progression and after drug treatment. *PLoS One* (2011) 6(3):e17550. doi:10.1371/journal.pone.0017550
18. Marakalala MJ, Raju RM, Sharma K, Zhang YJ, Eugenin EA, Prideaux B, et al. Inflammatory signaling in human tuberculosis granulomas is spatially organized. *Nat Med* (2016) 22(5):531–8. doi:10.1038/nm.4073
19. Yen CL, Stone SJ, Koliwad S, Harris C, Farese RV Jr. Thematic review series: glycerolipids. DGAT enzymes and triacylglycerol biosynthesis. *J Lipid Res* (2008) 49(11):2283–301. doi:10.1194/jlr.R800018-JLR200
20. Farese RV Jr, Walther TC. Lipid droplets finally get a little R-E-S-P-E-C-T. *Cell* (2009) 139(5):855–60. doi:10.1016/j.cell.2009.11.005
21. Smith J, Manoranjan J, Pan M, Bohsali A, Xu J, Liu J, et al. Evidence for pore formation in host cell membranes by ESX-1-secreted ESAT-6 and its role in *Mycobacterium marinum* escape from the vacuole. *Infect Immun* (2008) 76(12):5478–87. doi:10.1128/IAI.00614-08
22. Lee J, Repasy T, Papavinasasundaram K, Sassetti C, Kornfeld H. *Mycobacterium tuberculosis* induces an atypical cell death mode to escape from infected macrophages. *PLoS One* (2011) 6(3):e18367. doi:10.1371/journal.pone.0018367
23. Simeone R, Bobard A, Lippmann J, Bitter W, Majlessi L, Brosch R, et al. Phagosomal rupture by *Mycobacterium tuberculosis* results in toxicity and host cell death. *PLoS Pathog* (2012) 8(2):e1002507. doi:10.1371/journal.ppat.1002507
24. Conrad WH, Osman MM, Shanahan JK, Chu F, Takaki KK, Cameron J, et al. Mycobacterial ESX-1 secretion system mediates host cell lysis through bacterium contact-dependent gross membrane disruptions. *Proc Natl Acad Sci U S A* (2017) 114(6):1371–6. doi:10.1073/pnas.1620133114
25. Mahairas GG, Sabo PJ, Hickey MJ, Singh DC, Stover CK. Molecular analysis of genetic differences between *Mycobacterium bovis* BCG and vir ulent *M. bovis*. *J Bacteriol* (1996) 178(5):1274–82. doi:10.1128/jb.178.5.1274-1282.1996
26. Dobos KM, Spotts EA, Quinn FD, King CH. Necrosis of lung epithelial cells during infection with *Mycobacterium tuberculosis* is preceded by cell permeation. *Infect Immun* (2000) 68(11):6300–10. doi:10.1128/IAI.68.11.6300-6310.2000
27. Riendeau CJ, Kornfeld H. THP-1 cell apoptosis in response to mycobacterial infection. *Infect Immun* (2003) 71(1):254–9. doi:10.1128/IAI.71.1.254-259.2003
28. Dodo K, Katoh M, Shimizu T, Takahashi M, Sodeoka M. Inhibition of hydro gen peroxide-induced necrotic cell death with 3-amino-2-indolylmaleimide derivatives. *Bioorg Med Chem Lett* (2005) 15(12):3114–8. doi:10.1016/j.bmcl.2005.04.016
29. Jaishy B, Abel ED. Lipids, lysosomes, and autophagy. *J Lipid Res* (2016) 57(9):1619–35. doi:10.1194/jlr.R067520
30. Ruth RC, Owens K, Weglicki WB. Inhibition of lysosomal lipases by chlorpromazine: a possible mechanism of stabilization. *J Pharmacol Exp Ther* (1980) 212(3):361–7.
31. Listenberger LL, Han X, Lewis SE, Cases S, Farese RV Jr, Ory DS, et al. Triglyceride accumulation protects against fatty acid-induced lipotoxicity. *Proc Natl Acad Sci U S A* (2003) 100(6):3077–82. doi:10.1073/pnas.0630588100

32. Cao J, Zhou Y, Peng H, Huang X, Stahler S, Suri V, et al. Targeting acyl-CoA:-diacylglycerol acyltransferase 1 (DGAT1) with small molecule inhibitors for the treatment of metabolic diseases. *J Biol Chem* (2011) 286(48):41838–51. doi:10.1074/jbc.M111.245456
33. Tall AR, Yvan-Charvet L. Cholesterol, inflammation and innate immunity. *Nat Rev Immunol* (2015) 15(2):104–16. doi:10.1038/nri3793
34. Lee JY, Zhao L, Youn HS, Weatherill AR, Tapping R, Feng L, et al. Saturated fatty acid activates but polyunsaturated fatty acid inhibits Toll-like receptor 2 dimerized with toll-like receptor 6 or 1. *J Biol Chem* (2004) 279(17):16971–9. doi:10.1074/jbc.M312990200
35. Shi H, Kokoeva MV, Inouye K, Tzameli I, Yin H, Flier JS. TLR4 links innate immunity and fatty acid-induced insulin resistance. *J Clin Invest* (2006) 116(11):3015–25. doi:10.1172/JCI28898
36. Schwartz EA, Zhang WY, Karnik SK, Borwege S, Anand VR, Laine PS, et al. Nutrient modification of the innate immune response: a novel mechanism by which saturated fatty acids greatly amplify monocyte inflammation. *Arterioscler Thromb Vasc Biol* (2010) 30(4):802–8. doi:10.1161/ATVBAHA.109.201681
37. Nascimento EBM, Manneras-Holm L, Chibalin AV, Bjornholm M, Zierath JR. Diacylglycerol kinase alpha deficiency alters inflammation markers in adipose tissue in response to a high-fat diet. *J Lipid Res* (2018) 59(2):273–82. doi:10.1194/jlr.M079517
38. Chen M, Divangahi M, Gan H, Shin DS, Hong S, Lee DM, et al. Lipid mediators in innate immunity against tuberculosis: opposing roles of PGE2 and LXA4 in the induction of macrophage death. *J Exp Med* (2008) 205(12):2791–801. doi:10.1084/jem.20080767
39. Tobin DM, Vary JC Jr, Ray JP, Walsh GS, Dunstan SJ, Bang ND, et al. The lta4h locus modulates susceptibility to mycobacterial infection in zebrafish and humans. *Cell* (2010) 140(5):717–30. doi:10.1016/j.cell.2010.02.013
40. Zaslona Z, Palsson-McDermott EM, Menon D, Haneklaus M. The induction of pro-IL-1beta by lipopolysaccharide requires endogenous prostaglandin E2 production. *J Immunol* (2017) 198(9):3558–64.
41. Divangahi M, Chen M, Gan H, Desjardins D, Hickman TT, Lee DM, et al. *Mycobacterium tuberculosis* evades macrophage defenses by inhibiting plasma membrane repair. *Nat Immunol* (2009) 10(8):899–906. doi:10.1038/ni.1758
42. Dorhoi A, Yeremeev V, Nouailles G, Weiner J III, Jorg S, Heinemann E, et al. Type I IFN signaling triggers immunopathology in tuberculosis-susceptible mice by modulating lung phagocyte dynamics. *Eur J Immunol* (2014) 44(8):2380–93. doi:10.1002/eji.201344219
43. Leitinger N. The role of phospholipid oxidation products in inflammatory and autoimmune diseases: evidence from animal models and in humans. *Subcell Biochem* (2008) 49:325–50. doi:10.1007/978-1-4020-8830-8_12
44. Nixon GF. Sphingolipids in inflammation: pathological implications and potential therapeutic targets. *Br J Pharmacol* (2009) 158(4):982–93. doi:10.1111/j.1476-5381.2009.00281.x
45. Keestra-Gounder AM, Byndloss MX, Seyffert N, Young BM, Chavez-Arroyo A, Tsai AY, et al. NOD1 and NOD2 signalling links ER stress with inflammation. *Nature* (2016) 532(7599):394–7. doi:10.1038/nature17631
46. Missiroli S, Patergnani S, Caroccia N, Pedriali G, Perrone M, Previati M, et al. Mitochondria-associated membranes (MAMs) and inflammation. *Cell Death Dis* (2018) 9(3):329. doi:10.1038/s41419-017-0027-2
47. Saitoh T, Satoh T, Yamamoto N, Uematsu S, Takeuchi O, Kawai T, et al. Antiviral protein Viperin promotes toll-like receptor 7- and toll-like receptor 9-mediated type I interferon production in plasmacytoid dendritic cells. *Immunity* (2011) 34(3):352–63. doi:10.1016/j.immuni.2011.03.010
48. Peyron P, Vaubourgeix J, Poquet Y, Levillain F, Botanch C, Bardou F, et al. Foamy macrophages from tuberculous patients' granulomas constitute a nutrient-rich reservoir for *M. tuberculosis* persistence. *PLoS Pathog* (2008) 4(11):e1000204. doi:10.1371/journal.ppat.1000204
49. Dkhar HK, Nanduri R, Mahajan S, Dave S, Saini A, Somavarapu AK, et al. *Mycobacterium tuberculosis* keto-mycolic acid and macrophage nuclear receptor TR4 modulate foamy biogenesis in granulomas: a case of a heterologous and noncanonical ligand-receptor pair. *J Immunol* (2014) 193(1):295–305. doi:10.4049/jimmunol.1400092
50. Caire-Brandli I, Papadopoulos A, Malaga W, Marais D, Canaan S, Thilo L, et al. Reversible lipid accumulation and associated division arrest of *Mycobacterium avium* in lipoprotein-induced foamy macrophages may resemble key events during latency and reactivation of tuberculosis. *Infect Immun* (2014) 82(2):476–90. doi:10.1128/IAI.01196-13
51. Ouimet M, Koster S, Sakowski E, Ramkhelawon B, van Solingen C, Oldebeken S, et al. *Mycobacterium tuberculosis* induces the miR-33 locus to reprogram autophagy and host lipid metabolism. *Nat Immunol* (2016) 17(6):677–86. doi:10.1038/ni.3434
52. Holla S, Prakhar P, Singh V, Karnam A, Mukherjee T, Mahadik K, et al. MUSASHI-mediated expression of JMJD3, a H3K27me3 demethylase, is involved in foamy macrophage generation during mycobacterial infection. *PLoS Pathog* (2016) 12(8):e1005814. doi:10.1371/journal.ppat.1005814
53. Knight M, Braverman J, Asfaha K, Gronert K, Stanley S. Lipid droplet formation in *Mycobacterium tuberculosis* infected macrophages requires IFN-gamma/HIF-1alpha signaling and supports host defense. *PLoS Pathog* (2018) 14(1):e1006874. doi:10.1371/journal.ppat.1006874
54. Repasy T, Lee J, Marino S, Martinez N, Kirschner DE, Hendricks G, et al. Intracellular bacillary burden reflects a burst size for *Mycobacterium tuberculosis* in vivo. *PLoS Pathog* (2013) 9(2):e1003190. doi:10.1371/journal.ppat.1003190
55. Junqueira-Kipnis AP, Basaraba RJ, Gruppo V, Palanisamy G, Turner OC, Hsu T, et al. Mycobacteria lacking the RD1 region do not induce necrosis in the lungs of mice lacking interferon-gamma. *Immunology* (2006) 119(2):224–31. doi:10.1111/j.1365-2567.2006.02427.x
56. Stutz MD, Ojaimi S, Allison C, Preston S, Arandjelovic P, Hildebrand JM, et al. Necroptotic signaling is primed in *Mycobacterium tuberculosis*-infected macrophages, but its pathophysiological consequence in disease is restricted. *Cell Death Differ* (2017) 25(5):951–65. doi:10.1038/s41418-017-0031-1
57. Bloch H, Segal W. Biochemical differentiation of *Mycobacterium tuberculosis* grown in vivo and in vitro. *J Bacteriol* (1956) 72(2):132–41.
58. Ehrt S, Rhee K, Schnappinger D. Mycobacterial genes essential for the pathogen's survival in the host. *Immunol Rev* (2015) 264(1):319–26. doi:10.1111/imr.12256
59. Daniel J, Maamar H, Deb C, Sirakova TD, Kolattukudy PE. *Mycobacterium tuberculosis* uses host triacylglycerol to accumulate lipid droplets and acquires a dormancy-like phenotype in lipid-loaded macrophages. *PLoS Pathog* (2011) 7(6):e1002093. doi:10.1371/journal.ppat.1002093
60. Lee W, VanderVen BC, Fahey RJ, Russell DG. Intracellular *Mycobacterium tuberculosis* exploits host-derived fatty acids to limit metabolic stress. *J Biol Chem* (2013) 288(10):6788–800. doi:10.1074/jbc.M112.445056
61. VanderVen BC, Fahey RJ, Lee W, Liu Y, Abramovitch RB, Memmott C, et al. Novel inhibitors of cholesterol degradation in *Mycobacterium tuberculosis* reveal how the bacterium's metabolism is constrained by the intracellular environment. *PLoS Pathog* (2015) 11(2):e1004679. doi:10.1371/journal.ppat.1004679
62. Prieur X, Mok CY, Velagapudi VR, Nunez V, Fuentes L, Montaner D, et al. Differential lipid partitioning between adipocytes and tissue macrophages modulates macrophage lipotoxicity and M2/M1 polarization in obese mice. *Diabetes* (2011) 60(3):797–809. doi:10.2337/db10-0705
63. Chinetti-Gbaguidi G, Colin S, Staels B. Macrophage subsets in atherosclerosis. *Nat Rev Cardiol* (2015) 12(1):10–7. doi:10.1038/nrcardio.2014.173
64. Boven LA, Van Meurs M, Van Zwam M, Wierenga-Wolf A, Hintzen RQ, Boot RG, et al. Myelin-laden macrophages are anti-inflammatory, consistent with foam cells in multiple sclerosis. *Brain* (2006) 129(Pt 2):517–26. doi:10.1093/brain/awh707
65. Koliwad SK, Streeper RS, Monetti M, Cornelissen I, Chan L, Terayama K, et al. DGAT1-dependent triacylglycerol storage by macrophages protects mice from diet-induced insulin resistance and inflammation. *J Clin Invest* (2010) 120(3):756–67. doi:10.1172/JCI36066
66. Malandrino MI, Fucho R, Weber M, Calderon-Dominguez M, Mir JF, Valcarcel L, et al. Enhanced fatty acid oxidation in adipocytes and macrophages reduces lipid-induced triglyceride accumulation and inflammation. *Am J Physiol Endocrinol Metab* (2015) 308(9):E756–69. doi:10.1152/ajpendo.00362.2014

67. Kiss RS, Maric J, Marcel YL. Lipid efflux in human and mouse macrophagic cells: evidence for differential regulation of phospholipid and cholesterol efflux. *J Lipid Res* (2005) 46(9):1877–87. doi:10.1194/jlr.M400482-JLR200
68. Rigamonti E, Chinetti-Gbaguidi G, Staels B. Regulation of macrophage functions by PPAR-alpha, PPAR-gamma, and LXRs in mice and men. *Arterioscler Thromb Vasc Biol* (2008) 28(6):1050–9. doi:10.1161/ATVBAHA.107.158998
69. Jaisinghani N, Dawa S, Singh K, Nandy A, Menon D, Bhandari P, et al. Necrosis triggered by *Mycobacterium tuberculosis* alters macrophage triglyceride metabolism and inflammatory response in a DGAT1-dependent manner. *BioRxiv* (2017). doi:10.1101/187104

2

Human Metapneumovirus: Mechanisms and Molecular Targets used by the Virus to Avoid the Immune System

Jorge A. Soto[1], Nicolás M. S. Gálvez[1], Felipe M. Benavente[1], Magdalena S. Pizarro-Ortega[1], Margarita K. Lay[2], Claudia Riedel[3], Susan M. Bueno[1], Pablo A. Gonzalez[1] and Alexis M. Kalergis[1,4]*

[1] Millennium Institute on Immunology and Immunotherapy, Departamento de Genética Molecular y Microbiología, Facultad de Ciencias Biológicas, Pontificia Universidad Católica de Chile, Santiago, Chile, [2] Departamento de Biotecnología, Facultad de Ciencias del Mar y Recursos Biológicos, Universidad de Antofagasta, Antofagasta, Chile, [3] Departamento de Ciencias Biológicas, Facultad de Ciencias de la Vida, Universidad Andrés Bello, Santiago, Chile, [4] Departamento de Endocrinología, Facultad de Medicina, Pontificia Universidad Católica de Chile, Santiago, Chile

***Correspondence:**
Alexis M. Kalergis
akalergis@bio.puc.cl

Human metapneumovirus (hMPV) is a respiratory virus, first reported the year 2001. Since then, it has been described as one of the main etiological agents that causes acute lower respiratory tract infections (ALRTIs), which is characterized by symptoms such as bronchiolitis, wheezing and coughing. Susceptible population to hMPV-infection includes newborn, children, elderly and immunocompromised individuals. This viral agent is a negative-sense, single-stranded RNA enveloped virus, that belongs to the *Pneumoviridae* family and *Metapneumovirus* genus. Early reports—previous to 2001—state several cases of respiratory illness without clear identification of the responsible pathogen, which could be related to hMPV. Despite the similarities of hMPV with several other viruses, such as the human respiratory syncytial virus or influenza virus, mechanisms used by hMPV to avoid the host immune system are still unclear. In fact, evidence indicates that hMPV induces a poor innate immune response, thereby affecting the adaptive immunity. Among these mechanisms, is the promotion of an anergic state in T cells, instead of an effective polarization or activation, which could be induced by low levels of cytokine secretion. Further, the evidences support the notion that hMPV interferes with several pattern recognition receptors (PRRs) and cell signaling pathways triggered by interferon-associated genes. However, these mechanisms reported in hMPV are not like the ones reported for hRSV, as the latter has two non-structural proteins that are able to inhibit these pathways. Several reports suggest that viral glycoproteins, such as G and SH, could play immune-modulator roles during infection. In this work, we discuss the state of the art regarding the mechanisms that underlie the poor immunity elicited by hMPV. Importantly, these mechanisms will be compared with those elicited by other common respiratory viruses.

Keywords: human metapneumovirus, immune system, evasion, cytokines, respiratory virus

INTRODUCTION

Human Metapneumovirus (hMPV) is a respiratory virus discovered by van Den Hoogen et al. the year 2001, in samples from Dutch children with acute lower respiratory tract illness (ALRTI) (1). This virus is known to present a similar pathology and clinical symptoms as the ones reported for the human orthopneumovirus, previously known as human respiratory syncytial virus (hRSV) (2). Clinical symptoms of hMPV-infection can be manifested in both upper and lower respiratory tracts with a predominance for the latter. These symptoms are mainly associated with the appearance of coughing, bronchitis, bronchiolitis and respiratory manifestations related to the absence of airflow (2–4). Symptomatology induced by hMPV-infection is caused by a typical Th17-like immune response, characterized by the secretion of interleukin (IL)-6 and TNF-α in the lungs (5). This immune response is also accompanied by an inadequate Th2-like profile, which is characterized by the early secretion of IL-4, IL-5, IL-8, and other pro-inflammatory cytokines (6–8). Particularly, the thymic stromal lymphopoietin (TSLP), a cytokine known to impair T cell activation, promotes a delay in the Th1-like immunity and triggers the secretion of cytokines related to a Th2-like profile, resulting in high infiltration of neutrophils in the lung of infected mice (9). This abnormal response, along with an excessive mucus production by goblet cells, triggers the collapse of the respiratory airways (3, 10). Infection with hMPV in children under 2-years-old is a risk factor for the development of asthma later in life, as reported for hRSV (11, 12). It has also been reported that, in some of the most severe cases, hMPV promotes chronic obstructive pulmonary disease (COPD) and an exacerbated response, as asthma, in humans (10, 13). It has been estimated that about 10–12% of the respiratory illness in children are associated to hMPV, being considered as one of the most prevalent viruses causing hospitalization in young children (4, 14). It has also been described that hMPV is involved in hospitalizations at a rate of 1 out of 1,000 children under the age of 5 year; and 3 out of 1,000 infants under the age of 6 months. Additionally, it has been reported that prevalence of hMPV infection is equivalent to influenza virus and parainfluenza virus types 1-3 (15).

HMPV belongs to the *Pneumoviridae* family and *Metapneumovirus* genus. It has a negative-sense, single-stranded RNA genome of about 13 Kb of length, encoding 9 structural proteins that go as follows: 3′-N-P-M-F-M2-SH-G-L-5′ (**Figure 1**) (16). The different effects of these proteins on the immune system of the host are not fully characterized. The attachment G protein, one of the two proteins responsible for viral entry, has been widely studied, as it exhibits a role in the evasion of the immune response, inhibiting the interferon (IFN) pathways (17). For hRSV, this IFN pathway inhibition has been demonstrated to be caused by the non-structural proteins 1 and 2 (NS1 and NS2) (18). Remarkably, and as stated above, hMPV genome does not encode for any homolog of these NS proteins. Therefore, this shared ability to inhibit IFN pathway observed in both viruses, in the case of hMPV, is associated with the G glycoprotein, suggesting a possible gain of function for this protein, as compared with hRSV.

Despite increased incidence of hMPV infections in the last years and its impact on health care centers worldwide, neither vaccines nor effective treatments are commercially available to control or prevent infections caused by this viral agent. This is mainly due to the unclear knowledge and lack of characterization of the infection and evasion mechanisms of the immune system used by hMPV. Nonetheless, a candidate vaccine using a recombinant *Mycobacterium bovis* Bacillus Calmette-Guerin (rBCG) that expresses the P protein of hMPV has recently been developed (19). This rBCG candidate vaccine has shown promising results in mouse studies, inducing a protective adaptive immunity—both cellular and humoral—against hMPV-infection with an effective viral clearance (19–21). In this article we will discuss different evasion mechanisms developed by hMPV to prevent the generation of an adequate immune response and the role of different viral proteins involved in these virulence mechanisms.

PERSISTENCE OF HMPV IN EPITHELIAL CELLS

It has been described that hMPV is able to persist in respiratory infected cells after the replicative viral cycle is completed. Indeed, hMPV persistence has been demonstrated in infected mice (22, 23). Measurement of plaque forming units (PFUs) from homogenized lungs of hMPV-infected mice evidenced a biphasic infection cycle, with a peak of viral particles at 7 days post-infection (dpi) and a second peak at 14 dpi. Nevertheless, the authors also reported the appearance of PFUs from the samples obtained from lungs during 28 and 60 days post-infection (22). Additionally, viral RNA was detected by Reverse-Transcription quantitative Polymerase Chain Reaction (RT-qPCR) even after 180 days post-infection. These observations suggest that hMPV may have developed mechanisms that allow its persistence inside of the host cell, resisting viral clearance until, at least, 2 months after the initial infection (22, 23).

Moreover, a study performed by Hamelin et al. found that hMPV-infected mice exhibit a strong pulmonary inflammation associated with airway obstruction (10). Further, higher viral loads were found after 5 days of infection, and these titers were still detected 12 days after, when homogenized lungs from these mice were used to infect LLC-MK2 cells *in vitro*. Similarly, detection of viral copy numbers from infected lung by RT-qPCR indicated that the highest value was detected after 5 days of the initial infection, with a considerable decrease after 21 days. Interestingly, the number of copies of the viral genetic material increased after 42 days of infection and it was still detectable until day 154. All these evidences support the idea of a chronic infection in mice. These results could suggest a relationship with the development of asthma in children infected with this virus, as chronic pulmonary disease is hallmark for the appearance of these condition that could be probably be caused by a chronic infection with this virus (11). However, further studies are require to determine if such models of infection could represent the complexity of hMPV infections in humans (10).

Despite the gaps of knowledge regarding hMPV persistence, a possible mechanism of how this virus may survive in epithelial

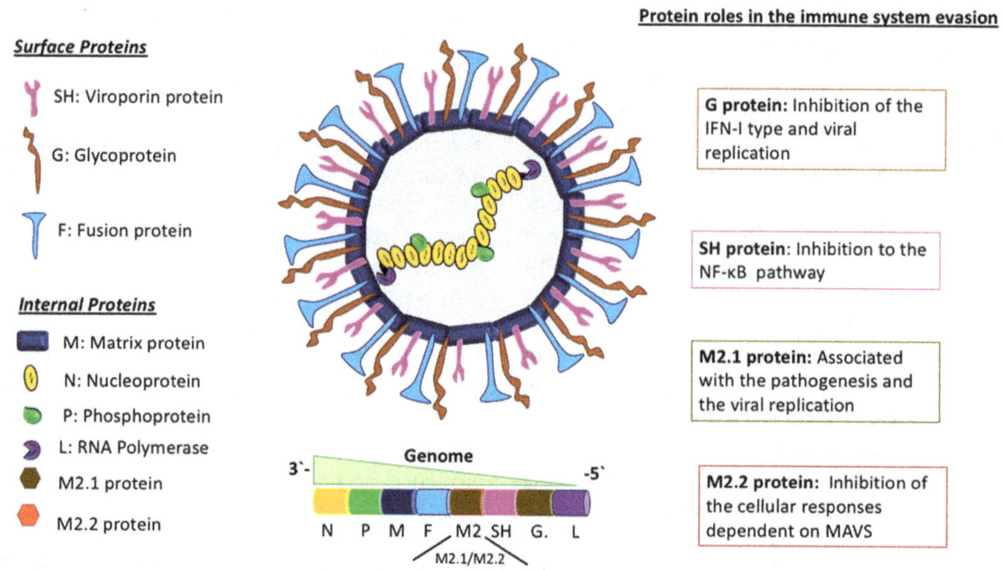

FIGURE 1 | Molecular description of hMPV and the role of viral proteins in the evasion of the immune response. Schematics of the hMPV viral particle in the center and its genomic organization. In the left panel are depicted the viral proteins synthetized by hMPV, separated in two different groups: "surface proteins" and "internal proteins." The right panel describes the main roles of some viral proteins involved in the evasion of the immune response. The proteins M2.1 and M2.2 are expressed only during the replicative viral cycle.

cells for such long periods of time has been recently suggested. Typically, death of infected host cells implies a reduction in viral replication and an increase in the capacity of antigen presentation by immune cells. A study performed by Marsico et al. described in human alveolar epithelial A549 cells that hMPV is able to persist through the inhibition of the apoptosis machinery (24). This effect was associated with an increase in the expression of Bcl-2, an antiapoptotic factor from the Bcl-2 family, in the surface of hMPV-infected cells after 14 days of infection. In addition, the authors postulated a direct correlation between cellular survival and viral replication, suggesting that hMPV starts its infective cycle with a strong peak of replication and a significant increase in cellular apoptosis, followed by a decrease in viral infective rates, promoting a slow cellular proliferation, overcoming apoptosis and inducing cell cycle arrest in G2/M (24). On the other hand, hRSV-infection has been associated with an early induction of Mcl-1 -another antiapoptotic factor that belongs to the Bcl-2 family- along with more antiapoptotic factors (Bcl-W, Bcl-xL) and pro-apoptotic factors (Bid, Bax, Bak), which all could be mediated by the NF-κB pathway (25), suggesting that hMPV could also be using others factor from the Bcl-2 family.

ROLE AND EFFECT OF THE HMPV-PROTEINS IN AVOIDING THE IMMUNE RESPONSE

Currently, the mechanisms of immune evasion used by hMPV are unclear. However, the ability of some hMPV structural proteins to inhibit some cellular pathways required to enhance viral infection have been described. Among these, the attachment or G glycoprotein has the function to recognize and promote the first interaction with the host (26). It has also been described that the G protein has the ability to inhibit the IFN-I response not only *in vitro* (17), but also in an *in vivo* model (27). The latter study showed that the G protein is associated with the recruitment of neutrophils into the alveolar space in lungs of mice infected with hMPV (27). The authors propose that this phenomenon is due to the inhibition of the IFN response, detecting important changes in molecules involved in the recruitment of neutrophils such as; CCL3, CCL4, VEGF, TNF, IL-17, and CXCL2 (27). Also, it has been demonstrated that hMPV activates the TSLP pathway and, therefore, promotes the recruitment of polymorphonuclear cells (PMNs) that secrete cytokines such as IL-13 and IL-5 (9).

A study performed by Le Nouen et al. associated a lower capacity of hMPV infected- human monocyte-derived dendritic cells (MDDCs) to present hMPV antigens to naïve T cells (28). This study described that hMPV-infected MDDCs showed lower maturation levels in flow cytometry assays. Consequently, this effect induced a poor T cell activation, as compared with MDDCs infected with a mutant hMPV that lacked both SH and G glycoprotein genes (ΔSHG). Remarkably, this effect was not observed when a mutant virus deficient in either SH or G genes was used (ΔSH or ΔG, respectively) (28). The MDDCs infected with ΔSHG virus showed an increased maturation rate, promoting the activation of naïve T cells into activated T CD4+ cells, with a Th1-like profile (28).

Interestingly, the infection rate detected in MDDCs was lower than the one identified in epithelial cells. The G protein has also been shown to induce enhanced viral replication in airway epithelial cells (AECs), but poorly in MDDCs (28). However, an *in vivo* study using the ΔG hMPV mutant virus, demonstrated that the viral replication of this mutant was impaired, promoting a small increase in the type I IFN secretion (27). Another study showed that the ΔSH hMPV mutant strain did not affect viral replication capacity when compared to the WT virus, but it did exhibit an inhibition of the NF-kB pathway in human lung epithelial cells (29). The deletion of both viral G and SH genes is related to an increase in the number of effective immunological synapses between DCs stimulated by hMPV and memory CD4+ T cells, therefore promoting the activation of these memory T cells. Altogether, it has been shown that G and SH proteins might reduce the ability of hMPV-infected DCs to activate CD4+ T cells, since both proteins are associated with decreased internalization of the virus into DCs (28). The G protein of hRSV has been described to modulate the host immune response in several ways. It has been shown that hRSV-G protein induces a biased Th2-like immune response in mice, although it can be reverted by using anti-G protein monoclonal antibodies (30). Also, hRSV-G protein can diminish the activation of DCs via interaction with DC/L-SIGN (transmembrane proteins that recognize mannose- and fucose-containing oligosaccharides), which promotes phosphorylation of ERK1 and ERK2 *in vitro* (31).

Nevertheless, some studies suggest that G protein promotes the inhibition of toll-like receptor 4 (TLR4) signaling in MDDCs, affecting the type I IFN secretion (32). The expression of type I IFN and several chemokines can be blocked by down-regulating TLR4 with siRNA, demonstrating that TLR4 is important for the activation of MDDCs induced by hMPV (32). In addition, it has been described that the G protein is also able to inhibit cellular responses induced by hMPV, by interfering with the TLR4-dependent signaling and affecting the production of cytokines and chemokines (32). Therefore, the G protein of this virus negatively modulates the immune response of the host. A study performed with TLR4-deficient mice conducted by Velayutham et al. showed that TLR4 not only plays an important role in the activation of the innate immune response to hMPV, but also contributes to disease pathogenesis (33). Inflammatory response and disease severity were seen to be diminished in hMPV-infected mice lacking TLR4, which was related to significantly lower levels of pro-inflammatory cytokines (TNF-α, IL-1β, IL-6) and chemokines in these mice. Inflammatory cells in BAL, lungs and lymph nodes were also significantly reduced in TLR4-deficient mice when compared with WT mice. Lastly, parameters like body weight loss, hyperresponsiveness and airway obstruction associated with clinical disease severity were reduced in TLR4-deficient mice (33). Similarly, immune response to hRSV induces the activation of the NF-κB pathway dependent on the expression of TLR4, however, the inflammatory response of the airway is not dependent on TLR4 (34).

The negative regulation of the type I IFN signaling pathway observed upon hMPV infection, can also be explained by the activity of the SH protein of the virus. Indeed, the deletion of hMPV SH protein is associated with an increase in the production of IL-6, IL-8 and the expression of other genes dependent of the NF-κB pathway (29). Furthermore, it has been recently determined that SH inhibits the phosphorylation of STAT1, impairing its subsequent signaling (35). Once the IFN-α receptor (IFNAR) is activated, STAT1 is needed downstream of the pathway for the expression of antiviral effector molecules (36–38). The SH protein from hRSV has been shown to prevent apoptosis in hRSV-infected cells, as this protein can inhibit TNF-α-induced death and also inhibit NF-κB activation induced by TNF-α (39). More recently, it has been proposed that hRSV-SH protein could be part of a signaling pathway that induces activation of inflammasomes, by increasing permeability and disrupting membrane architecture, which could be associated with a viral ion channel formation (40).

Although the G and SH are the most studied proteins regarding hMPV capacities to evade immunity, other proteins have also been associated to these processes. Among those, the M2-2 protein has been shown to inhibit MAVS (mitochondrial antiviral signaling), thus contributing to hMPV immune evasion, silencing the cellular responses dependent on MAVS (41). Since MAVS is needed for activation of NF-κB and IRF3, the inhibition of this protein results in enhanced viral replication and cell death, while its overexpression augments the production of IFN (activated by NF-κB and IRF3) and results in an antiviral state (42). NF-κB and IRF3 are activated by hMPV through TRAF5, TRAF6, and TRAF3, which are recruited by MAVS, thus, when suppressed by M2-2, the immune response dependent on MAVS is also inhibited, as it has been recently described (43).

Moreover, a recent *in vitro* study indicated that DCs infected with hMPV lacking the M2-2 gene produce a greater amount of cytokines, chemokines and IFNs, suggesting that the M2-2 protein has an inhibitory role on the innate immune response (44). In addition, in the same study, it was pointed out that M2-2 is capable of inhibiting the expression of genes that are dependent on MyD88 (myeloid differentiation protein response 88), an essential adapter for some TLRs, critical for the immune responses of DCs (44). hRSV strains lacking the M2-2 protein do not grow as efficiently as WT virus (45, 46). Also, it has been suggested that this protein works regulating the RNA synthesis, as infected cells with hRSV lacking M2-2 gene accumulate mRNA beyond the levels detected on cells infected with WT virus (45). The hRSV M2-2 gene has been deleted as an approach for the development of vaccine against hRSV (RSV MEDI ΔM2-2) (46).

Little is known about the role of the M2-1 protein in hMPV evasion mechanisms. However, this protein presents a critical role in hMPV pathogenesis and viral replication (47, 48). One possible characteristic suggested for the protein's role is its Zinc binding activity. Some studies suggest that mutations in this zinc binding protein can affect the infective capacity of hMPV, promoting an attenuated infection in cotton rats (47). The M2-1 protein from hRSV has a transcriptional function, as it can prevent early termination of the viral RNA transcription, which requires the formation of the RdRp complex and the interaction with RNA and the hRSV P protein. Remarkably, the hRSV M2-1 protein increases the processivity of the viral RNA polymerase (49, 50).

The matrix (M) protein is mainly associated with the assembly of the hMPV viral particle (16). It is also known that this protein promotes the production of inflammatory cytokines in MDDCs, such as IL-1β, TNF-α, IL-6, and IL-8 (4, 51).

Lastly, the retinoic acid inducible gene (RIG-I) can sense hMPV infection and induce a type I IFN response, however, the hMPV-B1 strain has been described to avoid this IFN response thanks to the phosphoprotein (P), which prevents RIG-I activation (52). The M protein from hRSV is essential for viral replication and proliferation. This protein interacts with the nucleocapsids under the plasma membrane and with the envelope glycoproteins, suggesting participation in virus assembly and inhibition of transcription (53). Mice infected with hRSV lacking the M protein exhibited reduced weight loss, viral titters, and pulmonary dysfunction, as compared to control groups. Also, an important memory immune response is seen on the M-null hRSV-infected mice (54).

More studies are needed to determine the interactions between hMPV proteins and different host factors associated with the immune response, in order to understand the immune modulation during the infective process and pathogenesis, which will improve the design of efficient therapies and prophylactic approaches against this pathogen.

INEFFICIENT CYTOKINE PROFILE SECRETION

Several studies have been performed to characterize the immune response associated with hMPV infection—particularly, by assessing the profile of secreted cytokines (55). It has been reported that DCs obtained from mice can reduced their migratory capacity, cytokine production, and CD4+ T cell activation, when infected with hMPV, similarly as observed in hRSV infections (56–61). However, the cytokine profile induced by hMPV in humans is different from the cytokine profile induced by hRSV or influenza virus (55).

The recognition of hMPV by the innate immune system is associated with pattern recognition receptors (PRRs). This recognition in the upper and lower respiratory tract is performed by AECs, hMPV main target cells for infection, and by phagocytic cells, such as DCs and macrophages, that express PRRs and can recognize several pathogen-associated molecular patterns (PAMPs) (62). These PAMPs include double-stranded RNA and viral proteins produced during the replication cycle. The activation of PRRs renders immune cells able to promote the activation of several pro-inflammatory cytokines and chemokines (62).

Recently, it has been reported that hMPV infection induces the production of thymic stromal lymphopoietin (TSLP) as an early response to the viral infection by AECs (9). This upregulation induces an allergic-like innate immune response that drives the expression of Th1- and Th2-like cytokine such as TNF-α, IL-5, and IL-13, as a part of a late antiviral response that eventually promotes an increase in polymorphonuclear cells recruitment and an induction of mucus secretion in the mouse lung (9). In turn, a pronounced pulmonary inflammatory response and an increase in viral replication is produced upon hMPV infection.

As hRSV and hMPV exhibit similar pathologies, they have been continuously misdiagnosed among them (63). Accordingly, it has been described that the cytokine profile is similar between the two viruses, although with some differences. Indeed, Herd et al. described that the transcript levels associated with Th1-like cytokines (i.e., IL-12) and Th2-associated cytokines (i.e., IL-4 and IL-10) were significantly enhanced upon infection with either hMPV or hRSV, when compared with the respective controls in a BALB/c mouse model (64). However, levels of IL-12 were significantly higher in hMPV-infected mice when compared with hRSV-infected mice. This report also describes an increase in the secretion of IFN-γ and IFN-β (both Th1-like cytokines), along with MIP-1a and CXCL-10 (chemokines associated with the activation of granulocytes, and the chemoattraction of macrophages and T cells after the hMPV and hRSV infection) (64). Moreover, several others signaling molecules, particularly Mig, CXCL1, MIP-1β, and IP-10, are upregulated in infected mice when compared with non-infected animals.

Recently, *in vitro* studies performed by Tzannou et al., described that the immunodominant antigens of hMPV are the F, N, M2-1, M and P proteins (65). These authors also indicated that the polyclonal CD4+ T cells repertoire produced during infection was mainly associated with the secretion of IFN-γ, TNF-α, GM-CSF, and granzyme B. However, contrary to what was described above, no secretion of IL-6 or IL-10 was detected. Interestingly, mice models of hMPV-infection show that CD8+ T cells, but not CD4+ T cells nor neutralizing antibodies, are involved in the protection from reinfection. The opposite phenomena is seen in the case of hRSV-infections, where CD4+ T cells are shown to be required for protection against reinfections (66).

An increase in the secretion of IFN-γ, IL-1β, IL-2, IL-4, and IL-6 has been described in nasopharyngeal aspirates of children infected with either hMPV or hRSV that exhibit also acute respiratory tract infection symptoms; this in line with what has been previously reported in some works with mouse model (67). Remarkably, IL-2 and IL-1β secretions were higher in hMPV-infected children, when compared to those infected with hRSV. Likewise, IL-4 secretion was higher in hRSV-infected children, as compared with hMPV-infected children. These findings may imply that the robust Th2-like response that has previously been observed and extensively characterized for hRSV is not exhibited in a similar magnitude by hMPV (67). Moreover, the authors indicate that, along with this IL-1β and IL-6 increase, a Th17-like immune response associated with neutrophil-mediated asthma could be elicited during hMPV infection (67).

A study performed in Argentina using samples from newborns and children under 1-year-old, showed that low levels of IL-1β, TNF-α, IL-6, IL-8, and IL-12 were detected in samples from hMPV-infected children, as compared with children infected with hRSV or influenza virus (55). This study suggests that, despite the fact that infection caused by hMPV shares similarities with those caused by hRSV—including symptoms and pathology—hMPV induces significantly lower levels of respiratory inflammatory cytokines, as compared with the response observed in hRSV-infected children (55). Interestingly, the data obtained in this study are different to those obtained in a study performed by Jartti et al., where IL-8 levels induced by hMPV were higher than the ones induced by hRSV

(68). Considering all these, it is unclear how hMPV is able to induce lung collapse in a similar way than hRSV.

It has been previously reported that many viruses are able to induce the activation of the type-I IFN pathway (i.e., IFN-α and IFN-β), promoting the proliferation and differentiation of adaptive immunity cells (69). Particularly, IFN-α and IFN-β bind to the IFNAR, prompting a signaling cascade that is mainly associated with the phosphorylation of STAT1, and its consequent dimerization with STAT2. This dimer is able to reach the nucleus and activate the transcription of several anti-viral genes that may promote viral clearance (69). *In vitro* studies have reported that hMPV is able to avoid the type-I IFN pathway, as it can modulate the first steps in the signaling cascade associated with this network. As seen for other viruses, such as influenza A virus (IAV) and hRSV, modulation of this pathway is performed by several virulence factors (69).

It has been reported for IAV that hemagglutinin, one of the surface proteins of this pathogen, is capable of inducing degradation of IFNAR, therefore inhibiting autocrine signaling associated with these molecules (69). Likewise, the NS1 protein of hRSV is able to target STAT proteins so that they are degraded through the proteasome, as described by Ramaswamy et al. (70). Particularly, for hMPV it was recently reported that the modulation of this pathway seems to be mainly through the inhibition of STAT1 phosphorylation, induced by the SH protein of this virus. The lack of phosphorylation of this protein seems to be related to a desensitization of the IFNAR to IFN-α. Moreover, other proteins have been associated with this modulation, such as G and M2.2 proteins (41, 71). Therefore, even though hMPV does seem to induce a similar response as the ones seen for other respiratory viruses, the mechanisms associated to this induction seem to be different (35, 55, 67).

Another possible reason to explain the IFN pathway inhibition are the defective interfering (DI) RNA produced during the viral replication process. It has been reported that an increase in the DI RNA can promote type-I IFN secretion in epithelial cells, where it was described that a high multiplicity of infection (MOI) of hMPV promotes an increase in the DI RNA, but a low MOI decreases the production of DI RNA and hence, an absence of type-I IFN response is observed (72). This phenomenon has only been identified in culture cell lines, such as A549 and Vero cells (72). Remarkably, this strategy to activate the type I-IFN pathway has been also described in other viruses, such as the Sendai virus (SeV), Measles virus Edmonston strain (MeVEdm), and hRSV (73).

TLRS AND THEIR EFFECTS OVER THE IMMUNE RESPONSE INDUCED BY HMPV

TLRs are a type of receptor associated with the activation of different pathways of the immune system, mainly the innate immune system (74–78). This activation occurs by the recognition of different pathogen associated molecular patterns (PAMPs) that promote an intracellular signaling pathway in the cell. As a consequence, cytokines and chemokines are secreted in response to stimuli.

Some TLRs involved with hMPV-infection have been studied (**Figure 2**), suggesting that the absence of TLR4 in mice infected with hMPV results in a decrease in the production of cytokines,

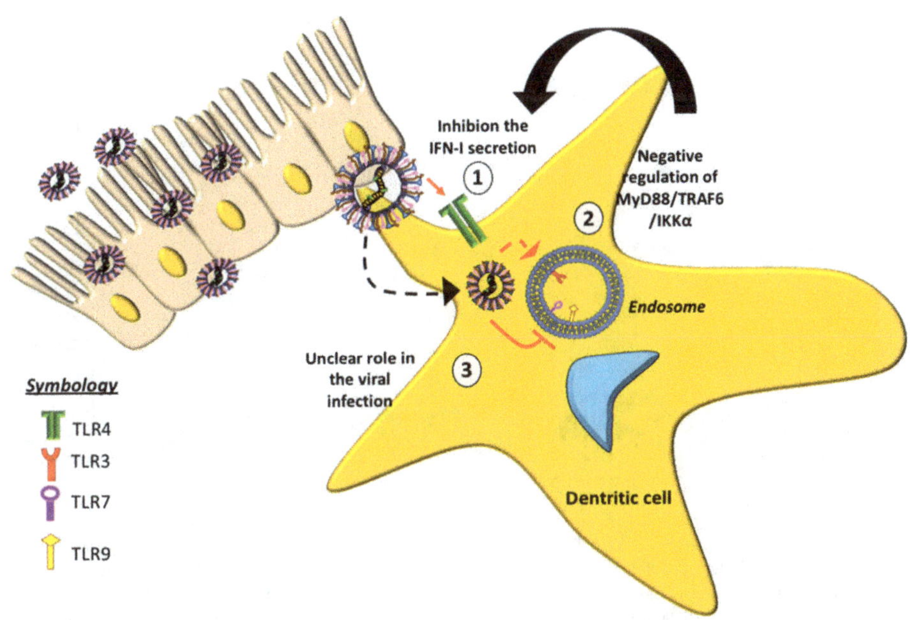

FIGURE 2 | Toll-like receptors (TLRs) and their role in the evasion of the immune response induced by hMPV. The figure shows the effect of different TLRs in response to hMPV-infection. (1) At the surface of the host cell, TLR4 (green receptor) is associated with the inhibition of type-I IFN. (2) In the intracellular space, TLR3 (red receptor) is involved in the negative regulation of the MyD88/TRAF6/IKKα pathway. (3) The roles of TLRs 7 and 9 (purple and yellow receptor, respectively) in hMPV infection are currently unclear.

such as IFN-α/β, as well as reduced inflammatory response and disease severity (33). Similarly, a reduction in lung inflammation and disease severity has been reported in mice lacking MyD88 (79). The absence of MyD88 negatively affects the production of cytokines and chemokines and the recruitment of DCs, CD4+ and CD8+ T cells into the lungs of infected animals (79). These data indicate that both TLR4 and MyD88 are involved in the pathogenesis of the disease, the pathogenic response against the virus and in the lung inflammation.

Another role associated with MyD88 is its participation in one of the two pathways involved in the production of type-I IFN in response to *in vitro* hMPV infection, when the virus is detected by TLR3 and TLR7. Once TLR3 detects hMPV, it is able to activate IFN regulatory factor 3 (IRF3) through TRIF, whereas TLR7 activates IRF7 through MyD88 (41, 52). RIG-I and MDA5 are two helicases from the RIG-I-like receptor (RLR) family that induce signaling downstream to MAVS after detecting viral dsRNA in the cytosol (48, 56, 57). Subsequently, MAVS activates IRF3, and this in turn activates the production of type-I IFN and the up-regulation of IRF7 and NF-κB, thus producing proinflammatory cytokines and type-III IFNs (80). The absence of MDA5 in mutant mice is related with a more severe disease caused by hMPV (i.e., increased pulmonary inflammation and cellular infiltration, and a more sustained weight loss over time). This phenomenon is accompanied by an increase in viral replication and decreased production of type I-IFN, which suggests an altered antiviral response (81).

In an epithelial cell model, hMPV elicits the expression of both, RIG-I and MDA5, however, it has been suggested a more important role for RIG-I, as its inhibition results in a negative regulation of both downstream transcription factors NF-κB and IRF (**Figure 3**). This in turn results in a diminished production of IFN and pro-inflammatory cytokines, and an increase in viral replication, which highlights the role of RIG-I contribution to an antiviral state. This study also suggests that MDA5 seems to play a non-significant role in cellular responses induced by hMPV (80). Similarly, during early hRSV-infection (6 h post-infection), viral N protein colocalizes with RIG-I and MDA5, and later (12 h post-infection) N protein appears in close proximity to MAVS and MDA5, suggesting that the decreased IFN response -and thus the inefficient innate response observed in the experiment- is due to an interaction between the N protein and MAVS and MDA5 (82).

Once DCs have recognized the pathogen through their TLR7 and TLR9 receptors, the signaling pathways induce the activation

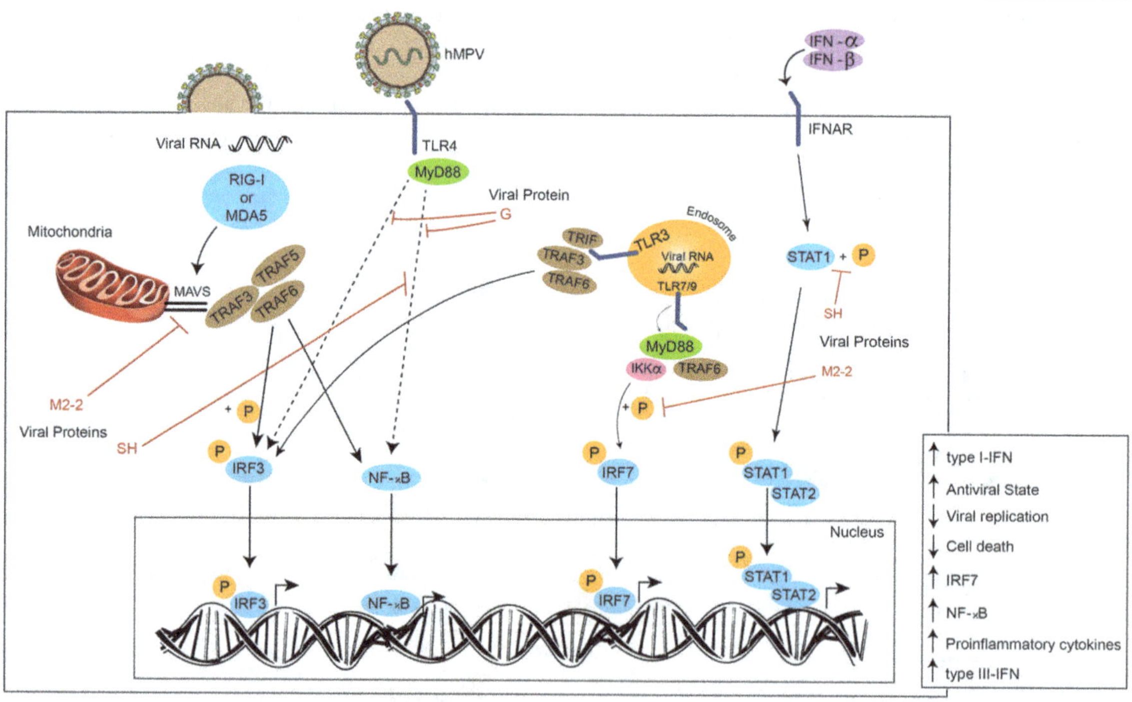

FIGURE 3 | Effects of hMPV proteins on signaling pathways. Once the viral particle has fused with the plasmatic membrane, the viral RNA is delivered to the cytoplasm and recognized by MDA5 or RIG-I (PRRs), activating the IRF3 and NF-κB pathways through TRAF3, TRAF5, and TRAF6 after these factors are recruited by MAVS. After the viral proteins are translated from viral RNA inside the host cell, the M2-2 viral protein can inhibit MAVS and thus, the MAVS-dependent immune response. Viral particles are also detected by TLR4, initiating the signaling which ends in the translocation of both transcription factors IRF3 and NF-κB to the nucleus, promoting an antiviral state and the expression of type-I IFN. The G viral protein interferes with the TLR4-dependent signaling, negatively modulating the immune response of the host and promoting viral replication. The SH viral protein can inhibit the NF-κB signaling as well. Viral RNA detected inside endosomes by TLR3 and TLR7/9 results in the phosphorylation of both transcriptional factors IRF3 and IRF7, and their entry to the nucleus to promote the expression of type-III IFN and proinflammatory cytokines. The M2-2 viral protein inhibits the phosphorylation of IRF7, preventing its translocation to the nucleus. The SH viral protein induces the same effect on IFNAR signaling by preventing the phosphorylation of STAT1.

of genes encoding for IFN-α (83–86). The M2-2 protein has also been proposed to be a potent negative regulator of the TLR7/9-dependent production of IFN-α in pDCs, since it is suggested that it is capable of inhibiting phosphorylation of Ser477-IRF7 induced by MyD88/TRAF6/IKKα (**Figure 3**) (87).

In addition, a study performed in neonatal mice showed that the absence of IRF3 and IRF7 is a critical factor involved in hMPV clearance. However, this response was only observed when both transcription factors were absent. It was determined through a KO mice model that the absence of IRF3 induced a decrease in IFN-β, IFN-λ2/3, and IFN-γ secretion, although IFN-α expression was not affected. Consequently, this triggered an increase in the viral loads detected in the lungs (88). Regarding IRF7, it was found that its absence decreased the expression of only four cytokines, but that viral loads in the lungs were not affected and a Th2-like profile was promoted with its characteristic increase in the eosinophil population (88). IPS-1 (IFN-β promoter stimulator 1) levels correlated positively with IFN-β secretion, and its absence resulted in an increase in IFN-a4 secretion (88). This is similar to what was observed in the IRF-7-lacking model, suggesting that IFN- α could likely be an IPS-1/IRF3-independent activation pathway of TLR7-MyD88 in plasmacytoid dendritic cells.

A recent study by Baños-Lara et al. showed a differential miRNA pattern expression in Monocyte derived DCs (MoDCs) induced by hMPV- and hRSV-infection. Therein, they report that hMPV induces a higher expression of has-miR-185–5p, a miRNA that affects different genes such as FOXO1, PDCD4 and RECK, among others; but the effect in the dysregulation of these genes is not reported (89). On the other hand, hRSV induces the expression of miR-4448, that is associated with the Akt/mTOR pathway, inhibiting apoptosis and, as a consequence, increasing cell survivor (90).

CONCLUSION

hMPV is an emergent respiratory virus that each year increases its incidence and burden. Furthermore, despite its similarities with hRSV at a genomic and clinical level, the immune response triggered by both viruses are not identical. Likewise, the immune responses elicited in humans and mouse models exhibit significant differences in the cytokine secretion profile. In addition, hMPV mechanisms to escape the immune system are mostly unknown and yet to be described, although more studies regarding the understanding of this viral agent are emerging. Currently, it is known that SH and G glycoprotein are the most important proteins involved in evasion of the immune response, promoting the inhibition of an antiviral immune response triggered by type-I IFN. Also, the modulation of different intracellular TLR involved in the immune response against viral particles or intracellular pathogens is clearly a mechanism that needs to be characterized in detail. Remarkably, hamsters, mice, and even non-human primates used as animal models of hMPV-infection are, in different degrees, semi-permissive to viral infection (91), thus t is highly important to perform more studies to determine if such models are representative of an hMPV-infection in humans.

AUTHOR CONTRIBUTIONS

JS, NG, FB, and MP-O are responsible for the writing of this review article. ML, CR, SB, and PG are responsible for reviewing the article and AK is the leading investigator and assisted in the organization and revision of the manuscript.

ACKNOWLEDGMENTS

We would also like to thank Trinidad Celis for her support in the elaboration of the manuscript's figures.

REFERENCES

1. van den Hoogen BG, de Jong JC, Groen J, Kuiken T, de Groot R, Fouchier RA, Osterhaus AD. A newly discovered human pneumovirus isolated from young children with respiratory tract disease. *Nat Med.* (2001) 7:719–24. doi: 10.1038/89098
2. Schildgen V, van den Hoogen B, Fouchier R, Tripp RA, Alvarez R, Manoha C, et al. Human metapneumovirus: lessons learned over the first decade. *Clin Microbiol Rev.* (2011) 24:734–54. doi: 10.1128/CMR.00015-11
3. Boivin G, De Serres G, Côté S, Gilca R, Abed Y, Rochette L, at al. Human metapneumovirus infections in hospitalized children. *Emerg Infect Dis.* 9:634–40. doi: 10.3201/eid0906.030017
4. Feuillet F, Lina B, Rosa-Calatrava M, Boivin G. Ten years of human metapneumovirus research. *J Clin Virol.* (2012) 53:97–105. doi: 10.1016/j.jcv.2011.10.002
5. Huck B, Neumann-Haefelin D, Schmitt-Graeff A, Weckmann M, Mattes J, Ehl S, et al. Human metapneumovirus induces more severe disease and stronger innate immune response in BALB/c mice as compared with respiratory syncytial virus. *Respir Res.* (2007) 8:6. doi: 10.1186/1465-9921-8-6
6. Romagnani S. Regulation of the T cell response. *Clin Exp Allergy* (2006) 36:1357–66. doi: 10.1111/j.1365-2222.2006.02606.x
7. Fietta P, Delsante G. The effector T helper cell triade. *Riv Biol.* (2010) 102:61–74.
8. Ito T, Amakawa R, Inaba M, Hori T, Ota M, Nakamura K, et al. Plasmacytoid dendritic cells regulate Th cell responses through OX40 ligand and Type I IFNs. *J Immunol.* (2004) 172:4253–9. doi: 10.4049/jimmunol.172.7.4253
9. Lay MK, Céspedes PF, Palavecino CE, León MA, Díaz RA, Salazar FJ, et al. Human metapneumovirus infection activates the TSLP pathway that drives excessive pulmonary inflammation and viral replication in mice. *Eur J Immunol.* (2015) 45:1680–95. doi: 10.1002/eji.201445021
10. Hamelin M, Prince GA, Gomez AM, Kinkead R, Boivin G. Human metapneumovirus infection induces long-term pulmonary inflammation associated with airway obstruction and hyperresponsiveness in mice. *J Infect Dis.* (2006) 193:1634–42. doi: 10.1086/504262

11. García-García ML, Calvo C, Casas I, Bracamonte T, Rellán A, Gozalo F, et al. Human metapneumovirus bronchiolitis in infancy is an important risk factor for asthma at age 5. *Pediatr Pulmonol.* (2007) doi: 10.1002/ppul.20597
12. Sigurs N, Aljassim F, Kjellman B, Robinson PD, Sigurbergsson F, Bjarnason R, et al. Asthma and allergy patterns over 18 years after severe RSV bronchiolitis in the first year of life. *Thorax* (2010) 65:1045–52. doi: 10.1136/thx.2009.121582
13. Peiris JSM, Tang W-H, Chan K-H, Khong P-L, Guan Y, Lau Y-L, Chiu SS. Children with respiratory disease associated with metapneumovirus in Hong Kong. *Emerg Infect Dis.* (2003) 9:628–33. doi: 10.3201/eid0906.030009
14. Prado SMA, Perret PC, Montecinos PL, Veloz BA, Le Corre PN, Habash AL, et al. [Human metapneumovirus as hospitalization cause in children under 3 years old with acute respiratory infections during 2004]. Metapneumovirus Hum como causa Hosp en ninos bajo 3 anos edad, con Infecc Respir aguda, durante el ano 2004. *Rev Chilena Infectol.* (2007) 24:19–26.
15. Edwards KM, Zhu Y, Griffin MR, Weinberg GA, Hall CB, Szilagyi PG, et al. Burden of human metapneumovirus infection in young children. *N Engl J Med.* (2013) 368:633–43. doi: 10.1056/NEJMoa1204630
16. van den Hoogen BG, Bestebroer TM, Osterhaus ADME, Fouchier RAM. Analysis of the genomic sequence of a human metapneumovirus. *Virology* (2002) 295:119–32. doi: 10.1006/viro.2001.1355
17. Bao X, Liu T, Shan Y, Li K, Garofalo RP, Casola A. Human metapneumovirus glycoprotein G inhibits innate immune responses. *PLoS Pathog.* (2008) 4:e1000077. doi: 10.1371/journal.ppat.1000077
18. Barik S. Respiratory syncytial virus mechanisms to interfere with type 1 interferons. *Curr Top Microbiol Immunol.* (2013) 372:173–91. doi: 10.1007/978-3-642-38919-1-9
19. Palavecino CE, Cespedes PF, Gomez RS, Kalergis AM, Bueno SM. Immunization with a recombinant bacillus calmette-guerin strain confers protective Th1 immunity against the Human Metapneumovirus. *J Immunol.* (2014) 192:214–23. doi: 10.4049/jimmunol.1300118
20. Bueno SM, Gonzalez PA, Cautivo KM, Mora JE, Leiva ED, Tobar HE, et al. Protective T cell immunity against respiratory syncytial virus is efficiently induced by recombinant BCG. *Proc Natl Acad Sci USA.* (2008) 105:20822–7. doi: 10.1073/pnas.0806244105
21. Cautivo KM, Bueno SM, Cortes CM, Wozniak A, Riedel CA, Kalergis AM. Efficient lung recruitment of respiratory syncytial virus-specific Th1 cells induced by recombinant bacillus calmette-guerin promotes virus clearance and protects from infection. *J Immunol.* (2010) 185:7633–45. doi: 10.4049/jimmunol.0903452
22. Alvarez R, Harrod KS, Shieh WJ, Zaki S, Tripp RA. Human metapneumovirus persists in BALB/c mice despite the presence of neutralizing antibodies. *J Virol.* (2004) 78:14003–11. doi: 10.1128/Jvi.78.24.14003-14011.2004
23. Alvarez R, Tripp RA. The immune response to human metapneumovirus is associated with aberrant immunity and impaired virus clearance in BALB/c Mice. *J Virol.* (2005) 79:5971–8. doi: 10.1128/JVI.79.10.5971-5978.2005
24. Marsico S, Caccuri F, Mazzuca P, Apostoli P, Roversi S, Lorenzin G, et al. Human lung epithelial cells support human metapneumovirus persistence by overcoming apoptosis. *Pathog Dis.* (2018) 76:fty013. doi: 10.1093/femspd/fty013
25. Kotelkin A, Prikhod 'ko EA, Cohen JI, Collins PL, Bukreyev A. Respiratory syncytial virus infection sensitizes cells to apoptosis mediated by tumor necrosis factor-related apoptosis-inducing ligand. *J Virol.* (2003) 77:9156–72. doi: 10.1128/JVI.77.17.9156–9172.2003
26. Levine S, Kaliaber-Franco R, Paradiso PR. Demonstration that glycoprotein G is the attachment protein of respiratory syncytial virus. *J Gen Virol.* (1987) 68:2521–4. doi: 10.1099/0022-1317-68-9-2521
27. Cheemarla NR, Guerrero-Plata A. Human metapneumovirus attachment protein contributes to neutrophil recruitment into the airways of infected mice. *Viruses* (2017) 9:E310. doi: 10.3390/v9100310
28. Le Nouen C, Hillyer P, Brock LG, Winter CC, Rabin RL, Collins PL, et al. Human metapneumovirus SH and G glycoproteins inhibit macropinocytosis-mediated entry into human dendritic cells and reduce CD4+ T Cell activation. *J Virol.* (2014) 88:6453–69. doi: 10.1128/JVI.03261-13
29. Bao X, Kolli D, Liu T, Shan Y, Garofalo RP, Casola A. Human metapneumovirus small hydrophobic protein inhibits NF- B transcriptional activity. *J Virol.* (2008) 82:8224–9. doi: 10.1128/JVI.02584-07
30. Boyoglu-Barnum S, Chirkova T, Todd SO, Barnum TR, Gaston KA, Jorquera P, et al. Prophylaxis with a Respiratory Syncytial Virus (RSV) Anti-G protein monoclonal antibody shifts the adaptive immune response to RSV rA2-line19F infection from Th2 to Th1 in BALB/c Mice. *J Virol.* (2014) 88:10569–83. doi:10.1128/JVI.01503-14
31. Johnson TR, McLellan JS, Graham BS. Respiratory syncytial virus glycoprotein G interacts with DC-SIGN and L-SIGN to activate ERK1 and ERK2. *J Virol.* (2012) 86:1339–47. doi: 10.1128/JVI.06096-11
32. Kolli D, Bao X, Liu T, Hong C, Wang T, Garofalo RP, Casola A. Human metapneumovirus glycoprotein G inhibits TLR4-dependent signaling in monocyte-derived dendritic cells. *J Immunol.* (2011) 187:47–54. doi: 10.4049/jimmunol.1002589
33. Velayutham TS, Kolli D, Ivanciuc T, Garofalo RP, Casola A. Critical role of TLR4 in human metapneumovirus mediated innate immune responses and disease pathogenesis. *PLoS ONE* (2013) 8:e78849. doi: 10.1371/journal.pone.0078849
34. Haeberle H A, Takizawa R, Casola A, Brasier AR, Dieterich H-J, Van Rooijen N, et al. Respiratory syncytial virus-induced activation of nuclear factor-kappaB in the lung involves alveolar macrophages and toll-like receptor 4-dependent pathways. *J Infect Dis.* (2002) 186:1199–206. doi: 10.1086/344644
35. Hastings AK, Amato KR, Wen SC, Peterson LS, Williams J V. Human metapneumovirus small hydrophobic (SH) protein downregulates type I IFN pathway signaling by affecting STAT1 expression and phosphorylation. *Virology* (2016) 494:248–56. doi: 10.1016/j.virol.2016.04.022
36. Sadler AJ, Williams BRG. Interferon-inducible antiviral effectors. *Nat Rev Immunol.* (2008) 8:559–68. doi: 10.1038/nri2314
37. Biron CA. Interferons α and β as immune regulators—a new look. *Immunity* (2001) 14:661–4. doi: 10.1016/S1074-7613(01)00154-6
38. Barber GN. Host defense, viruses and apoptosis. *Cell Death Differ.* (2001) 8:113–26. doi: 10.1038/sj.cdd.4400823
39. Fuentes S, Tran KC, Luthra P, Teng MN, He B. Function of the respiratory syncytial virus small hydrophobic protein. *J Virol.* (2007) 81:8361–6. doi: 10.1128/JVI.02717-06
40. Triantafilou K, Kar S, Vakakis E, Kotecha S, Triantafilou M. Human respiratory syncytial virus viroporin SH: a viral recognition pathway used by the host to signal inflammasome activation. *Thorax* (2013) 68:66–75. doi: 10.1136/thoraxjnl-2012-202182
41. Ren J, Wang Q, Kolli D, Prusak DJ, Tseng C-TK, Chen ZJ, et al. Human Metapneumovirus M2-2 protein inhibits innate cellular signaling by targeting MAVS. *J Virol.* (2012) 86:13049–61. doi: 10.1128/JVI.01248-12
42. Seth RB, Sun L, Ea CK, Chen ZJ. Identification and characterization of MAVS, a mitochondrial antiviral signaling protein that activates NF-κB and IRF3. *Cell* (2005) 122:669–82. doi: 10.1016/j.cell.2005.08.012
43. Chen Y, Deng X, Deng J, Zhou J, Ren Y, Liu S, et al. Functional motifs responsible for human metapneumovirus M2-2-mediated innate immune evasion. *Virology* (2016) 499:361–8. doi: 10.1016/j.virol.2016.09.026
44. Ren J, Liu G, Go J, Kolli D, Zhang G, Bao X. Human metapneumovirus M2-2 protein inhibits innate immune response in monocyte-derived dendritic cells. *PLoS ONE* (2014) 9:e91865. doi: 10.1371/journal.pone.0091865
45. Bermingham A, Collins PL. The M2-2 protein of human respiratory syncytial virus is a regulatory factor involved in the balance between RNA replication and transcription. *Proc Natl Acad Sci USA.* (1999) 96:11259–64. doi: 10.1073/pnas.96.20.11259
46. Karron RA, Luongo C, Thumar B, Loehr KM, Englund JA, Collins PL, et al. A gene deletion that up-regulates viral gene expression yields an attenuated RSV vaccine with improved antibody responses in children. *Sci Transl Med.* (2015) 7:312ra175. doi: 10.1126/scitranslmed.aac8463
47. Cai H, Zhang Y, Ma Y, Sun J, Liang X, Li J. Zinc binding activity of human metapneumovirus M2-1 protein is indispensable for viral replication and pathogenesis *in vivo*. *J Virol.* (2015) 89:6391–5. doi: 10.1128/JVI.03488-14
48. Cai H, Zhang Y, Lu M, Liang X, Jennings R, Niewiesk S, Li J. Phosphorylation of human metapneumovirus M2-1 protein upregulates viral replication and pathogenesis. *J Virol.* (2016) 90:7323–38. doi: 10.1128/JVI.00755-16
49. Blondot M-L, Dubosclard V, Fix J, Lassoued S, Aumont-Nicaise M, Bontems F, et al. Structure and functional analysis of the RNA- and viral phosphoprotein-binding domain of respiratory syncytial virus M2-1 protein. *PLoS Pathog.* (2012) 8:e1002734. doi: 10.1371/journal.ppat.1002734

50. Cartee TL, Wertz GW. Respiratory syncytial virus M2-1 protein requires phosphorylation for efficient function and binds viral RNA during infection. *J Virol.* (2001) 75:12188–97. doi: 10.1128/JVI.75.24.12188-12197.2001
51. Bagnaud-Baule A, Reynard O, Perret M, Berland J-L, Maache M, Peyrefitte C, et al. The human metapneumovirus matrix protein stimulates the inflammatory immune response *in vitro*. *PLoS ONE* (2011) 6:e17818. doi: 10.1371/journal.pone.0017818
52. Goutagny N, Jiang Z, Tian J, Parroche P, Schickli J, Monks BG, et al. Cell type-specific recognition of human metapneumoviruses (HMPVs) by retinoic acid-inducible gene I (RIG-I) and TLR7 and viral interference of RIG-I ligand recognition by HMPV-B1 phosphoprotein. *J Immunol.* (2010) 184:1168–79. doi: 10.4049/jimmunol.0902750
53. Ghildyal R, Ho A, Jans DA. Central role of the respiratory syncytial virus matrix protein in infection. *FEMS Microbiol Rev.* (2006) 30:692–705. doi: 10.1111/j.1574-6976.2006.00025.x
54. Schmidt ME, Oomens AGP, Varga SM. Single-cycle respiratory syncytial virus infection induces robust adaptive immune responses and reduces disease severity in mice. *J Immunol.* (2018) 200. Available online at: http://www.jimmunol.org/content/200/1_Supplement/60.2
55. Laham FR, Israele V, Casellas JM, Garcia AM, Lac Prugent CM, Hoffman SJ, et al. Differential production of inflammatory cytokines in primary infection with human metapneumovirus and with other common respiratory viruses of infancy. *J Infect Dis.* (2004) 189:2047–56. doi: 10.1086/383350
56. Le Nouën C, Munir S, Losq S, Winter CC, McCarty T, Stephany DA, et al. Infection and maturation of monocyte-derived human dendritic cells by human respiratory syncytial virus, human metapneumovirus, and human parainfluenza virus type 3. *Virology* (2009) 385:169–82. doi: 10.1016/j.virol.2008.11.043
57. Guerrero-Plata A, Kolli D, Hong C, Casola A, Garofalo RP. Subversion of pulmonary dendritic cell function by paramyxovirus infections. *J Immunol.* (2009) 182:3072–83. doi: 10.4049/jimmunol.0802262
58. Guerrero-Plata A, Casola A, Suarez G, Yu X, Spetch LA, Peeples ME, et al. Differential response of dendritic cells to human metapneumovirus and respiratory syncytial virus. *Am J Respir Cell Mol Biol.* (2006) 34:320–9. doi: 10.1165/rcmb.2005-0287OC
59. Céspedes PF, Gonzalez PA, Kalergis AM. Human metapneumovirus keeps dendritic cells from priming antigen-specific naive T cells. *Immunology* (2013) 139:366–76. doi: 10.1111/imm.12083
60. Le Nouën C, Hillyer P, Winter CC, McCarty T, Rabin RL, Collins PL, et al. Low CCR7-mediated migration of human monocyte derived dendritic cells in response to human respiratory syncytial virus and human metapneumovirus. *PLoS Pathog.* (2011) 7:e1002105. doi: 10.1371/journal.ppat.1002105
61. Le Nouen C, Hillyer P, Munir S, Winter CC, McCarty T, Bukreyev A, et al. Effects of human respiratory syncytial virus, metapneumovirus, parainfluenza virus 3 and influenza virus on CD4+ T cell activation by dendritic cells. *PLoS ONE* (2010) 5:e15017. doi: 10.1371/journal.pone.0015017
62. Kolli D, Velayutham T, Casola A. Host-viral interactions: role of pattern recognition receptors (PRRs) in human pneumovirus infections. *Pathogens* (2013) 2:232–63. doi: 10.3390/pathogens2020232
63. Boivin G, Abed Y, Pelletier G, Ruel L, Moisan D, Côté S, et al. Virological features and clinical manifestations associated with human metapneumovirus: a new paramyxovirus responsible for acute respiratory-tract infections in all age groups. *J Infect Dis.* (2002) 186:1330–4. doi: 10.1086/344319
64. Herd KA, Nelson M, Mahalingam S, Tindle RW. Pulmonary infection of mice with human metapneumovirus induces local cytotoxic T-cell and immunoregulatory cytokine responses similar to those seen with human respiratory syncytial virus. *J Gen Virol.* (2010) 91:1302–10. doi: 10.1099/vir.0.015396-0
65. Tzannou I, Nicholas SK, Lulla P, Aguayo-Hiraldo PI, Misra A, Martinez CA, et al. Immunologic profiling of human metapneumovirus for the development of targeted immunotherapy. *J Infect Dis.* 216:678–87. doi: 10.1093/infdis/jix358
66. Kolli D, Bataki EL, Spetch L, Guerrero-Plata A, Jewell AM, Piedra PA, et al. T lymphocytes contribute to antiviral immunity and pathogenesis in experimental human metapneumovirus infection. *J Virol.* (2008) 82:8560–9. doi: 10.1128/JVI.00699-08
67. Park J-S, Kim Y-H, Kwon E, Callaway Z, Fujisawa T, Kim C-K. Comparison of nasal cytokine profiles of human metapneumovirus and respiratory syncytial virus. *Asia Pac Allergy* (2017) 7:206. doi: 10.5415/apallergy.2017.7.4.206
68. Jartti T, Van Den Hoogen B, Garofalo RP, Osterhaus ADME, Ruuskanen O. Metapneumovirus and acute wheezing in children. *Lancet* (2002) 360:1393–4. doi: 10.1016/S0140-6736(02)11391-2
69. Xia C, Vijayan M, Pritzl CJ, Fuchs SY, McDermott AB, Hahm B. Hemagglutinin of influenza a virus antagonizes type i interferon (IFN) responses by inducing degradation of type I IFN receptor 1. *J Virol.* (2016) 90:2403–17. doi: 10.1128/JVI.02749-15
70. Ramaswamy M, Shi L, Monick MM, Hunninghake GW, Look DC. Specific inhibition of type I interferon signal transduction by respiratory syncytial virus. *Am J Respir Cell Mol Biol.* (2004) 30:893–900. doi: 10.1165/rcmb.2003-0410OC
71. Bao X, Kolli D, Ren J, Liu T, Garofalo RP, Casola A. Human metapneumovirus glycoprotein g disrupts mitochondrial signaling in airway epithelial cells. *PLoS ONE* (2013) 8: e62568. doi: 10.1371/journal.pone.0062568
72. van den Hoogen BG, van Boheemen S, de Rijck J, van Nieuwkoop S, Smith DJ, Laksono B, et al. Excessive production and extreme editing of human metapneumovirus defective interfering RNA is associated with type I IFN induction. *J Gen Virol.* (2014) 95:1625–33. doi: 10.1099/vir.0.066100-0
73. Manzoni TB, López CB. Defective (interfering) viral genomes re-explored: impact on antiviral immunity and virus persistence. *Future Virol.* (2018) 13:493–503. doi: 10.2217/fvl-2018-0021
74. Kawai T, Akira S. Innate immune recognition of viral infection. *Nat Immunol.* (2006) 7:131–7. doi: 10.1038/ni1303
75. Akira S, Uematsu S, Takeuchi O. Pathogen recognition and innate immunity. *Cell* (2006) 124:783–801. doi: 10.1016/j.cell.2006.02.015
76. Aderem A, Ulevitch RJ. Toll-like receptors in the induction of the innate immune response. *Nature* (2000) 406:782–7. doi: 10.1038/35021228
77. Akira S, Takeda K. Functions of toll-like receptors: Lessons from KO mice. *Comptes Rendus Biol.* (2004) 327:581–9. doi: 10.1016/j.crvi.2004.04.002
78. Takeda K, Akira S. Toll-like receptors in innate immunity. *Int Immunol.* (2005) 17:1–14. doi: 10.1093/intimm/dxh186
79. Ren J, Kolli D, Deng J, Fang R, Gong B, Xue M, et al. MyD88 controls human metapneumovirus-induced pulmonary immune responses and disease pathogenesis. *Virus Res.* (2013) 176:241–50. doi: 10.1016/j.virusres.2013.06.014
80. Liao S, Bao X, Liu T, Lai S, Li K, Garofalo RP, Casola A. Role of retinoic acid inducible gene-I in human metapneumovirus-induced cellular signalling. *J Gen Virol.* (2008) 89:1978–86. doi: 10.1099/vir.0.2008/000778-0
81. Baños-Lara MDR, Ghosh A, Guerrero-Plata A. Critical role of MDA5 in the interferon response induced by human metapneumovirus infection in dendritic cells and *in vivo*. *J Virol.* (2013) 87:1242–51. doi: 10.1128/JVI.01213-12
82. Lifland AW, Jung J, Alonas E, Zurla C, Crowe JE, Santangelo PJ. Human respiratory syncytial virus nucleoprotein and inclusion bodies antagonize the innate immune response mediated by MDA5 and MAVS. *J Virol.* (2012) 86:8245–58. doi: 10.1128/JVI.00215-12
83. Kumar H, Kawai T, Akira S. Toll-like receptors and innate immunity. *Biochem Biophys Res Commun.* (2009) 388:621–5. doi: 10.1016/j.bbrc.2009.08.062
84. Kawai T, Akira S. The roles of TLRs, RLRs and NLRs in pathogen recognition. *Int Immunol.* (2009) 21:317–37. doi: 10.1093/intimm/dxp017
85. Ning S, Pagano JS, Barber GN. IRF7: Activation, regulation, modification and function. *Genes Immun.* (2011) 12:399–414. doi: 10.1038/gene.2011.21
86. Blasius AL, Beutler B. Intracellular toll-like receptors. *Immunity* (2010) 32:305–15. doi: 10.1016/j.immuni.2010.03.012
87. Kitagawa Y, Sakai M, Funayama M, Itoh M, Gotoh B. Human metapneumovirus M2-2 protein acts as a negative regulator of alpha interferon production by plasmacytoid dendritic cells. *J Virol.* (2017) 91:e00579-17. doi: 10.1128/JVI.00579-17
88. Spann KM, Loh Z, Lynch JP, Ullah A, Zhang V, Baturcam E, et al. IRF-3, IRF-7, and IPS-1 promote host defense against acute human

metapneumovirus infection in neonatal mice. *Am J Pathol.* (2014) 184:1795–806. doi: 10.1016/j.ajpath.2014.02.026

89. Baños-Lara MDR, Zabaleta J, Garai J, Baddoo M, Guerrero-Plata A. Comparative analysis of miRNA profile in human dendritic cells infected with respiratory syncytial virus and human metapneumovirus. *BMC Res Notes* (2018) 11:432. doi: 10.1186/s13104-018-3541-0
90. Groskreutz DJ, Monick MM, Yarovinsky TO, Powers LS, Quelle DE, Varga SM, et al. Respiratory syncytial virus decreases p53 protein to prolong survival of airway epithelial cells. *J Immunol.* (2007) 179:2741–7. doi: 10.4049/jimmunol.179.5.2741
91. MacPhail M, Schickli JH, Tang RS, Kaur J, Robinson C, Fouchier RAM, Osterhaus et al. Identification of small-animal and primate models for evaluation of vaccine candidates for human metapneumovirus (hMPV) and implications for hMPV vaccine design. *J Gen Virol.* (2004) 85:1655–63. doi: 10.1099/vir.0.79805-0

3

Phage Lysins for Fighting Bacterial Respiratory Infections: A New Generation of Antimicrobials

Roberto Vázquez[1,2]*, Ernesto García*[1,2] *and Pedro García*[1,2*]

[1] *Centro de Investigaciones Biológicas (CSIC), Madrid, Spain,* [2] *Centro de Investigación Biomédica en Red de Enfermedades Respiratorias (CIBERES), Madrid, Spain*

***Correspondence:**
Pedro García
pgarcia@cib.csic.es

Lower respiratory tract infections and tuberculosis are responsible for the death of about 4.5 million people each year and are the main causes of mortality in children under 5 years of age. *Streptococcus pneumoniae* is the most common bacterial pathogen associated with severe pneumonia, although other Gram-positive and Gram-negative bacteria are involved in respiratory infections as well. The ability of these pathogens to persist and produce infection under the appropriate conditions is also associated with their capacity to form biofilms in the respiratory mucous membranes. Adding to the difficulty of treating biofilm-forming bacteria with antibiotics, many of these strains are becoming multidrug resistant, and thus the alternative therapeutics available for combating this kind of infections are rapidly depleting. Given these concerns, it is urgent to consider other unconventional strategies and, in this regard, phage lysins represent an attractive resource to circumvent some of the current issues in infection treatment. When added exogenously, lysins break specific bonds of the peptidoglycan and have potent bactericidal effects against susceptible bacteria. These enzymes possess interesting features, including that they do not trigger an adverse immune response and raise of resistance is very unlikely. Although Gram-negative bacteria had been considered refractory to these compounds, strategies to overcome this drawback have been developed recently. In this review we describe the most relevant *in vitro* and *in vivo* results obtained to date with lysins against bacterial respiratory pathogens.

Keywords: phage lysins, pneumonia, respiratory infection, antibacterials, antibiotic resistance, endolysins

THE IMPACT OF BACTERIAL RESPIRATORY DISEASES ON HUMAN HEALTH

Lower respiratory tract infections remain the most deadly communicable diseases, and caused 3.2 million deaths worldwide in 2015 (1). Tuberculosis is still to date among the top 10 death causes, and community-acquired pneumonia is the single largest bacterial infectious cause of death in children worldwide (2). *Streptococcus pneumoniae* (pneumococcus) accounts for most of the bacterial pneumonia cases in children, followed by *Haemophilus influenzae* type b, and other bacterial pathogens: *Streptococcus pyogenes* (group A *Streptococcus*), non-typeable *H. influenzae*, *Staphylococcus aureus*, *Mycoplasma pneumoniae, Moraxella catarrhalis*, and *Klebsiella pneumoniae* (3). Pneumococcus is also a common cause of community-acquired pneumonia in elderly patients with comorbidities (4). On the other hand, hospital-acquired pneumonia and ventilator-associated pneumonia are among the leading nosocomial infections worldwide, with an increasing frequency of multidrug resistant (MDR) Gram-negative bacteria (G−) as the bacteriologic cause (5).

Indeed, antimicrobial resistance (AMR) and associated morbidity and mortality have been increasing globally. A recent study estimated that AMR could produce 10 million deaths a year by 2050 (6), although this prediction should be taken with care (7). Accordingly, economic simulations predict that the world will suffer an annual shortfall loss of between $1 and $3.4 trillion by 2030 because of AMR (8). In this scenario, the World Health Organization (WHO) has called for global action on AMR (9). This has encouraged several actions: (a) prevention and control actions in healthcare facilities (10); (b) widespread antimicrobial stewardship programs (11); (c) reduction of antibiotic use in livestock production and the environment (12); and (d) the search for alternatives to the currently used antibiotics (13), particularly against a group of MDR bacteria having a global impact (14). Among these priority pathogens, *S. pneumoniae*, *H. influenzae* and those referred to as "the ESKAPE bugs" (15), are of particular concern. Of note, *Mycobacterium tuberculosis* was not included in the above list as it is already in a globally established priority for which innovative new treatments are urgently needed (16). A few decades ago, phage therapy revived as an alternative to conventional antibiotics and, since the beginning of twenty-first century, phage lytic enzymes have also been extensively tested as antibacterials. This area of research is the focus of this review and the most relevant results of certain enzymes against respiratory pathogens will be discussed. Extensive details on the issue can be found in other recent reviews (17–26).

GENERAL CHARACTERISTICS OF LYSINS

Endolysins, or more simply lysins, are phage-encoded enzymes capable of hydrolyzing the bacterial cell wall (CW) and that are synthesized at the end of the phage replication cycle. The peptidoglycan (PG) polymer is the basic component of the CW, and is composed of chains of a disaccharide repeat made up of *N*-acetylglucosamine and *N*-acetylmuramic acid, linked by $\beta(1\rightarrow4)$ glycosidic bonds. Glycan strands are cross-linked by tetra/pentapeptide side stems attached to muramic acid residues through amide bonds. Lysins are usually classified as glycosidases [glucosaminidases, transglycosylases, and lysozymes (or muramidases)], if they break any of the bonds of the glycan chain, *N*-acetylmuramoyl-L-alanine amidases (NAM-amidases), if they break the amide bonds between the glycan strands and peptide chains, or endopeptidases if they hydrolyze different bonds within peptide chains. When purified lysins are added exogenously, their CW-degrading activity can lead to rapid osmotic lysis and bacterial death. The enzymatic activity of lysins was the basis for their exploration as antibacterial agents and they were also named "enzybiotics" (27). Lysins possess several advantages over antibiotics: (a) they rapidly kill bacteria, practically upon contact; (b) they can be specific to the target pathogen, particularly against Gram-positive (G+) bacteria (28–31), which allows to preserve the normal microbiota (32); (c) development of resistance seems very unlikely (33, 34), probably because these enzymes directly target an essential and well-conserved structural component such as the PG, which cannot be easily modified without compromising fitness (35); (d) with few exceptions (36, 37), lysins are active independently of the bacterial physiological state (38, 39); (e) they are effective against MDR bacteria (20, 34, 40–42); (f) they can act synergistically with other lysins or antibiotics and thus theoretically reduce the development of resistance while increasing therapeutic efficiency; and (g) lysins are also effective killing colonizing pathogens growing on mucosal surfaces and/or in biofilms (**Tables 1, 2**).

Lysins encoded by phages infecting G+ bacteria generally display a modular structure, comprising one or more catalytic domains (CDs) and one or more CW binding domains (CWBD). Although the species specificity of a lysin is generally assigned to its CWBD, there are some data suggesting that combined interactions of CD and CWBD with unknown CW receptors may play a significant role (129). On the other hand, phages from G– bacteria usually encode globular lysins with a single CD, with several exceptions (31, 111, 128).

Concerning their systemic, therapeutic use, it has been alleged that lysins, as foreign proteins, could be expected to trigger the production of neutralizing antibodies that might hinder their antibacterial action in subsequent administrations. However, early studies addressing this potential drawback, strongly suggested that highly immune serum slows down—but does not block—lysins (46, 130). Pre-clinical and clinical trials with the antistaphylococcal lysin SAL-1 have been performed in animal models and, lately, in humans. An immune response was indeed elicited after repeated intravenous injections of SAL200, as demonstrated by the presence of specific antibodies and reduced C3 complement levels in the animal blood samples (80). Still, pharmacokinetic, pharmacodynamic, and tolerance studies of SAL200 in monkeys and humans did not show any serious adverse effects or clinically significant alterations even at the highest dose tested (81, 82). Anyhow, host immune responses to specific lysin formulations must always be considered concerning safety and improving the therapeutic potential of lysins.

The antibacterial efficacy of lysins can be improved by several means including: (a) replacement of certain amino acids to modify the net charge of the enzyme (53, 131) or allow dimerization (132); (b) deletion of entire domains (75, 133); (c) construction of chimeric proteins by domain shuffling (41); (d) fusion to cationic peptides (or other domains) to render lysins capable to cross the outer membrane (OM), a widely recognized drawback of lysin therapy against G– bacteria (122, 134, 135), or to increase CW affinity (136); (e) co-administration of lysins with membrane destabilizing agents (EDTA, carvacrol, etc.), especially in G– pathogens (53, 112).

LYSINS AGAINST GRAM-POSITIVE BACTERIA

Streptococcus pneumoniae

The key aspect of the *S. pneumoniae* system is the role of the aminoalcohol choline in the enzymatic activity of the bacterial autolysin LytA, and the pneumococcal phage lysins. Choline forms part of the (lipo)teichoic acids and constitutes an absolute requirement for the binding of these enzymes—members of the choline-binding family of proteins (CBPs) (137)—to the CW substrate. This peculiarity explains the extreme specificity

TABLE 1 | Selected lysins active against Gram-positive bacteria and acid-fast mycobacteria.

Species	Lysin/phage	Susceptible bacteria tested	Methodology used		Acc. No.; comments	References
			In vitro	*in vivo*		
S. pneumoniae						
	Pal/Dp-1	Pneumococci and relatives	Biofilm; synergy with Cpl-1	Colonization and sepsis (mice)	O03979	(40, 43–45)
	Cpl-1/Cp-1	Pneumococci and relatives	Biofilm; synergy with Pal and antibiotics; cell culture	Colonization, otitis, pneumonia, sepsis (mice)	P15057	(43–52)
	LytA	Pneumococci and relatives	Biofilm	Sepsis (mice)	P06653; major autolysin	(45, 53)
	Cpl-7/Cp-7	Streptococci; other G+	Biofilm		P19385	(45, 53)
	Cpl-7S	Streptococci; other G+	Cell culture	Colonization (mice), pneumococcal infection (zebrafish)	Engineered protein	(51, 53)
	Cpl-711	Pneumococci and relatives	Biofilm; synergy with antibiotics; cell culture	Colonization and sepsis (mice), pneumococcal infection (zebrafish)	Chimera of Cpl-7 and Cpl-1	(41, 51, 54)
	PL3	Pneumococci and relatives	Biofilm	Pneumococcal infection (zebrafish)	Chimera of Pal and LytA	(38)
***S. pyogenes* (GAS)**						
	PlyC/C_1	GAS and other streptococci	Biofilm; cell culture (intracellular killing of GAS)	Colonization (mice)	J7M5V6	(27, 55–57)
	PlyPy/MGAS315 prophage	GAS and other streptococci		Sepsis (mice)	AAM79913	(58)
***S. agalactiae* (GBS)**						
	PlyGBS	GAS, GBS and other streptococci		Colonization (mice)	Q5MY96	(59, 60)
S. aureus						
	Lysostaphin	Staphylococci	Biofilm; synergy with LysK; $CHAP_K$ and antibiotics; controlled release	Sepsis and colonization (mice, rats)	P10547; from *S. simulans*	(35, 61–72)
	LysK/K	Staphylococci	Biofilm; complex with polycationic peptides		Q6Y7T6	(61, 73, 74)
	$CHAP_K$	Staphylococci	Biofilm; synergy with lysostaphin; controlled release	Colonization (mice)	CHAP domain of LysK	(64, 75–78)
	ClyS	Staphylococci	Synergy with oxacillin and vancomycin	Colonization and septicemia (mice)	Chimera of Twort phage lysin (O56788) and φNM3 phage lysin (Q2FWV2)	(79)

(Continued)

TABLE 1 | Continued

Species	Lysin/phage	Susceptible bacteria tested	Methodology used		Acc. No.; comments	References
			In vitro	*in vivo*		
	SAL-1/SAP-1	Staphylococci	Biofilm	Bacteremia (mouse), toxicity and pharmacokinetics (rats, dogs, monkeys), pharmacokinetics and pharmacodynamics (healthy humans)	SAL200 is a drug formulation of SAL-1	(80–84)
	P128	Staphylococci	Biofilm; cell culture; synergy with antibiotics	Colonization and sepsis (rats)	Chimera of Gp57 (Q6Y7R1) and lysostaphin; under clinical testing	(85–92)
	LysGH15/GH15	Staphylococci	Biofilm	Sepsis and pneumonia (mice)	D6QY02	(93–97)
	CF-301 (PlySs2)/*S. suis* 9/1591 prophage	*S. aureus, S. pyogenes, S. pneumoniae*; other G+	Biofilm; synergy with antibiotics	Sepsis (mice)	M1NS67; under clinical testing	(33, 98, 99)
	ClyF	Staphylococci	Biofilm	Sepsis (mice)	Chimera of Ply187 (O56785) and PlySs2	(100)
***Mycobacterium* sp.**						
	LysB/Ms6	Mycobacteria	Growth inhibition with surfactants		Q9ZX49; esterase	(101, 102)
	LysB/Bxz2	Mycobacteria	Growth inhibition with surfactants		Q9FZR9; esterase	(101)
	LysA/BTCU-1	Mycobacteria	Cell culture		O64203; intracellular killing of *M. smegmatis*	(103)
	LysB/BTCU-1	Mycobacteria	Cell culture		R9R591; intracellular killing of *M. smegmatis*; esterase	(103)

TABLE 2 | Selected lysins active against Gram-negative bacteria.

Species	Lysin/phage	Susceptible bacteria	Methodology used	Acc. No.; comments	References
P. aeruginosa					
	Lys1521/*B. amyloliquefaciens* phage	G–	Activity on intact bacteria	Q94ML9	(104–107)
	EL188/EL	G–	Activity on permeabilized bacteria	CAG27282	(108–110)
	KZ144/φKZ	G–	Activity on permeabilized bacteria	AAL83045	(108, 110)
	OBPgp279/OBP	G–	Activity on intact bacteria	YP_004958186	(111)
	Art-175	G–	Activity on intact bacteria	Chimera of KZ144 and SMAP-29 peptide	(34, 112)
	LysPA26/JD010	G–	Activity on intact bacteria, biofilm	A0A1V0EFL1	(113)
A. baumannii					
	LysAB2/*Φ*AB2	G– and *S. aureus*	Activity on intact bacteria *in vivo*: sepsis (mice)	F1BCP4	(114, 115)
	LysABP-01/ØABP-01	G–	Activity on intact bacteria; synergy with colistin	KF548002	(116)
	PlyAB1/Abp1	*A. baumannii*	Activity on intact bacteria	YP_008058242	(117)
	PlyF307/RL-2015	*A. baumannii*; otros G–	Activity on intact bacteria, biofilm *in vivo*: sepsis (mice)	AJG41873	(36, 118)
	LysAB3/*A. baumannii* ATCC 17978 prophage	*A. baumannii*	Activity on intact bacteria	ABO12027	(119)
	LysAB4/*A. baumannii* ATCC 17978 prophage	*A. baumannii*	Activity on intact bacteria	CP000521	(119)
E. coli					
	Lysep3/Ep3	*E. coli, P. aeruginosa*	Activity on permeabilized bacteria	A0A088FRS5	(120)
	Lysep3-D8	G–, *Streptococcus* sp.	Activity on intact bacteria	Chimera of Lysep3 and Lys1521 (Q94ML9)	(121)
	Colicin-lysep3	*E. coli*	Activity on intact bacteria *in vivo*: intestinal infection	Chimera of Lysep3 and colicin A (Q47108)	(122)
	EndoT5/T5	*E. coli*	Activity on permeabilized bacteria	Q6QGP7	(123)
	PlyE146/*E. coli* 8.0569 prophage	G–	Activity on intact bacteria	EKK47578	(37)
K. pneumoniae					
	K11gp3.5/K11	G–	Activity on permeabilized bacteria	B3VCZ3	(124)
	KP32gp15/KP32	G–	Activity on permeabilized bacteria	D1L2U8	(124)
	KP27 lysin/KP27	G–	Activity on permeabilized bacteria; cell culture	K7NPX3	(125)
C. freundii					
	CfP1 lysin/CfP1	*Citrobacter* sp.	Activity on intact bacteria	A0A1B1IXL3	(126)
S. maltophilia					
	P28	G– and some G+	Activity on intact bacteria	Lytic enzyme from a bacteriocin system	(127)
***Burkholderia* sp.**					
	AP3gp15/AP3	G–	Activity on permeabilized bacteria	A0A1S5NV50	(128)

of CBPs for pneumococci. The first article reporting the use of a CBP as an enzybiotic demonstrated the capacity of the NAM-amidase Pal to kill pneumococci of every serotype tested, including penicillin-resistant isolates (40). These results were confirmed in a mouse model of nasopharyngeal carriage (27). The Cpl-1 lysozyme has also been successfully tested in several *in vitro* assays and in different animal models of infection (46–48), and a synergistic effect was found when Cpl-1 was used together with several antibiotics (49, 50), or in combination with Pal (43, 44). The Cpl-7 lysozyme represents an exception to choline-recognizing pneumococcal lysins, since it harbors a different CWBD (138–140) that allows it to recognize and kill a broader range of bacteria. Moreover, the bactericidal effect of Cpl-7 has been improved in the engineered Cpl-7S by inverting the net charge of its CWBD (53). To date, the most powerful killing lysins tested against *S. pneumoniae* are nonetheless chimeric proteins: Cpl-711, a chimera of Cpl-7 and Cpl-1 (41), and PL3, a fusion protein between Pal and LytA [**Table 1**; (38)]. Treatment with Cpl-711 strongly reduced the attachment of *S. pneumoniae* to human epithelial cells, and a single intranasal dose of Cpl-711 significantly reduced nasopharyngeal colonization in a mouse model (51).

Staphylococcus aureus

Although *S. aureus* is frequently carried asymptomatically in humans, it is also the cause of a variety of diseases and, particularly, methicillin-resistant strains (MRSA) are responsible for a great percentage of all infections, up to 80% in some countries (141). The *S. aureus* PG displays a characteristic pentaglycine interpeptide cross-linking the glycan strands (142). Most tested lysins in the *S. aureus* system contain two CDs (endopeptidase and NAM-amidase) together with an SH3b CWBD (61, 143, 144). Although the exact interaction between the CWBD and the structures to which these domains bind remains to be demonstrated in many cases, it has been proposed that some CWBDs recognize the pentaglycine peptide cross-bridge (145) or the CW-associated glycopolymers (79). Of note, the vast majority of studies reporting the therapeutic use of lysins are directed to fight *S. aureus* infections (20, 21). Together with lysostaphin (produced by *Staphylococcus simulans*), LysK and its derivatives seem to be the most lethal lysins against *S. aureus*, including MRSA (73, 76, 146, 147) as well as vancomycin-intermediate and -resistant isolates [see reference (21) and references therein]. Other examples of anti-staphylococcal lysins include several engineered proteins such as chimeric or truncated proteins (76, 85, 100, 148, 149) or fusion proteins with short cationic peptides able to cross the eukaryotic membrane and kill intracellular *S. aureus* (150, 151). Nevertheless, lysin-based studies that consider *S. aureus* as a respiratory pathogen are scarce and only include some decolonization assays (62, 63, 75, 85) and a single example of endolysin efficacy in a mouse *S. aureus* pneumonia model (93).

Other Gram-Positive Pathogens and Mycobacteria

S. pyogenes is a major causative agent of upper respiratory tract infections (152). The most relevant example of a lysin targeting this pathogen is PlyC, a peculiar multimeric enzyme that kills group A streptococci with high efficiency (27, 55). In addition, the ability of PlyC to penetrate respiratory tract epithelial cells to eliminate intracellular *S. pyogenes* cells has also been proven (56). This intracellular activity overcomes one of the major drawbacks of antibiotic therapy against streptococcal throat infections, which is bacterial self-protection by cellular invasion. Other lysins reported to kill *S. pyogenes* are PlyPy (58) and the broad range, pneumococcal phage-derived Cpl-7S (53). Besides, group B streptococci are known to cause severe pneumonia in newborns (153). At least one attempt has been conducted in mice toward oropharyngeal decolonization of group B streptococci using PlyGBS lysin (59).

The acid-fast *M. tuberculosis* is still rather unexplored for the development of lysin-based therapy. This might be due to the peculiarity of *Mycobacterium* CW structure, which comprises a thick PG layer covalently attached to arabinogalactan sterified with mycolic acids (154). Because of this architecture, the lytic cassette of mycobacteriophages comprises two different lytic enzymes: a classical PG hydrolase (usually named LysA) and mycolyl-arabinogalactan esterase (LysB), which cleaves the ester bond linking mycolic acid to the arabinogalactan-PG layer. As a result, the mycolic acid layer detaches from the cell, rendering vulnerable to osmotic shock and, finally, lysis (155). Some *in vitro* assays have been conducted with both mycobacteriophage-derived hydrolases, yielding, in general, promising results that show either growth arrest (101) or a bactericidal effect (103), but further research is still required. The mycobacterial endolysins and their therapeutical potential have been recently reviewed (156).

LYSINS AGAINST GRAM-NEGATIVE BACTERIA

Pseudomonas aeruginosa

The first lysins tested against *P. aeruginosa*, for example, EL188, only killed bacteria when membrane permeabilizers (e.g., polycationic agents, EDTA) were co-administered (108, 109). Due to the potential difficulties of therapies based on the co-administration of lysins and permeabilizing agents, some of the most recent efforts have been directed toward the engineering of the enzymes themselves, giving rise to the "artilysin" concept (134). In this study, lysins were fused to cationic, antimicrobial peptides (AMPs), and these fusions were able to exert a permeabilizing activity that allowed them to cross *P. aeruginosa* OM to degrade the PG layer both *in vitro* and *in vivo* (134). Art-175 is an artilysin that was constructed by fusing lysin KZ144 and the sheep myeloid AMP 29 (SMAP-29), and further optimizing the thermostability of the resulting chimera by point mutation of several cysteine residues (34). Art-175 was able to efficiently kill either antibiotic-susceptible or MDR *P. aeruginosa* strains. Of note, Art-175 also controlled the appearance of persisters, i.e., bacterial subpopulations transiently tolerant to antibiotics that often appear upon antiinfective chemotherapy (157).

Despite the engineering efforts mentioned above, lysins able to lyse G− bacteria on their own are also currently available.

Typically, this intrinsic activity from without relies on non-enzymatic mechanisms, which were first described for the T4 phage lysozyme (158) and then in several *P. aeruginosa* phage lysins (159). These lysins harbor AMP-like elements (peptides with an amphipathic secondary structure and a positive net charge) that destabilize the OM. In some cases, as for T4 lysozyme, these regions account for the bactericidal activity of the enzyme to a higher extent than the enzymatic activity itself (158). One of the first examples of a lysin with a natural cationic peptide exploited as an enzybiotic was the *Bacillus amyloliquefaciens* phage lysin Lys1521, which was indeed able to lyse *P. aeruginosa* cells (104). Other examples of *P. aeruginosa* lysins with intrinsic anti-G− activity include OBPgp279 (124) and LysPA26 (113). Although active research is being performed to deal with the OM barrier issue, no extensive *in vivo* experimental evidence has been provided for the clearance, upon lysin treatment, of *P. aeruginosa* from respiratory infections.

Acinetobacter baumannii

In general, lysins against G− bacteria appear to be less specific than their G+ counterparts, possibly due to the (apparently) simpler organization of the former sacculi (160). This broader spectrum allows some lysins to kill several pathogenic genera, like the already mentioned lysin LysPA26, which besides *P. aeruginosa* can also lyse other G− pathogens such as *E. coli*, *K. pneumoniae* or *A. baumannii* (113), or Art-175, which also kills *A. baumannii* (112). This bacterium is a potential respiratory pathogen (particularly for immunocompromised and debilitated patients) that is receiving great attention in recent years due to its worrisome increased antibiotic resistance (161). Thus, several enzybiotics have also been developed with emphasis in their *A. baumannii* killing capacity, such as LysAB3 and LysAB4 (119), PlyAB1 (117), and LysABP-01 (116).

PlyF307 was capable of killing *A. baumannii* isolates, including MDR strains, both in planktonic and biofilm cultures (36) and represents the first example of an intact lysin with intrinsic anti-G− activity tested in a mammalian (mouse bacteremia) model. Unsurprisingly, it was later determined that such intrinsic activity from without partly resided in a cationic peptide located in the C-terminal domain of the lysin (118). Further studies revealed that this region contains sub-domain structural motifs with membrane permeabilizing ability, but lacking enzymatic activity; similar motifs have also been found in other lysins. For example, lysin LysAB2 (114) represents a broad-spectrum enzybiotic, both active against G+ and G− bacteria (*A. baumannii*, *Escherichia coli* and, surprisingly, *S. aureus*). Based on its permeabilizing properties (114), AMPs based on the C-terminal region of LysAB2 have been synthesized and demonstrated high antimicrobial activity when tested in mice infected with *A. baumannii* (115).

Other Gram-Negative Pathogens

In spite of being a prominent member of the ESKAPE group (162), there are only few reports of lysins active against *K. pneumoniae*. As already mentioned, LysPA26 also showed bactericidal activity against *K. pneumoniae* (113). Consequently, it is conceivable that some of the other broad spectrum anti-G− lysins would kill *K. pneumoniae*. As for specific *Klebsiella* phage lysins, some examples of lysins with proven lytic activity are those from phages K11, KP32, and KP27 (124, 125, 163), but only KP32 and KP27 were tested for their anti-*Klebsiella* activity. Although usually associated with intestinal infections, *E. coli* is also a frequent cause of nosocomial pneumonia (164). Again, some of the other G− lysins are also active against *E. coli* (105, 113, 114, 116, 124). Specifically from an *E. coli* phage, Lysep3 lysin has demonstrated noticeable activity against permeabilized *E. coli* cells (120). Moreover, a chimeric construction between Lysep3 and a colicin was able to traverse the OM via specific recognition by OM transporters (122, 165).

CONCLUDING REMARKS AND FUTURE TRENDS

As MDR bacterial respiratory pathogens are increasingly prevalent, alternative therapeutics are urgently needed. Lysins represent more than a hope in this scenario and may be a perfect counterpart to therapies based on standard antibiotics. The potential for lysin development is seemingly endless. For example, thousands of putative lysins, many of which displaying novel domain architectures, have been recently described using bioinformatic techniques (166). All this huge amount of information, together with the crystal structures of lysins and a more detailed knowledge on the bacterial CW structure, will provide better insights to design and construct "tailor-made lysins" potentially directed against any desired pathogen. Drug delivery and other added-value systems involving lysins are now also being researched by setting up different approaches (167–170). Several polymers have been studied as potential drug release vehicles not only for research but also for clinical purposes. Particularly interesting is the case of poly(*N*-isopropylacrylamide) (PNIPAM) that has been used for the coadministration of the $CHAP_K$ lysin and lysostaphin through a thermally triggered release event (the temperature increase due to infection) (64).

Although a limited number of endolysins have entered clinical trials and some of them are already available in the market [reviewed in reference (18)], phages and phage-based products are subjected to strict regulatory measures (171). Moreover, in spite of their demonstrated specificity and lack of resistance development, the use of phage endolysins in humans raises several concerns. Among them, the relatively short plasma life of lysins, their immunogenicity and possible toxicity, the proinflammatory response to bacterial debris, and the difficulties to attack intracellular bacteria have been mentioned. Although only limited data of phage lysin interactions with the human body, e.g., pharmacokinetic/pharmacodynamic studies, have been published, it is encouraging that most (if not all) of the above mentioned potential limitations lack current experimental support (18, 23, 25). Although this scenario seems favorable toward hitting the clinic in the short term, further evidence is still due, especially when bacterial respiratory diseases—in particular, those caused by G− bacteria—are considered. Additional efforts to cover the currently unmet therapeutic requirements are warranted.

AUTHOR CONTRIBUTIONS

RV, EG, and PG wrote, edited, and approved the final manuscript.

ACKNOWLEDGMENTS

We acknowledge support of the publication fee by the CSIC Open Access Publication Support Initiative through its Unit of Information Resources for Research (URICI).

REFERENCES

1. World Health Organization. *The Top 10 Causes of Death* (2017). Available online at: http://www.who.int/mediacentre/factsheets/fs310/en/ (Accessed April 18, 2018).
2. World Health Organization. *Pneumonia* (2016). Available online at: http://www.who.int/mediacentre/factsheets/fs331/en (Accessed April 24, 2018).
3. Rodrigues CMC, Groves H. Community-acquired pneumonia in children: the challenges of microbiological diagnosis. *J Clin Microbiol.* (2018) 56:e01318-17. doi: 10.1128/JCM.01318-17
4. Torres A, Cillóniz C, Blasi F, Chalmers JD, Gaillat J, Dartois N, et al. Burden of pneumococcal community-acquired pneumonia in adults across Europe: a literature review. *Respir Med.* (2018) 137:6–13. doi: 10.1016/j.rmed.2018.02.007
5. Kidd JM, Kuti JL, Nicolau DP. Novel pharmacotherapy for the treatment of hospital-acquired and ventilator-associated pneumonia caused by resistant Gram-negative bacteria. *Expert Opin Pharmacother.* (2018) 19:397–408. doi: 10.1080/14656566.2018.1438408
6. O'Neill J. *Review on Antimicrobial Resistance. Antimicrobial Resistance: Tackling a Crisis for the Health and Wealth of Nations* (2014). Available online at: https://amr-review.org/sites/default/files/AMR%20Review%20Paper%20-%20Tackling%20a%20crisis%20for%20the%20health%20and%20wealth%20of%20nations_1.pdf. (Accessed April 24, 2018).
7. de Kraker MEA, Stewardson AJ, Harbarth S. Will 10 million people die a year due to antimicrobial resistance by 2050? *PLoS Med.* (2016) 13:e1002184. doi: 10.1371/journal.pmed.1002184
8. World Bank. *Drug-Resistant Infections: A Threat to our Economic Future* (2017). Available online at: http://www.worldbank.org/en/topic/health/publication/drug-resistant-infections-a-threat-to-our-economic-future (Accessed September 24, 2018).
9. World Health Organization. *Antimicrobial Resistance* (2018). Available online at: http://www.who.int/en/news-room/fact-sheets/detail/antimicrobial-resistance (Accessed April 25, 2018).
10. Pires D, de Kraker MEA, Tartari E, Abbas M, Pittet D. 'Fight antibiotic resistance—It's in your hands': call from the World Health Organization for 5th May 2017. *Clin Infect Dis.* (2017) 64:1780–3. doi: 10.1093/cid/cix226
11. Pulcini C. Antibiotic stewardship: a European perspective. *FEMS Microbiol Lett.* (2017) 364, fnx230. doi: 10.1093/femsle/fnx230
12. Holmes AH, Moore LSP, Sundsfjord A, Steinbakk M, Regmi S, Karkey A, et al. Understanding the mechanisms and drivers of antimicrobial resistance. *Lancet* (2016) 387:176–87. doi: 10.1016/S0140-6736(15)00473-0
13. Tacconelli E, Sifakis F, Harbarth S, Schrijver R, van Mourik M, Voss A, et al. Surveillance for control of antimicrobial resistance. *Lancet Infect Dis.* (2018) 18:E99–106. doi: 10.1016/S1473-3099(17)30485-1
14. World Health Organization. *Global Priority List of Antibiotic-Resistant Bacteria to Guide Research, Discovery, and Development of New Antibiotics* (2017). Available online at: http://www.who.int/medicines/publications/WHO-PPL-Short_Summary_25Feb-ET_NM_WHO.pdf (Accessed April, 26 2018).
15. Rice LB. Federal funding for the study of antimicrobial resistance in nosocomial pathogens: No ESKAPE. *J Infect Dis.* (2008) 197:1079–81. doi: 10.1086/533452
16. World Health Organization. *Global Tuberculosis Report 2018* (2018). Available online at: http://www.who.int/tb/publications/global_report/en/ (Accessed September 24, 2018).
17. Cooper CJ, Koonjan S, Nilsson AS. Enhancing whole phage therapy and their derived antimicrobial enzymes through complex formulation. *Pharmaceuticals* (2018) 11:34. doi: 10.3390/ph11020034
18. Gerstmans H, Criel B, Briers Y. Synthetic biology of modular endolysins. *Biotechnol Adv.* (2018) 36:624–40. doi: 10.1016/j.biotechadv.2017.12.009
19. Gu J, Xi H, Cheng M, Han W. Phage-derived lysins as therapeutic agents against multidrug-resistant Enterococcus faecalis. *Future Microbiol.* (2018) 13:275–8. doi: 10.2217/fmb-2017-0235
20. Gutiérrez D, Fernández L, Rodríguez A, García P. Are phage lytic proteins the secret weapon to kill *Staphylococcus aureus*? *mBio* (2018) 9:e01923-17. doi: 10.1128/mBio.01923-17
21. Haddad Kashani H, Schmelcher M, Sabzalipoor H, Seyed Hosseini E, Moniri R. Recombinant endolysins as potential therapeutics against antibiotic-resistant *Staphylococcus aureus*: current status of research and novel delivery strategies. *Clin Microbiol Rev.* (2018) 31:e00071-17. doi: 10.1128/CMR.00071-17
22. Love MJ, Bhandari D, Dobson RCJ, Billington C. Potential for bacteriophage endolysins to supplement or replace antibiotics in food production and clinical care. *Antibiotics* (2018) 7:17. doi: 10.3390/antibiotics7010017
23. Oliveira H, São-José C, Azeredo J. Phage-derived peptidoglycan degrading enzymes: challenges and future prospects for *in vivo* therapy. *Viruses* (2018) 10:292. doi: 10.3390/v10060292
24. São-José C. Engineering of phage-derived lytic enzymes: improving their potential as antimicrobials. *Antibiotics* (2018) 7:29. doi: 10.3390/antibiotics7020029
25. Sharma U, Vipra A, Channabasappa S. Phage-derived lysins as potential agents for eradicating biofilms and persisters. *Drug Discov Today* (2018) 23:848–56. doi: 10.1016/j.drudis.2018.01.026
26. Fischetti V. Development of phage lysins as novel therapeutics: a historical perspective. *Viruses* (2018) 10:310. doi: 10.3390/v10060310
27. Nelson D, Loomis L, Fischetti VA. Prevention and elimination of upper respiratory colonization of mice by group A streptococci by using a bacteriophage lytic enzyme. *Proc Natl Acad Sci USA* (2001) 98:4107–12. doi: 10.1073/pnas.061038398
28. López R, García E, García P, García JL. The pneumococcal cell wall degrading enzymes: a modular design to create new lysins? *Microb Drug Resist.* (1997) 3:199–211. doi: 10.1089/mdr.1997.3.199
29. Loessner MJ, Kramer K, Ebel F, Scherer S. C-terminal domains of Listeria monocytogenes bacteriophage murein hydrolases determine specific recognition and high-affinity binding to bacterial cell wall carbohydrates. *Mol Microbiol.* (2002) 44:335–49. doi: 10.1046/j.1365-2958.2002.02889.x
30. Schuch R, Nelson D, Fischetti VA. A bacteriolytic agent that detects and kills *Bacillus anthracis*. *Nature* (2002) 418:884–9. doi: 10.1038/nature01026
31. Briers Y, Schmelcher M, Loessner MJ, Hendrix J, Engelborghs Y, Volckaert G, et al. The high-affinity peptidoglycan binding domain of *Pseudomonas* phage endolysin KZ144. *Biochem Biophys Res Commun.* (2009) 383:187–91. doi: 10.1016/j.bbrc.2009.03.161
32. Cheng M, Zhang Y, Li X, Liang J, Hu L, Gong P, et al. Endolysin LysEF-P10 shows potential as an alternative treatment strategy for

multidrug-resistant *Enterococcus faecalis* infections. *Sci Rep.* (2017) 7:10164. doi: 10.1038/s41598-017-10755-7

33. Gilmer DB, Schmitz JE, Euler CW, Fischetti VA. Novel bacteriophage lysin with broad lytic activity protects against mixed infection by *Streptococcus pyogenes* and methicillin-resistant *Staphylococcus aureus*. *Antimicrob Agents Chemother.* (2013) 57:2743–50. doi: 10.1128/AAC.02 526-12
34. Briers Y, Walmagh M, Grymonprez B, Biebl M, Pirnay J-P, Defraine V, et al. Art-175 is a highly efficient antibacterial against multidrug-resistant strains and persisters of *Pseudomonas aeruginosa*. *Antimicrob Agents Chemother.* (2014) 58:3774–84. doi: 10.1128/AAC.02668-14
35. Kusuma C, Jadanova A, Chanturiya T, Kokai-Kun JF. Lysostaphin-resistant variants of *Staphylococcus aureus* demonstrate reduced fitness *in vitro* and *in vivo*. *Antimicrob Agents Chemother.* (2007) 51:475–82. doi: 10.1128/AAC.00786-06
36. Lood R, Winer BY, Pelzek AJ, Diez-Martinez R, Thandar M, Euler CW, et al. Novel phage lysin capable of killing the multidrug-resistant gram-negative bacterium *Acinetobacter baumannii* in a mouse bacteremia model. *Antimicrob Agents Chemother.* (2015) 59:1983–91. doi: 10.1128/AAC.04641-14
37. Larpin Y, Oechslin F, Moreillon P, Resch G, Entenza JM, Mancini S. *In vitro* characterization of PlyE146, a novel phage lysin that targets Gram-negative bacteria. *PLoS ONE* (2018) 13:e0192507. doi: 10.1371/journal.pone.0192507
38. Blázquez B, Fresco-Taboada A, Iglesias-Bexiga M, Menéndez M, García P. PL3 amidase, a tailor-made lysin constructed by domain shuffling with potent killing activity against pneumococci and related species. *Front Microbiol.* (2016) 7:1156. doi: 10.3389/fmicb.2016.01156
39. Vázquez R, Domenech M, Iglesias-Bexiga M, Menéndez M, García P. Csl2, a novel chimeric bacteriophage lysin to fight infections caused by Streptococcus suis, an emerging zoonotic pathogen. *Sci Rep.* (2017) 7:16506. doi: 10.1038/s41598-017-16736-0
40. Loeffler JM, Nelson D, Fischetti VA. Rapid killing of *Streptococcus pneumoniae* with a bacteriophage cell wall hydrolase. *Science* (2001) 294:2170–2. doi: 10.1126/science.1066869
41. Díez-Martínez R, De Paz HD, García-Fernández E, Bustamante N, Euler CW, Fischetti VA, et al. A novel chimeric phage lysin with high *in vitro* and *in vivo* bactericidal activity against *Streptococcus pneumoniae*. *J Antimicrob Chemother.* (2015) 70:1763–73. doi: 10.1093/jac/dkv038
42. Yang H, Wang M, Yu J, Wei H. Antibacterial activity of a novel peptide-modified lysin against *Acinetobacter baumannii* and *Pseudomonas aeruginosa*. *Frontiers Microbiol.* (2015) 6:1471. doi: 10.3389/fmicb.2015.01471
43. Loeffler JM, Fischetti VA. Synergistic lethal effect of a combination of phage lytic enzymes with different activities on penicillin-sensitive and -resistant *Streptococcus pneumoniae* strains. *Antimicrob Agents Chemother.* (2003) 47:375–7. doi: 10.1128/AAC.47.1.375-377.2003
44. Jado I, López R, García E, Fenoll A, Casal J, García P, et al. Phage lytic enzymes as therapy of antibiotic-resistant *Streptococcus pneumoniae* infection in a murine sepsis model. *J Antimicrob Chemother.* (2003) 52:967–73. doi: 10.1093/jac/dkg485
45. Domenech M, García E, Moscoso M. *In vitro* destruction of *Streptococcus pneumoniae* biofilms with bacterial and phage peptidoglycan hydrolases. *Antimicrob Agents Chemother.* (2011) 55:4144–8. doi: 10.1128/AAC.00492-11
46. Loeffler JM, Djurkovic S, Fischetti VA. Phage lytic enzyme Cpl-1 as a novel antimicrobial for pneumococcal bacteremia. *Infect Immun.* (2003) 71:6199–204. doi: 10.1128/IAI.71.11.6199-6204.2003
47. McCullers JA, Karlström Å, Iverson AR, Loeffler JM, Fischetti VA. Novel strategy to prevent otitis media caused by colonizing *Streptococcus pneumoniae*. *PLoS Pathog.* (2007) 3:e28. doi: 10.1371/journal.ppat.0030028
48. Doehn JM, Fischer K, Reppe K, Gutbier B, Tschernig T, Hocke AC, et al. Delivery of the endolysin Cpl-1 by inhalation rescues mice with fatal pneumococcal pneumonia. *J Antimicrob Chemother.* (2013) 68:2111–7. doi: 10.1093/jac/dkt131
49. Vouillamoz J, Entenza JM, Giddey M, Fischetti VA, Moreillon P, Resch G. Bactericidal synergism between daptomycin and the phage lysin Cpl-1 in a mouse model of *pneumococcal bacteraemia*. *Int J Antimicrob Agents* (2013) 42:416–21. doi: 10.1016/j.ijantimicag.2013.06.020
50. Djurkovic S, Loeffler JM, Fischetti VA. Synergistic killing of *Streptococcus pneumoniae* with the bacteriophage lytic enzyme Cpl-1 and penicillin or gentamicin depends on the level of penicillin resistance. *Antimicrob Agents Chemother.* (2005) 49:1225–8. doi: 10.1128/AAC.49.3.1225-1228.2005
51. Corsini B, Díez-Martínez R, Aguinagalde L, González-Camacho F, García-Fernández E, Letrado P, et al. Chemotherapy with phage lysins reduces pneumococcal colonization of the respiratory tract. *Antimicrob Agents Chemother.* (2018) 62:e02212–17. doi: 10.1128/AAC.02212-17
52. Witzenrath M, Schmeck B, Doehn JM, Tschernig T, Zahlten J, Loeffler JM, et al. Systemic use of the endolysin Cpl-1 rescues mice with fatal pneumococcal pneumonia. *Crit Care Med.* (2009) 37:642–9. doi: 10.1097/CCM.0b013e31819586a6
53. Díez-Martínez R, de Paz HD, Bustamante N, García E, Menéndez M, García P. Improving the lethal effect of Cpl-7, a pneumococcal phage lysozyme with broad bactericidal activity, by inverting the net charge of its cell wall-binding module. *Antimicrob Agents Chemother.* (2013) 57:5355–65. doi: 10.1128/AAC.01372-13
54. Letrado P, Corsini B, Díez-Martínez R, Bustamante N, Yuste JE, García P. Bactericidal synergism between antibiotics and phage endolysin Cpl-711 to kill multidrug-resistant pneumococcus. *Future Microbiol.* (2018) (in press).
55. Nelson D, Schuch R, Chahales P, Zhu S, Fischetti VA. PlyC: a multimeric bacteriophage lysin. *Proc Natl Acad Sci USA* (2006) 103:10765–70. doi: 10.1073/pnas.0604521103
56. Shen Y, Barros M, Vennemann T, Gallagher DT, Yin Y, Linden SB, et al. A bacteriophage endolysin that eliminates intracellular streptococci. *eLife* (2016) 5:e13152. doi: 10.7554/eLife.13152
57. Shen Y, Koller T, Kreikemeyer B, Nelson DC. Rapid degradation of *Streptococcus pyogenes* biofilms by PlyC, a bacteriophage-encoded endolysin. *J Antimicrob Chemother.* (2013) 68:1818–24. doi: 10.1093/jac/dkt104
58. Lood R, Raz A, Molina H, Euler CW, Fischetti VA. A highly active and negatively charged *Streptococcus pyogenes* lysin with a rare D-alanyl-L-alanine endopeptidase activity protects mice against streptococcal bacteremia. *Antimicrob Agents Chemother.* (2014) 58:3073–84. doi: 10.1128/AAC.00115-14
59. Cheng Q, Nelson D, Zhu S, Fischetti VA. Removal of group B streptococci colonizing the vagina and oropharynx of mice with a bacteriophage lytic enzyme. *Antimicrob Agents Chemother.* (2005) 49:111–7. doi: 10.1128/AAC.49.1.111-117.2005
60. Cheng Q, Fischetti VA. Mutagenesis of a bacteriophage lytic enzyme PlyGBS significantly increases its antibacterial activity against group B streptococci. *Appl Microbiol Biotechnol.* (2007) 74:1284–91. doi: 10.1007/s00253-006-0771-1
61. Schmelcher M, Shen Y, Nelson DC, Eugster MR, Eichenseher F, Hanke DC, et al. Evolutionarily distinct bacteriophage endolysins featuring conserved peptidoglycan cleavage sites protect mice from MRSA infection. *J Antimicrob Chemother.* (2015) 70:1453–65. doi: 10.1093/jac/dku552
62. Kokai-Kun JF, Walsh SM, Chanturiya T, Mond JJ. Lysostaphin cream eradicates *Staphylococcus aureus* nasal colonization in a cotton rat model. *Antimicrob Agents Chemother.* (2003) 47:1589–97. doi: 10.1128/AAC.47.5.1589-1597.2003
63. Walsh S, Kokai-Kun J, Shah A, Mond J. Extended nasal residence time of lysostaphin and an anti-staphylococcal monoclonal antibody by delivery in semisolid or polymeric carriers. *Pharm Res.* (2004) 21:1770–5. doi: 10.1023/B:PHAM.0000045227.16829.37
64. Hathaway H, Ajuebor J, Stephens L, Coffey A, Potter U, Sutton JM, et al. Thermally triggered release of the bacteriophage endolysin CHAPK and the bacteriocin lysostaphin for the control of methicillin resistant *Staphylococcus aureus* (MRSA). *J Control Release* (2017) 245:108–15. doi: 10.1016/j.jconrel.2016.11.030
65. Polak J, Della Latta P, Blackburn P. *In vitro* activity of recombinant lysostaphin-antibiotic combinations toward methicillin-resistant *Staphylococcus aureus*. *Diagn Microbiol Infect Dis.* (1993) 17:265–70. doi: 10.1016/0732-8893(93)90034-5
66. Climo MW, Ehlert K, Archer GL. Mechanism and suppression of lysostaphin resistance in oxacillin-resistant *Staphylococcus aureus*. *Antimicrob Agents Chemother.* (2001) 45:1431–7. doi: 10.1128/AAC.45.5.1431-1437.2001
67. Kiri N, Archer G, Climo MW. Combinations of lysostaphin with β-lactams are synergistic against oxacillin-resistant *Staphylococcus*

epidermidis. *Antimicrob Agents Chemother.* (2002) 46:2017–20. doi: 10.1128/AAC.46.6.2017-2020.2002

68. Wu JA, Kusuma C, Mond JJ, Kokai-Kun JF. Lysostaphin disrupts *Staphylococcus aureus* and *Staphylococcus epidermidis* biofilms on artificial surfaces. *Antimicrob Agents Chemother.* (2003) 47:3407–14. doi: 10.1128/AAC.47.11.3407-3414.2003
69. Walsh S, Shah A, Mond J. Improved pharmacokinetics and reduced antibody reactivity of lysostaphin conjugated to polyethylene glycol. *Antimicrob Agents Chemother.* (2003) 47:554–8. doi: 10.1128/AAC.47.2.554-558.2003
70. Kokai-Kun JF, Chanturiya T, Mond JJ. Lysostaphin as a treatment for systemic *Staphylococcus aureus* infection in a mouse model. *J Antimicrob Chemother.* (2007) 60:1051–9. doi: 10.1093/jac/dkm347
71. Becker SC, Foster-Frey J, Donovan DM. The phage K lytic enzyme LysK and lysostaphin act synergistically to kill MRSA. *FEMS Microbiol Lett.* (2008) 287:185–91. doi: 10.1111/j.1574-6968.2008.01308.x
72. Aguinaga A, Francés ML, Del Pozo JL, Alonso M, Serrera A, Lasa I, et al. Lysostaphin and clarithromycin: a promising combination for the eradication of *Staphylococcus aureus* biofilms. *Int J Antimicrob Agents* (2011) 37:585–7. doi: 10.1016/j.ijantimicag.2011.02.009
73. O'Flaherty S, Coffey A, Meaney W, Fitzgerald GF, Ross RP. The recombinant phage lysin LysK has a broad spectrum of lytic activity against clinically relevant staphylococci, including methicillin-resistant *Staphylococcus aureus. J Bacteriol.* (2005) 187:7161–4. doi: 10.1128/JB.187.20.7161-7164.2005
74. Filatova LY, Donovan DM, Becker SC, Lebedev DN, Priyma AD, Koudriachova HV, et al. Physicochemical characterization of the staphylolytic LysK enzyme in complexes with polycationic polymers as a potent antimicrobial. *Biochimie* (2013) 95:1689–96. doi: 10.1016/j.biochi.2013.04.013
75. Fenton M, Casey PG, Hill C, Gahan CGM, Ross RP, McAuliffe O, et al. The truncated phage lysin CHAPk eliminates *Staphylococcus aureus* in the nares of mice. *Bioeng Bugs* (2010) 1:404–7. doi: 10.4161/bbug.1.6.13422
76. Horgan M, O'Flynn G, Garry J, Cooney J, Coffey A, Fitzgerald GF, et al. Phage lysin LysK can be truncated to its CHAP domain and retain lytic activity against live antibiotic-resistant staphylococci. *Appl Environ Microbiol.* (2009) 75:872–4. doi: 10.1128/AEM.01831-08
77. Fenton M, Ross RP, McAuliffe O, O'Mahony J, Coffey A. Characterization of the staphylococcal bacteriophage lysin CHAPK. *J Appl Microbiol.* (2011) 111:1025–35. doi: 10.1111/j.1365-2672.2011.05119.x
78. Fenton M, Keary R, McAuliffe O, Ross RP, O'Mahony J, Coffey A. Bacteriophage-derived peptidase CHAPK eliminates and prevents staphylococcal biofilms. *Int J Microbiol.* (2013) 2013:625341. doi: 10.1155/2013/625341
79. Daniel A, Euler C, Collin M, Chahales P, Gorelick KJ, Fischetti VA. Synergism between a novel chimeric lysin and oxacillin protects against infection by methicillin-resistant *Staphylococcus aureus. Antimicrob Agents Chemother.* (2010) 54:1603–12. doi: 10.1128/AAC.01625-09
80. Jun SY, Jung GM, Yoon SJ, Choi Y-J, Koh WS, Moon KS, et al. Preclinical safety evaluation of intravenously administered SAL200 containing the recombinant phage endolysin SAL-1 as a pharmaceutical ingredient. *Antimicrob Agents Chemother.* (2014) 58:2084–8. doi: 10.1128/AAC.02232-13
81. Jun SY, Jung GM, Yoon SJ, Youm SY, Han H-Y, Lee J-H, et al. Pharmacokinetics of the phage endolysin-based candidate drug SAL200 in monkeys and its appropriate intravenous dosing period. *Clin Exp Pharmacol Physiol.* (2016) 43:1013–6. doi: 10.1111/1440-1681.12613
82. Jun SY, Jang IJ, Yoon S, Jang K, Yu K-S, Cho JY, et al. Pharmacokinetics and tolerance of the phage endolysin-based candidate drug SAL200 after a single intravenous administration among healthy volunteers. *Antimicrob Agents Chemother.* (2017) 61:e02629-16. doi: 10.1128/AAC.02 629-16
83. Jun SY, Jung GM, Son J-S, Yoon SJ, Choi Y-J, Kang SH. Comparison of the antibacterial properties of phage endolysins SAL-1 and LysK. *Antimicrob Agents Chemother.* (2011) 55:1764–7. doi: 10.1128/AAC.01097-10
84. Jun SY, Jung GM, Yoon SJ, Oh M-D, Choi Y-J, Lee WJ, et al. Antibacterial properties of a pre-formulated recombinant phage endolysin, SAL-1. *Int J Antimicrob Agents* (2013) 41:156–61. doi: 10.1016/j.ijantimicag.2012.10.011
85. Paul VD, Rajagopalan SS, Sundarrajan S, George SE, Asrani JY, Pillai R, et al. A novel bacteriophage Tail-Associated Muralytic Enzyme (TAME) from phage K and its development into a potent antistaphylococcal protein. *BMC Microbiol.* (2011) 11:226. doi: 10.1186/1471-2180-11-226
86. Vipra AA, Desai SN, Roy P, Patil R, Raj JM, Narasimhaswamy N, et al. Antistaphylococcal activity of bacteriophage derived chimeric protein P128. *BMC Microbiol.* (2012) 12:41. doi: 10.1186/1471-2180-12-41
87. George SE, Chikkamadaiah R, Durgaiah M, Joshi AA, Thankappan UP, Madhusudhana SN, et al. Biochemical characterization and evaluation of cytotoxicity of antistaphylococcal chimeric protein P128. *BMC Res Notes* (2012) 5:280. doi: 10.1186/1756-0500-5-280
88. Drilling AJ, Cooksley C, Chan C, Wormald PJ, Vreugde S. Fighting sinus-derived *Staphylococcus aureus* biofilms *in vitro* with a bacteriophage-derived muralytic enzyme. *Int Forum Allergy Rhinol.* (2016) 6:349–55. doi: 10.1002/alr.21680
89. Poonacha N, Nair S, Desai S, Tuppad D, Hiremath D, Mohan T, et al. Efficient killing of planktonic and biofilm-embedded coagulase-negative staphylococci by bactericidal protein P128. *Antimicrob Agents Chemother.* (2017) 61:e00457-17. doi: 10.1128/AAC.00457-17
90. Nair S, Desai S, Poonacha N, Vipra A, Sharma U. Antibiofilm activity and synergistic inhibition of *Staphylococcus aureus* biofilms by bactericidal protein P128 in combination with antibiotics. *Antimicrob Agents Chemother.* (2016) 60:7280–9. doi: 10.1128/AAC.01118-16
91. Nair S, Poonacha N, Desai S, Hiremath D, Tuppad D, Mohan T, et al. Restoration of sensitivity of a diverse set of drug-resistant *Staphylococcus* clinical strains by bactericidal protein P128. *J Med Microbiol.* (2018) 67:296–307. doi: 10.1099/jmm.0.000697
92. Channabasappa S, Durgaiah M, Chikkamadaiah R, Kumar S, Joshi A, Sriram B. Efficacy of novel antistaphylococcal ectolysin P128 in a rat model of methicillin-resistant *Staphylococcus aureus* bacteremia. *Antimicrob Agents Chemother.* (2018) 62:e01358-17. doi: 10.1128/AAC.01358-17
93. Xia F, Li X, Wang B, Gong P, Xiao F, Yang M, et al. Combination therapy of LysGH15 and apigenin as a new strategy for treating pneumonia caused by *Staphylococcus aureus. Appl Environ Microbiol.* (2016) 82:87–94. doi: 10.1128/AEM.02581-15
94. Gu J, Xu W, Lei L, Huang J, Feng X, Sun C, et al. LysGH15, a novel bacteriophage lysin, protects a murine bacteremia model efficiently against lethal methicillin-resistant *Staphylococcus aureus* infection. *J Clin Microbiol.* (2011) 49:111–7. doi: 10.1128/JCM.01144-10
95. Gu J, Zuo J, Lei L, Zhao H, Sun C, Feng X, et al. LysGH15 reduces the inflammation caused by lethal methicillin-resistant *Staphylococcus aureus* infection in mice. *Bioeng Bugs* (2011) 2:96–9. doi: 10.4161/bbug.2.2.14883
96. Zhang L, Li D, Li X, Hu L, Cheng M, Xia F, et al. LysGH15 kills *Staphylococcus aureus* without being affected by the humoral immune response or inducing inflammation. *Sci Rep.* (2016) 6:29344. doi: 10.1038/srep29344
97. Zhang Y, Cheng M, Zhang H, Dai J, Guo Z, Li X, et al. Antibacterial effects of phage lysin LysGH15 on planktonic cells and biofilms of diverse staphylococci. *Appl Environ Microbiol.* (2018) 84:e00886-18. doi: 10.1128/AEM.00886-18
98. Schuch R, Lee HM, Schneider BC, Sauve KL, Law C, Khan BK, et al. Combination therapy with lysin CF-301 and antibiotic is superior to antibiotic alone for treating methicillin-resistant *Staphylococcus aureus*-induced murine bacteremia. *J Infect Dis.* (2014) 209:1469–78. doi: 10.1093/infdis/jit637
99. Schuch R, Khan BK, Raz A, Rotolo JA, Wittekind M. Bacteriophage lysin CF-301, a potent antistaphylococcal biofilm agent. *Antimicrob Agents Chemother.* (2017) 61:e02666-16. doi: 10.1128/AAC.02666-16
100. Yang H, Zhang H, Wang J, Yu J, Wei H. A novel chimeric lysin with robust antibacterial activity against planktonic and biofilm methicillin-resistant *Staphylococcus aureus. Sci Rep.* (2017) 7:40182. doi: 10.1038/srep40182
101. Grover N, Paskaleva EE, Mehta KK, Dordick JS, Kane RS. Growth inhibition of *Mycobacterium smegmatis* by mycobacteriophage-derived enzymes. *Enzyme Microb Technol.* (2014) 63:1–6. doi: 10.1016/j.enzmictec.2014.04.018
102. Gil F, Grzegorzewicz AE, Catalão MJ, Vital J, McNeil MR, Pimentel M. Mycobacteriophage Ms6 LysB specifically targets the outer membrane of *Mycobacterium smegmatis. Microbiology* (2010) 156:1497–504. doi: 10.1099/mic.0.032821-0
103. Lai M-J, Liu C-C, Jiang S-J, Soo P-C, Tu M-H, Lee J-J, et al. Antimycobacterial activities of endolysins derived from a mycobacteriophage, BTCU-1. *Molecules* (2015) 20:19277–90. doi: 10.3390/molecules201019277

104. Morita M, Tanji Y, Mizoguchi K, Soejima A, Orito Y, Unno H. Antibacterial activity of *Bacillus amyloliquefaciens* phage endolysin without holin conjugation. *J Biosci Bioeng.* (2001) 91:469–73. doi: 10.1016/S1389-1723(01)80275-9
105. Morita M, Tanji Y, Orito Y, Mizoguchi K, Soejima A, Unno H. Functional analysis of antibacterial activity of *Bacillus amyloliquefaciens* phage endolysin against Gram-negative bacteria. *FEBS Lett.* (2001) 500:56–9. doi: 10.1016/S0014-5793(01)02587-X
106. Orito Y, Morita M, Hori K, Unno H, Tanji Y. *Bacillus amyloliquefaciens* phage endolysin can enhance permeability of *Pseudomonas aeruginosa* outer membrane and induce cell lysis. *Appl Microbiol Biotechnol.* (2004) 65:105–9. doi: 10.1007/s00253-003-1522-1
107. Muyombwe A, Tanji Y, Unno H. Cloning and expression of a gene encoding the lytic functions of *Bacillus amyloliquefaciens* phage: evidence of an auxiliary lysis system. *J Biosci Bioeng.* (1999) 88:221–5. doi: 10.1016/S1389-1723(99)80206-0
108. Briers Y, Volckaert G, Cornelissen A, Lagaert S, Michiels CW, Hertveldt K, et al. Muralytic activity and modular structure of the endolysins of *Pseudomonas aeruginosa* bacteriophages φKZ and EL. *Mol Microbiol.* (2007) 65:1334–44. doi: 10.1111/j.1365-2958.2007.05870.x
109. Briers Y, Walmagh M, Lavigne R. Use of bacteriophage endolysin EL188 and outer membrane permeabilizers against *Pseudomonas aeruginosa*. *J Appl Microbiol.* (2011) 110:778–85. doi: 10.1111/j.1365-2672.2010.04931.x
110. Briers Y, Cornelissen A, Aertsen A, Hertveldt K, Michiels CW, Volckaert G, et al. Analysis of outer membrane permeability of *Pseudomonas aeruginosa* and bactericidal activity of endolysins KZ144 and EL188 under high hydrostatic pressure. *FEMS Microbiol Lett.* (2008) 280:113–9. doi: 10.1111/j.1574-6968.2007.01051.x
111. Walmagh M, Briers Y, dos Santos SB, Azeredo J, Lavigne R. Characterization of modular bacteriophage endolysins from *Myoviridae* phages OBP, 201j2-1 and PVP-SE1. *PLoS ONE* (2012) 7:e36991. doi: 10.1371/journal.pone.0036991
112. Defraine V, Schuermans J, Grymonprez B, Govers SK, Aertsen A, Fauvart M, et al. Efficacy of artilysin Art-175 against resistant and persistent *Acinetobacter baumannii*. *Antimicrob Agents Chemother.* (2016) 60:3480–8. doi: 10.1128/AAC.00285-16
113. Guo M, Feng C, Ren J, Zhuang X, Zhang Y, Zhu Y, et al. A novel antimicrobial endolysin, LysPA26, against *Pseudomonas aeruginosa*. *Front Microbiol.* (2017) 8:293. doi: 10.3389/fmicb.2017.00293
114. Lai M-J, Lin N-T, Hu A, Soo P-C, Chen L-K, Chen L-H, et al. Antibacterial activity of *Acinetobacter baumannii* phage *Φ*FB2 endolysin (LysAB2) against both Gram-positive and Gram-negative bacteria. *Appl Microbiol Biotechnol.* (2011) 90:529–39. doi: 10.1007/s00253-011-3104-y
115. Peng S-Y, You R-I, Lai M-J, Lin N-T, Chen L-K, Chang K-C. Highly potent antimicrobial modified peptides derived from the *Acinetobacter baumannii* phage endolysin LysAB2. *Sci Rep.* (2017) 7:11477. doi: 10.1038/s41598-017-11832-7
116. Thummeepak R, Kitti T, Kunthalert D, Sitthisak S. Enhanced antibacterial activity of *Acinetobacter baumannii* bacteriophage ØABP-01 endolysin (LysABP-01) in combination with colistin. *Front Microbiol.* (2016) 7:1402. doi: 10.3389/fmicb.2016.01402
117. Huang G, Shen X, Gong Y, Dong Z, Zhao X, Shen W, et al. Antibacterial properties of *Acinetobacter baumannii* phage Abp1 endolysin (PlyAB1). *BMC Infect Dis.* (2014) 14:681. doi: 10.1186/s12879-014-0681-2
118. Thandar M, Lood R, Winer BY, Deutsch DR, Euler CW, Fischetti VA. Novel engineered peptides of a phage lysin as effective antimicrobials against multidrug-resistant *Acinetobacter baumannii*. *Antimicrob Agents Chemother.* (2016) 60:2671–9. doi: 10.1128/AAC.02972-15
119. Lai M-J, Soo P-C, Lin N-T, Hu A, Chen Y-J, Chen L-K, et al. Identification and characterisation of the putative phage-related endolysins through full genome sequence analysis in *Acinetobacter baumannii* ATCC 17978. *Int J Antimicrob Agents* (2013) 42:141–8. doi: 10.1016/j.ijantimicag.2013.04.022
120. Lv M, Wang S, Yan G, Sun C, Feng X, Gu J, et al. Genome sequencing and analysis of an *Escherichia coli* phage vB_EcoM-ep3 with a novel lysin, Lysep3. *Virus Genes* (2015) 50:487–97. doi: 10.1007/s11262-015-1195-8
121. Wang S, Gu J, Lv M, Guo Z, Yan G, Yu L, et al. The antibacterial activity of *E. coli* bacteriophage lysin lysep3 is enhanced by fusing the *Bacillus amyloliquefaciens* bacteriophage endolysin binding domain D8 to the C-terminal region. *J Microbiol.* (2017) 55:403–8. doi: 10.1007/s12275-017-6431-6
122. Yan G, Liu J, Ma Q, Zhu R, Guo Z, Gao C, et al. The N-terminal and central domain of colicin A enables phage lysin to lyse *Escherichia coli* extracellularly. *Antonie van Leeuwenhoek* (2017) 110:1627–35. doi: 10.1007/s10482-017-0912-9
123. Shavrina MS, Zimin AA, Molochkov NV, Chernyshov SV, Machulin AV, Mikoulinskaia GV. *In vitro* study of the antibacterial effect of the bacteriophage T5 thermostable endolysin on *Escherichia coli* cells. *J Appl Microbiol.* (2016) 121:1282–90. doi: 10.1111/jam.13251
124. Walmagh M, Boczkowska B, Grymonprez B, Briers Y, Drulis-Kawa Z, Lavigne R. Characterization of five novel endolysins from Gram-negative infecting bacteriophages. *Appl Microbiol Biotechnol.* (2013) 97:4369–75. doi: 10.1007/s00253-012-4294-7
125. Maciejewska B, Roszniowski B, Espaillat A, Kesik-Szeloch A, Majkowska-Skrobek G, Kropinski AM, et al. Klebsiella phages representing a novel clade of viruses with an unknown DNA modification and biotechnologically interesting enzymes. *Appl Microbiol Biotechnol.* (2017) 101:673–84. doi: 10.1007/s00253-016-7928-3
126. Oliveira H, Pinto G, Oliveira A, Oliveira C, Faustino MA, Briers Y, et al. Characterization and genome sequencing of a *Citrobacter freundii* phage CfP1 harboring a lysin active against multidrug-resistant isolates. *Appl Microbiol Biotechnol.* (2016) 100:10543–53. doi: 10.1007/s00253-016-7858-0
127. Dong H, Zhu C, Chen J, Ye X, Huang Y-P. Antibacterial activity of *Stenotrophomonas maltophilia* endolysin P28 against both Gram-positive and Gram-negative bacteria. *Front Microbiol.* (2015) 6:1299. doi: 10.3389/fmicb.2015.01299
128. Maciejewska B, Zrubek K, Espaillat A, Wiśniewska M, Rembacz KP, Cava F, et al. Modular endolysin of Burkholderia AP3 phage has the largest lysozyme-like catalytic subunit discovered to date and no catalytic aspartate residue. *Sci Rep.* (2017) 7:14501. doi: 10.1038/s41598-017-14797-9
129. Becker SC, Foster-Frey J, Stodola AJ, Anacker D, Donovan DM. Differentially conserved staphylococcal SH3b_5 cell wall binding domains confer increased staphylolytic and streptolytic activity to a streptococcal prophage endolysin domain. *Gene* (2009) 443:32–41. doi: 10.1016/j.gene.2009.04.023
130. López R, García E, García P. Enzymes for anti-infective therapy: phage lysins. *Drug Discov Today Ther Strateg.* (2004) 1:469–74. doi: 10.1016/j.ddstr.2004.09.002
131. Low LY, Yang C, Perego M, Osterman A, Liddington R. Role of net charge on the catalytic domain and the influence of the cell-wall binding domain on the bactericidal activity, specificity, and host-range of phage lysins. *J Biol Chem.* (2011) 286:34391–403. doi: 10.1074/jbc.M111.244160
132. Resch G, Moreillon P, Fischetti VA. A stable phage lysin (Cpl-1) dimer with increased antipneumococcal activity and decreased plasma clearance. *Int J Antimicrob Agents* (2011) 38:516–21. doi: 10.1016/j.ijantimicag.2011.08.009
133. Donovan DM, Foster-Frey J. LambdaSa2 prophage endolysin requires Cpl-7-binding domains and amidase-5 domain for antimicrobial lysis of streptococci. *FEMS Microbiol Lett.* (2008) 287:22–33. doi: 10.1111/j.1574-6968.2008.01287.x
134. Briers Y, Walmagh M, Van Puyenbroeck V, Cornelissen A, Cenens W, Aertsen A, et al. Engineered endolysin-based "Artilysins" to combat multidrug-resistant Gram-negative pathogens. *mBio* (2014) 5:e01379–14. doi: 10.1128/mBio.01379-14
135. Antonova NP, Balabanyan VY, Tkachuk AP, Makarov VV, Gushchin VA. Physical and chemical properties of recombinant KPP10 phage lysins and their antimicrobial activity against *Pseudomonas aeruginosa*. *Bull RSMU* (2018) 7:22–9. doi: 10.24075/brsmu.2018.010
136. Rodríguez-Rubio L, Chang W-L, Gutiérrez D, Lavigne R, Martínez B, Rodríguez A, et al. 'Artilysation' of endolysin lSa2lys strongly improves its enzymatic and antibacterial activity against *streptococci*. *Sci Rep.* (2016) 6:35382. doi: 10.1038/srep35382
137. López R, García E. Recent trends on the molecular biology of pneumococcal capsules, lytic enzymes, and bacteriophage. *FEMS Microbiol Rev.* (2004) 28:553–80. doi: 10.1016/j.femsre.2004.05.002
138. García P, García JL, García E, Sánchez-Puelles JM, López R. Modular organization of the lytic enzymes of *Streptococcus pneumoniae* and its bacteriophages. *Gene* (1990) 86:81–8. doi: 10.1016/0378-1119(90)90116-9

139. Bustamante N, Campillo NE, García E, Gallego C, Pera B, Diakun GP, et al. Cpl-7, a lysozyme encoded by a pneumococcal bacteriophage with a novel cell wall-binding motif. *J Biol Chem.* (2010) 285:33184–96. doi: 10.1074/jbc.M110.154559
140. Bustamante N, Iglesias-Bexiga M, Bernardo-García N, Silva-Martín N, García G, Campanero-Rhodes MA, et al. Deciphering how Cpl-7 cell wall-binding repeats recognize the bacterial peptidoglycan. *Sci Rep.* (2017) 7:16494. doi: 10.1038/s41598-017-16392-4
141. World Health Organization. *Antimicrobial Resistance: Global Report on Surveillance* (2014). Available online at: http://www.who.int/drugresistance/documents/surveillancereport/en/ (Accessed September 24, 2018).
142. Rajagopal M, Walker S. Envelope structures of Gram-positive bacteria. *Curr Top Microbiol Immunol.* (2017) 404:1–44. doi: 10.1007/82_2015_5021
143. Sass P, Bierbaum G. Lytic activity of recombinant bacteriophage φ11 and φ12 endolysins on whole cells and biofilms of *Staphylococcus aureus*. *Appl Environ Microbiol.* (2007) 73:347–52. doi: 10.1128/AEM.01616-06
144. Pritchard DG, Dong S, Baker JR, Engler JA. The bifunctional peptidoglycan lysin of *Streptococcus agalactiae* bacteriophage B30. *Microbiology* (2004) 150:2079–87. doi: 10.1099/mic.0.27063-0
145. Gründling A, Schneewind O. Cross-linked peptidoglycan mediates lysostaphin binding to the cell wall envelope of *Staphylococcus aureus*. *J Bacteriol.* (2006) 188:2463–72. doi: 10.1128/JB.188.7.2463-2472.2006
146. Idelevich EA, von Eiff C, Friedrich AW, Iannelli D, Xia G, Peters G, et al. *In vitro* activity against *Staphylococcus aureus* of a novel antimicrobial agent, PRF-119, a recombinant chimeric bacteriophage endolysin. *Antimicrob Agents Chemother.* (2011) 55:4416–9. doi: 10.1128/AAC.00217-11
147. Idelevich EA, Schaumburg F, Knaack D, Scherzinger AS, Mutter W, Peters G, et al. The recombinant bacteriophage endolysin HY-133 exhibits *in vitro* activity against different African clonal lineages of the *Staphylococcus aureus* complex, including *Staphylococcus schweitzeri*. *Antimicrob Agents Chemother.* (2016) 60:2551–3. doi: 10.1128/AAC.02859-15
148. Schmelcher M, Powell AM, Becker SC, Camp MJ, Donovan DM. Chimeric phage lysins act synergistically with lysostaphin to kill mastitis-causing *Staphylococcus aureus* in murine mammary glands. *Appl Environ Microbiol.* (2012) 78:2297–305. doi: 10.1128/AEM.07050-11
149. Mao J, Schmelcher M, Harty WJ, Foster-Frey J, Donovan DM. Chimeric Ply187 endolysin kills *Staphylococcus aureus* more effectively than the parental enzyme. *FEMS Microbiol Lett.* (2013) 342:30–6. doi: 10.1111/1574-6968.12104
150. Becker SC, Roach DR, Chauhan VS, Shen Y, Foster-Frey J, Powell AM, et al. Triple-acting lytic enzyme treatment of drug-resistant and intracellular *Staphylococcus aureus*. *Sci Rep.* (2016) 6:25063. doi: 10.1038/srep25063
151. Wang Z, Kong L, Liu Y, Fu Q, Cui Z, Wang J, et al. A phage lysin fused to a cell-penetrating peptide kills intracellular methicillin-resistant *Staphylococcus aureus* in keratinocytes and has potential as a treatment for skin infections in mice. *Appl Environ Microbiol.* (2018) 84:e00380–18. doi: 10.1128/AEM.00380-18
152. Brouwer S, Barnett Timothy C, Rivera-Hernandez T, Rohde M, Walker Mark J. *Streptococcus pyogenes* adhesion and colonization. *FEBS Lett.* (2016) 590:3739–57. doi: 10.1002/1873-3468.12254
153. Heath PT, Culley FJ, Jones CE, Kampmann B, Le Doare K, Nunes MC, et al. Group B streptococcus and respiratory syncytial virus immunisation during pregnancy: a landscape analysis. *Lancet Infect Dis.* (2017) 17:e223–34. doi: 10.1016/S1473-3099(17)30232-3
154. Squeglia F, Ruggiero A, Berisio R. Chemistry of peptidoglycan in *Mycobacterium tuberculosis* life cycle: an off-the-wall balance of synthesis and degradation. *Chemistry* (2018) 24:2533–46. doi: 10.1002/chem.201702973
155. Payne KM, Hatfull GF. Mycobacteriophage endolysins: diverse and modular enzymes with multiple catalytic activities. *PLoS ONE* (2012) 7:e34052. doi: 10.1371/journal.pone.0034052
156. Catalão MJ, Pimentel M. Mycobacteriophage lysis enzymes: targeting the mycobacterial cell envelope. *Viruses* (2018) 10:428. doi: 10.3390/v10080428
157. Fisher RA, Gollan B, Helaine S. Persistent bacterial infections and persister cells. *Nat Rev Microbiol.* (2017) 15:453–64. doi: 10.1038/nrmicro.2017.42
158. Düring K, Porsch P, Mahn A, Brinkmann O, Gieffers W. The non-enzymatic microbicidal activity of lysozymes. *FEBS Lett.* (1999) 449:93–100. doi: 10.1016/S0014-5793(99)00405-6
159. Rotem S, Radzishevsky I, Inouye RT, Samore M, Mor A. Identification of antimicrobial peptide regions derived from genomic sequences of phage lysins. *Peptides* (2006) 27:18–26. doi: 10.1016/j.peptides.2005.07.001
160. de Pedro MA, Cava F. Structural constraints and dynamics of bacterial cell wall architecture. *Front Microbiol.* (2015) 6:449. doi: 10.3389/fmicb.2015.00449
161. Elhosseiny NM, Attia AS. *Acinetobacter*: an emerging pathogen with a versatile secretome. *Emerg Microb Infect.* (2018) 7:33. doi: 10.1038/s41426-018-0030-4
162. Porreca AM, Sullivan KV, Gallagher JC. The epidemiology, evolution, and treatment of KPC-producing organisms. *Curr Infect Dis Rep.* (2018) 20:13. doi: 10.1007/s11908-018-0617-x
163. Junn HJ, Youn J, Suh KH, Lee SS. Cloning and expression of Klebsiella phage K11 lysozyme gene. *Protein Expr Purif.* (2005) 42:78–84. doi: 10.1016/j.pep.2005.03.026
164. Koulenti D, Tsigou E, Rello J. Nosocomial pneumonia in 27 ICUs in Europe: perspectives from the EU-VAP/CAP study. *Eur J Clin Microbiol Infect Dis.* (2017) 36:1999–2006. doi: 10.1007/s10096-016-2703-z
165. Lukacik P, Barnard TJ, Keller PW, Chaturvedi KS, Seddiki N, Fairman JW, et al. Structural engineering of a phage lysin that targets gram-negative pathogens. *Proc Natl Acad Sci USA* (2012) 109:9857–62. doi: 10.1073/pnas.1203472109
166. Fernández-Ruiz I, Coutinho FH, Rodríguez-Valera F. Thousands of novel endolysins discovered in uncultured phage genomes. *Front Microbiol.* (2018) 9:1033. doi: 10.3389/fmicb.2018.01033
167. Huang WC, Tsai PJ, Chen YC. Multifunctional Fe3O4@Au nanoeggs as photothermal agents for selective killing of nosocomial and antibiotic-resistant bacteria. *Small* (2009) 5:51–6. doi: 10.1002/smll.200801042
168. Kell AJ, Stewart G, Ryan S, Peytavi R, Boissinot M, Huletsky A, et al. Vancomycin-modified nanoparticles for efficient targeting and preconcentration of Gram-positive and Gram-negative bacteria. *ACS Nano* (2008) 2:1777–88. doi: 10.1021/nn700183g
169. Li Y, Krentz TM, Wang L, Benicewicz BC, Schadler LS. Ligand engineering of polymer nanocomposites: from the simple to the complex. *ACS Appl Mater Interfaces* (2014) 6:6005–21. doi: 10.1021/am405332a
170. Choi K-H, Lee H-J, Park BJ, Wang K-K, Shin EP, Park J-C, et al. Photosensitizer and vancomycin-conjugated novel multifunctional magnetic particles as photoinactivation agents for selective killing of pathogenic bacteria. *Chem Commun.* (2012) 48:4591–3. doi: 10.1039/c2cc17766h
171. Maciejewska B, Olszak T, Drulis-Kawa Z. Applications of bacteriophages versus phage enzymes to combat and cure bacterial infections: an ambitious and also a realistic application? *Appl Microbiol Biotechnol.* (2018) 102:2563–81. doi: 10.1007/s00253-018-8811-1

4

Immunity to the Dual Threat of Silica Exposure and *Mycobacterium tuberculosis*

Petr Konečný [1,2*], ***Rodney Ehrlich*** [1], ***Mary Gulumian*** [3,4,5] ***and Muazzam Jacobs*** [2,5,6]

[1] Centre for Environmental and Occupational Health, School of Public Health and Family Medicine, University of Cape Town, Cape Town, South Africa, [2] Division of Immunology, Department of Pathology and Institute of Infectious Disease and Molecular Medicine, Faculty of Health Sciences, University of Cape Town, Cape Town, South Africa, [3] National Health Laboratory Service, Department of Toxicology and Biochemistry, National Institute for Occupational Health, Johannesburg, South Africa, [4] Division of Molecular Medicine and Haematology, University of the Witwatersrand, Johannesburg, South Africa, [5] National Health Laboratory Service, Johannesburg, South Africa, [6] Immunology of Infectious Disease Research Unit, South African Medical Research Council, Cape Town, South Africa

***Correspondence:**
Petr Konečný
petr.kony@gmail.com

Exposure to silica and the consequent development of silicosis are well-known health problems in countries with mining and other dust producing industries. Apart from its direct fibrotic effect on lung tissue, chronic and immunomodulatory character of silica causes susceptibility to tuberculosis (TB) leading to a significantly higher TB incidence in silica-exposed populations. The presence of silica particles in the lung and silicosis may facilitate initiation of tuberculous infection and progression to active TB, and exacerbate the course and outcome of TB, including prognosis and survival. However, the exact mechanisms of the involvement of silica in the pathological processes during mycobacterial infection are not yet fully understood. In this review, we focus on the host's immunological response to both silica and *Mycobacterium tuberculosis*, on agents of innate and adaptive immunity, and particularly on silica-induced immunological modifications in co-exposure that influence disease pathogenesis. We review what is known about the impact of silica and *Mycobacterium tuberculosis* or their co-exposure on the host's immune system, especially an impact that goes beyond an exclusive focus on macrophages as the first line of the defense. In both silicosis and TB, acquired immunity plays a major role in the restriction and/or elimination of pathogenic agents. Further research is needed to determine the effects of silica in adaptive immunity and in the pathogenesis of TB.

Keywords: tuberculosis, silica, immunity, macrophages, granulomas, T cell

INTRODUCTION

It has long been hypothesized that inhaled silica dust contributes to TB development and progression via its physicochemical and biological properties (1–3). However, while recent research has explored the role of silica in immune response impairment, the mechanisms of reaction to the combination of silica particles and *Mycobacterium tuberculosis* (Mtb) are poorly understood (4). In this review, the immunological responses to silica exposure and to Mtb are reviewed, either as independent pathways, or where evidence is available, in the context of co-exposure and dual disease.

Silica and Silicosis

There are a number of pathologies associated with exposure to silica, including silicosis, lung malignancy, autoimmune disease and pulmonary infection, notably tuberculosis (5, 6).

Silicosis is a disease of the lower respiratory system caused by high dose and/or long-term inhalation of silica particles in mining and occupations involved in rock or sand processing, manufacturing of stone based products and utilization of sand as an abrasive agent (7–9). Silicosis results from the deposition of respirable silica particles in the lower respiratory tract, causing inflammation, collagen deposition, and fibrotic lesions. The outcome may vary from subclinical pathological changes to severe damage of lung tissue, diminished quality of life, and decreased lifespan (10). The development of a specific type of fibrotic granuloma the signal pathological lesion of silicosis is not restricted to the lungs but has also been observed in the liver, spleen, and bone marrow (11).

The prevalence of acute and severe silicosis due to very high exposures has decreased in the modern era and silicosis in general is uncommon in developed countries. However, silicosis remains prevalent in countries with extensive mining industries, such as China (6, 12, 13), South Africa (14, 15), Mexico (16), Brazil (17), and India (18), and continues to be recorded in the USA (19) and Australia (20). However, many countries do not register occupational diseases accurately and the enduring "residence time" of silica in the lungs after exposure, with a long asymptomatic phase, prevents early diagnosis (21).

The immune system response to silica particles has been extensively studied. Research has focused mainly on the initial interaction with cells residing in the lungs and the immunological modification of innate immune cellular responses. Special attention has been paid to the first encounters of silica with alveolar macrophages (AMs). In general, silica particles enter the alveolar space after inhalation and interact with macrophages, resulting in the engulfment of inhaled particles into the phagosome. The MARCO scavenger receptor has been described as the main molecule responsible for silica recognition and uptake (22), although other receptors from the group of Pattern Recognition receptors (PRRs) can be involved. It has been shown that CD204 may also interact with silica and inhibit the activity of macrophages. Some of the PRRs, such as Toll-like receptors (TLRs), are crucial in the response to bacterial infection. Significant downregulation of Toll-like receptor 2 (TLR2) following silica exposure might be one of the reasons contributing to higher TB susceptibility (23). Finally, the inability of macrophages to digest and eliminate phagocytized particles leads to persistent inflammation and modification of cellular responses (24).

The toxicity and pathogenicity profile of silica and thus the risk of silicosis vary with the size, physical and chemical properties of the inhaled particles (1, 25). A number of studies have focused on identification and characterization of specific toxic parameters (25–33). For example, different admixtures in dust can alter the biological activity of the silica particles (1, 34–38). While crystalline structure has long been accepted as conferring toxicity on silica (39, 40), recent research suggests that the number and distribution of silanol and siloxane groups rather than crystallinity feature as the primary toxic factors (41).

Silica and Tuberculosis

Tuberculosis remains one of the most dangerous diseases of the modern world, causing more than 1.3 million deaths, and with over 10 million new (incident) TB cases worldwide, in 2017 (42). Many risk co-factors for TB have been identified, including malnutrition, alcohol, diabetes and drug abuse (43–46). HIV infection is a potent co-factor (42, 47), while a higher incidence of TB has also been observed in individuals suffering from parasitic infections such as malaria (48) and leishmaniasis (49). Inhalant co-factors include smoking (50) and indoor air pollution (51, 52). The co-occurrence of silica exposure, silicosis, and TB has long been identified in populations exposed to silica-containing dust (53, 54) and progression of TB associated with silica exposure or silicosis has been of interest at least since the beginning of twentieth century (55). The spectrum of effect after exposure to the two agents is complex. It ranges from retained silica particles in the lung and TB infection without active disease, to dual disease, referred to as silicotuberculosis. The fibrotic phase of silicosis may be sub-radiological and thus not clinically evident (56), while significant host pathological changes may be observed in the pre-fibrotic stages as a result of silica particle activity (57).

The protection of silica-exposed and silicotic individuals against mycobacterial infection and TB in particular remains an important clinical and public health issue in the twenty-first century (58). Silica dust control, treatment of latent TB infection, early detection and effective treatment of TB are the main modalities of control. However, at the community level, a recent trial of mass treatment of latent TB infection in gold miners failed to show a reduction in TB incidence rates after treatment courses had ended (59). With respect to vaccination, the evidence does not support the use of Bacillus Calmette–Guérin (BCG) in tuberculin negative silica exposed workers or silicotics (60). For example, vaccination with BCG in guinea pigs exposed to silica-containing dust has been reported as causing an increase in fatal BCG infection, while an increased death rate from silicosis and silicotuberculosis has been observed in BCG vaccinated Bulgarian miners (61).

With the objective of understanding exposure-response effects, the risk as well as the progression and severity of mycobacterial infection in the presence of silica exposure have been investigated, using variable dust composition and concentrations of quartz (the most common crystalline silica polymorph), and various inoculation sites of different mycobacterial strains. While tracheal and, in particular, intravenous infection produce extensive pulmonary lesions, a subcutaneous introduction of bacilli did not show any pathological changes. It has also been confirmed that quartz represents the most toxic form and that there is a relationship between increasing dust/silica concentration, number of bacilli and development of tuberculous lesions (62). Co-exposure *in vivo* in guinea pig models has also provided information about the active role of Mtb in pneumoconio-tuberculous lesion formation, with the introduction of the antituberculotic drug rifampicin resulting in decreased formation or its elimination (63).

However, since activation of the immune system underlies disease activation and its accelerated progression, the factors targeting components of protective immune mechanisms and leading to impairment of defense against mycobacterial infections need to be understood. Exposure to silica decreases cellular function, reduces the capacity of dendritic cell activation and leads to a non-specific, impaired inflammatory response which compromises antibacterial mechanisms (64). These effects provide pathways for the promotion by silica exposure of increased susceptibility to bacterial infections, particularly *Mycobacterium tuberculosis* and other mycobacterial species (63, 65, 66).

Detailed mechanisms leading to disease in the presence of silica and Mtb are not yet understood, and multiple pathways are likely to be involved. For example, genetic polymorphism of tumor necrosis factor alpha (TNF-α), natural resistance-associated macrophage protein 1 (NRAMP1), and inducible nitric oxide synthase (iNOS) in macrophages have been shown to influence the response to both silica exposure or silicosis and TB in Chinese iron miners (67). Similar observations have been made in silicotic South African gold miners (68). Based on their specific single nucleotide polymorphism, different genotypes of the above-mentioned proteins showed intricate differential effects. These were either protective (variation of iNOS Ser608Leu genotype in silicosis) or had deleterious effects (G>C mutation of NRAMP1 intron 4 in silicosis, combined NRAMP1 D543N G/G and INT4 G/C+C/C, polymorphic site of G/A substitutions at positions−308 of TNF-α and TNF-a-308 G/G and NRAMP1 INT4 G/C+C/C genotype in TB) (67, 68).

Polymorphism of other genes related to the response to TB and silica such as transforming growth factor-beta 1 (TGF-β1) and cytokines interleukin 10 (IL-10) and interferon gamma (IFNγ) have been investigated, but no association found (69).

The following sections review the innate and adaptive cellular immune responses to silica and Mtb separately and with co-exposure, according to the immune cells or processes involved. The findings are summarized in **Table 1**, which also highlights the gaps in knowledge.

INNATE CELLULAR IMMUNE RESPONSES IN SILICOSIS AND TUBERCULOSIS

Alveolar Macrophages (AMs)

Alveolar macrophages represent the first line of defense against many airborne pathogens and inhaled environmental particles. The reaction of AMs after exposure to silica (70, 105–115) has been extensively studied. The tissue remodeling and formation of granulomas in response to exposure to both silica and Mtb suggest that similar mechanisms are involved in the elimination process in individuals exposed to silica or Mtb separately (116–118). Results from several studies have confirmed a noticeable difference in growth of Mtb in macrophages preloaded with silica particles; macrophages were more susceptible to infection represented by an increase in the number of infected macrophages and a higher number of bacilli present in each cell (119). Thus, silica particles facilitate intracellular replication and subsequent release from macrophages (61).

Using BCG vaccine inoculations, silicotic mice exhibited a higher accumulation of BCG colonies in harvested organs linearly correlating with the length of incubation than naïve counterparts. After 12 weeks, more than 40 times more colonies were observed in the spleen of silicotic mice, 70 times more in the liver and more than 6,000 times more in the lungs. Presence of silica particles significantly affects cellular response and bacterial growth properties (71). Higher Mtb burdens have been observed in murine lungs preloaded with silica compared to silica-free control animals (73). Also, extracted AMs contained more engulfed bacilli. The transplantation of AMs from silica-exposed into control, silica-unexposed mice, resulted in an increase of susceptibility to TB upon infection with Mtb. Thus, macrophages preloaded with silica particles exhibit a higher number of Mtb-phagocyting cells as well as higher rates of Mtb phagocytosis, leading to an increase in the number of bacteria engulfed in the macrophage (120). Silica-containing macrophages also display impaired capability to adhere and migrate compared to healthy controls (72).

Enhanced Mtb phagocytosis could be caused by an interaction with intracellularly located surfactant-associated protein A (SP-A) or its related proteins (121–123) A significantly higher release of SP-A has been shown to follow exposure to silica (124) and this increase was associated with reduced silica-related toxicity to AMs (62, 125) analyzed the impact of various types of dust particles on lung tissue after co-administration with inoculated BCG and specifically on the development of fibrotic lesions. They demonstrated that rats and guinea-pigs developed only mild fibrotic lesions after exposure to mine dust, anthracite, kaolin, and BCG alone but large destructive lesions with combined dust and BCG.

Dendritic Cells (DCs)

The influence of silica exposure on DCs function has been little investigated. Beamer and Holian (126) describe an increase of DCs accompanying the decrease in numbers of AMs after exposure to silica. It has been reported that viability of DCs is compromised after exposure to silica particles (74). The role of DCs in resistance is also not well-documented in cases of silica potentiated TB. It has been shown that mycobacteria are able to enter the intracellular spaces of DCs via the specific surface protein DC-specific intercellular adhesion molecule-3 grabbing non-integrin (DC-SIGN) (127). Although the main carriers of Mtb are macrophages, the most infected population of cells in lymph nodes are DCs. The evidence is that antigen presentation properties and migration of DCs play important roles in the establishment of long-term infection (75). They also increase their antigen-presenting properties after infection with mycobacteria, facilitate immune system responses through secretion of pro-inflammatory cytokines [tumor necrosis factor alpha (TNFα), IL-1] and up-regulation of co-stimulatory (CD54, CD40) molecules (76). DCs also specifically stimulate the production of IFNγ by T cells after exposure to Mtb (128).

TABLE 1 | Basic summary of acquired knowledge about specific components of the immune system after exposure to silica, Mtb, or both, highlighting the gaps and opportunities for future research.

	Silica	Mtb	Silica + Mtb
Macrophages	Dose-dependent Induction of apoptosis, fibrotic nodule formation, chronic activation of inflammatory and anti-inflammatory pathways, ROS, and RNI production (6)	Granuloma formation, chronic inflammation, survival mechanisms: ROS and RNI detoxification, blockade of phagosome maturation, granuloma formation (70)	Increase in Mtb uptake (71); impairment of adhesion and migration (72, 73)
Dendritic cells	Lower viability (74)	Cells with the highest bacterial burden in lymph nodes (75); increase in antigen presentation and secretion of pro-inflammatory cytokines (76); activation of adaptive immunity (77)	Yet to be investigated
Neutrophils	Decreased phagocytosis and viability (78, 79)	Control of Mtb replication, prolonged activation—tissue damage (80); trapping of bacilli (81); facilitation of disease progression (82)	Yet be investigated
NKs	Decrease in NKs (83, 84); silica nanoparticles cause increase in NKs (85)	Protective role of NKs—production of IFNγ (86)	Yet to be investigated
Antigens	Inconsistent evidence, increase in antigen-presenting properties of AMs (87)	CD1 mediated T cell activation (88, 89); signaling for APCs (90)	Yet to be investigated
T cells CD4+, CD8+, γδ T cells	Increase in FAS ligand—higher rate of apoptosis (91); shift between Th1/Th2 response (92–96); Tregs and Tresps activation (97); reduced inhibitory activity of T cells (98)	Bacteriostatic and bactericidal effect (77); IFNγ production—phagocytic properties of macrophages, Th2 response activation and Tregs production (99, 100)	Sporadic and contradictory evidence
Antibody-mediated immunity (B cells)	Increase and decrease in B cell activity (101); increase in autoantibodies (97)	B cells are the producers of antibodies, modulators of T cell activity and T cell memory, influencing function of dendritic cells (102); association with containment of Mtb (103); CD4+ T cell regulation (104)	Yet to be investigated

Neutrophils

Neutrophils rapidly respond to pathogen challenge and contribute to control of Mtb replication. However, apart from its protective properties, the cell's prolonged oxidative and proteolytic activity also lead to tissue damage (80). Neutrophils possess the direct ability to restrict Mtb by engulfment of bacilli (129, 130). Increased influx of neutrophils into Mtb-infected tissue has been observed although in this study no bacteria were found inside these cells. This might point to antibacterial activity independent of phagocytosis (131). Their detailed role in disease is thus not yet fully understood.

It has been found that low concentrations of neutrophils in the peripheral blood cause incapability to restrict or kill introduced Mtb (132). Its oxidative phagocytic properties may kill some of the bacteria after phagocyting the dying macrophage (133). Antimicrobial extracellular traps (NETs) formed by neutrophils are also able to contribute to antimycobacterial activity by trapping bacilli, but not often by killing them (81). Neutrophil-related restriction of mycobacterial growth can also be caused by their role in specific T helper 1 (Th1) and Th17 cell production (134). In contrast, it has been argued that neutrophils possess only poor direct antimycobacterial activity and that they instead facilitate the progression of infection (82). Silica particles are known to harm neutrophils in similar ways to that of their effect on macrophages, by decreasing their viability and phagocytic properties (78, 79).

Other Cells [Basophils, Eosinophils, Natural Killer (NK) Cells]

Detailed information about other components of the innate immune system in patients with silica-related TB is almost non-existent. A protective role for NK cells has been observed in mouse lung and splenic cultures infected with Mtb. In this study, production of IFNγ by NK cells significantly contributed to limiting mycobacterial infection, independently of IFNγ produced by T cells. Higher mycobacterial burden and granulocytic activity have been observed after depletion of Interleukin 12 (IL-12), which generally promotes NK cell cytotoxic activity (86). A decrease in NK cell number has been observed after the introduction of silica particles (83, 84). Detailed understanding of silica effects on NK cells is still lacking, but it has been observed that silica particles inhibit Toxoplasma-induced NK cell activity (135). By contrast, silica nanoparticles induce a significant increase in NK cells in mouse spleen, which may indicate a size-dependent effect of the particles on NK cells (85).

ADAPTIVE CELLULAR IMMUNE RESPONSES IN SILICOSIS AND TUBERCULOSIS

Antigen Presentation

Antigen presentation is generally described as the presentation of lysed proteins on the surface of antigen-presenting cells (APCs) via the Major Histocompatibility Complexes (MHC), which is recognized by T cell receptors leading to their activation. Mycobacterial phospholipids activate CD1-mediated T cells (88, 89), and it has been observed that Mtb provides signaling for both T cells (lipid antigens) and APCs (polar lipids via TLR-2) (90).

Silica, as a pro-inflammatory agent, causes primarily induction of apoptosis of AMs. Various studies indicate that silica does not act as an antigen (136). Rather, silica particles support the increase of antigen-presenting properties of macrophages (87). Enhanced activation of AMs could also be related to autoimmune disease as a result of silica exposure. No significant differences were detected in the expression of MHC II molecules on AMs between silicosis and other diseases, such as sarcoidosis and allergic alveolitis (137). However, Pfau et al. (138) observed that silica-related antigens presented by apoptotic AMs are recognized by autoantibodies in mice. The question of how silica particles modulate presentation of antigen in the relationship with mycobacterial infection remains unanswered.

T Lymphocytes—CD4+, CD8+, γδ T Cells

T cells activation occurs on exposure to an antigen which is presented by APCs. The major APCs responsible for defense against mycobacterial infection and activators of adaptive immunity are macrophages and dendritic cells. Broad antimycobacterial activity is provided by different subsets of T cells targeting a wide range of specific mycobacterial antigens. It is known, for example, that CD4+, CD8+, γδ T cells, and CD1 restricted T cells response to infection, contributing to bacteriostatic and bactericidal effects (77). CD4+ and CD8+ T cells act as IFNγ producers and facilitate the phagocytic properties of macrophages (**Figure 1**). The activity of these subsets might be independent of each other, although their combined activity shows the strongest anti-mycobacterial effects (139). The onset of adaptive immunity is initiated with a significant delay after initial exposure to the pathogen. The restrictive activity of T cells is sufficient for bacterial arrest but not sufficient to kill mycobacteria, which might contribute to prolonged incubation and consequent re-activation of disease (140). In case of T cells response, a number of studies have confirmed that mycobacterial infection triggers Th2 response and T regulatory cells (Tregs) production rather than Th1 response. Deficiency in Th1 response may contribute to poor elimination and successful proliferation of Mtb in the host (99, 100).

The response of adaptive immunity components to silica particles is related to the cascade of activities mediated by the interaction with cells involved in innate immunity, particularly macrophages. However, direct interaction of T cells with silica cannot be excluded. It has been observed, that T cells acquire higher expression of FAS receptor and its ligands in lymphocytes obtained from bronchoalveolar lavage (BAL) fluid from silica-exposed individuals. This includes an over 20% increase in Fas receptor and more than 30% in Fas ligand on CD4+, CD8+ CD56+, and CD45RO+ cells, corresponding to the higher rate of apoptosis (30%) (91). Both inflammatory and anti-inflammatory responses have been induced after exposure to silica. However, conflicting results in specific cytokine production have been reported, suggesting that there is a shift between Th1/Th2 responses during disease progression. There is noticeable inconsistency for another cytokine involved in Th1 response, IFN-γ. Its levels in lungs and lymph nodes have been reported as both elevated and undetected in silica-exposed mice. As a result of Th2 response, an increase in production of IL-12 mRNA and IgG_1 has been reported in silicotic mice and *in vitro* (92, 96).

More recently, attention has been paid to the role of silica in autoimmune responses, in which autoimmune cells are activated by signals from silica-induced apoptotic macrophages (141). Following silica exposure, Tregs and Responder T cells (Tresps) are chronically activated and infiltrate the peripheral T cell population. By increased production of Fas ligand, Treg cells induce apoptosis and impair the immune response (97). Therefore, the overall number and inhibitory activity of T cells are reduced, with Tresps surviving due to an expression of apoptosis inhibitors (98). A closer look at cellular quantitative evaluation shows a silica-induced reduction of a number of macrophages and a consequential decrease of macrophage-dependent activity of T- and NK cells (142).

Some of the features related to the leukocyte response modulation after silica exposure entail inconsistent and contradictory mechanistic effects regarding silica-TB co-occurrence. For example, increased production of TGF-β as a reaction to silica (143) should assist in the process of elimination of Mtb, not its potentiation (144, 145). There is other evidence for a protective effect of silica in its interaction with the immune system, for example in protecting against the development of diabetes (146, 147).

Antibody-Mediated Immunity

B lymphocytes mediate specific immunological responses against pathogens via the production of specific antibodies. They can modulate responses to infection independent of antibodies; however, the mechanism(s) of such activity is not yet understood (148). The proliferation of plasma cells in patients with silicosis was discovered early (149, 150). Silica particles can cause both an increase and inhibition of B cell activity. Reduced and increased numbers of antibodies have been observed after exposure to silica in animal models. Moseley et al. (101) observed complete inhibition of immunoglobulin-secreting cells (ISCs) after the addition of silica in low- and high-density cultures depleted of monocytes. In contrast, in high-density cultures of unfractionated mononuclear cells, silica caused a significant increase in ISCs. It, therefore, seems that the number of immunoglobulin secreting cells is dependent not just on silica particles but also on other factors such as density of culture and presence of monocytes. A significant reduction in B cells was observed in mouse spleens treated

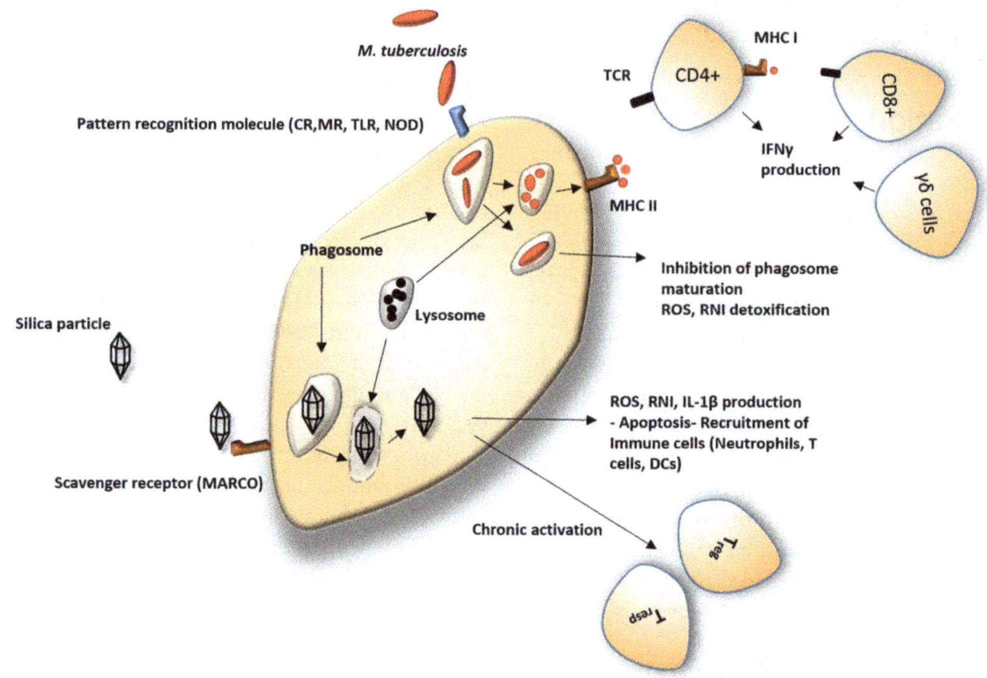

FIGURE 1 | Response of macrophage to silica and *Mycobacterium*. CR, Complement receptors; MR, Mannose receptors; TLR, Toll like receptors; NOD, Nod-like receptors; ROS, Reactive oxygen species; RNI, Reactive nitrogen intermediates; IL-1β, Interleukin 1 beta; MHC I, major histocompatibility complex 1; MHC II, major histocompatibility complex 2; IFNγ, Interferon gamma; TCR, T-cell receptor; DCs, dendritic cells; CD4+/CD8+, effector T cells; T_{regs}, regulatory T cells; T_{resps}, responder T cells; γδ cells, gamma delta T cells. Silica particles are usually recognized by scavenger receptors and engulfed by macrophages. Owing to the poor capability of the cell in eliminating the particle by standard lysosomal proteolytic enzymes, silica particles remain in the cell and initiate a cascade of pro- and anti-inflammatory processes, leading to a number of pathological modifications in the immune response. Mycobacterium is identified by a different set of cellular receptors but undergoes a similar process upon its ingestion. The physiological response of the immune system consists of digestion of bacilli and its antigen presentation on the cell surface leading to recruitment of effector cells such as CD4+ and CD8+ T cells. Mycobacterial evasive mechanisms frequently manage to avoid elimination, leading to pathological.

with silica nanoparticles (85). The most common effect of silica was an increase of autoantibodies such as rheumatoid factor (anti IgG), and anti-nuclear antibodies related to autoimmune diseases such as Caplan's syndrome, scleroderma, (ANCA)-related vasculitis/nephritis, and systemic lupus erythematosus (97).

In response to mycobacterial infection, B cells do not simply act as producers of antibodies but also as modulators of T cell activity and development of T cell memory. They also influence the function of other effector cells such as DCs. The importance of B cells during mycobacterial infection is based on the co-operation and co-stimulation with other components of the immune system, suggesting more complex involvement in the immunological response (102). Antibodies in lymphocyte supernatants have been studied to obtain information about its diagnostic potential in pediatric TB patients. The findings indicated that antibodies were present at higher concentrations only during acute disease in TB positive patients compared to controls (151). Proliferating B cells are mostly present in sites of granulomas actively secreting TB-specific antibodies (103, 152) observed that abnormally located B cells in patients with TB are associated with a containment of Mtb and with IL-17 and IL-22 production. The same group also described inhibitory effect of TB-related B cells on Th17 cell activation and therefore its involvement in CD4+ T cell regulation (104). While the overall role of B cells in the immune response to *M. tuberculosis* has been studied extensively (153, 154), its relationship with silica exposure has not yet been documented.

CONCLUSION

It is evident that the human immune system plays a central role in pathophysiological processes initiated after silica exposure and which have an impact on the development of TB. A detailed description of silica's involvement in TB infection, course, progression, re-activation and outcome has yet to be properly described. Existing research confirms the substantial role of the innate immune system in both direct defense and in the mobilization of other components of the immune system as a response to TB infection. Such findings are likely to underlie the higher susceptibility of silica-exposed and silicotic individuals to TB. However, there remain a number of gaps in knowledge, as summarized in **Table 1**.

Recent findings suggest a more complex involvement of adaptive immunity in the containment and elimination of Mtb and its activation in latent infection. The effects of the immune response to silica exposure are complex and do not always lead to increased susceptibility to TB; some promote the elimination of mycobacteria rather than their proliferation. For example, silica-induced Th1 response activation, mediating TNFα and IFNγ production, should in theory contribute to resistance to or elimination of Mtb. An increase in Th2 response after exposure to silica might be one of the contributing factors for successful propagation of Mtb. Discrepancies in evidence of pro- and anti-inflammatory pathway involvement, however, suggest more intricate reactions promoting fibrogenesis which might make a direct contribution to predisposition to TB.

The subject of this review has clinical relevance. The pathological activity of silica is important in the susceptibility to and prognosis of associated TB in silica-exposed populations globally. The considerations in this review should inform studies that aim to investigate outcomes of standard TB treatment regimens as they apply to silicotuberculosis by providing insight into mechanisms relevant to drug efficacy.

Finally, knowledge gained from the study of the silica-TB interaction could provide information relevant to the understanding of other pathological processes associated with silica exposure.

AUTHOR CONTRIBUTIONS

The subject of the review was co-conceived by all the authors. PK conducted the literature search and drafted the manuscript. RE, MG, and MJ contributed substantial intellectual content to the contents of the review and its finalization. All authors take responsibility for the final manuscript.

REFERENCES

1. Allison AC, Harington JS, Birbeck M. An examination of the cytotoxic effects of silica on macrophages. *J Exp Med.* (1966) 124:141–54. doi: 10.1084/jem.124.2.141
2. Gulumian M, Borm PJ, Vallyathan V, Castranova V, Donaldson K, Nelson G, et al. Mechanistically identified suitable biomarkers of exposure, effect, and susceptibility for silicosis and coal-worker's pneumoconiosis: a comprehensive review. *J Toxicol Environ Health B Crit Rev.* (2006) 9:357–95. doi: 10.1080/15287390500196537
3. Chavez-Galan L, Ramon-Luing LA, Torre-Bouscoulet L, Perez-Padilla R, Sada-Ovalle I. Pre-exposure of *Mycobacterium tuberculosis*-infected macrophages to crystalline silica impairs control of bacterial growth by deregulating the balance between apoptosis and necrosis. *PLoS ONE* (2013) 8:e80971. doi: 10.1371/journal.pone.0080971
4. Balmes JR. Commentary from JOEM forum- silicosis: then and now. *J Occup Environ Med.* (2017) 59:222–233. doi: 10.1097/JOM.00000000000009
5. Ding M, Chen F, Shi X, Yucesoy B, Mossman B, Vallyathan V. Diseases caused by silica: mechanisms of injury and disease development. *Int Immunopharmacol.* (2002) 2:173–82. doi: 10.1016/S1567-5769(01)00170-9
6. Leung CC, Yu IT, Chen W. Silicosis. *Lancet* (2012) 379:2008–18. doi: 10.1016/S0140-6736(12)60235-9
7. Cocco P, Rice CH, Chen JQ, McCawley MA, McLaughlin JK, Dosemeci M. Lung cancer risk, silica exposure, and silicosis in Chinese mines and pottery factories: the modifying role of other workplace lung carcinogens. *Am J Ind Med.* (2001) 40:674–82. doi: 10.1002/ajim.10022
8. Rimal B, Greenberg AK, Rom WN. Basic pathogenetic mechanisms in silicosis: current understanding. *Curr Opin Pulm Med.* (2005) 11:169–73. doi: 10.1097/01.mcp.0000152998.11335.24
9. Greenberg MI, Waksman J, Curtis J. Silicosis: a review. *Dis Mon.* (2007) 53:394–416. doi: 10.1016/j.disamonth.2007.09.020
10. Collis EL. Recent views on pneumonoconioses. *Proc R Soc Med.* (1931) 24:531–42.
11. Eide J, Gylseth B, Skaug V. Silicotic lesions of the bone marrow: histopathology and microanalysis. *Histopathology* (1984) 8:693–703. doi: 10.1111/j.1365-2559.1984.tb02381.x
12. Chen W, Zhuang Z, Attfield MD, Chen BT, Gao P, Harrison JC, et al. Exposure to silica and silicosis among tin miners in China: exposure-response analyses and risk assessment. *Occup Environ Med.* (2001) 58:31–7. doi: 10.1136/oem.58.1.31
13. Deng H, Xu H, Zhang X, Sun Y, Wang R, Brann D, et al. Protective effect of Ac-SDKP on alveolar epithelial cells through inhibition of EMT via TGF-beta1/ROCK1 pathway in silicosis in rat. *Toxicol Appl Pharmacol.* (2016) 294:1–10. doi: 10.1016/j.taap.2016.01.010
14. Stanton DW, Belle BK, Dekker KJJ, Du Plessis JJL. *South African Mining Industry Best Practice on the Prevention of Silicosis.* Mine Health and Safety Council (2006). Available online at: http://www.oit.org/wcmsp5/groups/public/---ed_protect/---protrav/---safework/documents/publication/wcms_118101.pdf
15. Nelson G, Girdler-Brown B, Ndlovu N, Murray J. Three decades of silicosis: disease trends at autopsy in South African gold miners. *Environ Health Perspect.* (2010) 118:421–6. doi: 10.1289/ehp.0900918
16. Mendez-Vargas MM, Baez-Revueltas FB, Lopez-Rojas P, Tovalin-Ahumada JH, Zamudio-Lara JO, Marin-Cotonieto IA, et al. [Silicosis and industrial bronchitis by exposure to silica powders and cement]. *Rev Med Inst Mex Seguro Soc.* (2013) 51:384–9.
17. Antao VC, Pinheiro GA, Kavakama J, Terra-Filho M. High prevalence of silicosis among stone carvers in Brazil. *Am J Ind Med.* (2004) 45:194–201. doi: 10.1002/ajim.10331
18. Jindal SK. Silicosis in India: past and present. *Curr Opin Pulm Med.* (2013) 19:163–8. doi: 10.1097/MCP.0b013e32835bb19e
19. Nasrullah M, Mazurek JM, Wood JM, Bang KM, Kreiss K. Silicosis mortality with respiratory tuberculosis in the United States, 1968-2006. *Am J Epidemiol.* (2011) 174:839–48. doi: 10.1093/aje/kwr159
20. Zosky GR, Hoy RF, Silverstone EJ, Brims FJ, Miles S, Johnson AR, et al. Coal workers' pneumoconiosis: an Australian perspective. *Med J Aust.* (2016) 204:414–8. doi: 10.5694/mja16.00357
21. Gibson GJ, Loddenkemper R, Lundback B, Sibille Y. Respiratory health and disease in Europe: the new European Lung White Book. *Eur Respir J.* (2013) 42:559–63. doi: 10.1183/09031936.00105513
22. Hamilton RF Jr, Thakur SA, Mayfair JK, Holian A. MARCO mediates silica uptake and toxicity in alveolar macrophages from C57BL/6 mice. *J Biol Chem.* (2006) 281:34218–26. doi: 10.1074/jbc.M605229200
23. Beamer GL, Seaver BP, Jessop F, Shepherd DM, Beamer CA. Acute exposure to crystalline silica reduces macrophage activation in response to bacterial lipoproteins. *Front Immunol* (2016) 7:49. doi: 10.3389/fimmu.2016.00049
24. Shkurupy VA, Nadeev AP, Karpov MA, Bugrimova YS. Experimental cytomorphological studies of the reaction of mononuclear phagocyte system in granulomatosis of mixed (silicotic and tuberculous) etiology. *Bull Exp Biol Med.* (2010) 149:462–5. doi: 10.1007/s10517-010-0971-7
25. Fenoglio I, Croce A, Di Renzo F, Tiozzo R, Fubini B. Pure-silica zeolites (Porosils) as model solids for the evaluation of the physicochemical features determining silica toxicity to macrophages. *Chem Res Toxicol.* (2000) 13:489–500. doi: 10.1021/tx990169u

26. Denny JJ, Robson WD, Irwin DA. The prevention of silicosis by metallic aluminum: I. A preliminary report. *Can Med Assoc J.* (1937) 37:1–11.
27. Nash T, Allison AC, Harington JS. Physico-chemical properties of silica in relation to its toxicity. *Nature* (1966) 210:259–61. doi: 10.1038/210259a0
28. Stöber W, Brieger H. On the theory of silicosis. IV. The topochemical interaction. *Arch Environ Health* (1968) 16:706–8.
29. Huggins CW, Meyers GT. *Report of Investigations 9053 Particle Size Distribution of Quartz and Other Respirable Dust Particles Collected at Metal Mines, Nonmetal Mines, and Processing Plants.* US Department of the Interior. Bureau of Mines Report of Investigations (1986). Available online at: https://stacks.cdc.gov/view/cdc/10618
30. Hlavay J, Polyák K, Wesemann G. Particle size distribution of mineral phases and metals in dusts collected at different workplaces. *Fresenius' J Analyt Chem.* (1992) 344:319–21.
31. Lin W, Huang YW, Zhou XD, Ma Y. *In vitro* toxicity of silica nanoparticles in human lung cancer cells. *Toxicol Appl Pharmacol.* (2006) 217:252–9. doi: 10.1016/j.taap.2006.10.004
32. Fubini B, Ghiazza M, Fenoglio I. Physico-chemical features of engineered nanoparticles relevant to their toxicity. *Nanotoxicology* (2010) 4:347–63. doi: 10.3109/17435390.2010.509519
33. Wang Z, Wang C, Liu S, He W, Wang L, Gan J, et al. Specifically formed corona on silica nanoparticles enhances transforming growth factor beta1 activity in triggering lung fibrosis. *ACS Nano* (2017) 11:1659–72. doi: 10.1021/acsnano.6b07461
34. Ghio AJ, Kennedy TP, Schapira RM, Crumbliss AL, Hoidal JR. Hypothesis: is lung disease after silicate inhalation caused by oxidant generation? *Lancet* (1990) 336:967–9. doi: 10.1016/0140-6736(90)92421-D
35. Borm PJ. Toxicity and occupational health hazards of coal fly ash (CFA). A review of data and comparison to coal mine dust. *Ann Occup Hyg.* (1997) 41:659–76. doi: 10.1016/S0003-4878(97)00026-4
36. Flynn JL, Chan J. Immunology of tuberculosis. *Annu Rev Immunol.* (2001) 19:93–129. doi: 10.1146/annurev.immunol.19.1.93
37. Fubini B, Hubbard A. Reactive oxygen species (ROS) and reactive nitrogen species (RNS) generation by silica in inflammation and fibrosis. *Free Radic Biol Med.* (2003) 34:1507–16. doi: 10.1016/S0891-5849(03)00149-7
38. Brown JM, Swindle EJ, Kushnir-Sukhov NM, Holian A, Metcalfe DD. Silica-directed mast cell activation is enhanced by scavenger receptors. *Am J Respir Cell Mol Biol.* (2007) 36:43–52. doi: 10.1165/rcmb.2006-0197OC
39. Nagelschmidt G. The relation between lung dust and lung pathology in pneumoconiosis. *Br J Ind Med.* (1960) 17:247–59. doi: 10.1136/oem.17.4.247
40. Castranova V, Vallyathan V. Silicosis and coal workers' pneumoconiosis. *Environ Health Perspect.* (2000) 108(Suppl. 4):675–84. doi: 10.1289/ehp.00108s4675
41. Pavan C, Fubini B. Unveiling the variability of "quartz hazard" in light of recent toxicological findings. *Chem Res Toxicol.* (2017) 30:469–85. doi: 10.1021/acs.chemrestox.6b00409
42. WHO. *Global Tuberculosis Report* (2018).
43. Narasimhan P, Wood J, MacIntyre CR, Dilip M. Risk factors for tuberculosis. *Pulmon Med.* (2013) 2013:828939. doi: 10.1155/2013/828939
44. Lönnroth K, Williams BG, Stadlin S, Jaramillo E, Dye C. Alcohol use as a risk factor for tuberculosis - a systematic review. *BMC Public Health* (2008) 8:289. doi: 10.1186/1471-2458-8-289
45. Jeon CY, Murray MB. Diabetes mellitus increases the risk of active tuberculosis: a systematic review of 13 observational studies. *PLoS Med.* (2008) 5:e152. doi: 10.1371/journal.pmed.005015
46. Deiss RG, Rodwell TC, Garfein RS. Tuberculosis and illicit drug use: review and update. *Clin Infect Dis.* (2009) 48:72–82. doi: 10.1086/594126
47. Low A, Gavriilidis G, Larke N, B-Lajoie MR, Drouin O, Stover J, et al. Incidence of opportunistic infections and the impact of antiretroviral therapy among HIV-infected adults in low- and middle-income countries: a systematic review and meta-analysis. *Clin Infect Dis.* (2016) 62:1595–603. doi: 10.1093/cid/ciw125
48. Khor CC, Chapman SJ, Vannberg FO, Dunne A, Murphy C, Ling EY, et al. A Mal functional variant is associated with protection against invasive pneumococcal disease, bacteremia, malaria and tuberculosis. *Nat Genet.* (2007) 39:523–8. doi: 10.1038/ng1976
49. Shweta SB, Bhatnagar S, Gupta AK, Murti K, Pandey K. Co-infection of visceral leishmaniasis and pulmonary tuberculosis: a case study. *Asian Pac J Trop Dis.* (2014) 4:57–60. doi: 10.1016/S2222-1808(14)60315-7
50. Bates MN, Khalakdina A, Pai M, Chang L, Lessa F, Smith KR. Risk of tuberculosis from exposure to tobacco smokea systematic review and meta-analysis. *Arch Intern Med.* (2007) 167:335–42. doi: 10.1001/archinte.167.4.335
51. Kurmi OP, Sadhra CS, Ayres JG, Sadhra SS. Tuberculosis risk from exposure to solid fuel smoke: a systematic review and meta-analysis. *J Epidemiol Commun Health* (2014) 68:1112–8. doi: 10.1136/jech-2014-204120
52. Öztürk AB, Kiliçaslan Z, Işsever H. Effect of smoking and indoor air pollution on the risk of tuberculosis: smoking, indoor air pollution and tuberculosis. *Tuberk Toraks* (2014) 62:1-6. doi: 10.5578/tt.7013
53. Cowie RL. The epidemiology of tuberculosis in gold miners with silicosis. *Am J Respir Crit Care Med.* (1994) 150(5 Pt 1):1460–2. doi: 10.1164/ajrccm.150.5.7952577
54. Barboza CE, Winter DH, Seiscento M, Santos Ude P, Terra Filho M. Tuberculosis and silicosis: epidemiology, diagnosis and chemoprophylaxis. *J Bras Pneumol.* (2008) 34:959–66. doi: 10.1590/S1806-37132008001100012
55. Gye WE, Kettle EH. Silicosis and Miners' phthisis. *Br J Exp Pathol.* (1922) 3:241–51.
56. Hnizdo E, Murray J, Sluis-Cremer GK, Thomas RG. Correlation between radiological and pathological diagnosis of silicosis: an autopsy population based study. *Am J Ind Med.* (1993) 24:427–45. doi: 10.1002/ajim.4700240408
57. Mossman BT, Churg A. Mechanisms in the pathogenesis of asbestosis and silicosis. *Am J Respir Crit Care Med.* (1998) 157(5 Pt 1):1666–80. doi: 10.1164/ajrccm.157.5.9707141
58. Sherson D. Silicosis in the twenty first century. *Occup Environ Med.* (2002) 59: 721–2. doi: 10.1136/oem.59.11.721
59. Churchyard GJ, Fielding KL, Grant AD. A trial of mass isoniazid preventive therapy for tuberculosis control. *N Engl J Med.* (2014) 370:1662–3. doi: 10.1056/NEJMoa1214289
60. Parker J, Wagner GR. Silicosis. In: *ILO Encyclopaedia of Occupational Health and Safety, Part I, Respiratory Disease.* International Labour Organisation (2012).
61. Snider DE Jr. The relationship between tuberculosis and silicosis. *Am Rev Respir Dis.* (1978) 118:455–60.
62. Attygalle D, Harrison CV, King EJ, Mohanty GP. Infective pneumoconiosis. I. The influence of dead tubercle bacilli (BCG) on the dust lesions produced by anthracite, coal-mine dust, and kaolin in the lungs of rats and guinea-pigs. *Br J Ind Med.* (1954) 11:245–59.
63. Gernez-Rieux C, Tacquet A, Devulder B, Voisin C, Tonnel A, Aerts C, et al. Experimental study of interactions between pneumoconiosis and mycobacterial infections. *Ann NY Acad Sci.* (1972) 200:106–26.
64. Beamer CA, Holian A. Silica suppresses Toll-like receptor ligand-induced dendritic cell activation. *FASEB J.* (2008) 22:2053–63. doi: 10.1096/fj.07-095299
65. De Oliveira Abrão C, de Araújo Filho, JA. *Mycobacterium sherrisii* lung infection in a Brazilian patient with silicosis and a history of pulmonary tuberculosis. *Case Rep Infect Dis.* (2015) 2015:498608. doi: 10.1155/2015/498608
66. Blanco Pérez JJ, Pérez González A, Morano Amado LE, Guerra Vales JL, Vázquez Gallardo R, Salgado Barreira Á, et al. Clinical significance of environmental mycobacteria isolated from respiratory specimens of patients with and without silicosis. *Arch. Bronconeumol.* (2016) 52:145–50. doi: 10.1016/j.arbres.2015.07.007
67. Qu Y, Tang Y, Cao D, Wu F, Liu J, Lu G, et al. Genetic polymorphisms in alveolar macrophage response-related genes, and risk of silicosis and pulmonary tuberculosis in Chinese iron miners. *Int J Hyg Environ Health* (2007) 210:679–89. doi: 10.1016/j.ijheh.2006.11.010
68. Corbett EL, Mozzato-Chamay N, Butterworth AE, De Cock KM, Williams BG, Churchyard GJ, et al. Polymorphisms in the tumor necrosis factor-alpha gene promoter may predispose to severe silicosis in black South African miners. *Am J Respir Crit Care Med.* (2002) 165:690–3. doi: 10.1164/ajrccm.165.5.2010050
69. Wu F, Qu Y, Tang Y, Cao D, Sun P, Xia Z. Lack of association between cytokine gene polymorphisms and silicosis and pulmonary

tuberculosis in Chinese iron miners. *J Occup Health* (2008) 50:445–54. doi: 10.1539/joh.L8006

70. Longhi G, Hanifi-Moghaddam P, Touabassy R, Saleh M. Macrophage infection by mycobacteria. *Mycobact Dis.* (2016) 6:1–11. doi: 10.4172/2161-1068.1000197
71. Ebina T, Takahashi Y, Hasuike T. Effect of quartz powder on tubercle bacilli and phagocytes. *Am Rev Respir Dis.* (1960) 82:516–27.
72. Dauber JH, Rossman MD, Daniele RP. Pulmonary fibrosis: bronchoalveolar cell types and impaired function of alveolar macrophages in experimental silicosis. *Environ Res.* (1982) 27:226–36. doi: 10.1016/0013-9351(82)90074-3
73. Pasula R, Britigan BE, Turner J, Martin WJ II. Airway delivery of silica increases susceptibility to mycobacterial infection in mice: potential role of repopulating macrophages. *J Immunol.* (2009) 182:7102–9. doi: 10.4049/jimmunol.0803642
74. Vallhov H, Gabrielsson S, Stromme M, Scheynius A, Garcia-Bennett AE. Mesoporous silica particles induce size dependent effects on human dendritic cells. *Nano Lett.* (2007) 7:3576–82. doi: 10.1021/nl0714785
75. Wolf AJ, Linas B, Trevejo-Nunez GJ, Kincaid E, Tamura T, Takatsu K, et al. *Mycobacterium tuberculosis* infects dendritic cells with high frequency and impairs their function *in vivo*. *J Immunol.* (2007) 179:2509–19. doi: 10.4049/jimmunol.179.4.2509
76. Henderson, RA, Watkins SC, Flynn JL. Activation of human dendritic cells following infection with *Mycobacterium tuberculosis*. *J Immunol.* (1997) 159:635–43.
77. Boom WH, Canaday DH, Fulton SA, Gehring AJ, Rojas RE, Torres M. Human immunity to *M. tuberculosis*: T cell subsets and antigen processing. *Tuberculosis (Edinb)* (2003) 83:98–106. doi: 10.1016/S1472-9792(02)00054-9
78. Zimmerman BT, Canono BP, Campbell PA. Silica decreases phagocytosis and bactericidal activity of both macrophages and neutrophils *in vitro*. *Immunology* (1986) 59:521–5.
79. Leigh J, Wang H, Bonin A, Peters M, Ruan X. Silica-induced apoptosis in alveolar and granulomatous cells *in vivo*. *Environ Health Perspect.* (1997) 105(Suppl. 5):1241–5.
80. Zay K, Loo S, Xie C, Devine DV, Wright J, Churg A. Role of neutrophils and alpha1-antitrypsin in coal- and silica-induced connective tissue breakdown. *Am J Physiol.* (1999) 276(2 Pt 1):L269–79.
81. Ramos-Kichik V, Mondragon-Flores R, Mondragon-Castelan M, Gonzalez-Pozos S, Muniz-Hernandez S, Rojas-Espinosa O, et al. Neutrophil extracellular traps are induced by *Mycobacterium tuberculosis*. *Tuberculosis (Edinb)* (2009) 89:29–37. doi: 10.1016/j.tube.2008.09.009
82. Eruslanov EB, Lyadova IV, Kondratieva TK, Majorov KB, Scheglov IV, Orlova MO et al. Neutrophil responses to *Mycobacterium tuberculosis* infection in genetically susceptible and resistant mice. *Infect Immun.* (2005) 73:1744–53. doi: 10.1128/IAI.73.3.1744-1753.2005
83. Kiessling R, Hochman PS, Haller O, Shearer GM, Wigzell H, Cudkowicz G. Evidence for a similar or common mechanism for natural killer cell activity and resistance to hemopoietic grafts. *Eur J Immunol.* (1977) 7:655–63. doi: 10.1002/eji.1830070915
84. Riccardi C, Santoni A, Barlozzari T, Herberman RB. *In vivo* reactivity of mouse natural killer (NK) cells against normal bone marrow cells. *Cell Immunol.* (1981) 60:136–43. doi: 10.1016/0008-8749(81)90254-9
85. Park EJ, Park K. Oxidative stress and pro-inflammatory responses induced by silica nanoparticles *in vivo* and *in vitro*. *Toxicol Lett.* (2009) 184:18–25. doi: 10.1016/j.toxlet.2008.10.012
86. Feng CG, Kaviratne M, Rothfuchs AG, Cheever A, Hieny S, Young HA, et al. NK cell-derived IFN-gamma differentially regulates innate resistance and neutrophil response in T cell-deficient hosts infected with *Mycobacterium tuberculosis*. *J Immunol.* (2006) 177:7086–93. doi: 10.4049/jimmunol.177.10.7086
87. Migliaccio CT, Hamilton RF Jr, Holian A. Increase in a distinct pulmonary macrophage subset possessing an antigen-presenting cell phenotype and *in vitro* APC activity following silica exposure. *Toxicol Appl Pharmacol.* (2005) 205:168–76. doi: 10.1016/j.taap.2004.11.005
88. Matsunaga I, Bhatt A, Young DC, Cheng TY, Eyles SJ, Besra GS, et al. *Mycobacterium tuberculosis* pks12 produces a novel polyketide presented by CD1c to T cells. *J Exp Med.* (2004) 200:1559–69. doi: 10.1084/jem.20041429
89. Ulrichs T, Moody DB, Grant E, Kaufmann SH, Porcelli SA. T-cell responses to CD1-presented lipid antigens in humans with *Mycobacterium tuberculosis* infection. *Infect Immun.* (2003) 71:3076–87. doi: 10.1128/IAI.71.6.3076-3087.2003
90. Roura-Mir C, Wang L, Cheng TY, Matsunaga I, Dascher CC, Peng SL, et al. *Mycobacterium tuberculosis* regulates CD1 antigen presentation pathways through TLR-2. *J Immunol.* (2005) 175:1758–66. doi: 10.4049/jimmunol.175.3.1758
91. Hamzaoui A, Ammar J, Grairi H, Hamzaoui K. Expression of Fas antigen and Fas ligand in bronchoalveolar lavage from silicosis patients. *Mediators Inflamm.* (2003) 12:209–14. doi: 10.1080/09629350310001599648
92. Huaux F, Lardot C, Arras M, Delos M, Many MC, Coutelier JP, et al. Lung fibrosis induced by silica particles in NMRI mice is associated with an upregulation of the p40 subunit of interleukin-12 and Th-2 manifestations. *Am J Respir Cell Mol Biol.* (1999) 20:561–72. doi: 10.1165/ajrcmb.20.4.3342
93. Garn H, Friedetzky A, Kirchner A, Jager R, Gemsa D. Experimental silicosis: a shift to a preferential IFN-gamma-based Th1 response in thoracic lymph nodes. *Am J Physiol Lung Cell Mol Physiol.* (2000) 278:L1221–30. doi: 10.1152/ajplung.2000.278.6.L1221
94. Davis GS, Pfeiffer LM, Hemenway DR. Interferon-gamma production by specific lung lymphocyte phenotypes in silicosis in mice. *Am J Respir Cell Mol Biol.* (2000) 22:491–501. doi: 10.1165/ajrcmb.22.4.3599
95. Barbarin V, Xing Z, Delos M, Lison D, Huaux F. Pulmonary overexpression of IL-10 augments lung fibrosis and Th2 responses induced by silica particles. *Am J Physiol Lung Cell Mol Physiol.* (2005) 288:L841–8. doi: 10.1152/ajplung.00329.2004
96. Huaux F. New developments in the understanding of immunology in silicosis. *Curr Opin Allergy Clin Immunol.* (2007) 7:168–73. doi: 10.1097/ACI.0b013e32802bf8a5
97. Lee S, Hayashi H, Maeda M, Matsuzaki H, Kumagai-Takei N, Chen Y, et al. Chapter 9: Immunostimulation by silica particles and the development of autoimmune dysregulation. In: *Immune Response Activation*. Croatia: InTech Open Access Publisher (2014), 249–265. Available online at: https://www.intechopen.com/books/immune-response-activation/immunostimulation-by-silica-particles-and-the-development-of-autoimmune-dysregulation
98. Lee S, Hayashi H, Maeda M, Chen Y, Matsuzaki H, Kumagai-Takei N, et al. Environmental factors producing autoimmune dysregulation–chronic activation of T cells caused by silica exposure. *Immunobiology* (2012) 217:743–8. doi: 10.1016/j.imbio.2011.12.009
99. Lienhardt C, Azzurri A, Amedei A, Fielding K, Sillah J, Sow OY, et al. Active tuberculosis in Africa is associated with reduced Th1 and increased Th2 activity *in vivo*. *Eur J Immunol.* (2002) 32:1605–13. doi: 10.1002/1521-4141(200206)32:6<1605::AID-IMMU1605>3.0.CO;2-6
100. He XY, Xiao L, Chen HB, Hao J, Li J, Wang YJ, et al. T regulatory cells and Th1/Th2 cytokines in peripheral blood from tuberculosis patients. *Eur J Clin Microbiol Infect Dis.* (2010) 29:643–50. doi: 10.1007/s10096-010-0908-0
101. Moseley PL, Monick M, Hunninghake GW. Divergent effects of silica on lymphocyte proliferation and immunoglobulin production. *J Appl Physiol.* (1988) 65:350–7. doi: 10.1152/jappl.1988.65.1.350
102. Kozakiewicz L, Phuah J, Flynn J, Chan J. The role of B cells and humoral immunity in *Mycobacterium tuberculosis* infection. In: Divangahi M, editor. *The New Paradigm of Immunity to Tuberculosis. Advances in Experimental Medicine and Biology, Vol. 783*. New York, NY: Springer (2013). p. 225–50. doi: 10.1007/978-1-4614-6111-1_12
103. Zhang M, Wang Z, Graner MW, Yang L, Liao M, Yang Q, et al. B cell infiltration is associated with the increased IL-17 and IL-22 expression in the lungs of patients with tuberculosis. *Cell Immunol.* (2011) 270:217–23. doi: 10.1016/j.cellimm.2011.05.009
104. Zhang M, Zheng X, Zhang J, Zhu Y, Zhu X, Liu H, et al. CD19(+)CD1d(+)CD5(+) B cell frequencies are increased in patients with tuberculosis and suppress Th17 responses. *Cell Immunol.* (2012) 274:89–97. doi: 10.1016/j.cellimm.2012.01.007
105. Harington JS. Some biological actions of silica: their part in the pathogenesis of silicosis. *S Afr Med J.* (1963) 37:451–6.
106. Adamis Z, Timar M. Studies on the effect of quartz, bentonite and coal dust mixtures on macrophages *in vitro*. *Br J Exp Pathol.* (1978) 59:411–5.
107. Dubois CM, Bissonnette E, Rola-Pleszczynski M. Asbestos fibers and silica particles stimulate rat alveolar macrophages to release tumor necrosis factor.

Autoregulatory role of leukotriene B4. *Am Rev Respir Dis.* (1989) 139:1257–64. doi: 10.1164/ajrccm/139.5.1257
108. Hamilton RF Jr, Thakur SA, Holian A. Silica binding and toxicity in alveolar macrophages. *Free Radic Biol Med.* (2008) 44:1246–58. doi: 10.1016/j.freeradbiomed.2007.12.027
109. Liang D, Wang Y, Zhu Z, Yang G, An G, Li X, et al. BMP-7 attenuated silica-induced pulmonary fibrosis through modulation of the balance between TGF-beta/Smad and BMP-7/Smad signaling pathway. *Chem Biol Interact.* (2016) 243:72–81. doi: 10.1016/j.cbi.2015.11.012
110. De Voss JJ, Rutter K, Schroeder BG, Su H, Zhu Y, Barry CE III. The salicylate-derived mycobactin siderophores of *Mycobacterium tuberculosis* are essential for growth in macrophages. *Proc Natl Acad Sci USA.* (2000) 97:1252–7. doi: 10.1073/pnas.97.3.1252
111. Berrington WR, Hawn TR. *Mycobacterium tuberculosis*, macrophages, and the innate immune response: does common variation matter? *Immunol Rev.* (2007) 219:167–86. doi: 10.1111/j.1600-065X.2007.00545.x
112. Pieters J. *Mycobacterium tuberculosis* and the macrophage: maintaining a balance. *Cell Host Microbe* (2008) 3:399–407. doi: 10.1016/j.chom.2008.05.006
113. Guirado E, Schlesinger LS, Kaplan G. Macrophages in tuberculosis: friend or foe. *Semin Immunopathol.* (2013) 35:563–83. doi: 10.1007/s00281-013-0388-2
114. Podinovskaia M, Lee W, Caldwell S, Russell DG. Infection of macrophages with *Mycobacterium tuberculosis* induces global modifications to phagosomal function. *Cell Microbiol.* (2013) 15:843–59. doi: 10.1111/cmi.12092
115. Neyrolles O, Wolschendorf F, Mitra A, Niederweis M. Mycobacteria, metals, and the macrophage. *Immunol Rev.* (2015) 264:249–63. doi: 10.1111/imr.12265
116. Mukhopadhyay S, Gal AA. Granulomatous lung disease: an approach to the differential diagnosis. *Arch Pathol Lab Med.* (2010) 134:667–90. doi: 10.1043/1543-2165-134.5.667
117. Huynh KK, Joshi SA, Brown EJ. A delicate dance: host response to mycobacteria. *Curr Opin Immunol.* (2011) 23:464–72. doi: 10.1016/j.coi.2011.06.002
118. Guirado E, Schlesinger LS. Modeling the *Mycobacterium tuberculosis* granuloma - the critical battlefield in host immunity and disease. *Front Immunol.* (2013) 4:98. doi: 10.3389/fimmu.2013.00098
119. Allison AC, Hart PD. Potentiation by silica of the growth of *Mycobacterium tuberculosis* in macrophage cultures. *Br J Exp Pathol.* (1968) 49:465–76.
120. Arkhipov SA, Shkurupy VA, Bugrimova YS. Effect of preliminary load of macrophages with silicium dioxide on phagocytosis of BCG strain micobacteria by macrophages and antimicrobial activity. *Bull Exp Biol Med.* (2010) 149:534–6. doi: 10.1007/s10517-010-0986-0
121. Gaynor CD, McCormack FX, Voelker DR, McGowan SE, Schlesinger LS. Pulmonary surfactant protein A mediates enhanced phagocytosis of *Mycobacterium tuberculosis* by a direct interaction with human macrophages. *J Immunol.* (1995) 155:5343–51.
122. Downing JF, Pasula R, Wright JR, Twigg HL III, Martin WJ II. Surfactant protein a promotes attachment of *Mycobacterium tuberculosis* to alveolar macrophages during infection with human immunodeficiency virus. *Proc Natl Acad Sci USA.* (1995) 92:4848–52.
123. Pasula R, Downing JF, Wright JR, Kachel DL, Davis TE Jr, Martin WJ II. Surfactant protein A (SP-A) mediates attachment of *Mycobacterium tuberculosis* to murine alveolar macrophages. *Am J Respir Cell Mol Biol.* (1997) 17:209–17.
124. Viviano CJ, Rooney SA. Early increase in expression of surfactant protein A gene in type II cells from silica-treated rats. *Am J Physiol.* (1997) 273(2 Pt 1):L395–400.
125. Spech RW, Wisniowski P, Kachel DL, Wright, JR, Martin WJ II. Surfactant protein A prevents silica-mediated toxicity to rat alveolar macrophages. *Am J Physiol Lung Cell Mol Physiol.* (2000) 278:L713–8. doi: 10.1152/ajplung.2000.278.4.L713
126. Beamer CA, Holian A. Antigen-presenting cell population dynamics during murine silicosis. *Am J Respir Cell Mol Biol.* (2007) 37:729–38. doi: 10.1165/rcmb.2007-0099OC
127. Tailleux L, Schwartz O, Herrmann JL, Pivert E, Jackson M, Amara A, et al. DC-SIGN is the major *Mycobacterium tuberculosis* receptor on human dendritic cells. *J Exp Med.* (2003) 197:121–7. doi: 10.1084/jem.20021468
128. Giacomini E, Iona E, Ferroni L, Miettinen M, Fattorini L, Orefici G, et al. Infection of human macrophages and dendritic cells with *Mycobacterium tuberculosis* induces a differential cytokine gene expression that modulates T cell response. *J Immunol.* (2001) 166:7033–41. doi: 10.4049/jimmunol.166.12.7033
129. Eum SY, Kong JH, Hong MS, Lee YJ, Kim JH, Hwang SH, et al. Neutrophils are the predominant infected phagocytic cells in the airways of patients with active pulmonary TB. *Chest* (2010) 137:122–8. doi: 10.1378/chest.09-0903
130. Sugawara I, Udagawa T, Yamada H. Rat neutrophils prevent the development of tuberculosis. *Infect Immun.* (2004) 72:1804–6. doi: 10.1128/IAI.72.3.1804-1806.2004
131. Pedrosa J, Saunders BM, Appelberg R, Orme IM, Silva MT, Cooper AM. Neutrophils play a protective nonphagocytic role in systemic *Mycobacterium tuberculosis* infection of mice. *Infect Immun.* (2000) 68:577–83. doi: 10.1128/IAI.68.2.577-583.2000
132. Martineau AR, Newton SM, Wilkinson KA, Kampmann B, Hall BM, Nawroly N, et al. Neutrophil-mediated innate immune resistance to mycobacteria. *J Clin Invest.* (2007) 117:1988–94. doi: 10.1172/JCI31097
133. Yang CT, Cambier CJ, Davis JM, Hall CJ, Crosier PS, Ramakrishnan L. Neutrophils exert protection in the early tuberculous granuloma by oxidative killing of mycobacteria phagocytosed from infected macrophages. *Cell Host Microbe* (2012) 12:301–12. doi: 10.1016/j.chom.2012.07.009
134. Trentini MM, de Oliveira FM, Kipnis A, Junqueira-Kipnis AP. The role of neutrophils in the induction of specific Th1 and Th17 during vaccination against tuberculosis. *Front Microbiol.* (2016) 7:1–13. doi: 10.3389/fmicb.2016.00898
135. Hauser WE Jr, Sharma SD, Remington JS. Natural killer cells induced by acute and chronic toxoplasma infection. *Cell Immunol.* (1982) 69:330–46. doi: 10.1016/0008-8749(82)90076-4
136. Weirich U, Friemann J, Rehn B, Henkeludecke U, Lammers T, Sorg C, et al. Silicotic lymph node reactions in mice: genetic differences, correlation with macrophage markers, and independence from T lymphocytes. *J Leukoc Biol.* (1996) 59:178–88. doi: 10.1002/jlb.59.2.178
137. Bretana A, Goihman-Yahr M, Tapia FJ, Isturiz G, Viloria N, Carrasquero M, et al. Comparative ultrastructure and immunolabeling of MHC-II antigens of alveolar macrophages obtained from patients with paracoccidioidomycosis and other lung diseases. *J Leukoc Biol.* (1995) 57:101–9.
138. Pfau JC, Brown JM, Holian A. Silica-exposed mice generate autoantibodies to apoptotic cells. *Toxicology* (2004) 195:167–76. doi: 10.1016/j.tox.2003.09.011
139. Tufariello JM, Chan J, Flynn JL. Latent tuberculosis: mechanisms of host and bacillus that contribute to persistent infection. *Lancet Infect Dis.* (2003) 3:578–90. doi: 10.1016/S1473-3099(03)00741-2
140. Ernst JD. The immunological life cycle of tuberculosis. *Nat Rev Immunol.* (2012) 12:581–91. doi: 10.1038/nri3259
141. Kumagai-Takei N, Hayashi H, Maeda M, Miura I, Matsuzaki H, Lee S, et al. Chapter 9: Immunological effects of silica and related dysregulation of autoimmunity. In: Mavragani CP, editor. *Autoimmune Disorders-Pathogenetic Aspects. Immunological Effects of Silica and Related Altered Regulation of Autoimmunity.* Croatia: InTech Open Access Publisher (2011), 157–174.
142. Amano K, Yoon JW. Studies on autoimmunity for initiation of beta-cell destruction. V. Decrease of macrophage-dependent T lymphocytes and natural killer cytotoxicity in silica-treated BB rats. *Diabetes* (1990) 39:590–6. doi: 10.2337/diab.39.5.590
143. Jagirdar J, Begin R, Dufresne A, Goswami S, Lee TC, Rom WN. Transforming growth factor-beta (TGF-beta) in silicosis. *Am J Respir Crit Care Med.* (1996) 154(4 Pt 1):1076–81. doi: 10.1164/ajrccm.154.4.8887610
144. Champsi J, Young LS, Bermudez LE. Production of TNF-alpha, IL-6 and TGF-beta, and expression of receptors for TNF-alpha and IL-6, during murine *Mycobacterium avium* infection. *Immunology* (1995) 84:549–54.
145. Toossi Z, Gogate P, Shiratsuchi H, Young T, Ellner JJ. Enhanced production of TGF-beta by blood monocytes from patients with active tuberculosis and presence of TGF-beta in tuberculous granulomatous lung lesions. *J Immunol.* (1995) 154:465–73.

146. Oschilewski U, Kiesel U, Kolb H. Administration of silica prevents diabetes in BB-rats. *Diabetes* (1985) 34:197–9. doi: 10.2337/diab.34.2.197
147. Charlton B, Bacelj A, Mandel TE. Administration of silica particles or anti-Lyt2 antibody prevents beta-cell destruction in NOD mice given cyclophosphamide. *Diabetes* (1988) 37:930–5. doi: 10.2337/diab.37.7.930
148. Maglione PJ, Chan J. How B cells shape the immune response against *Mycobacterium tuberculosis*. *Eur J Immunol.* (2009) 39:676–86. doi: 10.1002/eji.200839148
149. Vigliani EC, Pernis B. Immunological factors in the pathogenesis of the hyaline tissue of silicosis. *Ind Med Surg.* (1958) 27:643–5. doi: 10.1136/oem.15.1.8
150. Vigliani EC, Pernis B. An immunological approach to silicosis. *J Occup Environ Med.* (1959) 1:319–28.
151. Raqib R, Mondal D, Karim MA, Chowdhury F, Ahmed S, Luby S, et al. Detection of antibodies secreted from circulating *Mycobacterium tuberculosis*-specific plasma cells in the diagnosis of pediatric tuberculosis. *Clin Vaccine Immunol.* (2009) 16:521–7. doi: 10.1128/CVI.00391-08
152. Phuah JY, Mattila JT, Lin PL, Flynn JL. Activated B cells in the granulomas of nonhuman primates infected with *Mycobacterium tuberculosis*. *Am J Pathol.* (2012) 181:508–14. doi: 10.1016/j.ajpath.2012.05.009
153. Chan J, Mehta S, Bharrhan S, Chen Y, Achkar JM, Casadevall A, et al. The role of B cells and humoral immunity in *Mycobacterium tuberculosis* infection. *Semin Immunol.* (2014) 26:588–600. doi: 10.1016/j.smim.2014.10.005
154. Rao M, Valentini D, Poiret T, Dodoo E, Parida S, Zumla A, et al. B in TB: B cells as mediators of clinically relevant immune responses in Tuberculosis. *Clin Infect Dis.* (2015) 61(Suppl. 3):S225–34. doi: 10.1093/cid/civ614

5

The Role of Mucosal Immunity in Pertussis

Luis Solans[1,2,3,4†] *and Camille Locht*[1,2,3,4*]

[1] *Center of Infection and Immunity of Lille, Institut Pasteur de Lille, Lille, France,* [2] *Inserm U1019, Lille, France,* [3] *CNRS UMR8204, Lille, France,* [4] *Center for Infection and Immunity of Lille, Univ. Lille, Lille, France*

***Correspondence:**
Camille Locht
camille.locht@pasteur-lille.fr

Pertussis or whooping cough, mainly caused by *Bordetella pertussis*, is a severe respiratory disease that can affect all age groups but is most severe and can be life-threatening in young children. Vaccines against this disease are widely available since the 1950s. Despite high global vaccination coverage, the disease is not under control in any country, and its incidence is even increasing in several parts of the world. Epidemiological and experimental evidence has shown that the vaccines fail to prevent *B. pertussis* infection and transmission, although they are very effective in preventing disease. Given the high infection rate of *B. pertussis*, effective control of the disease likely requires prevention of infection and transmission in addition to protection against disease. With rare exceptions *B. pertussis* infections are restricted to the airways and do not usually disseminate beyond the respiratory epithelium. Therefore, protection at the level of the respiratory mucosa may be helpful for an improved control of pertussis. Yet, compared to systemic responses, mucosal immune responses have attracted relatively little attention in the context of pertussis vaccine development. In this review we summarize the available literature on the role of mucosal immunity in the prevention of *B. pertussis* infection. In contrast to vaccination, natural infection in humans and experimental infections in animals induce strong secretory IgA responses in the naso-pharynx and in the lungs. Several studies have shown that secretory IgA may be instrumental in the control of *B. pertussis* infection. Furthermore, studies in mouse models have revealed that *B. pertussis* infection, but not immunization with current acellular pertussis vaccines induces resident memory T cells, which may also contribute to protection against colonization by *B. pertussis*. As these resident memory T cells are long lived, vaccines that are able to induce them should provide long-lasting immunity. As of today, only one vaccine designed to induce potent mucosal immunity is in clinical development. This vaccine is a live attenuated *B. pertussis* strain delivered nasally in order to mimic the natural route of infection. Due to its ability to induce mucosal immunity it is expected that this approach will contribute to improved control of pertussis.

Keywords: pertussis, secretory IgA, tissue-resident memory T cells, mucosal vaccine, live attenuated vaccine

INTRODUCTION

Whooping cough, also referred to as pertussis, is a severe respiratory disease that can be life threatening in newborns and non-vaccinated young children. The disease can also occur in older children, adolescents and adults. Although it is usually not fatal in these age groups, it represents a risk of various serious complications, including pneumothorax, and rib fractures

(1). The main causative agent of whooping cough is *Bordetella pertussis* (2), a gram negative coccobacillus which is able to colonize the human upper respiratory tract by attaching to the ciliated cells. Other *Bordetella* species, such as *Bordetella parapertussis* (3) and *Bordetella holmesii* (4), can cause diseases similar to pertussis, albeit usually with much less severe symptoms than typical whooping cough caused by *B. pertussis*.

It is estimated that whooping cough causes globally around 200,000 deaths per year and more than 24 million new pertussis cases in children younger than 5 years were reported in 2014 (5), in spite of the wide usage of efficacious pertussis vaccines (6). Although the pertussis incidence has dramatically decreased since the first introduction of these vaccines (7), whooping cough remains a major global public health problem, mostly in resource-poor countries. However, surprisingly, its prevalence is also strongly increasing in westernized countries (8), especially since the switch from the first-generation, whole-cell vaccines to the new-generation, acellular pertussis vaccines. Several reasons may account for this resurgence, including faster waning of immunity through acellular compared to whole-cell vaccines and potential strain adaptation to escape vaccine-induced immunity (9). Although the use of the current pertussis vaccines have certainly led to a spectacular reduction in whooping cough disease incidence, the vaccines did not appear to interrupt the circulation of *B. pertussis* in susceptible populations, and several studies have shown that symptom-less carriage of *B. pertussis* in adults is more common than previously appreciated (10–14). In fact, asymptomatic transmission may be a major driver of the resurgence of pertussis in highly vaccinated populations, as suggested by mathematical modeling studies (15). Studies with non-human primates have shown that both the whole-cell and acellular vaccines provide strong protection against pertussis disease, but none of them prevents infection by *B. pertussis* (16). Therefore, it seems logical to assume that optimal control of pertussis requires the use of vaccines that prevent both whooping cough disease and infection by *B. pertussis*. Only vaccines that prevent or strongly limit infection of a causative infectious agent will induce sufficient herd immunity to eventually eradicate the respective disease.

MUCOSAL IMMUNE RESPONSES INDUCED BY *B. PERTUSSIS* INFECTION

B. pertussis as a Strictly Mucosal Pathogen

B. pertussis is known to be mainly an upper respiratory tract pathogen, but lower respiratory tract infections can also occur, especially in severe pertussis cases (2). However, dissemination outside of the respiratory tract is almost unheard of. Disseminated *B. pertussis* infection has only rarely been described and has been seen exclusively in severely immune-compromised individuals (17). In mice *B. pertussis* also remains in the respiratory tract and disseminates to other organs, such as liver and spleen, only in mice with severe immune defects, such as IFN-γ-receptor deficient mice (18). It is therefore likely that the local immunity in the respiratory tract may be important for the control of *B. pertussis* infection. Yet, today, all commercially available vaccines are given parenterally and do not induce local immune responses. Systemic immune responses have been extensively studied in several models [summarized in the review by (19)], whereas comparatively little is known about the role of local immune responses in the control of whooping cough. Unlike immunization with current pertussis vaccines, infection with *B. pertussis* appears to induce sterilizing immunity in the airways of non-human primates (16) and it is conceivable that this is linked to a potent mucosal immune response to the infection. Strong IL-17 induction was seen in the nasopharyngeal washes 5–7 days after *B. pertussis* infection of baboons (20). This was paralleled by the strong induction of IL-6 and IL-23 in convalescent baboons and followed by the increase in Th-17-associated chemokines and cytokines, such as GCSF, important for neutrophil differentiation, IL-8, MCP-1, and MIP-1a, important for the regulation of influx of various cell types involved in the clearance of respiratory pathogens. In mice IL-17 has been shown to also play an important role in the production of secretory IgA (sIgA) in the mucosal lumen by the induction of the poly-Ig receptor on the basal side of the epithelial cells (21, 22) and by facilitating the recruitment of B cells upon infection (22). However, mucosal IgA responses could not be measured in the nasopharyngeal washes of *B. pertussis*-infected baboons, due to the lack of suitable antibodies that can recognize baboon IgA. The source of the mucosal IL-17, innate cells or $CD4^+$ Th17 cells, has also yet to be determined in the convalescent baboons.

Secretory IgA Responses Induced by Infection With *B. pertussis*

In humans *B. pertussis* infection has long been shown to lead to potent anti-*B. pertussis* IgA production in nasal secretions (23). They appear during week 2–3 of illness and can often still be found when the *B. pertussis* organism can no longer be recovered. They can persist for several months after the onset of symptoms, but usually decline to low levels after 6 months. Anti-*B. pertussis* sIgA from nasal washes and serum IgA of convalescent patients have been shown to inhibit adherence of *B. pertussis* to human respiratory epithelial cells (24). These antibodies are preferentially induced during convalescence and much less so after vaccination. In addition to inhibiting *B. pertussis* adherence to epithelial cells, anti-*B. pertussis* IgA from convalescent subjects can also enhance *B. pertussis* uptake by human polymorphonuclear leukocytes *in vitro* via the myeloid IgA receptor FcαRI (CD89) and lead to subsequent bacterial killing (25). However, this study was done using serum IgA, and it remains to be seen whether similar observations can be made with sIgA.

The effect of IgA on the course of infection by *B. pertussis* has been investigated by the use of IgA-deficient mice (26). Surprisingly, when wild type or IgA-deficient mice were intranasally challenged with 5×10^5 colony-forming units (CFU) of virulent *B. pertussis*, similar amounts of CFUs were recovered for both mouse strains from the lungs, trachea, and nasal cavities at each time point, up to 105 days post-inoculation, suggesting that IgA plays no critical role in clearing *B. pertussis* from the murine respiratory tract. Furthermore, a first infection by *B.*

pertussis appeared to protect wild-type and IgA-deficient mice alike against a secondary infection in the lungs, trachea, and the noses, suggesting that IgA is not required neither to prevent a secondary infection of the upper and lower respiratory tract of *B. pertussis*-primed mice. Interestingly, this is in contrast to *Bordetella bronchiseptica* infections, for which IgA appeared to play a critical role in protection of the upper, but not of the lower respiratory tract. However, these findings are in conflict with recent data obtained from mice vaccinated with BPZE1, a live attenuated nasal pertussis vaccine (27). BPZE1 is a *B. pertussis* TohamaI derivative containing mutations in its genome that eliminate or inactivate three major *B. pertussis* toxins: tracheal cytotoxin, dermonecrotic toxin, and pertussis toxin (PTx) (28). In contrast to vaccination with acellular pertussis vaccines, nasal administration of BPZE1 protects mice against nasal as well as lung colonization by virulent *B. pertussis*, and BPZE1-induced protection in the nose was strongly diminished in IgA-deficient mice (27). The reasons for these conflicting findings are not clear, but the most important difference between the two studies is the use of a virulent *B. pertussis* in the former and of an attenuated strain in the latter study. As the attenuated strain lacks two toxins and produces inactive PTx, could it be that one or several of these toxins produced by the virulent strain overrides the need for IgA? Whether this or other technical differences between the two studies may explain the different outcomes between them remains to be investigated.

In humans, there is no published evidence so far that IgA deficiency may be associated with enhanced *B. pertussis* infection. However, epidemiological studies addressing specifically *B. pertussis* infection are scarce, and most studies focus on pertussis disease. It may thus very-well be possible that IgA deficiency increases the likelihood of being infected by *B. pertussis*, without necessarily impacting on pertussis disease, against which other immune mechanisms, such as PTx neutralization by serum IgG, may be at play.

Local Cellular Responses Induced by Infection With *B. pertussis*

In addition to mucosal antibodies, especially sIgA, *B. pertussis* infection also induces cellular immune mechanisms in the airways (see **Figure 1**). As such, neutrophils, and macrophages, but also $CD4^+$ T cells, and γδ T cells infiltrate the lungs of mice after *B. pertussis* infection (29). Neutrophils may kill phagocytosed bacteria, but their role in early *B. pertussis* clearance from the respiratory tract has not been established (30), although they may be important at later stages of the infection via induced opsonizing antibodies. Furthermore, PTx produced by *B. pertussis* during infection inhibits neutrophil recruitment into the lungs, which may delay the clearance of the organism by opsonizing antibodies (31), suggesting that they are important at certain stages of the infection, and that *B. pertussis* uses its toxin to subvert its neutrophil-mediated elimination. Airway macrophages may also contribute to clearance of *B. pertussis*, as their depletion in mice by the administration of liposome-encapsulated clodronate enhanced the infection despite the influx of neutrophils (32).

For obvious reasons detailed data on local immune cell responses to *B. pertussis* infection in humans are not available, but they have been studied in mice. *B. pertussis*-specific $CD4^+$ T cells can be detected in the lungs of mice ~3 weeks post-infection and have been shown to secrete IFN-γ and/or IL-17 (33, 34). IFN-γ-deficient mice show a higher bacterial burden and clear the infection later than wild-type mice (35), indicating an important role of this cytokine in the control of *B. pertussis* infection.

At least some of these *B. pertussis*-specific IFN-γ- and/or IL-17-producing $CD4^+$ T cells that can be found in the mouse lungs after infection may be tissue-resident memory T (Trm) cells, as characterized by the expression of CD44, CD69, and/or CD103 and the lack of expression of CD62L. These cells reside only in peripheral tissues and do not re-circulate. When induced by a first encounter with a pathogen at a mucosal site, they respond rapidly to a second infection with the same organism. Wilk et al. (36) have shown that $CD4^+CD69^+$ and/or $CD103^+$ T cells are indeed induced in the lungs of mice upon *B. pertussis* infection, and their increase in numbers was associated with *B. pertussis* clearance. These cells persisted for several months in the lung tissues and expanded rapidly and significantly *in situ* upon re-infection. They produced IFN-γ and/or IL-17, and were thus of the Th1 and Th17 type, although most of the cells were of the Th17 type. The specific role of Trm cells can be examined in mice by a treatment with the sphingosine-1-phosphage receptor agonist FTY720 (fingolimod), an inhibitor of lymphocyte migration from the lymph nodes to the mucosal tissues (37). Upon treatment with FTY720, the only T cells present in the mucosa are almost exclusively Trm cells. When mice were treated with FTY720, primary infection with *B. pertussis* was significantly prolonged, whereas the drug had no effect on the course of a secondary infection (36), suggesting that the locally residing T cells developed during the primary infection and rapidly expanding during the secondary infection play a critical role in clearance of the secondary infection. This was confirmed by the adoptive transfer of the lung $CD4^+$ T cells from convalescent mice to naïve, sub-lethally irradiated mice, which significantly reduced the bacterial burden after infection of these mice with *B. pertussis*. This was not seen when lung $CD4^+$ T cells from naïve mice were transferred.

In addition to $CD4^+$ Trm cells, *B. pertussis* infection also leads to the expansion of γδ Trm cells in the lungs of mice (38). Although γδ T cells are usually involved in innate immune responses, they can also mount antigen-specific responses, feature memory-like phenotypes and express CD69 and/or CD103, like $CD4^+$ Trm. IL-17-secreting γδ T cells appear in the lungs of *B. pertussis*-infected mice within hours after aerosol exposure, providing an early innate source of IL-17. Their frequency then rapidly declines and rises again 1 week later. The cells of the first wave are predominantly $V\gamma4^-\gamma1^-$ cells, whereas those of the second wave are $V\gamma4^+$ cells. In the presence of antigen-presenting cells, but not in their absence, these latter cells respond *in vitro* to *B. pertussis* antigens by the secretion of IL-17. Moreover, they further expand upon re-infection with *B. pertussis*, suggesting that the primary infection had induced

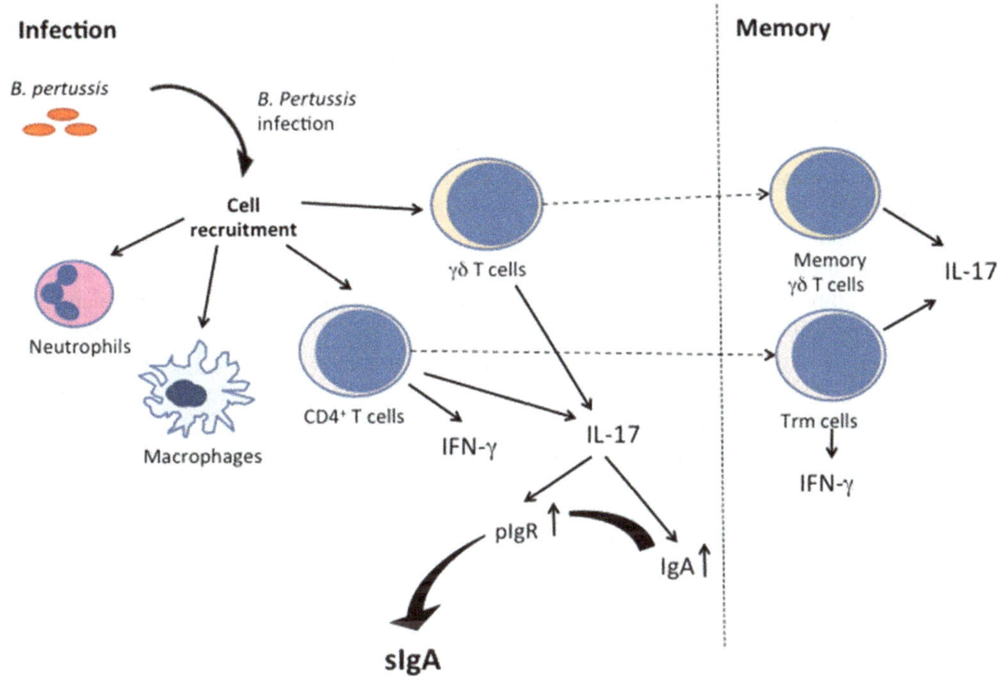

FIGURE 1 | Cellular immune responses and induction of sIgA by *B. pertussis* infection. *B. pertussis* infection induces innate immune cell (such as neutrophils and macrophages) activation, as well as IFN-γ-producing and IL-17-producing T cells. The Th-17 T cells are instrumental for sIgA production. The infection also results in resident memory T cells (γδ and CD4$^+$ T cells).

memory γδ T cells that persist for prolonged periods of time in the lungs. However, to what extend these cells contribute to the control of *B. pertussis* infection has not yet been established.

As these Trm cells are induced by infection but not by acellular pertussis vaccination, their induction may be linked to long-lived immunity, as seen after natural infection in contrast to immunization with pertussis vaccines, especially with acellular vaccines (39). However, recent data indicate that intranasal administration of acellular pertussis vaccines formulated with TLR2 and STING agonists is also very effective in inducing IL-17-secreting Trm cells and long-term protection against nasal colonization by *B. pertussis* (40).

Transcriptomic analyses of *B. pertussis*-infected mouse lungs showed that already 4 h post-infection, the gene expression profile started to change. The changes were maximal 14 days post-infection, after which the profile slowly returned to basal levels (41). As could be expected, acute phase responses and chemotaxis were observed at the early time points, followed by innate immune responses, phagocytosis, complement activation, antigen processing, and presentation, and finally genes involved in the adaptive immune responses at later time points. Infection induced the expression of cytokine and chemokine genes involved in chemotaxis, cell recruitment, and Th1/Th17 responses, as well as genes coding for membrane receptors, including Fc receptors, pIgR, and mucosal homing receptors, B-cell receptor signaling and antibody formation.

Infection by *B. pertussis* also induces local regulatory T cell responses in mice (42). These cells secret high levels of IL-10 and suppress Th-1 responses in the lungs, which may lead to subversion of protective immunity against *B. pertussis* and may also limit inflammatory pathology in the lungs (43).

PERTUSSIS VACCINATION VIA MUCOSAL ROUTES

Since natural *B. pertussis* infection induces potent mucosal immune responses and sterilizing immunity, in contrast to immunization with currently available vaccines, and since infection provides longer lasting protection than vaccination, it seems logical to use the mucosal, especially the nasal route to vaccinate against *B. pertussis* colonization and disease. Attempts to explore the mucosal routes for vaccination against pertussis have been undertaken in humans and in mice and have initially been focused on the oral route.

Oral Vaccination Against Pertussis

One to three oral administrations of a killed *B. pertussis* suspension to newborn babies were well-tolerated and able to induce agglutinating serum antibodies (44). It is not known whether this immunization regimen induced mucosal antibodies, especially in the nasal cavity, nor whether it effectively protected these newborns against *B. pertussis* infection and disease. However, in a subsequent study, oral immunization of newborn infants with a whole-cell pertussis vaccine was shown to result in a rise in anti-*B. pertussis* antibody titers in saliva, and these antibody titers were higher in the saliva than in the serum

(45), indicating the induction of mucosal immune responses. A study involving more than 20,000 newborns, who received orally 10^{12} killed bacterial cells on days 2, 3, 4, and 5 after birth confirmed that oral immunization with whole-cell pertussis vaccines induces serum and mucosal antibodies in the saliva against *B. pertussis* antigens (46). Although there was a lower frequency of pertussis disease in the orally vaccinated compared to the non-vaccinated children during the first year of life, this difference disappeared after the first year.

With the advent of recombinant DNA technologies, several bacterial vectors that can be administered orally have been engineered to produce individual protective *B. pertussis* antigens, mostly those antigens that are components of the acellular pertussis vaccines, such as PTx, filamentous hemagglutinin (FHA), and pertactin. Live attenuated *Salmonella* strains have been extensively evaluated as recombinant vehicles for the presentation of heterologous antigens to the mucosal immune system by oral administration. The *B. pertussis* pertactin gene has been successfully expressed in a *Salmonella typhimurium aro* vaccine strain (47). Oral vaccination with this strain resulted in a significant decrease of *B. pertussis* burden in the lungs after aerosol infection, as compared to non-vaccinated mice, or mice that had received the non-recombinant *Salmonella* strain. However, antibody levels to pertactin were undetectable after vaccination with the recombinant *Salmonella* strain, but were slightly higher after challenge than for the non-vaccinated mice, suggesting that the vaccination had primed the antibody response. Antibodies against FHA could however be detected after the oral administration of a recombinant *Salmonella dublin aroA* mutant (48). Both anti-FHA serum antibodies, including IgA, as well as anti-FHA IgA in gut wash fluids could be readily detected after feeding mice with the recombinant strain. Another study has shown that feeding of mice with a recombinant FHA-producing *S. typhimurium aroA* mutant or invasive *Escherichia coli* strain resulted in the appearance of anti-FHA IgA in the bronchoalveolar lavage fluids (49).

PTx is a complex multimeric protein composed of five different subunits [for review see (50)]. It is a protective antigen and included in all pertussis vaccines. Monoclonal antibodies directed against the S1 subunit of PTx (PTxA) have been shown to have strong protective potential in mouse models (51). Therefore, the *S. typhimurium aroA* and the invasive *E. coli* strains were also engineered to produce PTxA (52). Oral administration of these strains again resulted in high anti-PTxA antibody titers in the serum and anti-PTxA IgA in the lung lavages. However, the protective potential of these recombinant *Salmonella* and *E. coli* strains against *B. pertussis* challenge had not been addressed in any of these studies. Protection has been evaluated, however, against a recombinant *S. typhimurium aroA* mutant producing all five PTx subunits. Although this strain induced significant anti-PTx antibodies, it failed to protect mice from *B. pertussis* challenge (53).

In addition to attenuated pathogenic bacteria commensal bacteria, such as *Streptococcus gordonii*, have also been tested as delivery vehicles of *B. pertussis* antigens. A recombinant *S. gordinii* strain that presents PTxA on its surface via the transport by the *Streptococcus mutants* major surface protein P1 was found to elicit sIgA against PTx in the saliva and bronchoalveolar lavage fluids of mice upon oral feeding (54). However, again, protection was not assessed in this study.

In addition to mucosal delivery via recombinant bacterial vectors, *B. pertussis* antigens can also be formulated in nanoparticles to stabilize the antigens and to prevent degradation during transit through the digestive tract. When FHA and inactivated PTx were entrapped in poly-lactide-co-glycolide (PLG) nanoparticles and delivered orally multiple times to mice, T-cell responses were induced, as evidenced by IL-5, and low levels of IFN-γ secretion by splenocytes stimulated with FHA or PTx (55). However, the levels of these responses were highly variable between the animals. Orally immunized mice also induced antigen-specific IgA in the lungs, but their levels were not higher than those induced with the same antigens in solution. When the mice were aerosol challenged with virulent *B. pertussis*, a certain level of protection was observed, which was slightly stronger in the mice immunized with the encapsulated antigens. Although these studies provide a proof of concept that oral immunization may induce protective immunity to *B. pertussis*, at least in mice, strong oral adjuvants are certainly needed to enhance these responses.

Nasal Vaccination Against Pertussis

As *B. pertussis* is a respiratory pathogen, the induction of immune responses in the respiratory tract may be more effective to protect against this pathogen than oral immunization. The protective effect of intranasal vaccination against pulmonary *B. pertussis* infection in mice has already been shown in the 1940s (56, 57), at a time when the first whole-cell vaccines started to come in use and was suggested to be due to both systemic and local immune responses induced by the vaccination. However, intranasal vaccination with whole-cell vaccines provided no protection in the intracerebral challenge model (58), the classical mouse protection assays routinely used for the lot release of whole-cell pertussis vaccines (59). One of the first studies to administer pertussis vaccines via the respiratory tract to humans was published by Gerald Thomas in 1975 (60). He administered a whole-cell preparation by aerosol inhalation into the nostrils of 8 adult volunteers as a single dose. The aerosol vaccination was well-tolerated, better than intramuscular whole-cell vaccination in adults, and increased the IgA levels to *B. pertussis* antigens by ~2-fold in the respiratory secretions, but it did not induce serum antibody responses.

Human nasal vaccination with whole-cell pertussis vaccines were more recently followed up by vaccinating six adult volunteers, who had been immunized in their childhood, with a whole-cell vaccine consisting of 250 μg of *B. pertussis* protein in a 0.5 ml volume, given four times at weekly intervals. The nasal vaccine was overall well-tolerated and induced a significant increase in nasal IgA, as well as systemic IgA and IgG to *B. pertussis* antigens (61). The vaccination did not induce any appreciable level of anti-PTx antibodies, except for one subject, and only a modest increase in nasal anti-FHA IgA in five out of the six individuals. Enhanced T-cell responses could also be measured in these individuals, as evidenced by increased T-cell proliferation to *B. pertussis* whole-cell extracts (62). All six individuals showed a >2-fold increase in T cell proliferation. All vaccines also responded to FHA and four out of the six responded to PTx with a significant rise in T cell proliferation. Although there was no significant correlation between the concentrations of specific serum IgG and T cell proliferation, a significant correlation was found between T cell proliferation, and sIgA in the nasal fluids to whole-cell extracts. Whether intranasal vaccination with whole-cell pertussis vaccines indeed protects humans from *B. pertussis* infection and whooping cough disease remains unknown so far.

Protection against *B. pertussis* infection through nasal vaccination using defined antigens has been evaluated in mouse models. However, purified soluble antigens are usually poorly immunogenic when delivered nasally. Therefore, they have to be combined with mucosal adjuvants to elicit strong antigen-specific sIgA responses. Some of the most potent mucosal adjuvants are cholera toxin (CT) and *E. coli* heat-labile entertoxin (LT). These toxins are A-B toxins, in which the A subunit carries an enzymatic activity whereas the B moiety is responsible for the toxin binding to its receptors. As the CT B subunit has adjuvant properties even in the absence of the A subunit, a hybrid protein was constructed consisting of two copies of PTxA fused to the C-terminal portion of CTA and to CTB (63). This chimeric toxin induced anti-PTx serum IgG and mucosal IgA in the bronchoalveolar lavage fluids, the saliva, and vaginal washes after 6 intranasal immunizations with each 25 μg of the purified hybrid toxin. The serum anti-PTx antibodies were able to neutralize PTx action on Chinese Hamster Ovary cells. When the immunized mice were challenged with virulent *B. pertussis*, the bacterial counts in the lungs were more than 10-fold lower than in the non-vaccinated mice 7 days after challenge.

Instead of genetically fusing *B. pertussis* antigens to CTB or LTB, detoxified CT, or LT can also be mixed with acellular pertussis vaccines to enhance immunogenicity when given nasally. This was shown in a murine study, in which an acellular pertussis vaccine was mixed with genetically inactivated LT and given nasally twice at a 4-week interval (64). This resulted in enhanced antigen-specific serum IgG and sIgA, as well as local and systemic T-cell responses, and was associated with accelerated clearance of *B. pertussis* bacteria from the lungs after challenge.

Interestingly, whereas the addition of enzymatically inactive LT clearly enhanced protective immunity to acellular pertussis vaccine given nasally, this was not the case when whole-cell vaccines were mixed with CT and administered nasally up to four times to mice. Neither the levels of serum IgG or IgA, nor of IgA in saliva or bronchoalveolar lavage fluids to *B. pertussis* extracts were enhanced by the addition of CT (65). Instead, the IgA levels were significantly reduced when CT was given intranasally together with whole-cell pertussis vaccine. This may be due to the fact that whole-cell pertussis vaccines are already potent immunogens and have intrinsic adjuvant activity when given nasally (66) and/or that CT is toxic to the mucosal membrane of the respiratory tract (67). Furthermore, CTB and LTB may cause Bell's Palsy (68), which precludes their widespread use in humans.

However, potent immune responses to *B. pertussis* antigens can also be induced nasally when the vaccines are formulated with different adjuvants. When the cationic polysaccharide chitosan was combined with FHA and genetically detoxified PTx and administered intranasally, high serum IgG, and sIgA levels in lung lavages and nasal washes were observed to both antigens and were considerably higher than when the two antigens were given without chitosan (69). Other nasal adjuvants are onjisaponins from the roots of *Polygala tenuifolia*. When onjisaponins were given nasally together with a pertussis vaccine, a significant increase in serum IgG, and nasal IgA levels to *B. pertussis* antigens were seen compared to the pertussis vaccine alone (70). However, the effect of these adjuvant formulations on protection was not examined in any of the two studies. CpG-containing oligodeoxynucleotides have also been shown to enhance systemic and local antibody responses to PTx, FHA, and pertactin when administered nasally and increased the protection against *B. pertussis* challenge in mice (71), as did the addition of poly[di(sodium carboxylatophenoxy)phosphazene] (72).

More recently, bacterium-like particles (BLP) based on the food-grade bacterium *Lactococcus lactis* have been explored for intranasal vaccination (73). These BLP are generated by the treatment of *L. lactis* with hot acid, which retains the peptidoglycan matrix, and therefore the shape of the organism. When mixed with an acellular pertussis vaccine and administered intranasally, these particles strongly increased the serum IgG titers to the *B. pertussis* antigens and elicited *B. pertussis*-specific IgA responses in the nasal washes. This was associated with a significant level of protection compared to mice that were intranasally vaccinated with the acellular pertussis vaccine in the absence of BLP.

Outer membrane vesicles (OMV) are yet another promising approach for respiratory immunization. Ten years ago, Roberts et al. (74) showed that intransal administration of OMV prepared from *B. pertussis* and containing among others surface antigens, PTx, adenylate cyclase toxin, and lipooligosaccharide, to mice resulted in significant protection against pulmonary colonization by virulent *B. pertussis* upon intranasal challenge. More recently, aerosol vaccination with *B. pertussis* OMV has been shown to provide superior protection against *B. pertussis* challenge than subcutaneous vaccination with the same OMV, especially in the trachea and in the nose (75). Aerosol vaccination with the OMVs led to pulmonary anti-*B. pertussis* IgA, IgA-producing plasma cells, and Th17 cells in the lungs, as well as a rapid induction of pro-inflammatory cytokines and chemoattractants, such as IL-6 and CXCL10. Spray dried OMV with improved stability especially at high temperatures delivered twice by aerosol have also been shown to provide protection against *B. pertussis* colonization of the lungs, trachea, and nasal cavity (76). Importantly, the spray dried formulation was more protective in the nose than the same OMV in a liquid formulation.

Although some of these novel avenues show promise as mucosal vaccine candidates against pertussis disease and infection, none of them have yet entered clinical evaluation. So far, the most effective way to induce protective immunity against *B. pertussis* infection and disease is infection itself, as seen in both mouse and non-human primate studies (16). Furthermore, immunity induced by natural infection is longer lasting than that induced by immunization (39). These observations have led to the concept of live attenuated pertussis vaccines. The first live attenuated vaccine candidate was an *aroA* mutant of *B. pertussis* (77). This strain did not persist in the lung and induced protection against challenge after repeated intranasal administrations. A more recent *aroQ* mutant of *B. pertussis* persisted longer than the *aroA* mutant and provided protection against challenge already after a single nasal administration (78). A different strategy to engineer a live attenuated pertussis vaccine was based on the genetic elimination or inactivation of PTx, tracheal cytotoxin, and dermonecrotic toxin, which led to the vaccine candidate BPZE1. This vaccine candidate is highly attenuated, even in immune-compromised hosts, yet very immunogenic, and protective in mice after a single intranasal administration [for review see (79)]. Recently it was also shown to be immunogenic in baboons and to elicit high levels of IgG and IgA against PTx, FHA, and pertactin and to protect these baboons from severe pertussis induced by challenge with a very high dose of a highly virulent *B. pertussis* clinical isolate (80). Furthermore, upon challenge with this highly virulent isolate it reduced the overall bacterial burden by 99.998% over the non-vaccinated animals. BPZE1 is the most advanced novel pertussis vaccine candidate and has successfully completed phase I trials, where it was found to be safe in young human adults, able to transiently colonize the human nasopharynx, and to induce antibodies to PTx, FHA, pertactin and fimbriae after a single nasal administration (81). This vaccine candidate is currently entering a clinical phase II trial. Human monocyte-derived dendritic cells *in vitro* stimulated with BPZE1 were shown to polarize T cells toward a Th17 response (82).

In mice a single nasal administration of BPZE1 protected against challenge colonization of both the lungs and the noses, whereas two administration of 1/5 of a human dose of an acellular vaccine only induced protection in the lungs, but not in the nose (27). In addition, only BPZE1 induced *B. pertussis*-specific sIgA in the nasal cavity, and transfer of the nasal IgA was able to protect recipient mice against nasal colonization after *B. pertussis* challenge. These protective nasal IgA were not produced when poly-Ig-receptor-deficient mice were vaccinated with BPZE1, indicating that they were genuine sIgA. Furthermore, IgA-deficient or poly-Ig-receptor-deficient mice were much less protected by BPZE1 against nasal colonization by virulent *B. pertussis*, illustrating the critical role for IgA, and its secretion into the nasal cavity in protection. Moreover, protection against *B. pertussis* infection of both the lungs (83) and the noses (27) was long lived. BPZE1 also induced $CD4^{+}CD69^{+}CD103^{+}$ Trm cells in the nasal mucosa of mice, and these cells produced high levels of IL-17, but also appreciable levels of IFN-γ. The important role of IL-17 in the protection against nasal colonization by virulent *B. pertussis* was demonstrated by the fact that IL-17-deficient mice were no longer protected by intranasal vaccination with BPZE1 and also produced lower levels of sIgA than the wild-type mice after BPZE1 administration. Thus, BPZE1 protects mice against nasal infection by virulent *B. pertussis* via an IL-17-dependent sIgA-mediated mechanism.

CONCLUDING REMARKS

B. pertussis is a strictly respiratory pathogen, mainly found attached to the ciliated cells of the upper respiratory tract. Yet, routine vaccination is done parenterally, inducing circulating antibodies, and systemic cell-mediated immunity. Local mucosal immunity is not induced by the current vaccination regimens, which is likely the main reason why pertussis vaccination fails to control *B. pertussis* infection and only induces at best modest herd immunity. The fact that in many countries, in which high coverage with acelullar vaccines containing pertactin is achieved, pertactin-deficient *B. pertussis* strains are increasingly isolated (84–86), most likely due to vaccine pressure, suggests that some degree of anti-infection immunity is induced by some acellular vaccines. However, this is not sufficient to effectively control *B. pertussis* circulation even in highly vaccinated populations. It is most likely that local immunity is required for effective protection against infection by *B. pertussis.* Potent local antibody and T-cell responses are indeed induced upon natural infection in humans and experimental infection in mice and non-human primates. Since infection induces sterilizing immunity, these responses are likely to play a critical role in infection control. Several attempts have been made in both humans and animal models to induce local immunity by vaccination via the oral or nasal route. However, none of them have reached the stage of mass vaccination regimens. With a deeper understanding on protective local immunity, as it has emerged over the years, mucosal, especially nasal vaccination has recently attracted interest again, especially by using novel approaches, such as nasal delivery of live attenuated *B. pertussis* vaccines. One such candidate, BPZE1, is currently in clinical development and shows promise for providing durable local immunity and improved control of pertussis. It will of course be important to know whether nasal vaccines such as BPZE1 will protect against infection by the various *B. pertussis* clades currently circulating, as allelic variations of protective antigens have been proposed to contribute to the current pertussis resurgence in several countries. Furthermore, the effect of maternal antibodies transmitted to the offspring on immunity induced by mucosal vaccines is not yet known. This is of particular importance, as maternal immunization against pertussis is now recommended in several countries, based on the high effectiveness of this strategy to protect infants against severe pertussis in the first months of life (87).

AUTHOR CONTRIBUTIONS

LS prepared the first draft of the paper and critically revised the final draft. CL prepared the final draft of the paper.

REFERENCES

1. Hewlett EL, Edwards KM. Clinical practice. Pertussis–not just for kids. *N Engl J Med.* (2005) 352:1215–22. doi: 10.1056/NEJMcp041025
2. Mattoo S, Cherry JD. Molecular pathogenesis, epidemiology, and clinical manifestations of respiratory infections due to *Bordetella pertussis* and other *Bordetella* subspecies. *Clin Microbiol Rev.* (2005) 18:326–82. doi: 10.1128/CMR.18.2.326-382.2005
3. Heininger U, Stehr K, Schmitt-Grohe S, Lorenz C, Rost R, Christenson PD, et al. Clinical characteristics of illness caused by *Bordetella parapertussis* compared with illness caused by *Bordetella pertussis*. *Pediatr Infect Dis J.* (1994) 13:306–9 doi: 10.1097/00006454-199404000-00011
4. Mazengia E, Silva EA, Peppe JA, Timperi R, George H. Recovery of *Bordetella holmesii* from patients with pertussis-like symptoms: use of pulsed-field gel electrophoresis to characterize circulating strains. *J Clin Microbiol.* (2000) 38:2330–3.
5. Yeung KHT, Duclos P, Nelson EAS, Hutubessy RCW. An update of the global burden of pertussis in children younger than 5 years: a modelling study. *Lancet Infect Dis.* (2017) 17:974–80. doi: 10.1016/S1473-3099(17)30390-0
6. Feldstein LR, Mariat S, Gacic-Dobo M, Diallo MS, Conklin LM, Wallace AS. Global routine vaccination coverage, 2016. *MMWR Morb Mortal Wkly Rep.* (2017) 66:1252–5. doi: 10.15585/mmwr.mm6645a3
7. Black S. Epidemiology of pertussis. *Pediatr Infect Dis J.* (1997) 16(Suppl. 4):S85–9. doi: 10.1097/00006454-199704001-00003
8. von Konig CH, Halperin S, Riffelmann M, Guiso N. Pertussis of adults and infants. *Lancet Infect Dis.* (2002) 2:744–50. doi: 10.1016/S1473-3099(02)00452-8
9. Burns DL, Meade BD, Messionnier NE. Pertussis resurgence: perspectives from the Working Group Meeting on pertussis on the causes, possible paths forward, and gaps in our knowledge. *J Infect Dis.* (2014) 209(Suppl. 1):S32–5. doi: 10.1093/infdis/jit491
10. Zhang Q, Yin Z, Li Y, Luo H, Shao Z, Gao Y, et al. Prevalence of asymptomatic *Bordetella pertussis* and *Bordetella parapertussis* infections among school children in China as determined by pooled real-time PCR: a cross-sectional study. *Scand J Infect Dis.* (2014) 46:280–7. doi: 10.3109/00365548.2013.878034
11. de Greeff SC, de Melker HE, van Gageldonk PG, Schellekens JF, van der Klis FR, Mollema L, et al. Seroprevalence of pertussis in The Netherlands: evidence for increased circulation of *Bordetella pertussis*. *PLoS ONE* (2010) 5:e14183. doi: 10.1371/journal.pone.0014183
12. Hodder SL, Cherry JD, Mortimer Jr EA, Ford AB, Gornbein J, Papp K. Antibody responses to *Bordetella pertussis* antigens and clinical correlations in elderly community residents. *Clin Infect Dis.* (2000) 31:7–14. doi: 10.1086/313913
13. Moriuchi T, Otsuka N, Hiramatsu Y, Shibayama K, Kamachi K. A high seroprevalence of antibodies to pertussis toxin among Japanese adults: qualitative and quantitative analyses. *PLoS ONE* (2017) 12:e0181181. doi: 10.1371/journal.pone.0181181
14. Scott S, van der Sande M, Faye-Joof T, Mendy M, Sanneh B, Jallow FB, et al. Seroprevalence of pertussis in the Gambia: evidence for continued circulation of *Bordetella pertussis* despite high vaccination rates. *Pediatr Infect Dis J.* (2015) 34:333–8. doi: 10.1097/INF.0000000000000576
15. Althouse BM, Scarpino SV. Asymptomatic transmission and the resurgence of *Bordetella pertussis*. *BMC Med.* (2015) 13:146. doi: 10.1186/s12916-015-0382-8
16. Warfel JM, Zimmerman LI, Merkel TJ. Acellular pertussis vaccines protect against disease but fail to prevent infection and transmission in a nonhuman primate model. *Proc Natl Acad Sci USA.* (2014) 111:787–92. doi: 10.1073/pnas.1314688110
17. Janda WM, Santos E, Stevens J, Celig D, Terrile L, Schreckenberger PC. Unexpected isolation of *Bordetella pertussis* from a blood culture. *J Clin Microbiol.* (1994) 32:2851–3.
18. Mahon, BP, Sheahan BJ, Griffin F, Murphy G, Mills KH. Atypical disease after *Bordetella pertussis* respiratory infection of mice with targeted disruptions of interferon-gamma receptor or immunoglobulin μchain genes. *J Exp Med.* (1997) 186:1843–51. doi: 10.1084/jem.186.11.1843
19. Higgs R, Higgins SC, Ross PJ, Mills KH. Immunity to the respiratory pathogen *Bordetella pertussis*. *Mucosal Immunol.* (2012) 5:485–500. doi: 10.1038/mi.2012.54
20. Warfel JM, Merkel TJ. *Bordetella pertussis* infection induces a mucosal IL-17 response and long-lived Th17 and Th1 immune memory cells in nonhuman primates. *Mucosal Immunol.* (2013) 6:787–96. doi: 10.1038/mi.2012.117
21. Jaffar Z, Ferrini ME, Herritt LA, Roberts K. Cutting edge: lung mucosal Th17-mediated responses induce polymeric Ig receptor expression by the airway epithelium and elevate secretory IgA levels. *J Immunol.* (2009) 182:4507–11. doi: 10.4049/jimmunol.0900237
22. Christensen D, Mortensen R, Rosenkrands I, Dietrich J, Andersen P. Vaccine-induced Th17 cells are established as resident memory cells in the lung and promote local IgA responses. *Mucosal Immunol.* (2017) 10:260–70. doi: 10.1038/mi.2016.28
23. Goodman YE, Wort AJ, Jackson FL. Enzyme-linked immunosorbent assay for detection of pertussis immunoglobulin A in nasopharyngeal secretions as an indicator of recent infection. *J Clin Microbiol.* (1981) 13:286–92.
24. Tuomanen EI, Zapiain LA, Galvan P, Hewlett EL. Characterization of antibody inhibiting adherence of *Bordetella pertussis* to human respiratory epithelial cells. *J Clin Microbiol.* (1984) 20:167–70.
25. Hellwig SM, van Spriel AB, Schellekens JF, Mooi FR, van de Winkel JG. Immunoglobulin A-mediated protection against *Bordetella pertussis* infection. *Infect Immun.* (2001) 69:4846–50. doi: 10.1128/IAI.69.8.4846-4850.2001
26. Wolfe DN, Kirimanjeswara GS, Goebel EM, Harvill ET. Comparative role of immunoglobulin A in protective immunity against the Bordetellae. *Infect Immun.* (2007) 75:4416–22. doi: 10.1128/IAI.00412-07
27. Solans L, Debrie AS, Borkner L, Aguilo N, Thiriard A, Coutte L, et al. IL-17-dependent sIgA-mediated protection against nasal *Bordetella pertussis* infection by live attenuated BPZE1 vaccine. *Mucosal Immunol.* (2018) 11:1753–62. doi: 10.1038/s41385-018-0073-9
28. Mielcarek N, Debrie AS, Raze D, Bertout J, Rouanet C, Younes AB, et al. Live attenuated *B. pertussis* as a single-dose nasal vaccine against whooping cough. *PLoS Pathog.* (2006) 2:e65. doi: 10.1371/journal.ppat.0020065
29. McGuirk P, Mahon BP, Griffin F, Mills KHG. Compartmentalization of T cell responses following respiratory infection with *Bordetella pertussis*: hyporesponsiveness of lung T cells is associated with modulated expression of the co-stimulatory molecule CD28. *Eur J Immunol.* (1998) 28:153–63. doi: 10.1002/(SICI)1521-4141(199801)28:01<153::AID-IMMU153>3.0.CO;2-#
30. Andreasen C, Carbonetti NH. Role of neutrophils in response to *Bordetella pertussis* infection in mice. *Infect Immun.* (2009) 77:1182–8. doi: 10.1128/IAI.01150-08
31. Kirimanjeswara GS, Agosto LM, Kennett MJ, Bjornstad ON, Harvill ET. Pertussis toxin inhibits neutrophil recruitment to delay antibody-mediated clearance of *Bordetella pertussis*. *J Clin Invest.* (2005) 115:3594–601. doi: 10.1172/JCI24609
32. Carbonetti NH, Artamonova GV, Van Rooijen N, Ayala VI. Pertussis toxin targets airway macrophages to promote *Bordetella pertussis* infection of the respiratory tract. *Infect Immun.* (2007) 75:1713–20. doi: 10.1128/IAI.01578-06
33. Mills KH, Barnard A, Watkins J, Redhead K. Cell-mediated immunity to *Bordetella pertussis*: role of Th1 cells in bacterial clearance in a murine respiratory infection model. *Infect Immun.* (1993) 61:399–410.
34. Dunne A, Ross PJ, Pospisilova E, Masin J, Meaney A, Sutton CE, et al. Inflammasome activation by adenlyate cyclase toxin directs Th17 responses and protection against *Bordetella pertussis*. *J Immunol.* (2010) 185:1711–9. doi: 10.4049/jimmunol.1000105
35. Barbic J, Leef MF, Burns DL, Shahin RD. Role of gamma interferon in natural clearance of *Bordetella pertussis* infection. *Infect Immun.* (1997) 65:4904–8.
36. Wilk MM, Misiak A, McManus RM, Allen AC, Lynch MA, Mills KH. Lung CD4 tissue-resident memory T cells mediate adaptive immunity induced by previous infection of mice with *Bordetella pertussis*. *J Immunol.* (2017) 199:233–43. doi: 10.4049/jimmunol.1602051
37. Turner DL, Bickham KL, Thome JJ, Kim CY, D'Ovidio F, Wherry EJ, et al. Lung niches for the generation and maintenance of tissue-resident memory T cells. *Mucosal Immunol.* (2014) 7:501–10. doi: 10.1038/mi.2013.67
38. Misiak A, Wilk MM, Raverdeau M, Mills KH. IL-17-Producing innate and pathogen-specific tissue resident memory gammadelta T cells expand in the lungs of *Bordetella pertussis*-infected mice. *J Immunol.* (2017) 198:363–74. doi: 10.4049/jimmunol.1601024
39. Wearing HJ, Rohani P. Estimating the duration of pertussis immunity using epidemiological signatures. *PLoS Pathog.* (2009) 5:e1000647. doi: 10.1371/journal.ppat.1000647

40. Allen AC, Wilk MM, Misiak A, Borkner L, Murphy D, Mills KHG. Sustained protective immunity against *Bordetella pertussis* nasal colonization by intranasal immunization with a vaccine-adjuvant combination that induces IL-17-secreting T_{RM} cells. *Mucosal Immunol.* (2018) 11:1763–76. doi: 10.1038/s41385-018-0080-x
41. Raeven RH, Brummelman J, Pennings JL, Nijst OE, Kuipers B, Blok LE, et al. Molecular signatures of the evolving immune response in mice following a *Bordetella pertussis* infection. *PLoS ONE* (2014) 9:e104548. doi: 10.1371/journal.pone.0104548
42. McGuirk P, McCann C, Mills KH. Pathogen-specific T regulatory 1 cells induced in the respiratory tract by a bacterial molecule that stimulates interleukin 10 production by dendritic cells: a novel strategy for evasion or protective T helper type 1 responses by *Bordetella pertussis. J Exp Med.* (2002) 195:221–31. doi: 10.1084/jem.20011288
43. Higgins SC, Lavelle EC, McCann C, Keogh B, NcNeela E, Byrne P, et al. Toll-like receptor 4-mediated innate IL-10 activates antigen-specific regulatory T cells and confers resistance to *Bordetella pertussis* by inhibiting inflammatory pathology. *J Immunol.* (2003) 171:3119–27. doi: 10.4049/jimmunol.171.6.3119
44. Weigl B, Meitinger C, van Thiel D, Janetschek R. Oral immunization of newborn infants against pertussis. *Monat Kinder.* (1979) 127:461–3.
45. Maurer H, Höfler KH, Hilbe W, Huber EG. Preliminary findings with oral whooping cough vaccination in young infants. *Wien Klin Wochenschr.* (1979) 91:717–20.
46. Baumann E, Binder BR, Falk W, Huber EG, Kurz R, Rosanelli K. Development and clinical use of an oral heat-inactivated whole cell pertussis vaccine. *Dev Biol Stand.* (1985) 61:511–6.
47. Strugnell R, Dougan G, Chatfield S, Charles I, Fairweather N, Tite J, et al. Characterization of a *Salmonella typhimurmium aro* vaccine strain expressing the P.69 antigen of *Bordetella pertussis. Infect Immun.* (1992) 60:3994–4002.
48. Molina NC, Parker CD. Murine antibody response to oral infection with live *aroA* recombinant *Salmonella dublin* vaccine strains expressing filamentous hemagglutinin antigen from *Bordetella petussis. Infect Immun.* (1990) 58:2523–8.
49. Guzman CA, Brownlie RM, Kadurugamuwa J, Walker MJ, Timmis KN. Antibody responses in the lungs of mice following oral immunization with *Salmonella typhimurium aroA* and invasive *Escherichia coli* strains expressing the filamentous hemagglutinin of *Bordetella pertussis. Infect Immun.* (1991) 59:4391–7.
50. Sato H, Ito A, Chiba J, Sato Y. Monoclonal antibody against pertussis toxin: effect on toxin activity and pertussis infections. *Infect Immun.* (1984) 46:422–8.
51. Locht C, Coutte L, Mielcarek N. The ins and outs of pertussis toxin. *FEBS J.* (2011) 278:4668–82. doi: 10.1111/j.1742-4658.2011.08237.x
52. Walker MJ, Rohde M, Timmis KN, Guzman CA. Specific lung mucosal and systemic immune responses of mice with *Salmonella typhimurium aroA*, *Salmonella typhi* Ty21a, and invasive *Escherichia coli* expressing recombinant pertussis toxin S1 subunit. *Infect Immun.* (1992) 60:4260–8.
53. Dalla Pozza T, Yan H, Meek D, Gutzman CA, Walker MJ. Construction and characterization of *Salmonella typhimurium aroA* simultaneously expressing the five pertussis toxin subunts. *Vaccine* (1998) 16:522–9. doi: 10.1016/S0264-410X(97)80006-0
54. Lee SF, Halperin SA, Wang H, MacArthur A. Oral colonization and immune responses to *Streptococcus gordonii* expressing a pertussis toxin S1 fragment in mice. *FEMS Microbiol Lett.* (2002) 208:175–8. doi: 10.1111/j.1574-6968.2002.tb11078.x
55. Conway MA, Madrigal-Estebas L, McClean S, Brayden DJ, Mills KHG. Protection against *Bordetella pertussis* infection following parenteral or oral immunization with antigens entrapped in biodegradable particles: effect of formulation and route of immunization on induction of Thland Th2 cells. *Vaccine* (2001) 19:1940–50. doi: 10.1016/S0264-410X(00)00433-3
56. Dow RP. Active immunisation by the intranasal route. *Can J Publ Health* (1940) 31:370.
57. North EA, Anderson G. Active immunisation by the intranasal route in experimental pertussis. *Med J Aust.* (1942) 228–32.
58. Cooper GN. Active immunity in mice following the intranasal injection of sub-lethal doses of living *Haemophilus pertussis. J Pathol Bacteriol.* (1952) 64:65–74. doi: 10.1002/path.1700640109
59. Shapiro-Shapin CG. Pearl Kendrick, Grace Eldering, and the pertussis vaccine. *Emerg Infect Dis.* (2010) 16:1273–8. doi: 10.3201/eid1608.100288
60. Thomas G. Respiratory and humoral immune response to aerosol and intramuscular pertussis vaccine. *J Hyg Camb.* (1975) 74:233–7. doi: 10.1017/S0022172400024293
61. Berstad AKH, Holst J, Froholm LO, Haugen IL, Wedege E, Oftung F, et al. A nasal whole-cell pertussis vaccine induces specific systemic and cross-reactive mucosal antibody responses in human volunteers. *J Med Microbiol.* (2000) 49:157–63. doi: 10.1099/0022-1317-49-2-157
62. Berstad AKH, Oftung F, Korsvold GE, Haugen IL, Froholm LO, Holst J, et al. Induction of antigen-specific T cell responses in human volunteers after intranasal immunization with a whole-cell pertussis vaccine. *Vaccine* (2000) 18:2323–30. doi: 10.1016/S0264-410X(00)00024-4
63. Lee SF, Halperin SA, Salloum DF, MacMillan A, Morris A. Mucosal immunization with a genetically engineered pertussis toxin S1 fragment-cholera toxin subunit B chimeric protein. *Infect Immun.* (2003) 71:2272–5. doi: 10.1128/IAI.71.4.2272-2275.2003
64. Ryan EJ, McNeela E, Murphy GA, Stewart H, O'hagan D, Pizza M, et al. Mutants of *Escherichia coli* heat-labile toxin act as effective mucosal adjuvants for nasal delivery of an acellular pertussis vaccine: differential effects of the nontoxic AB complex and enzyme activity on Th1 and Th2 cells. *Infect Immun.* (1999) 67:6270–80.
65. Berstad AK, Holst J, Mogster B, Haugen IL, Haneberg B. A nasal whole-cell pertussis vaccine can induce strong systemic and mucosal antibody responses which are not enhanced by cholera toxin. *Vaccine* (1997) 15:1473–8. doi: 10.1016/S0264-410X(97)00064-9
66. Berstad AK, Andersen SR, Dalseg R, Dromtorp S, Holst J, Namork E, et al. Inactivated meningococci and pertussis bacteria are immunogenic and act as mucosal adjuvants for a nasal inactivated influenza vaccine. *Vaccine* (2000) 18:1910–9. doi: 10.1016/S0264-410X(99)00442-9
67. Gizurarson S, Tamura S, Kurata T, Hasiguchi K, Ogawa H. The effect of cholera toxin and cholera toxin B subunit on the nasal mucosal membrane. *Vaccine* (1991) 9:825–32. doi: 10.1016/0264-410X(91)90220-Z
68. Couch RB. Nasal vaccination, *Escherichia coli* enterotoxin, and Bell's palsy. *N Engl J Med.* (2004) 350:860–1. doi: 10.1056/NEJMp048006
69. Jabbal-Gill I, Fisher AN, Rappuoli R, Davis SS, Illum L. Stimulation of mucosal and systemic antibody responses against *Bordetella pertussis* filamentous haemagglutinin and recombinant pertussis toxin after nasal administration with chitosan in mice. *Vaccine* (1998) 16:2039–46. doi: 10.1016/S0264-410X(98)00077-2
70. Nagai T, Suzuki Y, Kiyohara H, Susa E, Kato T, Nagamine T, et al. Onjisaponins, from the root of *Polygala tenuifolia* Willdenow, as effective adjuvants for nasal influenza and diphtheria-pertussis-tetanus vaccines. *Vaccine* (2001) 19:4824–34. doi: 10.1016/S0264-410X(01)00215-8
71. Asokanathan C, Corbel M, Xing D. A CpG-containing oligodeoxynucleotide adjuvant for acellular pertussis vaccine improves the protective response against *Bordetella pertussis. Hum Vaccin Immunother.* (2013) 9:325–31. doi: 10.4161/hv.22755
72. Shim DH, Ko HJ, Volker G, Potter AA, Mutwiri G, Babiuk LA, et al. Efficacy of poly[di(sodium carboxylatophenoxy)phosphazene] (PCPP) as mucosal adjuvant to induce protective immunity against respiratory pathogens. *Vaccine* (2010) 28:2311–7. doi: 10.1016/j.vaccine.2009.12.069
73. Shi W, Kou Y, Jiang H, Gao F, Kong W, Su W, et al. Novel intranasal pertussis vaccine based on bacterium-like particles as a mucosal adjuvant. *Immunol Lett.* (2018) 198:26–32. doi: 10.1016/j.imlet.2018.03.012
74. Roberts R, Moreno G, Bottero D, Gaillard ME, Fingermann M, Graieb A, et al. Outer membrane vesicles as acellular vaccine against pertussis. *Vaccine* (2008) 26:4639–70. doi: 10.1016/j.vaccine.2008.07.004
75. Raeven RH, Brummelman J, Pennings J, van der Maas L, Helm K, Tilstra W, et al. Molecular and cellular signatures underlying superior immunity against *Bordetella pertussis* upon pulmonary vaccination. *Mucosal Immunol.* (2017) 11:979–93. doi: 10.1038/mi.2017.81
76. Kanojia G, Raeven RHM, van der Maas L, Bindels THE, van Riet E, Metz B, et al. Development of a thermostable spray dried outer membrane vesicle pertussis vaccine for pulmonary immunization. *J Control Release* (2018) 286:167–78. doi: 10.1016/j.jconrel.2018.07.035

77. Roberts M, Maskell D, Novotny P, Dougan G. Construction and characterization *in vivo* of *Bordetella pertussis aroA* mutants. *Infect Immun.* (1990) 58:732–9.
78. Cornford-Nairns R, Daggard G, Mukkur T. Novel, non-reverting, intranasal live attenuated whooping cough vaccine candidate. *J Microbiol Biotechnol.* (2012) 22:856–65. doi: 10.4014/jmb.1108.08003
79. Locht C. Live pertussis vaccines: will they protect against carriage and spread of pertussis? *Clin Microbiol Infect.* (2016) 22(Suppl. 5):S96–102. doi: 10.1016/j.cmi.2016.05.029
80. Locht C, Papin JF, Lecher S, Debrie AS, Thalen M, Solovay K, et al. Live attenuated pertussis vaccine BPZE1 protects baboons against *B. pertussis* disease and infection. *J Infect Dis.* (2017) 216:117–24. doi: 10.1093/infdis/jix254
81. Thorstensson R, Trollfors B, Al-Tawil N, Jahnmatz M, Bergström J, Ljungman M, et al. A phase I clinical study of a live attenuated *Bordetella pertussis* vaccine – BPZE1; a single centre, double-blind, placebo-controlled, dose-escalating study of BPZE1 given intranasally to healthy adult male volunteers. *PLoS ONE* (2014) 9:e83449. doi: 10.1371/journal.pone.0083449
82. Fedele G, Bianco M, Debrie AS, Locht C, Ausiello CM. Attenuated *Bordetella pertussis* vaccine candidate BPZE1 promotes human dendritic cell CCL21-induced migration and drives a Th1/Th17 response. *J Immunol.* (2011) 186:5388–96. doi: 10.4049/jimmunol.1003765
83. Feunou PF, Kammoun H, Debrie AS, Mielcarek N, Locht C. Long-term immunity against pertussis induced by a single nasal administration of live attenuated *B. pertussis* BPZE1. *Vaccine* (2010) 28:7047–53. doi: 10.1016/j.vaccine.2010.08.017
84. Otsuka N, Han HJ, Toyoizumi-Ajisaka H, Nakamura Y, Arakawa Y, Shibayama K, et al. Prevalence and genetic characterization of pertactin-deficient *Bordetella pertussis* in Japan. *PLoS ONE* (2012) 7:e31985. doi: 10.1371/journal.pone.0031985
85. Queenan AM, Cassiday PK, Evangelista A. Pertactin-negative variants of *Bordetella pertussis* in the United States. *N Engl J Med.* (2013) 368:583–4. doi: 10.1056/NEJMc1209369
86. Lam C, Octavia S, Ricafort L, Sintchenki V, Gilbert GL, Wood N, et al. Rapid increase in pertactin-deficient *Bordetella pertussis* isolates, Australia. *Emerg Infect Dis.* (2014) 20:626–33. doi: 10.3201/eid2004.131478
87. Campbell H, Gupta S, Dolan GP, Kapadia SJ, Kumar Singh A, Andrews N, et al. Review of vaccination in pregnancy to prevent pertussis in early infancy. *J Med Microbiol.* (2018) 67:1426–56. doi: 10.1099/jmm.0.000829

6

The Interplay Between Immune Response and Bacterial Infection in COPD: Focus Upon Non-Typeable *Haemophilus influenzae*

Yu-Ching Su[1], *Farshid Jalalvand*[2], *John Thegerström*[1] *and Kristian Riesbeck*[1]*

[1] *Clinical Microbiology, Department of Translational Medicine, Faculty of Medicine, Lund University, Malmö, Sweden,*
[2] *Department of Biology, Centre for Bacterial Stress Response and Persistence, University of Copenhagen, Copenhagen, Denmark*

Correspondence:
Kristian Riesbeck
kristian.riesbeck@med.lu.se

Chronic obstructive pulmonary disease (COPD) is a debilitating respiratory disease and one of the leading causes of morbidity and mortality worldwide. It is characterized by persistent respiratory symptoms and airflow limitation due to abnormalities in the lower airway following consistent exposure to noxious particles or gases. Acute exacerbations of COPD (AECOPD) are characterized by increased cough, purulent sputum production, and dyspnea. The AECOPD is mostly associated with infection caused by common cold viruses or bacteria, or co-infections. Chronic and persistent infection by non-typeable *Haemophilus influenzae* (NTHi), a Gram-negative coccobacillus, contributes to almost half of the infective exacerbations caused by bacteria. This is supported by reports that NTHi is commonly isolated in the sputum from COPD patients during exacerbations. Persistent colonization of NTHi in the lower airway requires a plethora of phenotypic adaptation and virulent mechanisms that are developed over time to cope with changing environmental pressures in the airway such as host immuno-inflammatory response. Chronic inhalation of noxious irritants in COPD causes a changed balance in the lung microbiome, abnormal inflammatory response, and an impaired airway immune system. These conditions significantly provide an opportunistic platform for NTHi colonization and infection resulting in a "vicious circle." Episodes of large inflammation as the consequences of multiple interactions between airway immune cells and NTHi, accumulatively contribute to COPD exacerbations and may result in worsening of the clinical status. In this review, we discuss in detail the interplay and crosstalk between airway immune residents and NTHi, and their effect in AECOPD for better understanding of NTHi pathogenesis in COPD patients.

Keywords: airway, COPD, exacerbation, immune response, infection, inflammation, non-typeable *Haemophilus influenza*

INTRODUCTION

The lungs are vital organs involved in gas exchange between the vascular system and the external environment, thus they are greatly exposed to the environment-derived microorganisms, including fungi, viruses, and bacteria. The bronchial tree and parenchymal tissues of the lungs, that until recently were considered as sterile, are colonized by phylogenetically-diverse microbes.

The genera of *Firmicutes, Bacteroidetes,* and *Proteobacteria* are the most common phyla identified and represent 60% of the total bacterial microbiome in the healthy airway (1, 2). The majority of the lung microbiota belongs to the normal flora that play an important role in the pulmonary epithelial integrity, colonization resistance, and homeostasis of the immune system in the respiratory tract (3). A small fraction of them are, however, potentially pathogenic microorganisms that are involved in a variety of lung diseases, as exemplified by the genus *Haemophilus.* Non-typeable *Haemophilus influenzae* (NTHi) is a Gram-negative coccobacillus that are commonly residing in the human airways. Uniquely and yet unexplained, NTHi is a commensal when colonizing the nasopharynx or throat, but pathogenic in the lower airways triggering a robust inflammatory response [for reviews see (4, 5)]. NTHi is considered a potential opportunistic pathogen as it frequently infects the lower respiratory tract of lungs with structural damage as a consequence of non-infectious lung diseases or mechanical injuries. Moreover, NTHi occasionally causes bronchitis and pneumonia (6). In addition, lower airway colonization by NTHi has been associated with disease progression of several more or less non-infectious lung diseases such as bronchiectasis (7), cystic fibrosis (8), interstitial lung diseases (9, 10), but mostly in chronic obstructive pulmonary disease (COPD) (11, 12). COPD is a severe inflammatory lung disease characterized by airflow limitation with a range of pathological changes. Both genetics and environmental factors trigger the onset of COPD, however, microbes including NTHi play an important role in the acute exacerbations. This review describes the disease progression of COPD in the context of host immune-interactions linked to NTHi, and the overall impact in disease exacerbation.

THE PATHOPHYSIOLOGY OF COPD

COPD is the third leading cause of morbidity and mortality worldwide expected to affect more than 210 million people by 2030 (13, 14). According to the Global Initiative for Chronic Obstructive Lung Disease (GOLD), COPD is a pulmonary disease that is manageable, but significant exacerbations and co-morbidities may, however, contribute to the overall severity in individual patients (15). COPD is characterized by chronic airflow limitation of the peripheral airways with a range of pathological changes in the lung that are not fully reversible, and usually become progressively worse over time. The progression of COPD is associated with an abnormal inflammatory response of the lung to noxious particles or gases.

From a pathological point of view, COPD comprises a group of pulmonary abnormalities related to the inflammatory reaction of the airways, alveoli, and pulmonary vessels (16–19). These include (i) pulmonary emphysema, (ii) chronic bronchitis, and (iii) disease in the small airways. The pulmonary abnormalities progressively affect all parts of the lung, resulting in increased resistance of the conducting airways and thus chronic airflow obstruction that eventually will lead to a declined lung function. **Emphysema** is a permanent loss of elastic lung recoil caused by elastolytic destruction and enlargement of the alveolar wall distal to the terminal bronchioles. This consequently results in the loss of alveolar attachments to the small airways and thus limitation of airflow and gaseous exchanges. **Chronic bronchitis** is characterized by consecutive and chronic cough with expectorations that last for more than 3 months within 2 years. It is associated with inflammation of the bronchial walls with increased inflammatory infiltrates, hyperplasia of goblet cells, hypertrophy of tracheobronchial submucosa, increased mucous secretion and, finally, dilatation of the airway ducts (airways of about 2–4 mm in internal diameter). The majority of the ciliated epithelium lining the airways are also either compromised or dysfunctionnal, and may be replaced by non-ciliated squamous epithelial cells. **Small airway diseases,** on the other hand, involve hyperplasia and metaplasia of mucosal glands and goblet cells, hypersecretion of intraluminal mucus, macrophage bronchiolitis, and accumulation of lymphocytes in the small bronchioles (airways of ~2 mm or less in diameter and terminal bronchioles). In addition, distortion, fibrosis, stenosis, tortuosities, hyperplasia, and hypertrophia of the small airway smooth muscles also contribute to the loss of elasticity in the lung parenchyma. Although COPD mainly affects the lungs, it also produces significant extrapulmonary consequences as a results of an escalated inflammatory response orchestrated by airway cells and immune mediators (20, 21). The co-morbidities are commonly seen in COPD patients despite the actual mechanism responsible for the systemic inflammation remains to be elucidated.

THE RISK FACTORS OF COPD AND CONSEQUENCES FOR AIRWAY FUNCTION

The development of COPD is multifactorial, with cigarette or tobacco smoking being the primary cause of COPD (22, 23). Other risk factors that may promote the onset and progression of COPD includes prolonged occupational exposure to particles/gases in mining and textile industries, air pollution resulting from biomass combustion, and bronchial hyperresponsiveness (16, 18, 24). The variability of COPD incidences among smokers is also explained by a genetic pre-disposition, such as α1-antitrypsin deficiency and cutis laxa [mutation of the elastin gene *(ELN)*] (25, 26). The α1-antitrypsin deficiency is caused by deleterious homozygous mutations in SERPINA1 which contributes to 1–2% of COPD cases. The deficiency results in increased neutrophil elastase activity that ultimately leads to the degradation and collapse of the alveoli. Importantly, meta-analyses of genome-wide association studies (GWAS) and other genotyping studies have revealed that multiple single nucleotide polymorphism (SNPs) in at least 34 genes from different pulmonary genomic loci are associated with COPD susceptibility (27–30).

Airway epithelium exposed to cigarette or tobacco smoke has compromised tight junctions and delayed epithelial wound repair (31–34). Moreover, cigarette smoke alters basal cell differentiation and subepithelial extracellular matrix (ECM) composition, and thus causes airway remodeling (i.e., goblet cell hyperplasia and small airway squamous metaplasia) (35–37). This results in mucus hypersecretion, impaired mucocilliary clearance, and airway obstruction. Tobacco or cigarette smoke also enhances proliferation and ECM deposition by activating the extracellular signal related kinase (ERK) and the p38 signaling pathway (38). The alteration of major ECM components are widespread in all lung compartments in COPD patients with a total increase of type I and III collagens, fibronectin, and laminin in parallel with reduced concentrations of proteoglycans, perlecan decorin, versican, biglycan, tenascin and elastin (39, 40). Cigarette induced-overexpression of matrix metalloproteases (MMPs-1, 2, 7, 9, 12, and 28) and elastase has also been reported, and may contribute to the airway tissue destruction and fibrosis (41–43). In addition, harmful volatile chemicals derived from cigarette smoke (i.e., acetaldehyde, acrolein, and crotonaldehyde) are prone to form carcinogen adducts with DNA and various proteins (i.e., apoliprotein E and surfactant protein A). They also dysregulate airway epithelial ion transport, disrupt the phagocytic activity of airway phagocytes, and diminish the airway surface liquid volume (44–46).

Numerous proteomics and transcriptomic analyses have unveiled the crucial impact of cigarette or tobacco smoke and COPD disease progression on airway gene expression (47, 48). The differential gene expression studies were done using COPD experimental models or clinical samples [i.e., bronchial epithelial cells, sputum, plasma, blood, and bronchoalveolar lavage (BAL) fluid]. Collectively, most of the altered genes are involved in oxidative stress, xenobiotic metabolism, antioxidant responses, DNA repair, ECM remodeling, inflammatory responses, and immune defenses, which the latter two are our major interest of discussion in this review. The omics data aid in the increased knowledge of molecular mechanisms in COPD. They may reflect the dynamic response and attempts by the airway epithelial cells to repair the cytotoxic injury primarily triggered by inhaled irritants. Deleterious and irreversible alterations occurring and interfering with the airway epithelial homeostasis and immune defense may promote COPD development and progression. Notably, gene alterations in phagosomal- and leukocyte transendothelial migration pathways (LTM) are significantly correlated with the level of T cells and airway obstruction in smokers (49). The LTM, however, were found to be further dysregulated in COPD patients. Hence, in addition to clinical/physiology variables, a number of gene products with significant differential gene expression may be targeted as specific proteomic signatures or biomarkers for early COPD detection, patient monitoring, disease subgrouping, and finally treatment selection (50, 51).

ALTERATION OF AIRWAY GENE EXPRESSION AND IMMUNE RESPONSE IN COPD

Effects of Tobacco or Cigarette Smoking

Tobacco or cigarette smoke regulates airway gene expression via two main mechanisms, by altering the status of (i) chromatin remodeling, and (ii) DNA methylation of the target genes (**Figure 1**) (52–54).

Chromatin remodeling is a result of a disrupted balance in histone acetylation/deacetylation (55). Excessive activation of more than 20 transcription factors including NF-κB, and lipoprotein peroxidation products (peroxinitrite, acrolein, and 4HNE from tobacco smoking) contributes to such anomaly. NF-κB is a key inflammatory and redox-sensitive transcription factor that plays a direct role in cigarette smoke-induced airway inflammation. NF-κB has been described as a "smoke-sensor" due to its sensitive activation by tobacco residues (56). Stimulation of multiple signaling cascades [p38 mitogen-activated protein (MAPK) kinases, mitogen and stress-activated kinase 1 (MSK1), protein kinase C zeta (PKCζ), and IκB kinase (IKK) complex (IKKα, IKKβ, and NEMO)] by tobacco residues promotes the activation and nuclear translocation of transcription factor NF-κB RelA/p65 (54, 57–64). This is followed by a complex formation of NF-κB/CBP-p300 [coactivator, CREB-binding protein (CBP) or CBP/p300] at target DNA sequences. It should be noted that CBP/p300 also has intrinsic histone acetyltransferase (HAT) activity. Subsequent acetylation and phosphorylation of the subunit p65 in the NF-κB/CBP-p300 complex by the activated MSK1/PKCζ-signaling pathways (and other 11 different kinases), and CBP/p300, respectively, are required for the full activation of NF-κB (57, 60, 63). This enhances the DNA binding affinity of the complex. Histones H3 and H4 in the chromatin complex of target sequences are then being acetylated (histone H3 at Lys9; H4 at Lys8 and Lys12) and phosphorylated (histone H3 at Ser10) by the subunit CBP of the NF-κB/CBP-p300 complex, and the activated MSK1 and PKCζ, respectively. The hyperacetylated core histones, however, fail to be neutralized or deacetylated by a dysfunctional histone deacetylase (HDAC2). Peroxinitrite nitrates the tyrosine residues of the HDAC2 and causes inhibition of activation and reduced expression of the protein. Of note, peroxinitrite is a by-product generated from the immune cell-derived nitrite oxide (NO) and reactive oxygen species (ROS) of cigarette smoke (65, 66).

Cigarette or tobacco smoke disturbs the DNA methylation status of target genes through several mechanisms. Firstly, DNA damage caused by cigarette smoke stimulates the DNA methyltransferase 1 (DNMT) to actively induce CpGs methylation at the damaged site (67). The hypermethylation is prone to introduce error of methylation in some target genes, resulting in reduced gene expression. Secondly, activation of nicotine signaling pathway by tobacco smoke causes CaMKII/IV and ERK/MAPK pathway activation that subsequently induces the activity of CBP to suppress the expression of DNMT1. This may result in reduced DNA methylation and thus altered level of gene repression by DNMT (68–70). Finally, enhanced activities of transcription factors such as hypoxia inducible factor 1 due to the high level of carbon monoxide and hypoxia have also been reported to influence airway gene expression (71).

Consequently, the combinatorial effect from both aberrant acetylation of histone and DNA methylation promotes the transformation of chromatin from a condensed structure to an activated open conformation. This facilitates irregular accessibility of DNA for transcription machineries, hence

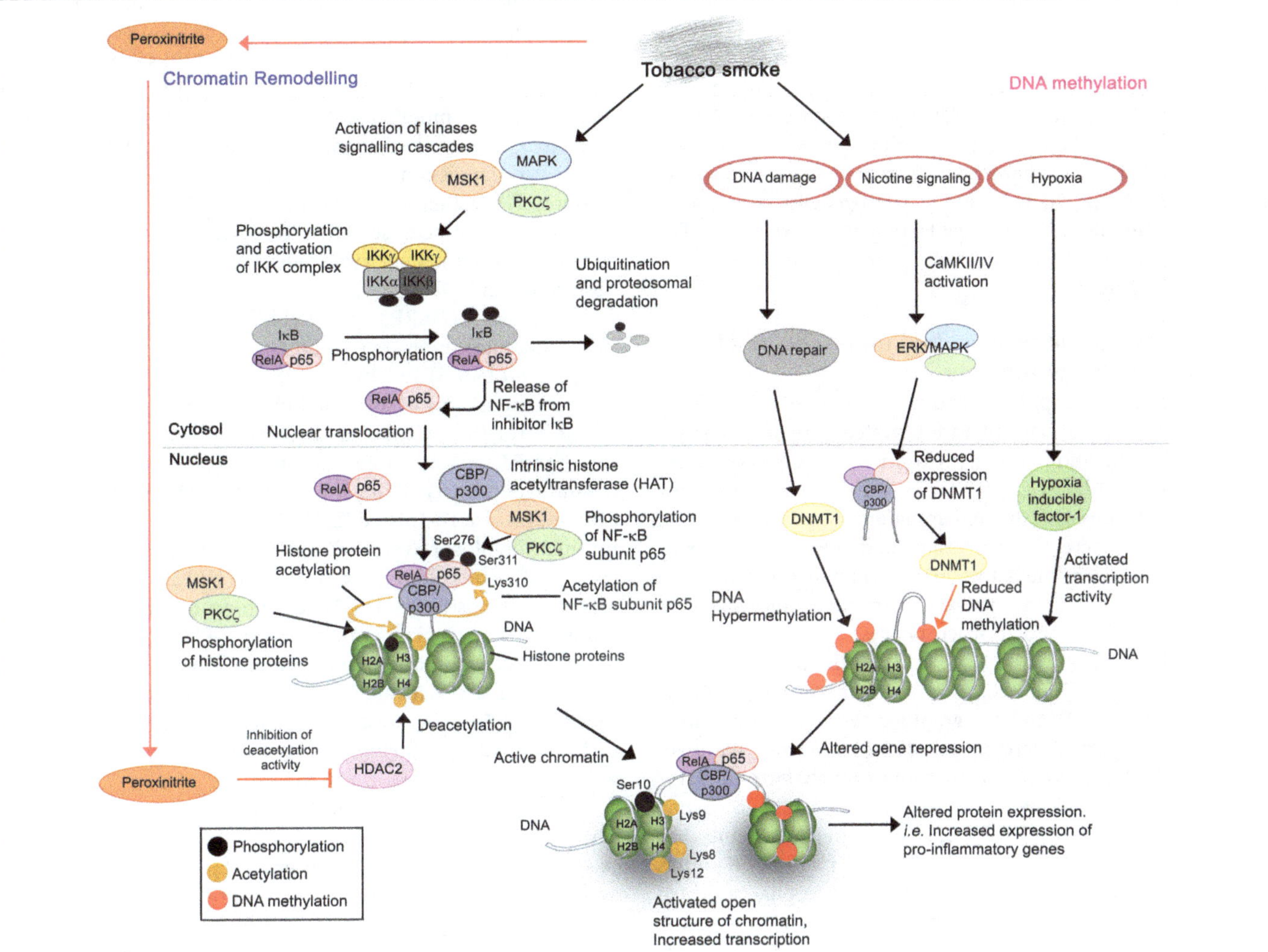

FIGURE 1 | Cigarette and tobacco smoke has several effects on gene regulation. Nicotine and other compounds in the smoke alter gene expression by two pathways, firstly, chromatin remodeling **(Left)** and secondly, DNA methylation **(Right)**. Chromatin remodeling involves activation of kinases signaling pathways, activation and nuclear translocation of transcription factor NF-κB (RelA/p65), and complex formation with CBP/p300 on specific DNA sites. CBP/p300 is intrinsically a histone acetyltransferase (HAT). Subunit p65 is further phosphorylated at Ser276 and Ser311, respectively, by MSK1 and PKCς, whereas CBP acetylates p65 at Lys310. The phosphorylation and acetylation enhance the interaction within the NF-κB/CBP/p300 complex while stabilizing the DNA binding of NF-κB. The complex of NF-κB/CBP/p300 then modifies the histones through CBP-mediated acetylations of histone H3 (at Lys9) and H4 at Lys 8 and Lys12, and phosphorylation of H3 at Ser10 by MSK1 and PKCς. This results in the structure change of chromatin, from a condensed structure (repressed) to an activated open conformation. The transcription of target genes is therefore increased. In the second mechanism, several side effects resulting from cigarette smoking such as DNA damage and nicotine signaling could trigger the hypermethylation or decreased methylation of target DNA. This may lead to DNA methylation anomalies and thus altered DNA expression. Resulting hypoxia due to high concentrations of carbon monoxide also contributes to altered gene expression. The aberrant gene expression by cigarette smoke mostly occurs in pro-inflammatory genes with resulting increased production of inflammatory mediators, and amplified inflammation in the COPD lung upon exposure.

irregular gene expression by various cell types in the airway. The mechanisms reported are responsible for increased expression of NF-κB-dependent proinflammatory gene products [i.e., IL-1β, IL-6, IL-8, CCL-5 cyclooxygenase (COX)-2, and MIP-2/CXCL2] in both pulmonary structural cells (bronchial, small airway, and alveolar epithelial cells) and immune cells (alveolar macrophages), increased VEGF and iNOS in nasal fibroblasts and lymphocytes (Jurkat T cells), respectively, and decreased activity of antioxidant transcription factor Nrf2 and α1-antitrypsin in bronchial epithelial cells (54, 56, 57, 59, 62–64, 72–79). These may contribute to the anatomical anomalies in the airway and excessive inflammatory responses among smokers during the course of COPD.

The Inflammatory Immune Response in COPD

COPD is associated with chronic inflammation in the peripheral airways orchestrated by both innate and adaptive immune responses that are interconnected via dendritic cells (80). Increasing numbers of inflammatory cells (neutrophils, macrophages, T and B lymphocytes, mast cell, eosinophils, and dendritic cells) and inflammatory mediators are accumulated in the airway lumen/wall in the lung parenchyma (19, 81). These immune cells and inflammatory mediators can hence be detected in the sputum and BAL fluid of COPD patients. The level of accumulation is positively correlated with disease severity. An increasing number of studies using animal models and clinical tissues have reported the nature of excessive airway inflammatory responses in COPD. Despite this, the heterogeneity in symptoms progression among COPD patients remain unexplained. The overall mechanism of COPD inflammatory immune response is depicted in **Figure 2.**

The First Line of Defense in the Lung—The Innate Immunity and Inflammasome

Lung structural cells (epithelial and endothelial cells, fibroblasts, and airway smooth muscle cells) are activated by inhaled irritants through the stimulation of several pattern recognitions receptors (PRRs), with Toll-like receptor (TLR)-4 being reported as the key player in most of the inflammatory responses (82–85). This causes an increased expression and release of an array of pro-inflammatory mediators and chemokines through the oxidative pathway by the activated bronchial epithelial cells and immune cells (alveolar macrophages). The inflammatory mediators [(interleukin (IL)-1β, IL-6, IL-8, IL-33, C-X-C motif chemokine ligand (CXCL) 10, granulocyte-macrophage colony-stimulating factor (GM-CSF), granulocyte-colony stimulating factor (G-CSF), tumor necrosis factor (TNF)-α, fibroblast growth factor 1 and 2 (FGF1/2), transforming growth factor (TGF)-β1, C-C motif chemokine ligand (CCL) 2, CCL20, and thymic stromal lymphopoietin (TSLP)] act on recruited immune cells and resident cells to initiate a series of innate immune responses (23, 86–90). Meanwhile, activated alveolar macrophages, which are usually patrolling the lung parenchyma, further release more pro-inflammatory mediators and chemokines [IL-1β, IL-6, IL-8, IL-23, TNF-α, CCL1, CXCL1, CXCL5 (ENA-78), CXCL9, CXCL10, CXCL11, CCL2, leukotriene B4 (LTB_4)], ROS, elastolytic enzyme [matrix metalloprotease protein (MMP)-2,−9, and−12; and cathepsin-K,- L, and -S], GM-CSF, and G-CSF (23, 91, 92). The enhanced levels of CCL2 and CXCL1 result in recruitement of blood monocytes expressing CCR2 and CXCR2 (receptors for CCL2 and CXCL1, respectively), to the lung and differentiate locally into macrophages. Interestingly, there are higher expression levels of the CCR2 and CXCR2 found on blood monocytes in COPD subjects (93). This may explain the rapid recruitment and excessive accumulation of monocyte-derived interstitial macrophages in the lung tissue of COPD patients (94, 95).

Upregulation of neutrophil chemoattractors (LTB_4, CXCL1, CXCL5, IL-8, and TNF-α) induces a massive migration of circulating neutrophils into the lung parenchyma (96). The transmigration of blood neutrophils occurs through adherence of the granulocytes to E-selectin of endothelial cells that is found to be upregulated in COPD (97). This results in airway neutrophilia in several COPD patients (96, 98, 99). The recruited neutrophils (to the lung) are then activated to secrete granule proteins [myeloperoxidase (MPO) and neutrophil lipocalin] while releasing its own IL-8 for further neutrophilic recruitment and amplification of the inflammation (100). In addition to the macrophage-derived proteases, neutrophils also secrete serine proteases [neutrophil elastase (NE), cathepsin G, proteinase-3, MMP-8, and MMP-9] that are associated with serious alveolar destruction in emphysema (101). The protease activity may be further enhanced in conditions with genetic deficiencies or suppressed expression of α1-antitrypsin by tobacco smoke. In addition, NE, cathepsin G, and proteinase-3 are involved in the stimulation of mucus secretion from submucosal glands and goblet cells, resulting in airway mucus hypersecretion and airway obstruction in COPD (101).

The NLRP3 (NLRP3: nucleotide-binding domain, leucine-rich-containing family, pyrin domain-containing-3 OR Nod-like receptor protein 3) inflammasome is a cytosolic multi-protein complex (consisting of the inflammation sensor protein NLRP3, adapter protein ASC, and the effector protein caspase-1) (102). The NLRP3 inflammasomes are involved in the COPD airway inflammation by regulating the production of pro-inflammatory cytokines IL-1α, IL-1β, and IL-18. These cytokines are important for neutrophil survival and activation of T helper (Th) 17 cells (103). Interestingly, local airway NLRP3 inflammasome activation is positively correlated with acute exacerbations and lower airway microbial colonization in COPD patients (103, 104). Moreover, in an elastase-induced emphysema model, the NLRP3 inflammasome is activated in addition to hyperproduction of mucin MUC5AC by diesel extract particles, extracellular ATP, and inflammatory protein S100 (105, 106).

The Adaptive Immunity in COPD

The adaptive immunity is initiated at a later stage, and is recognized by the increased number of T and B lymphocytes and pulmonary dendritic cells. Dendritic cells are the major antigen-presenting cells (APC) in the airways, and link the innate and adaptive immunity. Circulating dendritic cells (expressing receptors CCR2 and CCR6) are recruited to the airway via dendritic chemoattractants CCL2 and CCL20 released by activated airway epithelial cells in response to cigarette smoke (107, 108). Dendritic cells act by endocytosis of inhaled irritants that subsequently are processed into antigen peptides during maturation and further migration to lymph nodes.

Uncommitted T lymphocytes are thereafter primed by the presented antigen. These important cells are activated by IL-12 released from dendritic cells for subsequent commitment into antigen-specific T cell lineages, i.e., T helper 1 (Th1; $CD3^+CD4^+$) cells, whereas immature dendritic cells in the airway promote Th2 differentiation (23, 109). Interestingly, in COPD patients, pulmonary Th and cytotoxic T cells (Tc; $CD3^+CD8^+$) express more CXCR3 receptors compared to healthy individuals (110, 111). This enhances their migration toward chemoattractants CXCL9, CXCL10, and CXCL11 that are actively released by alveolar macrophages in COPD subjects. Activated $CD8^+$ T cell subset type 1 (Tc1) releases perforins, granzyme B, and TNF-α to induce alveolar cells apoptosis, contributing to the emphysema (112). In parallel, pulmonary Th17 T cells are activated by alveolar macrophage-derived IL-6 and IL-23 to secrete IL-17A and IL-22 causing neutrophilic inflammation (113, 114). Inflammatory cytokines are also released by type 3

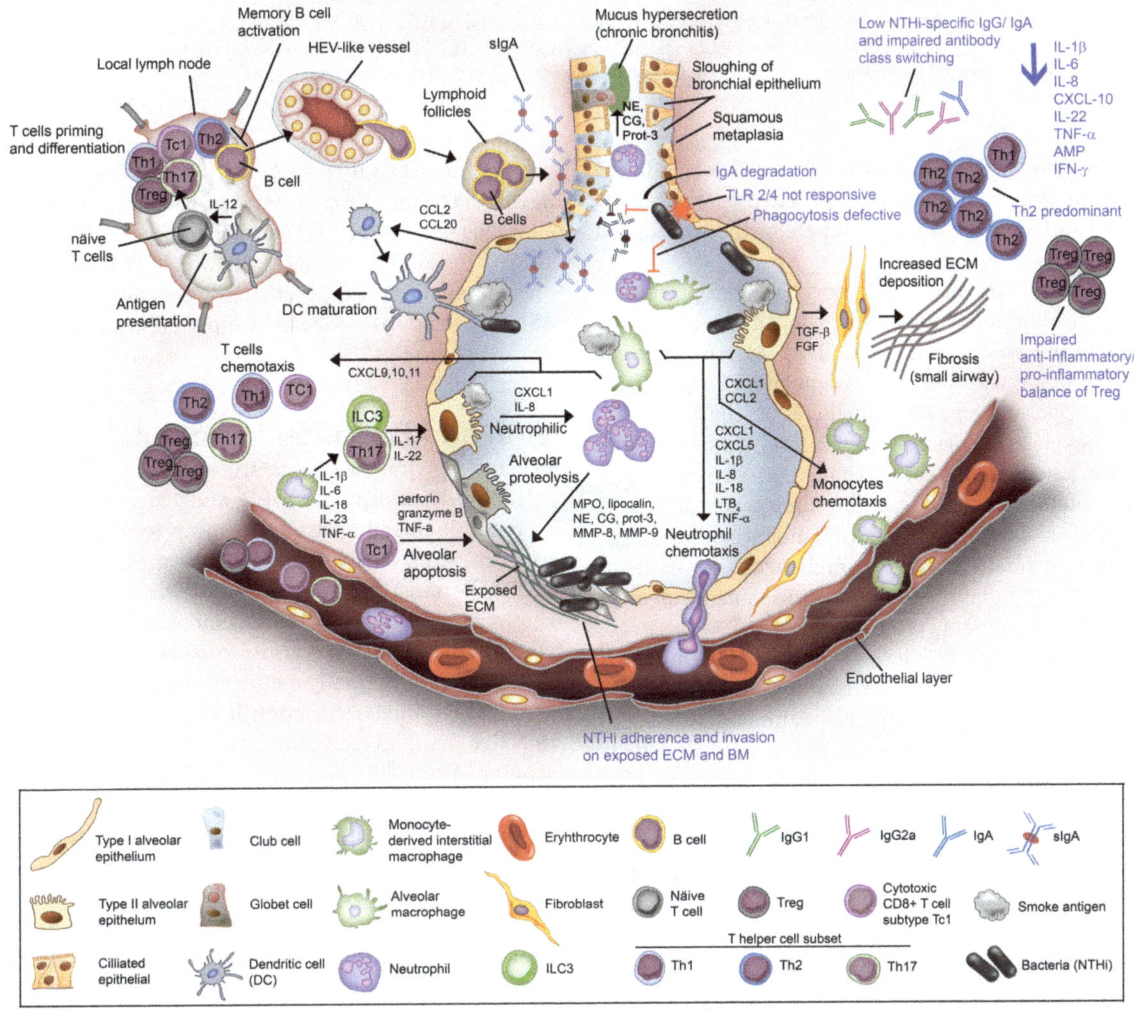

FIGURE 2 | Non-typeable *H. influenzae*-dependent immune responses in the lower airway of COPD patients result in inflammation. Airway epithelium exposed to cigarette or tobacco smoke display an increased permeability with compromised tight junctions, and airway remodeling (goblet cell hyperplasia and small airway squamous metaplasia). Cigarette smoke causes the activation of airway epithelium and alveolar macrophages. The activated airway structural and resident immune cells release an array of chemotactic factors responsible for recruitment of inflammatory and immune cells to the lung. Activated epithelium produces TGF-β and FGF that triggers the production of ECM molecules by fibroblasts. Increased deposition of ECM causes progression of fibrosis and air flow limitation. The chemokines CXCL1 and IL-8, and LTB$_4$ attract the circulating neutrophils through the receptors CXCR2 and BLT$_1$, respectively. Meanwhile, CXCL1 and CCL2 targeting the receptors CXCR2 and CCR2 on blood monocytes are also released. Recruited blood monocytes differentiate into macrophages in the airway tissue. Activated alveolar macrophage and epithelium cell also release inflammasome (1L-1β and IL-18) for neutrophils survival and activation of helper T cells Th17. The chemokine IL-23 are released by macrophages to attract T helper cell subset Th17, and ILC3. Both Th17 and ILC3 will release IL-17 and IL-22 that will act on the alveolar epithelium to release CXCL1 and IL-8 for enhanced recruitment of neutrophils, resulting in neutrophilic inflammation. Activated neutrophils are thereafter degranulated and release myeloperoxidase (MPO), lipocalin, neutrophil elastase (NE), cathepsin-G (CG), proteinase-3 (Prot-3), and matrix metalloprotease (MMP) 8 and 9. The granulated products are proteolytic and elastilolytic to aveolar, causing alveolar destruction and emphysema. In addition, NE, CG, and Prot-3 are also targeting goblet cells and submucosal glands to induce hypersecretion of mucus. Dendritic cells carrying the receptors CCR2 and CCR6 are recruited to airway tissue via chemottractants CCL2 and CCL20. The dendritic cells uptake the antigen (smoke residues), and present the antigens to the naïve T cells at lymph nodes. Uncommitted T lymphocytes are thereafter primed to the presented antigen and activated by IL-12 derived from dendritic cells (professional antigen presenting cells; APC). Mature/activated T cells expressing receptor CXCR3 are chemotactic toward CXCL9, CXCL10, and CXCL11 and are recruited to the lung tissue. Cytotoxic CD8+ T cell subtype Tc1 releases perforin and granzyme B resulting in epithelial apoptosis contributing to emphysema progression. For the humoral immune response, B cells are activated by Th2, enter the circulation via high-endothelial venule (HEV)-like vessel and transported to lung tissue, and organized into lymphoid follicles at peripheral airway. B cell-derived plasma cells from lymphoid follicles release IgA, and secreted into airway lumen as secretory IgA (sIgA) via the polymeric immunoglobulin receptor. Mucosal antibodies play an important role to eradicate pathogens and noxious antigens via immune exclusion. However, the airway defense by sIgA is diminished by NTHi IgA protease that degrade the antibodies. TLR2 and TLR4 of the airway phagocytes and epithelium following exposure to cigarette smoke are not responding to P6 and LOS of NTHi. This results in defective phagocytosis and delayed bacterial clearance from the airway. The suppressed TLR4 induction in T cells has also lead to Th2 predominant immune response, with low production of IFN-γ and reduced T cell-mediated immune killing of NTHi. Moreover, NTHi downregulates Foxp3 of Tregs and thus impairs the anti-inflammatory/pro-inflammatory balance of Tregs. The extensive immunosuppressive activity by Tregs diminishes the response of effector T to

(Continued)

FIGURE 2 | NTHi stimulation. Lastly, plasma cells from COPD patients fail to produce NTHi-specific antibodies and compromised immunoglobulin class switching. The impairment of the host immune response in COPD toward NTHi infection are labeled in blue. In total, NTHi infection in COPD lung adversely reduces the production of IL-1β, IL-6, IL-8, CXCL-10, IL-22, TNF-α, antimicrobial peptide (AMP), and IFN-γ. This may explain the inefficient eradication of airway pathogens in COPD patients whereby persistent NTHi infection concomitantly escalates the inflammation and thus exacerbation in COPD.

innate lymphoid cells (ILC3) (115). The ILCs are involved in the homeostasis of lung immunity and are regulated by epithelially produced IL-33 and TSLP (116, 117), and are further stimulated in response to cell damage.

The accumulation of B lymphocytes in the peripheral airway and within lymphoid follicles is associated with airway autoimmunity in the progression of COPD (118). Airway tissue damage in conjunction with impaired T-regulatory cells (Tregs), both related by cigarette smoke, contributes to the formation of autoantibodies against airway components. Autoantibodies against elastin, epithelial, endothelial, carbonylated, and citrullinated proteins are found in the circulation of COPD patients (119–124). The generation of autoantibodies might activate plasma exudate-derived complement components resulting in a chronic inflammation, and consequently damage of the airways with emphysema progression (124–127).

From a physiological point of view, a modulated inflammatory process is important for a protective and optimal immune response. However, the prolonged airway inflammation in COPD as a results of impaired homeostasis leads to serious side effects since it amplifies the tissue damage and impairs the local immune defenses. The abrogated local immune system may make the airways of COPD patients susceptible for opportunistic or recurrent infections by viruses and bacteria that in turn might exacerbate the disease.

ACUTE EXACERBATIONS OF COPD (AECOPD) AND ASSOCIATION WITH MICROBIAL COLONIZATION

Acute exacerbations of COPD (AECOPD) are episodes of acute symptom worsening that usually are associated with both respiratory (increased airway inflammation) and non-respiratory (system inflammation/co-morbidities) effects (128–130). The typical symptoms of an AECOPD include increased production of purulent sputum, dyspnea, cough, wheezing, and symptoms of a cold that may last from 7 days up to 12 weeks (15, 130, 131). It commonly occurs in patients with advanced COPD and results in additional therapy based on the level of exacerbations. Exacerbations are classified in three levels according to GOLD. There is the mild disease that can be treated with short acting bronchodilators (SAB); moderate disease with SAB combined with antibiotics and/ or oral corticosteroids; and finally severe exacerbations with acute respiratory failure which requires emergency room visit and eventually hospitalization (15, 130).

AECOPD is a complex yet multifactorial consequence of COPD. Most of the exacerbations could be triggered by infectious (up to 80%) or non-infectious agents (~10%) (AECOPD with known etiology), whereas up to 30% of cases are of unknown etiology (132, 133). Respiratory tract infections are the major causes for AECOPD with known etiology and are mainly attributed to infections by viruses, bacteria, and atypical bacteria (not detected with conventional Gram-staining) (11, 134, 135). Non-infectious causes of AECOPD include air pollution, environmental factors, meteorological effects, and comorbidities of the patients, all of which are partially contributing to COPD exacerbations (133, 135, 136).

Viral and Bacterial Infections in AECOPD

Respiratory viral infections are often the primary cause in the infection-dependent AECOPD, and virus was identified as single or multiple infecting strains from up to 64% of COPD patients with exacerbations recorded between years 2001–2017 (137–145). The most common infecting viruses are, by far, human rhinovirus, influenza virus A, and respiratory syncytial virus, whereas parainfluenza virus, coronavirus, echovirus, human metapneumovirus, and adenovirus are considerably rare.

Bacterial infections contribute to an average of 50% of infective acute exacerbations with a prevalence being reported ranging from 26 to 81% (132, 135, 146–148). The most commonly pathogenic bacterial species isolated from the lower airway of COPD patients during AECOPD are NTHi, *Moraxella catarrhalis, Streptococcus pneumoniae, Staphylococcus aureus, Pseudomonas aeruginosa*, and *Klebsiella pneumoniae* (11, 129, 133, 136, 149–152). It has been suggested that infection with new strains of the infecting species, rather than a new species, is highly associated with an increased risk of exacerbation (11, 153, 154). Atypical bacteria that cause exacerbations are *Chlamydia* spp., *Legionella pneumophilia*, and *Mycoplasma* spp.

In contrast to viral infections that are diagnosed in 5–45% of COPD patients with stable disease and increase to 39.3–64% during COPD exacerbations, bacterial colonization in the airways are more common with the same species during both stable disease (25–86%) and exacerbations (58.8–81%) (11, 132, 136, 137, 142, 155–158). Hence the precise or direct role of bacterial infection as the primary cause in triggering AECOPD remains controversial although a significantly increased bacterial load is observed during exacerbation in several patients. This further suggests that bacteria might be more involved as secondary invaders after an initial viral infection.

Viral infections have been reported to cause several physiological changes in the lung that in turn facilitates secondary bacterial invasion. The mechanism of bacterial superinfection has been described for *H. influenzae, S. pneumoniae, S. aureus,* and many other airway pathogens (159–161). Firstly, viral infections destroy the tight junctions of the airway epithelial barrier while inducing epithelium apoptosis. This results in the onset of airway epithelium lining repair whereby the sloughed off dead cells would become a rich nutrient source for growth of infecting bacteria. The damaged epithelium lining also enables bacterial adherence to the exposed basement membrane and ECM. Secondly, the demolished ciliated clearance as a result of the virus-damaged airway epithelium lining further promotes bacterial colonization and subsequent epithelial transmigration into deeper tissues (162–164). Lastly, viral infections are also detrimental to the airway immune defense by causing degradation of antimicrobial peptides (AMP), and by triggering IFN-γ secretion by immune cells. This results in suppressed macrophage and neutrophil responses to infecting bacteria, and thus enables bacterial evasion of the airway immune defense (165–168). Nevertheless, viral and bacterial coinfection have greater impact in the AECOPD airway inflammatory responses than bacteria or virus infection alone (168, 169). This is in parallel with the co-isolation of both respiratory viruses and bacteria from 6 to 30% of AECOPD patients (129, 133, 136, 170–174).

Infective AECOPD is also attributed to impaired functions of AMP, macrophages, and neutrophils triggered by inhaled irritants such as tobacco smoke. Expression of microbial-induced AMP (human β-defensin 2) is suppressed in airway epithelial cells when exposed to cigarette smoke (175, 176). Both the alveolar and monocyte-derived macrophages in patients with COPD are defective in phagocytosis of bacteria such as *H. influenzae* and *S. pneumoniae* (177, 178), and in efferocytosis of apoptotic neutrophils and epithelial cells. In addition, neutrophils from COPD patients are aberrant in chemotactic response with defective accuracy (179). All these factors contribute to the failure to resolve inflammation in COPD leading to facilitated chronic microbial colonization, also during exacerbations.

The Role of the Lung Microbiome in AECOPD

The low number of cultivable bacteria found in healthy individuals previously led to the conclusion that healthy and normal lungs are virtually sterile. This hypothesis is currently being revised, since the introduction of 16S rDNA based molecular diagnostics has shown that even healthy lungs have a distinct microbial community, different from that seen in the upper respiratory tract (180, 181). This has led to the concept of a core human lung microbiome which can be altered in COPD stable disease and during exacerbations (182). The role of the lung microbiome in the pathogenesis of COPD by influencing host immune response has also been suggested (151, 183–188).

The stability of the lung microbiome has profound impact on maintaining local immune homeostasis (189). According to the "vicious circle" hypothesis, airway inflammation and impaired immune defenses caused by either viral infections or irritant inhalation have ecological influence on the airway microenvironment and growth conditions that would eventually lead to dysbiosis of the lung microbiota (182, 190). The changed lung microbiome would then cause a maladaptive immunological response resulting in further inflammation and damage of the lung immune defenses, and additional alteration of the lung microbiome. The chain of events thus generates a vicious circle that contributes to COPD progression and exacerbation.

Several studies have documented that COPD progression from stable state to an exacerbation could induce microbiota shift in the lower airway (bronchioles), sputum, and throat (151, 190–196). Alteration in the microbiome complexity or richness is associated with the inflammatory process and changes in ECM protein expression in the lung, as observed in COPD (185, 197). Declined diversity in the lung microbiome has been reported to be related to disease severity, inflammation and decreased lung functions in COPD. This includes the increased emphysematous destruction, bronchial tissue remodeling, lymphoid follicle formation, elevated autoantibodies, and IL-17A production, and finally increased neutrophil extracellular traps (NET) formation in the airway of animal models or AECOPD patients (198–201). It has recently been reported that lung microbiome diversity is also associated with genetic factors. Mannose-binding lectin (MBL) deficiency has also been associated with disease severity and exacerbations in patients with cystic fibrosis and bronchiectasis (202). However, COPD patients with a genetic deficiency in MBL are less susceptible to *Haemophilus* spp. colonization, lowering the risk of exacerbations while their lung microbiota is more diverse than normal COPD patients (203).

THE CLINICAL ROLE OF NTHi IN COPD

In this review we will focus on NTHi, one of the dominant genera that is relatively abundant in the total COPD-dependent lung microbiome, due to its role of infection in COPD immunological responses (136, 149, 192–195, 198, 204–206).

The microbiology of *H. influenzae* has recently been reviewed in detail by our group and others (4, 5, 207). It is a Gram-negative coccobacillus that commonly colonizes the human nasopharynx, and is typed as capsulated (type a–f) or non-encapsulated strains (NTHi). *H. influenzae* may cause both invasive and mucosal disease (208). Since the introduction of capsule polysaccharide conjugate vaccines against type b (Hib), NTHi dominate, followed by capsule type f (Hif) (209, 210). Mucosal infections, including acute otitis media, sinusitis, and exacerbations in COPD, are nowadays mainly associated with NTHi. There has also been a significant shift in the epidemiology of severe invasive disease, from Hib infections in small children to NTHi in adults (210, 211). The most common principal infection focus by *H. influenzae* is now community acquired pneumonia (CAP), whereas the incidence of historically common diagnoses such as meningitis and epiglottitis have significantly decreased (210, 211). Patients with underlying conditions, notably COPD, seem to be at higher risk for invasive infections (209).

There is consensus that *H. influenzae* is one of the key bacterial pathogens involved in pathogenesis of both stable COPD disease and acute exacerbations (207). However, the relative abundance and significance of NTHi in COPD varies between different studies. Several factors, such as sampling methodology, choice of microbiological analysis and, if the patient has a stable disease or an exacerbation, or has been subject to previous antibiotic therapies, tend to affect the outcome of the studies (212).

Common sampling methods from the lower respiratory tract include both bronchoscopy techniques such as protected specimen brush (PSB) and collection of BAL fluid as well as non-invasive methods like sputum sampling (213). All of these methods, particularly sputum, are to some extent subject to the risk of contamination from the normal microbial flora of the oro- and nasopharynx, which might reduce their specificity (213). However, several studies still show a distinct association between lower respiratory tract samples and clinical parameters in COPD patients, making the information valuable (214).

Cultivable bacteria are seldom found in the lower airways of healthy individuals (215), whereas COPD patients show bacterial growth in 30–50% of cases even during stable disease (**Table 1**). On top of that, several studies have shown a significant increase in the *Proteobacteria* phylum, which includes *Haemophilus* spp., in individuals with both stable disease and AECOPD (**Table 2**). NTHi is consistently one of the predominating bacterial species isolated in those cultures; other important pathogens include *S. pneumoniae, M. catarrhalis,* and *P. aeruginosa* (219). During AECOPD, the bacterial load is increased even further, and NTHi continues to be the predominating species (208). Furthermore, acquisition of a new NTHi strain has, in one study, been linked to the onset of AECOPD (153). Moreover, the growth and dominance of *H. influenzae* following rhinovirus infection was observed in the sputum microbiome of patients with COPD (190).

COLONIZATION AND ADAPTATION OF NTHi IN THE LOWER AIRWAYS OF COPD PATIENTS

The chronic inflammation that characterizes COPD pathogenesis causes significant changes to the pulmonary tissue. The lower respiratory tract of patients suffering from this disease is marked by epithelial denuding, hypersecretion of mucus, disproportionate phagocyte presence and imbalances in antioxidant/oxidants (220). This altered *milieu* selects for specific bacterial species that are genetically equipped to competently address these environmental stressors (151, 195, 221). NTHi is the most common pathogen isolated from the sputum of COPD patients, and the primary cause of exacerbations (212), indicating a unique ability to colonize and persist in the chronically inflamed lower respiratory tract.

In recent years, great efforts have been made in understanding how NTHi colonizes the pulmonary tissue. In addition to the regular arsenal of virulence factors associated with NTHi (5), the bacterial pathogen undergoes specific adaptations to increase its fitness in the COPD setting. Specific genetic islands that include *ureABCEFGH, lic2b, hgbA, iga, hmw1,* and *hmw2* have been reported to be enriched in NTHi strains isolated from COPD patients compared to commensal NTHi (222). These genes are involved in raising the pH of the environment, lipooligosaccharide (LOS) synthesis, iron uptake, immune evasion, and attachment to host tissue. The validity of these findings is strengthened by previous work identifying upregulation of many of the same bacterial gene products during growth in COPD sputum (223). Moreover, peroxiredoxin-thioredoxin, an antioxidant enzyme, was found to be one of the most enriched proteins in NTHi during growth in COPD sputum, suggesting that the bacteria upregulate oxidative stress-countermeasures when facing oxidative imbalances in the diseased lung (223). Oxidative stress resistance has previously been shown to be vital for NTHi survival in infection models (224).

In a seminal investigation by Pettigrew et al., whole-genome sequencing (WGS) was conducted to follow the *in vivo* adaptation of NTHi to the COPD environment over time (225). Several interesting findings were reported in this work. Firstly, the median duration of persistence by the pathogen was found to be 161 days, but it could persist in patients for up to as many as 1,422 days. Secondly, slipped-strand mispairing-mediated phase variation was identified as the primary genetic adaptation to the niche. Poignantly, the genes affected by the regulation mechanism encoded for (among others) the HMW adhesins, LOS biosynthesis, and iron uptake, that is, the same processes identified in the previous studies as important for COPD adaptation (222, 223). Thirdly, and somewhat surprising, it was observed that a very limited number of genes were gained/lost during persistent colonization, meaning that selection for strains that thrive in the inflamed lower airways occurs at the very onset of colonization. Finally, the authors reported that genetic changes occurred in 8 of the 12 investigated vaccine antigens during persistent infections, a fact that might be taken into consideration for potential vaccine development against NTHi.

Another virulence factor that has been reported by Murphy and co-workers to play a pivotal role for NTHi survival in COPD settings is IgA-protease, a hydrolytic enzyme that cleaves secretory IgA (sIgA) antibodies in the mucosal epithelium (226–228). Four genes encode for the same number of different variants of the endopeptidase with various cleavage site specificities: two *igaA* (*igaA1* and *igaA2*) and two *igaB* (*igaB1* and *igaB2*). The *igaA* is present in all NTHi whereas *igaB* is present in ~40% of the strains (226). The *igaB1* gene has been reported to be more prevalent in COPD exacerbation-causing strains, although the *in vivo* expression levels did not differ from asymptomatic colonization strains that also carried the gene (226). However, IgA-protease B1 and B2 have been found to promote the intracellular survival of NTHi in human epithelial cells, providing a secondary function (in addition to hydrolysis of IgA antibodies) that could facilitate NTHi growth in inflamed environments (227). While a majority of the persistent NTHi strains that dwell in COPD patients continuously express one or more variants of the enzyme, it has recently been found that a phase variation to an OFF-state can occur via slipped-strand mispairing over time (228). This suggests that during certain conditions, there is a fitness benefit in not expressing *iga* in the airways of COPD patients, albeit the specifics of this process are currently unknown.

Another interesting aspect of NTHi colonization of COPD patients is with regard to biofilm formation (229). NTHi strains

TABLE 1 | Abundance and significance of NTHi and other potentially pathogenic bacteria in healthy individuals and various stages of COPD using culture-based methods.

Sample type	Microbiological analysis	Main findings			Study
		Healthy individuals	**AECOPD[b]**	**Stable COPD disease**	
PSB[a]	Quantitative culture	Potentially pathogenic bacteria found in 4% of patients	Potentially pathogenic bacteria found in 54% of patients	Potentially pathogenic bacteria found in 29% of patients	Rosell et al. (148)
		NTHi found in 3% of patients	NTHi found in 30% of patients (predominating species)	NTHi found in 17% of patients (predominating species)	
BAL[c]	Quantitative culture	Potentially pathogenic bacteria found in 0% of ex-smokers and in 20% of non-smokers (no NTHi)	N.A.[d]	Potentially pathogenic bacteria found in 34% of patients	Sethi et al. (216)
				NTHi predominating species	
Sputum/Throat swab/PSB /BAL	Culture and molecular typing of strains	NTHi recovered in 35% of patients at any respiratory site	NTHi recovered in 7% of intubated patients with respiratory exacerbation	NTHi recovered in 57% of patients at any respiratory site	Bandi et al (217)
Sputum	Culture and molecular typing of strains	N.A.	Isolation of a new strain of NTHi significantly associated with exacerbation	N.A.	Sethi et al. (153)
			Patients with a new NTHi-strain twice as likely to have AECOPD		
Sputum	Quantitative culture	N.A.	Potentially pathogenic bacteria found in 70% of exacerbations	Potentially pathogenic bacteria found in 48% of patients	Wilkinson et al. (172)
			NTHi predominating species (38%)	NTHi predominating species (14%)	
Sputum	Quantitative culture	N.A.	Potentially pathogenic bacteria found in 55% of exacerbations	Potentially pathogenic bacteria found in 38% of cultures	Papi et al. (171)
			NTHi predominating species	NTHi predominating species	

[a] *PSB, protected specimen brush.*
[b] *AECOPD, acute exacerbation of COPD.*
[c] *BAL, bronchoalveolar lavage.*
[d] *N.A., not applicable.*

that colonize the Eustachian tube causing otitis media are known to build up biofilms *in situ* (230). However, strains isolated from COPD patients tend to have significantly diminished ability to form biofilm compared to invasive strains or those isolated from otitis media patients (229), suggesting that this mechanism is not important for survival in the COPD niche. As biofilms tend to protect the bacterial community from external assaults, these findings could indicate that the hypermucoid milieu in the COPD airways is severely impaired in its ability to deliver an apt immune response for optimal clearance of residing microorganisms. In light of this impairment, biofilm formation might not be necessary for NTHi to persist in this particular environment.

Infections with NTHi have also been shown to reduce cellular levels of E-cadherin, a protein required for tight junction formation and epithelial cell integrity in human cells (231). Considering that perturbations in the epithelial cell barrier caused by the loss of E-cadherin is a common symptom of COPD, NTHi-mediated exacerbations likely contribute to this step of COPD pathogenesis. The subsequent denuding of the epithelium could facilitate microbial colonization of the basal lamina, a well-established virulence mechanism employed by NTHi and other pathogens (232). It is currently unknown which bacterial virulence factor(s) that induce the reduction of E-cadherin levels in the host.

In summary, investigations from recent years show that the environment of the lower respiratory tract of COPD patients selects for NTHi strains that can upregulate adhesins, modify LOS biosynthesis pathways, increase antioxidant stress responses and cellular invasion strategies, and, finally, trigger tolerance against acidic pH. These important colonization mechanisms thus provide researchers with viable targets for developing novel therapies.

NTHi-DEPENDENT AIRWAY IMMUNE RESPONSES IN COPD

NTHi is a commensal in the nasopharyngeal site but is often associated with strong inflammatory responses in the lower respiratory airways, especially in patients with COPD, bronchiectasis, cystic fibrosis, pneumonia, or idiopathic pulmonary fibrosis (11, 233). Colonization and subsequent

TABLE 2 | Abundance and significance of NTHi and other potentially pathogenic bacteria in healthy individuals and various stages of COPD using molecular methods.

Sample	Microbiological analysis	Main findings			Study
		Healthy individuals	**Stable COPD disease**	**AECOPD**	
Sputum	16S rDNA	N.A.	Baseline[a]	Significant increase of the Proteobacteria phylum (which includes *Haemophilus* spp.)	Huang et al. (195)
Sputum	16S rDNA	N.A.	Baseline[a]	An increase in relative abundance of *Haemophilus* spp. as well as other bacteria typically associated with exacerbations	Millares et al. (218)
Sputum	16S rDNA	No increase in numbers of proteobacterial sequences following rhinovirus infection	N.A.	Significant increase in numbers of proteobacterial sequences, mainly *H. influenzae*, following Rhinovirus infection	Molyneaux et al. (190)
Sputum	16S rDNA	N.A.	Baseline[a]	An increase in the relative abundance of *Haemophilus* spp. following exacerbation, an increase of *Haemophilus* following corticosteroid treatment but a decrease after antibiotic treatment	Wang et al. (149)
Sputum	16S rDNA	N.A.	A significant increase in the abundance of *Haemophilus* with increasing disease severity	No significant increase in abundance of *Haemophilus* genera during exacerbation	Mayhew et al. (151)

[a]*Comparison of the microbiota sampled from a patient during stable disease (defined as baseline) and during an exacerbation.*

infection of NTHi in the lower airways of COPD patients elicits episodes of immune responses orchestrated by both the innate and adaptive immunity. NTHi infection is thus commonly associated with inflammation that is mainly mediated by transcription factor NF-κB-dependent production of proinflammatory mediators. The activation of NF-κB requires induction of cross-signaling networks and cascades via activation of PRRs (pattern recognition receptors) of host innate immune cells (234). Unresolved or prolonged (chronic) inflammation or failure to restore the homeostatic inflammatory status potentially contributes to exacerbations. This is clearly shown in murine COPD simulation models with NTHi-triggered inflammation (235–237). Mice exposed to NTHi lysates display inflamed airways loaded with increased levels of inflammatory mediators and phagocyte infiltrates. Moreover, multiple exposures to bacterial lysates which may represent a chronic NTHi infection caused extremely high infiltration of phagocytes and lymphocytes in the airways of this particular mouse model. In addition, the airway walls of the infected animals were also thickened due to increased collagen deposition (fibrosis) that reflects the typical COPD features. The host immune response and specific interactions during NTHi infection in COPD is summarized in **Figure 2**.

NTHi Stimulation of PRRs in Immune Activation

The epithelium and alveolar macrophages are predominant cell types in the airway compartment. They comprise the first line of defense in the cellular immune response against potential inhaled pathogens and antigens. The sensing of bacteria, and particularly NTHi in the lower airways is initiated via PRRs expressed on innate immune cells and endothelium in addition to epithelial cells (238–240). TLRs are PRRs that sense stimulation by NTHi-derived pathogen-associated molecular patterns (PAMPs), and play a primary role in initiating effector cellular responses and intracellular signaling for NF-κB activation (238). Among the different TLRs, most of the studies on NTHi infection have by far been focused on TLR2 and 4. Lipoproteins including NTHi P6, and LOS are potent immunomodulators for activation of TLR2 and TLR4, respectively, and has been described in several studies on airway epithelial cells and alveolar macrophages (241–244).

Interaction of NTHi lipoprotein P6 with TLR2 on human epithelial cells [type II alveolar A549 and human middle ear epithelial cells (HMEE)] causes NF-κB-dependent activation via two distinct TLR-signaling pathways, that is, the NF-κB translocation-dependent, and -independent pathways (242). The NF-κB nuclear translocation-dependent pathway requires activation of NF-κB-inducing kinase IKK complex. In the second pathway, the MKK3/6-p38 MAPK signaling cascade is recruited for direct nuclear phosphorylation, and thus activation of NF-κB. The branching of both pathways may occur at the TGF-β activated kinase 1 (TAK1) signaling junction. NTHi stimulation via TLR2 and downstream activation of p38 MAPK/NF-κB-dependent pathways result in expression of COX-2 and prostaglandin (E2) (PGE2) that promote inflammatory responses (245).

TLR4 stimulation by NTHi LOS also contributes to the activation of NF-κB via two signaling pathways, the primary activating pathway of MyD88 cascade and the alternative pathway of Toll/IL-1R domain-containing adapter-inducing interferon-β (TRIF). Both pathways activate NF-κB through phosphorylation and degradation of inhibitor IκBα (243, 246). NTHi-TLR4 signaling mediates an effective innate immune response that leads to upregulation of TNF-α, IL-1β, IL-6, macrophage-inflammatory protein (MIP)-1α, MIP-2, and neutrophil infiltration in the airways of mice. The TLR4 response promotes efficient pulmonary clearance of bacteria in TLR4-expressing animals compared to CD14/TLR4 knockout mice (243, 244). A recent study by Jungnickel et al. revealed that, in parallel with the infection-induced pulmonary neutrophilic inflammation, NTHi-dependent stimulation of both TLR2 and TLR4 in a transgenic mouse [($Kras^{LA1}$) with oncogenic Kras allele in the lung epithelium] additionally promotes the proliferation of Kras-induced early adenomatous lesion in the lung in an TLR-dependent manner (247). The association or role of NTHi-induced airway inflammation in lung cancer progression, however, is not supported by another recent cohort study showing the lack of differences in NTHi specific-antibodies between cancer- and non-cancer COPD patients (12).

Lastly, Dectin-1 and the epidermal growth factor receptor (EFGR) pathway also have proinflammtory effects upon interaction with NTHi (248, 249). Activation of the Dectin-dependent proinflammatory response requires NTHi-induced phosphorylation of the Dectin-1 hem-immunoreceptor tyrosine-based activation motif (hemITAM) (248). Direct activation of EFGR in alveolar cells and HMEE by NTHi-derived EGF-like factor has been shown to contribute to NF-κB activation. The EFGR-dependent NF-κB activation is mediated via an NF-κB nuclear translocation-independent pathway, which involves both MKK3/6-p38 and PI3K/Akt signaling pathways (249). Surprisingly, the interaction of EFGR and NTHi also results in negative regulation and suppression of the induction of TLR2 via the Src-MKK3/6-p38 α/β MAP kinase-dependent signaling cascade, and this in turn may facilitate NTHi infection (250). The actual components of NTHi that exhibit the EGF-like factor activity have, however, yet to be defined. The EFGR-dependent negative regulation of TLR2 may thus suggest a novel mechanism targeted by NTHi for immune evasion by attenuating the responses of host PRR, despite the contradicted role of EFGR in proinflammatory and innate immune responses of the airway epithelium (251). NTHi infection also upregulates the NRLP3-inflammasome during NTHi-induced inflammation in the airway epithelium and alveolar macrophages, leading to increased secretion of IL-1β and IL-8, and thus neutrophilic influx to the lung (252).

Synergetic Action of NTHi and Inflammatory Mediators

Some of the endogenous inflammatory mediators that are produced in response to NTHi infection, including TNF-α, IL-1α, and TGF-β1, may act synergetically with NTHi on the airway epithelial and immune cells. The synergetic interaction drives a positive feedback loop to amplify the NF-κB transcriptional activity on proinflammatory genes and further augments airway inflammation.

The synergetic activation of NF-κB by NTHi and TNF-α in HMEE and normal human bronchial epithelial (NHBE) cells occurs via NF-κB nuclear translocation-dependent and independent pathways. The latter pathway involves MAPK/extracellular signal regulated kinase kinase kinase 1 (MEKK1)-dependent activation of MAPK kinase 3/6-p38 MAPK pathway (253). However, the synergetic action of NTHi with TGF-β1 is mediated by another mechanism which involves Smad3/4-protein kinase A (PKA)-p300-dependent signaling cascade. The pathway components, PKA and p300, phosphorylates residue Ser276 and acetylates Lys221 of the NF-κB subunit p65, respectively. This results in enhanced DNA-binding activity of NF-κB (254).

The synergetic action of NTHi with both TNF-α and TGF-β1 enhances the production of TNF-α, IL-1β, and IL-8 from airway epithelial cells and interstitial polymorphonuclear infiltrates. Recently, it has been reported that co-infection of human rhinovirus and NTHi on the airway epithelial cells (NHBE cells and the BEAS-2B cell line) also results in synergetic induction of CCL20 and IL-8, albeit the exact mechanism remains to be elucidated (255). Of note, activated macrophages also release increased concentrations of TNF-α and IL-1α (256), further enhancing the inflammatory synergetic effect of surrounding immune cells.

Finally, IL-1α acts synergetically with NTHi to upregulate the expression of AMP β-defensin 2 (DEFB-4) via the p38/MAPK pathway (257). Of note, IL-1α could also act individually to upregulate the expression of DEFB-4 via the Src-dependent MEK1/2-ERK1/2 signaling pathway (258). Taken together, the synergetic action may aid in the expansion of the inflammatory response and in some cases worsen the clinical outcome.

Phagocytosis of NTHi by Airway Phagocytes

Alveolar macrophages located in the air-parenchyma interface are the primary professional phagocytes in the lung (259, 260). These cells are responsible for infection eradication through its phagolysosomal machinery while releasing a plethora of inflammatory cytokines and chemokines for promoting a local inflammatory response and recruitment of neutrophils. Neutrophils are the first responder cells recruited from circulation to the airway for efficient killing of pathogens through an array of microbicidal strategies (261, 262). During NTHi lung infection, both alveolar macrophages and neutrophils are the main innate immune cells involved in the pulmonary bacterial clearance through phagocytosis. They are also an important source of cytokine secretion required for induction of other immune cells and enhanced bacterial killing. Eradication of NTHi by alveolar macrophages involves adhesion or contact, phagocytosis and phagolysosomal processing of bacteria, in addition to secretion of TNF-α. Phagocytic clearance of NTHi by alveolar macrophages is orchestrated through actin polymerization, plasma membrane lipid rafts, and phosphatidylinositol 3-kinase (PI3K) signaling cascade upon induction of macrophage PRRs by NTHi (256).

Interestingly, in response to NTHi infection, human alveolar macrophages, and blood neutrophils produce extensive amount of intracellular and extracellular ROS as a component of the antimicrobial defense. This leads to the formation of macrophage and neutrophil extracellular traps (METs and NETs, respectively), with co-expression of MMP-12 for enhanced bacterial killing (263, 264). Nevertheless, the overexpression of MMPs may adversely result in a protease imbalance and contribute to alveolar emphysematous destruction and bronchiectasis in COPD (265). Moreover, excessive endogenous ROS production could also introduce airway oxidative stress that is detrimental by causing chronic inflammation and tissue damage in the lung, and thus contributing to the COPD exacerbation (266, 267). The NET formation is elicited mainly by NTHi LOS in addition to other *Haemophilus* PAMPs (264).

Cellular and Humoral Immunity in NTHi Evasion

Several studies by King et al. have revealed that T cell-mediated adaptive immune responses against NTHi airway infection in patients with idiopathic bronchiectasis and COPD has been predominated by a Th2/Tc2 response (268–270). The activated T cells produce reduced level of the CD40 ligand and IFN-γ, and increased levels of TNF-α, IL-13, and IL-17, as well as altered IgG subclass production by plasma cells. It is to be noted that the Th2/Tc2-mediated immune response is less effective in suppressing NTHi infection. Redirecting the Th2/Tc2-mediated immune response to Thl/Tcl dominant (which is more protective) by adding the Thl/Tcl mediators (CD40 ligand and IFN-γ) has helped to restore the T cell-mediated immune killing of NTHi (269). However, a separate study in a COPD mouse model by Lu *et al.* reported that NTHi infection causes increased production of airway type 1 interferon (1-IFN) (271). It was further reported that DNA of NTHi acts as a PAMP in stimulating the STING/TBK1/IRF3 pathway, and thus the production of 1-IFN. The impact of the bacterial DNA-induced 1-IFN in host immune/inflammatory response, which may potentially induce a Thl/Tcl response requires further investigations.

COPD patients also have abnormally higher number of Treg cells, myeloid-derived suppressor cells (MDSC), and exhausted effector T cells (PD-1$^+$) than healthy individuals (272, 273). Cigarette smoke-induced anti-inflammatory activity of Tregs in a COPD model is further suppressed by NTHi infection. The pathogen causes downregulation of Foxp3 (biomarker of Tregs), and thus impairs the anti-inflammatory/pro-inflammatory balance of Tregs (273, 274). This may lead to the extensive immunosuppressive activity by Tregs on the proliferation of NTHi P6-specific effector T cells, causing a diminished response of effector T cells to sputum IL-6 and IL-8 induction, and increased levels of IL-10 and TGF-β1 (272, 275). Recently, it has been reported that mucosal-associated invariant T cells (MAIT) from COPD patients are more effective in response to NTHi stimulation and thus produce increased levels of IFN-γ, 3-, to 10-fold more than the COPD Th (CD4$^+$) and Tc (CD8$^+$) cells (276). However, the pulmonary MAIT cell immune responses are compromised in the presence of corticosteroids that are commonly used for the treatment of COPD. This may potentially prone the T cell-mediated immunity to a Th2/Tc2 response in COPD patients treated with corticosteroids (277). Interestingly, antigen-specific Th17 cells from NTHi-immunized non-COPD mice model recognize both homologous and heterologous strains of NTHi, and are able to confer protection upon adoptive transfer (278). However, it is unclear whether the Th17 cell which is prone to the inflammatory response could be "trained" to counteract the NTHi infection in COPD patients, particularly during exacerbations.

During the systemic humoral immune response in NTHi-infected COPD patients, greater concentrations of NTHi-specific IgG, IgA, IgM, and IgE serum antibodies are produced compared to non-infected controls (12, 279–281). Some of the NTHi-specific serum immunoglobulins are specific to P2, P5, and P6 (12, 282, 283). However, decreased mucosal antibodies associated with sIgA deficiency, or decreased total IgG in the small airways have been reported in COPD patients, and might be associated with disease severity (283, 284). Importantly, NTHi-specific mucosal sIgA has been found to be lower in the airways of NTHi-infected COPD patients than the non-colonized patients (285, 286).

The epithelial polymeric immunoglobulin receptor (pIgR) is essential for the generation of mucosal sIgA. It is, however, downregulated in COPD patients with a positive correlation to disease severity and increased level of TGF-β (287). The combinatorial effects of downregulated *pIg*R and elevated TGF-β1 contribute to an impaired mucosal IgA immunity in COPD patients. A mouse model lacking the *pIg*R ($^{-/-}$) is therefore devoid of sIgA and are susceptible to airway stimulation by an NTHi lysate resulting in increased inflammation and airway neutrophilia. Interestingly, introduction of exogenously added sIgA mitigated the airway inflammation (288). NTHi-infected COPD patients with greater airway inflammation have also decreased NTHi-specific mucosal IgG1 in the BAL fluid compared to the non-colonized patients (283). Interestingly, the phenomenon with decreased NTHi-specific antibodies seems to be restricted to the airways, since the specific serum antibodies are not affected. Therefore, the reduced mucosal IgG is unlikely to be associated with hypogammaglobulinemia (IgG deficiency), despite the latter was reported as a contributing factor in NTHi infection (289). Decreased airway IgA might be attributed to the expression of IgA proteases by NTHi. The bacterial IgA protease degrades the local airway IgA during airway colonization to avoid immune exclusion by sIgA (226, 228). Reduced mucosal antibodies might promote host immune evasion and resistance to complement-mediated killing of NTHi, thus enable persistent colonization of NTHi in the airways of COPD patients, in addition to a plethora of various other virulence mechanisms (4, 5, 207).

IMPAIRED IMMUNITY IN COPD IN RESPONSE TO NTHi INFECTION—CURRENTLY KNOWN MECHANISMS

In a cohort study of stable COPD patients, augmented airway inflammation and plasma fibrinogen, but not systemic inflammation, were found to be constantly correlated with the increased bacterial load (233). Higher numbers of NTHi has a greater impact than *S. pneumoniae* and *M. catarrhalis* in triggering inflammatory responses as measured by the augmented levels of inflammatory cytokines in sputum including IL-8, MPO, and 1L-1β. The increased inflammatory response in affected patients is potentially attributed to the persistent colonization of NTHi in the lower airway (207, 233). The compromised innate immune response in COPD, particularly the decreased microbicidal activity, has been regarded as one of the culprits for persistent airway colonization by NTHi, and is highly associated with COPD exacerbations (**Figure 2**).

TLR Tolerance: Unresponsive to NTHi Antigen Stimulation

Whilst the role of macrophage extracellular traps (MET) for killing of NTHi remains unknown, it has been reported that blood neutrophils and NET from COPD patients are defective in the killing of planktonic or biofilm/NET-entrapped NTHi, respectively (263, 264, 290). A series of studies by Berenson et al. revealed that alveolar macrophages derived from COPD patients are basically dysfunctional in eradication of NTHi (177, 291–293). Intriguingly, TLR2 and TLR4 expressed on alveolar macrophages from COPD patients are intrinsically unresponsive to the potent immunomodulatory lipoprotein P6 and LOS, respectively. This causes decreased LOS/P6-induced expression of TLRs, reduced NF-κB nuclear activation and consequently diminished IL-8, TNF-α, and IL-1β responses by alveolar macrophages from COPD patients. The compromised TLR expression and signaling potentially contribute to the defective complement-dependent and independent phagocytosis of NTHi. The defective phagocytosis is greater for NTHi than for *M. catarrhalis*, and correlates with disease severity. Interestingly, the phagocytosis disability was not detected in monocyte-derived macrophages in COPD. In contrast, however, Taylor et al. reported that monocyte-derived macrophages from COPD patients are also defective in phagocytosis of NTHi and *S. pneumoniae.* The author also suggested that the defective monocyte-derived macrophages are not attributed to the alteration in cell surface TLR2 or TLR4 expression, macrophage receptor with collagenous structure (MARCO), CD163, CD36 or the mannose receptor (178). The unresponsive TLR2 and TLR4 in COPD alveolar macrophages to NTHi lipoprotein and LOS might be explained by the recently reported phenomenon of TLR tolerance (294). Repetitive stimulation of COPD alveolar macrophages with the same TLR ligands, Pam3CSK4 and LPS desensitizes the TLR2 and TLR4, respectively, and generates TLR tolerance. Moreover, the repetitive TLR stimulation further reduced the production of TNF-α, CCL5, and IL-10 without affecting the constantly augmented level of IL-6 and IL-8 in alveolar macrophages. This may provide alternative explanations for diminished immune responses against the recurrent/repetitive infection by NTHi.

Altered and Abnormal TLR/PRR Expression: Inaccurate Responses to NTHi

The intrinsically reduced expression of TLRs in COPD patients may also contribute to the impaired pulmonary immune response thus facilitating NTHi persistent colonization. Expression of TLR2 or TLR4 are found to be lower on sputum neutrophils, alveolar macrophages, nasal epithelium, and T cells in COPD patients despite high concentrations of IL-8 and MMP-9 (295–298).

The lack of the more protective Thl/Tcl immune response in COPD patients against NTHi infection might be attributed to upregulated antagonists (A20, IRAK-M, and MyD88s) of the MyD88/IRAK/MAPK signaling pathway in COPD T cells (295). It should be noted that the MyD88/IRAK/MAPK pathway is required for expression of TLR4 in Thl, whereas production of IFN-γ in Thl/Tcl is TLR4-dependent via the TLR4/TRIF/IKKe/TBK1 signaling pathway. The antagonists prevent the NTHi LOS-induced TLR4 expression in Thl and Tcl and thus a reduced secretion of IFN-γ. In addition, unusual high numbers of Tregs in COPD patients have also contributed to effector T cell dysfunction or a Th2/Tc2 predominant immune response (272). However, Freeman et al. reported that Tc ($CD8^+$) cells from COPD patients have increased expression of TLR1, TLR2, TLR4, TLR6, and TLR2/1 as well as Tcl cytokines (IFN-γ and TNF-α) compared to healthy individuals that may imply the auto-aggressive response of lung Tc cells in COPD lung inflammation (299). However, the COPD Tc cells can only be stimulated by ligands for TLR2/1 (Pam3CSK4) yet tolerant to other agonists, indicating the dysfunctional TLRs or TLR tolerance on T cells despite their high level of receptor expression.

Inversely, peripheral blood neutrophils isolated from COPD patients have increased expression of TLR2, TLR4, and NLRP3 (298, 300). Nevertheless, the increased TLRs expression might not improve the microbicidal ability of COPD peripheral neutrophils probably due to the inaccurate responses to cytokines (179). In addition, certain types of SNPs (SNPs) in TLR2 and TLR4 have also been associated with decreased lung function, enhanced inflammatory responses and increased immune cell infiltration in COPD (301). Interestingly, the diminished IL-8 responsiveness of COPD alveolar macrophage to NTHi infection has a strong association with the carriage of TLR9 (T1237C) polymorphism instead of TLR2 (Arg753Gln), TLR4 (Thr399Ile; Asp299Gly), and TLR9 (T1486C) (302). The carriage of TLR9 (T1237C) is also positively correlated with diminished lung function. Of note, the activation of TLR9-signaling cascade in pro-inflammatory cytokine response requires stimulation from microbial DNA (303).

The Tobacco Smoke: Negative Effects on the Immune Defense Against NTHi

The microbicidal malfunction in both innate and adaptive immune cells is also potentially linked to the deleterious effect of tobacco smoke, the major risk factor for COPD. It has been reported that, exposure of tobacco or cigarette smoke can impair phagocytosis/engulfment of NTHi by alveolar macrophages isolated from COPD patients (256, 304). Moreover, the chemical exposure also suppressed the TLR-induced TNF-α, IL-6, and IL-10 production in COPD alveolar macrophages that have been pre-stimulated with TLR2, 4, or 5 ligands (Pam3CSK4, LPS, or phase I flagellin, respectively), or whole NTHi bacteria (305). This may potentially delay the macrophage-dependent bacterial clearance. The suppressive effect of cigarette smoke in macrophage-dependent phagocytosis is due to the suppression of the PI3K signaling cascade which is required for optimal phagocytic activity and movement (256). Meanwhile, the cigarette smoke also inhibits the activation of the p38-ERK signaling pathway and p65/NF-κB, thus dampens the NTHi LOS-induced cytokine production of COPD alveolar macrophages (305). The diminished alveolar macrophage responsiveness could also be related to anticholinergic agents used by COPD patients that results in lower concentrations of NTHi-induced TNF-α (306). Nevertheless, the impaired phagocytosis of NTHi by COPD alveolar macrophages could be improved in the presence of nuclear erythroid related factor 2 and microRNA MiR-328 (307, 308). Interestingly, in addition to the constant exacerbated inflammatory effect observed in different murine model studies, Gaschler et al. observed a rapid pulmonary clearance of NTHi in mice upon exposure to cigarette smoke, and this was positively correlated with an increased neutrophilia in the animal BAL fluid (236, 309–311). However, in other COPD animal studies, cigarette smoke also impaired the IL-22 production that has a potential anti-bacterial activity while delaying the airway clearance of NTHi (311–313). Interestingly, IL-22 might play a protective role in COPD exacerbation as supplementation of IL-22 manages to restore the homeostasis of airway immune response and improve NTHi clearance (313).

The increased airway neutrophilia might be due to the enhanced production of pulmonary IL-17 triggered by cigarette smoke (152, 236, 311, 314). This may imply the important microbicidal role of neutrophils (neutrophilia) in compensating the COPD- or cigarette smoke-associated dysfunctional alveolar macrophages (96, 315). However, such compensation may not be adequate to provide optimal immune defense to eradicate persistent NTHi lower airway colonization, since the cigarette smoke also has profound suppressive effect on the host adaptive immunity, thus constantly risking the COPD patients to episodes of exacerbation and relapsed infection. In adaptive immunity, cigarette smoke impairs the antigen-specific B and T cells responses to NTHi infection. It suppresses the secretion of IFN-γ and IL-4 by NTHi-specific T cells. Antibody production by B cells has also been attenuated, with lower levels of specific anti-P6 antibodies and compromised IgG1, IgG2a, and IgA class switching (311, 312).

A recent and some previous cohort studies revealed that the level of airway antimicrobial cathelicidin (hCAP18/LL-37) in COPD patients increase gradually from the stable disease to exacerbation states (176, 316). Moreover, higher levels of cathelicidin are positively associated with NTHi airway colonization, sputum neutrophilia, and higher concentrations of IL-8, particularly in the NTHi-infected COPD patients. Of note, cathelicidin and other AMPs play important roles in the innate immune defense against different pathogens and persist immunomodulatory properties (317–319). Ironically, it is plausible that the increased level of cathelicidin could diminish or alter the balance in lung microbiota, and the immune/inflammatory response. This might contribute to the "vicious circle," thus considerably increasing the risk for NTHi infection during COPD exacerbations (214, 320). Moreover, the microbicidal property of cathelicidin could be compromised by the inflammatory conditions in the airway, such as low pH, or the effect of cigarettes that causes peptide citrulination and modification (321, 322). Finally, expression of AMPs (human beta defensin 2 and S100A7) by COPD airway epithelium in response to NTHi infection, is also disturbed by cigarette smoke. The insulted airway cells have also a reduced expression of TLR4 and IL-8, and impaired NTHi-induced NF-κB activation (175, 296). Thus, a large body of evidence exists on the deleterious effects of tobacco smoke.

ANTIBIOTIC TREATMENT OF NTHi IN COPD

Antibiotic treatment of AECOPD has been shown to significantly reduce the risk of treatment failure, especially for in-patients with severe exacerbations and patients requiring intensive care (323). The efficacity of antibiotic treatment for out-patients with exacerbations is less clear (323, 324).

Recommendations on which empirical treatment to use for AECOPD varies between different countries, but common antimicrobial agents that are frequently used as definitive therapy against NTHi include aminopenicillins (with or without a beta-lactamase inhibitor), tetracyclines, trimethoprim-sulfamethoxazole, and fluoroquinolones. In addition, the Clinical and Laboratory Standards Institute (CLSI) has developed clinical breakpoints for the macrolides azithromycin and clarithromycin (325), whereas the European Committee on Antimicrobial Susceptibility Testing (EUCAST) have not set any clinical breakpoints against this class of antibiotics due to lack of clinical data (326). One study shows that NTHi frequently develops resistance to macrolides during prolonged treatment and that treatment failure may occur, making fluoroquinolones more reliable for eradication in COPD-patients (327). As for aminopenicillins, resistance is also common, with up to 10–20% of NTHi isolates expressing beta-lactamases and an additional 10–20% of the isolates having amino acid substitutions in penicillin-binding protein 3 (PBP3), which reduces their susceptibility to these agents (328, 329). The fraction of isolates expressing beta-lactamases has been stable during the last years, whereas an increase has been seen in isolates displaying altered PBP3 (330, 331). This is worrisome, since some of these amino acid substitutions also confer resistance to third generation cephalosporins (332). Moreover, there seems to be a correlation between isolates expressing altered PBP3 and increased invasiveness. Studies have shown that strains that express a mutated PBP3 with certain key amino acid substitution have a significantly higher rate of invasion of bronchial epithelial cells compared to strains with a wild type PBP3 (333). However, when such mutated PBP3 was cloned into a susceptible wild type strain, invasion efficacy did not increase, suggesting that PBP3 is only indirectly linked to invasion (334).

Besides using antibiotics for acute management of COPD exacerbations, some studies have considered the use of continuous prophylactic antibiotics in the management of patients with COPD (212). There is some evidence that continuous administration of macrolide antibiotics would prevent future exacerbations in a selected population of the most severely ill patients, but a Cochrane review revealed no support for a reduced all-cause mortality or less hospital readmissions (335). However, more recent studies have shown a significant decrease in both the frequency of exacerbations and hospitalizations when long-term azithromycin treatment was chosen (336).

The fact that macrolide antibiotics display not only antimicrobial effects, but also have anti-inflammatory and immunomodulatory properties, has made them interesting to use as prophylactic therapy (212). It has been shown that azithromycin inhibits mucus hypersecretion in the respiratory tract by significantly inhibiting TNF-α induction of the MUC5AC mucin secretion from human nasal epithelial cells (337). More specifically, it has been shown that azithromycin can reduce the NTHi-dependent induction of MUC5AC expression by suppressing the transcription factor activator protein-1 (338). Apart from affecting mucus secretion, it also seems that low-dose azithromycin has the ability to improve phagocytosis of bacteria by airway macrophages (339). One study showed that azithromycin concentrations that were unable to kill NTHi still increased the uptake rate of the bacteria into alveolar macrophages by enhancing their phagocytic function (340). However, the risk of development of antimicrobial resistance limits the use of low-dose azithromycin solely for its immunological properties. This has triggered an interest in finding new macrolide substances that lack antibiotic effect and solely interact with the airway immune system (341).

PERSPECTIVE IN NTHi VACCINE DEVELOPMENT

The considerable clinical problems caused by NTHi with regard to COPD exacerbations and otitis media has prompted the scientific community to investigate whether a vaccine can be developed against the pathogen (5, 58, 342). The search has been intensified due to a steady increase in antibiotic resistance and a trend of more invasive infections caused by NTHi over the last decade (5). Whereas, a highly efficient glycoconjugate vaccine has previously been developed against Hib, an identical strategy cannot be employed against NTHi due to the lack of a polysaccharide capsule. Vaccine developments efforts have thus been concentrated on identifying NTHi surface structures that are immunogenic, have low antigenic variability, and are conserved across this genetically highly heterogeneous species. Several promising vaccine candidates have been identified in the last 25 years, as excellently reviewed elsewhere (58, 342).

Two of these antigens, fused into one protein, Protein E-PilA, are together with Protein D currently being tested by GlaxoSmithKline in a phase IIb proof-of-concept clinical trial (randomized, observer-blind, placebo-controlled, and multicentric) for infection prophylaxis in COPD patients (50–70 years old) (5). Notably, the *M. catarrhalis* ubiquitous surface protein A2 (UspA2) is also included in the vaccine so that an immune response against both exacerbation-causing pathogens could be elicited by the same preparation. This clinical study (NCT03281876) is the only one currently being conducted on NTHi (and *M. catarrhalis*) according to clinicaltrials.gov, and as the investigations are on-going, the results are currently unknown.

Due to an increase in the difficulty to treat NTHi infections, an efficient and protective NTHi vaccine likely considerably raises the quality of life of COPD patients. Since NTHi-mediated exacerbations contribute to the progression of the disease and a steady deterioration of the pulmonary capacity of those patients, prevention against NTHi infections potentially slows down the debilitating effect of the disease. It is therefore critical to continue this line of research until such a vaccine has been obtained. It could also be worth targeting non-conventional structures with a vaccine, such as the secreted enzymes urease and IgA1-protease that have proven important for NTHi infections in COPD patients in several studies (222).

CONCLUSIONS

COPD is a multifaceted airway disease. Several factors influence the clinical outcome of COPD. Importantly, the crosstalk between intrinsic factors (the stability and integrity of the airway immune response and structure in addition to hereditary factors), and the extrinsic factors (lung microbiome, viral and bacterial infections, meteorological factors, and noxious inhalation) determines the fate of lower airway opportunistic infection by *H. influenzae*. Intriguingly, NTHi has been one of the most isolated pathogens at both stable and exacerbation states of COPD. Such persistent airway colonization of NTHi costs virulence fitness to counteract with the bactericidal effect of the host immune response. Adversely, the impaired defense mechanisms in COPD are not only unable to protect the lung structure from inhaled physical assaults, but they also fail to suppress NTHi infection. The disoriented immune response in COPD instead allows the pathogen to cause more harm and inflammation in the airways. The currently used bronchodilator and inhaled corticosteroid therapies have limited efficacy in preventing disease progression in COPD. Moreover, the inhaled corticosteroid therapies might have side effects that may weaken the immune response. Hence, more investigations are needed to garner a more adequate knowledge regarding the variabilities in immune networking of COPD. This knowledge will be an important platform for a more efficient drug design. In addition, a vaccine targeting NTHi is another important approach in controlling the infective exacerbations in COPD as the antibiotic treatment is also getting dampened by the emergence of NTHi antibiotic resistance.

AUTHOR CONTRIBUTIONS

Y-CS coordinated and drafted the major part of the manuscript, and prepared the figures; FJ participated in the literature study of virulence and vaccine research of NTHi; JT prepared the review section for NTHi epidemiology in COPD and antibiotic studies; Y-CS and KR edited and critically revised the manuscript. All authors read and approved the final manuscript.

ACKNOWLEDGMENTS

We thank the following funding agencies for their financial support during the preparation of the manuscript. They are the Alfred Österlund, the Anna and Edwin Berger, the Swedish Medical Research Council (grant number K2015-57X-03163-43-4, www.vr.se), the Physiographical Society (Forssman's Foundation and, Endowments for the Natural Sciences, Medicine and Technology), Skåne County Council's research and development foundation, and Heart Lung Foundation (KR: grant number 20150697, www.hjart-lungfonden.se).

REFERENCES

1. Charlson ES, Bittinger K, Haas AR, Fitzgerald AS, Frank I, Yadav A, et al. Topographical continuity of bacterial populations in the healthy human respiratory tract. *Am J Respir Crit Care Med.* (2011) 184:957–63. doi: 10.1164/rccm.201104-0655OC
2. Dickson RP, Erb-Downward JR, Freeman CM, McCloskey L, Falkowski NR, Huffnagle GB, et al. Bacterial topography of the healthy human lower respiratory tract. *MBio* (2017) 8:e02287-16. doi: 10.1128/mBio.02287-16
3. Man WH, de Steenhuijsen Piters WA, Bogaert D. The microbiota of the respiratory tract: gatekeeper to respiratory health. *Nat Rev Microbiol.* (2017) 15:259–70. doi: 10.1038/nrmicro.2017.14
4. Duell BL, Su YC, Riesbeck K. Host-pathogen interactions of nontypeable *Haemophilus influenzae*: from commensal to pathogen. *FEBS Lett.* (2016) 590:3840–53. doi: 10.1002/1873-3468.12351
5. Jalalvand F, Riesbeck K. Update on non-typeable *Haemophilus influenzae*-mediated disease and vaccine development. *Expert Rev Vaccines* (2018) 17:503–12. doi: 10.1080/14760584.2018.1484286
6. Slack MPE. The evidence for non-typeable *Haemophilus influenzae* as a causative agent of childhood pneumonia. *Pneumonia (Nathan)* (2017) 9:9. doi: 10.1186/s41479-017-0033-2
7. Pizzutto SJ, Hare KM, Upham JW. Bronchiectasis in children: current concepts in immunology and microbiology. *Front Pediatr.* (2017) 5:123. doi: 10.3389/fped.2017.00123
8. Cardines R, Giufre M, Pompilio A, Fiscarelli E, Ricciotti G, Di Bonaventura G, et al. *Haemophilus influenzae* in children with cystic fibrosis: antimicrobial susceptibility, molecular epidemiology, distribution of adhesins and biofilm formation. *Int J Med Microbiol.* (2012) 302:45–52. doi: 10.1016/j.ijmm.2011.08.003
9. Azadeh N, Limper AH, Carmona EM, Ryu JH. The role of infection in interstitial lung diseases: a review. *Chest* (2017) 152:842–52. doi: 10.1016/j.chest.2017.03.033
10. Garzoni C, Brugger SD, Qi W, Wasmer S, Cusini A, Dumont P, et al. Microbial communities in the respiratory tract of patients with interstitial lung disease. *Thorax* (2013) 68:1150–6. doi: 10.1136/thoraxjnl-2012-202917
11. Sethi S, Murphy TF. Infection in the pathogenesis and course of chronic obstructive pulmonary disease. *N Engl J Med.* (2008) 359:2355–65. doi: 10.1056/NEJMra0800353
12. Sriram KB, Cox AJ, Sivakumaran P, Singh M, Watts AM, West NP, et al. Non-typeable *Haemophilus influenzae* detection in the lower airways of patients with lung cancer and chronic obstructive pulmonary disease. *Multidiscip Respir Med.* (2018) 13:11. doi: 10.1186/s40248-018-0123-x
13. Ferkol T, Schraufnagel D. The global burden of respiratory disease. *Ann Am Thorac Soc.* (2014) 11:404–6. doi: 10.1513/AnnalsATS.201311-405PS
14. Diaz-Guzman E, Mannino DM. Epidemiology and prevalence of chronic obstructive pulmonary disease. *Clin Chest Med.* (2014) 35:7–16. doi: 10.1016/j.ccm.2013.10.002
15. GOLD-Report. Global strategy for diagnosis, management, and prevention of chronic obstructive pulmonary disease (2018 Report). in *Global Initiative for Chronic Obstructive Lung Disease.* Agusti AG, Vogelmeier C, editor (2018). Available online at: http://goldcopd.org
16. Chung KF, Adcock IM. Multifaceted mechanisms in COPD: inflammation, immunity, and tissue repair and destruction. *Eur Respir J.* (2008) 31:1334–56. doi: 10.1183/09031936.00018908
17. Barbu C, Iordache M, Man MG. Inflammation in COPD: pathogenesis, local and systemic effects. *Rom J Morphol Embryol.* (2011) 52:21–7.
18. Barnes PJ, Burney PG, Silverman EK, Celli BR, Vestbo J, Wedzicha JA, et al. Chronic obstructive pulmonary disease. *Nat Rev Dis Primers* (2015) 1:15076. doi: 10.1038/nrdp.2015.76
19. Rabe KF, Watz H. Chronic obstructive pulmonary disease. *Lancet* (2017) 389:1931–40. doi: 10.1016/S0140-6736(17)31222-9
20. Fabbri LM, Luppi F, Beghe B, Rabe KF. Complex chronic comorbidities of COPD. *Eur Respir J.* (2008) 31:204–12. doi: 10.1183/09031936.00114307
21. Huertas A, Palange P. COPD: a multifactorial systemic disease. *Ther Adv Respir Dis.* (2011) 5:217–24. doi: 10.1177/1753465811400490
22. Mannino DM, Buist AS. Global burden of COPD: risk factors, prevalence, and future trends. *Lancet* (2007) 370:765–73. doi: 10.1016/S0140-6736(07)61380-4
23. Strzelak A, Ratajczak A, Adamiec A, Feleszko W. Tobacco smoke induces and alters immune responses in the lung triggering inflammation, allergy, asthma and other lung diseases: a mechanistic review. *Int J Environ Res Public Health* (2018) 15:E1033. doi: 10.3390/ijerph15051033
24. Imaoka H, Hoshino T. Bronchial asthma: progress in diagnosis and treatments. Topics: II. Pathogenesis and pathophysiology; 1. The Dutch hypothesis and British hypothesis. *Nihon Naika Gakkai Zasshi* (2013) 102:1359–64. doi: 10.2169/naika.102.1359
25. Primhak RA, Tanner MS. Alpha-1 antitrypsin deficiency. *Arch Dis Child.* (2001) 85:2–5. doi: 10.1136/adc.85.1.2
26. Rodriguez-Revenga L, Iranzo P, Badenas C, Puig S, Carrio A, Mila M. A novel elastin gene mutation resulting in an autosomal dominant form of cutis laxa. *Arch Dermatol.* (2004) 140:1135–9. doi: 10.1001/archderm.140.9.1135
27. Cho MH, McDonald ML, Zhou X, Mattheisen M, Castaldi PJ, Hersh CP, et al. Risk loci for chronic obstructive pulmonary disease: a genome-wide association study and meta-analysis. *Lancet Respir Med.* (2014) 2:214–25. doi: 10.1016/S2213-2600(14)70002-5
28. Lee SR, Kim WT, Kim TN, Nam JK, Kim WJ, Leem SH. Association between the length of the MUC8-minisatellite 5 region and susceptibility to chronic obstructive pulmonary disease (COPD). *Genes Genomics* (2018) 40:123–7. doi: 10.1007/s13258-017-0630-8
29. Smith BM, Traboulsi H, Austin JHM, Manichaikul A, Hoffman EA, Bleecker ER, et al. Human airway branch variation and chronic obstructive pulmonary disease. *Proc Natl Acad Sci USA.* (2018) 115:E974–81. doi: 10.1073/pnas.1715564115
30. Jackson VE, Ntalla I, Sayers I, Morris R, Whincup P, Casas JP, et al. Exome-wide analysis of rare coding variation identifies novel associations with COPD and airflow limitation in MOCS3, IFIT3 and SERPINA12. *Thorax* (2016) 71:501–9. doi: 10.1136/thoraxjnl-2015-207876
31. D'Anna C, Cigna D, Di Sano C, Di Vincenzo S, Dino P, Ferraro M, et al. Exposure to cigarette smoke extract and lipopolysaccharide modifies cytoskeleton organization in bronchial epithelial cells. *Exp Lung Res.* (2017) 43:347–58. doi: 10.1080/01902148.2017.1377784
32. Aghapour M, Raee P, Moghaddam SJ, Hiemstra PS, Heijink IH. Airway epithelial barrier dysfunction in chronic obstructive pulmonary disease: role

of cigarette smoke exposure. *Am J Respir Cell Mol Biol.* (2018) 58:157–69. doi: 10.1165/rcmb.2017-0200TR

33. Lapperre TS, Sont JK, van Schadewijk A, Gosman MM, Postma DS, Bajema IM, et al. Smoking cessation and bronchial epithelial remodelling in COPD: a cross-sectional study. *Respir Res.* (2007) 8:85. doi: 10.1186/1465-9921-8-85
34. Perotin JM, Adam D, Vella-Boucaud J, Delepine G, Sandu S, Jonvel AC, et al. Delay of airway epithelial wound repair in COPD is associated with airflow obstruction severity. *Respir Res.* (2014) 15:151. doi: 10.1186/s12931-014-0151-9
35. Papi A, Casoni G, Caramori G, Guzzinati I, Boschetto P, Ravenna F, et al. COPD increases the risk of squamous histological subtype in smokers who develop non-small cell lung carcinoma. *Thorax* (2004) 59:679–81. doi: 10.1136/thx.2003.018291
36. Cosio M, Ghezzo H, Hogg JC, Corbin R, Loveland M, Dosman J, et al. The relations between structural changes in small airways and pulmonary-function tests. *N Engl J Med.* (1978) 298:1277–81. doi: 10.1056/NEJM197806082982303
37. Burgstaller G, Oehrle B, Gerckens M, White ES, Schiller HB, Eickelberg O. The instructive extracellular matrix of the lung: basic composition and alterations in chronic lung disease. *Eur Respir J.* (2017) 50:1601805. doi: 10.1183/13993003.01805-2016
38. Vogel ER, VanOosten SK, Holman MA, Hohbein DD, Thompson MA, Vassallo R, et al. Cigarette smoke enhances proliferation and extracellular matrix deposition by human fetal airway smooth muscle. *Am J Physiol Lung Cell Mol Physiol.* (2014) 307:L978–86. doi: 10.1152/ajplung.00111.2014
39. Kranenburg AR, Willems-Widyastuti A, Moori WJ, Sterk PJ, Alagappan VK, de Boer WI, et al. Enhanced bronchial expression of extracellular matrix proteins in chronic obstructive pulmonary disease. *Am J Clin Pathol.* (2006) 126:725–35. doi: 10.1309/JC477FAEL1YKV54W7
40. van Straaten JF, Coers W, Noordhoek JA, Huitema S, Flipsen JT, Kauffman HF, et al. Proteoglycan changes in the extracellular matrix of lung tissue from patients with pulmonary emphysema. *Mod Pathol.* (1999) 12:697–705.
41. Ahrman E, Hallgren O, Malmstrom L, Hedstrom U, Malmstrom A, Bjermer L, et al. Quantitative proteomic characterization of the lung extracellular matrix in chronic obstructive pulmonary disease and idiopathic pulmonary fibrosis. *J Proteomics* (2018) 2018:S1874-3919(18)30084-8. doi: 10.1016/j.jprot.2018.02.027
42. Churg A, Zhou S, Wright JL. Series "matrix metalloproteinases in lung health and disease": Matrix metalloproteinases in COPD. *Eur Respir J.* (2012) 39:197–209. doi: 10.1183/09031936.00121611
43. Sandhaus RA, Turino G. Neutrophil elastase-mediated lung disease. *COPD* (2013) 10(Suppl 1):60–3. doi: 10.3109/15412555.2013.764403
44. Moore PJ, Reidel B, Ghosh A, Sesma J, Kesimer M, Tarran R. Cigarette smoke modifies and inactivates SPLUNC1, leading to airway dehydration. *FASEB J.* (2018) 32:1–16. doi: 10.1096/fj.201800345R
45. Larstad M, Almstrand AC, Larsson P, Bake B, Larsson S, Ljungstrom E, et al. Surfactant protein A in exhaled endogenous particles is decreased in chronic Obstructive pulmonary disease (COPD) patients: a pilot study. *PLoS ONE* (2015) 10:e0144463. doi: 10.1371/journal.pone.0144463
46. Takamiya R, Uchida K, Shibata T, Maeno T, Kato M, Yamaguchi Y, et al. Disruption of the structural and functional features of surfactant protein A by acrolein in cigarette smoke. *Sci Rep.* (2017) 7:8304. doi: 10.1038/s41598-017-08588-5
47. Kopa PN, Pawliczak R. Effect of smoking on gene expression profile - overall mechanism, impact on respiratory system function, and reference to electronic cigarettes. *Toxicol Mech Methods* (2018) 28:397–409. doi: 10.1080/15376516.2018.1461289
48. Kan M, Shumyatcher M, Himes BE. Using omics approaches to understand pulmonary diseases. *Respir Res.* (2017) 18:149. doi: 10.1186/s12931-017-0631-9
49. Yang M, Kohler M, Heyder T, Forsslund H, Garberg HK, Karimi R, et al. Long-term smoking alters abundance of over half of the proteome in bronchoalveolar lavage cell in smokers with normal spirometry, with effects on molecular pathways associated with COPD. *Respir Res.* (2018) 19:40. doi: 10.1186/s12931-017-0695-6
50. Damera G, Pham TH, Zhang J, Ward CK, Newbold P, Ranade K, et al. A sputum proteomic signature that associates with increased IL-1β levels and bacterial exacerbations of COPD. *Lung* (2016) 194:363–9. doi: 10.1007/s00408-016-9877-0
51. Fujii K, Nakamura H, Nishimura T. Recent mass spectrometry-based proteomics for biomarker discovery in lung cancer, COPD, and asthma. *Expert Rev Proteomics* (2017) 14:373–86. doi: 10.1080/14789450.2017.1304215
52. Philibert RA, Sears RA, Powers LS, Nash E, Bair T, Gerke AK, et al. Coordinated DNA methylation and gene expression changes in smoker alveolar macrophages: specific effects on VEGF receptor 1 expression. *J Leukoc Biol.* (2012) 92:621–31. doi: 10.1189/jlb.1211632
53. Wan ES, Qiu W, Baccarelli A, Carey VJ, Bacherman H, Rennard SI, et al. Cigarette smoking behaviors and time since quitting are associated with differential DNA methylation across the human genome. *Hum Mol Genet.* (2012) 21:3073–82. doi: 10.1093/hmg/dds135
54. Zhao J, Harper R, Barchowsky A, Di YP. Identification of multiple MAPK-mediated transcription factors regulated by tobacco smoke in airway epithelial cells. *Am J Physiol Lung Cell Mol Physiol.* (2007) 293:L480–90. doi: 10.1152/ajplung.00345.2006
55. Geiman TM, Robertson KD. Chromatin remodeling, histone modifications, and DNA methylation-how does it all fit together? *J Cell Biochem.* (2002) 87:117–25. doi: 10.1002/jcb.10286
56. Ahn KS, Aggarwal BB. Transcription factor NF-kappaB: a sensor for smoke and stress signals. *Ann N Y Acad Sci.* (2005) 1056:218–33. doi: 10.1196/annals.1352.026
57. Sundar IK, Chung S, Hwang JW, Lapek JD, Jr., Bulger M, Friedman AE, et al. Mitogen- and stress-activated kinase 1 (MSK1) regulates cigarette smoke-induced histone modifications on NF-kappaB-dependent genes. *PLoS ONE* (2012) 7:e31378. doi: 10.1371/journal.pone.0031378
58. Khan MN, Ren D, Kaur R, Basha S, Zagursky R, Pichichero ME. Developing a vaccine to prevent otitis media caused by nontypeable *Haemophilus influenzae*. *Expert Rev Vaccines* (2016) 15:863–78. doi: 10.1586/14760584.2016.1156539
59. Marumo S, Hoshino Y, Kiyokawa H, Tanabe N, Sato A, Ogawa E, et al. p38 mitogen-activated protein kinase determines the susceptibility to cigarette smoke-induced emphysema in mice. *BMC Pulm Med.* (2014) 14:79. doi: 10.1186/1471-2466-14-79
60. Herlaar E, Brown Z. p38 MAPK signalling cascades in inflammatory disease. *Mol Med Today* (1999) 5:439–47.
61. Viatour P, Merville MP, Bours V, Chariot A. Phosphorylation of NF-kappaB and IkappaB proteins: implications in cancer and inflammation. *Trends Biochem Sci.* (2005) 30:43–52. doi: 10.1016/j.tibs.2004.11.009
62. Yang SR, Valvo S, Yao H, Kode A, Rajendrasozhan S, Edirisinghe I, et al. IKK alpha causes chromatin modification on pro-inflammatory genes by cigarette smoke in mouse lung. *Am J Respir Cell Mol Biol.* (2008) 38:689–98. doi: 10.1165/rcmb.2007-0379OC
63. Yao H, Hwang JW, Moscat J, Diaz-Meco MT, Leitges M, Kishore N, et al. Protein kinase C zeta mediates cigarette smoke/aldehyde- and lipopolysaccharide-induced lung inflammation and histone modifications. *J Biol Chem.* (2010) 285:5405–16. doi: 10.1074/jbc.M109.041418
64. Anto RJ, Mukhopadhyay A, Shishodia S, Gairola CG, Aggarwal BB. Cigarette smoke condensate activates nuclear transcription factor-kappaB through phosphorylation and degradation of IkappaB(alpha): correlation with induction of cyclooxygenase-2. *Carcinogenesis* (2002) 23:1511–8. doi: 10.1093/carcin/23.9.1511
65. Morgan MJ, Liu ZG. Crosstalk of reactive oxygen species and NF-kappaB signaling. *Cell Res.* (2011) 21:103–15. doi: 10.1038/cr.2010.178
66. Schmidt P, Youhnovski N, Daiber A, Balan A, Arsic M, Bachschmid M, et al. Specific nitration at tyrosine 430 revealed by high resolution mass spectrometry as basis for redox regulation of bovine prostacyclin synthase. *J Biol Chem.* (2003) 278:12813–9. doi: 10.1074/jbc.M208080200
67. Lee MK, Hong Y, Kim SY, London SJ, Kim WJ. DNA methylation and smoking in Korean adults: epigenome-wide association study. *Clin Epigenetics* (2016) 8:103. doi: 10.1186/s13148-016-0266-6
68. Satta R, Maloku E, Zhubi A, Pibiri F, Hajos M, Costa E, et al. Nicotine decreases DNA methyltransferase 1 expression and glutamic acid

decarboxylase 67 promoter methylation in GABAergic interneurons. *Proc Natl Acad Sci USA.* (2008) 105:16356–61. doi: 10.1073/pnas.0808699105
69. Shen JX, Yakel JL. Nicotinic acetylcholine receptor-mediated calcium signaling in the nervous system. *Acta Pharmacol Sin.* (2009) 30:673–80. doi: 10.1038/aps.2009.64
70. Benowitz NL. Nicotine addiction. *N Engl J Med.* (2010) 362:2295–303. doi: 10.1056/NEJMra0809890
71. Daijo H, Hoshino Y, Kai S, Suzuki K, Nishi K, Matsuo Y, et al. Cigarette smoke reversibly activates hypoxia-inducible factor 1 in a reactive oxygen species-dependent manner. *Sci Rep.* (2016) 6:34424. doi: 10.1038/srep34424
72. Mercado N, Thimmulappa R, Thomas CM, Fenwick PS, Chana KK, Donnelly LE, et al. Decreased histone deacetylase 2 impairs Nrf2 activation by oxidative stress. *Biochem Biophys Res Commun.* (2011) 406:292–8. doi: 10.1016/j.bbrc.2011.02.035
73. Shin JM, Park JH, Kim HJ, Park IH, Lee HM. Cigarette smoke extract increases vascular endothelial growth factor production via TLR4/ROS/MAPKs/NF-kappaB pathway in nasal fibroblast. *Am J Rhinol Allergy* (2017) 31:78–84. doi: 10.2500/ajra.2017.31.4415
74. Reynolds PR, Kasteler SD, Schmitt RE, Hoidal JR. Receptor for advanced glycation end-products signals through Ras during tobacco smoke-induced pulmonary inflammation. *Am J Respir Cell Mol Biol.* (2011) 45:411–8. doi: 10.1165/rcmb.2010-0231OC
75. Alam S, Li Z, Janciauskiene S, Mahadeva R. Oxidation of Z alpha1-antitrypsin by cigarette smoke induces polymerization: a novel mechanism of early-onset emphysema. *Am J Respir Cell Mol Biol.* (2011) 45:261–9. doi: 10.1165/rcmb.2010-0328OC
76. Pandey KC, De S, Mishra PK. Role of proteases in chronic obstructive pulmonary disease. *Front Pharmacol.* (2017) 8:512. doi: 10.3389/fphar.2017.00512
77. Yang SR, Chida AS, Bauter MR, Shafiq N, Seweryniak K, Maggirwar SB, et al. Cigarette smoke induces proinflammatory cytokine release by activation of NF-kappaB and posttranslational modifications of histone deacetylase in macrophages. *Am J Physiol Lung Cell Mol Physiol.* (2006) 291:L46–57. doi: 10.1152/ajplung.00241.2005
78. Moretto N, Bertolini S, Iadicicco C, Marchini G, Kaur M, Volpi G, et al. Cigarette smoke and its component acrolein augment IL-8/CXCL8 mRNA stability via p38 MAPK/MK2 signaling in human pulmonary cells. *Am J Physiol Lung Cell Mol Physiol.* (2012) 303:L929–38. doi: 10.1152/ajplung.00046.2012
79. Hasnis E, Bar-Shai M, Burbea Z, Reznick AZ. Mechanisms underlying cigarette smoke-induced NF-kappaB activation in human lymphocytes: the role of reactive nitrogen species. *J Physiol Pharmacol.* (2007) 58 (Suppl 5 Pt 1):275–87.
80. Givi ME, Redegeld FA, Folkerts G, Mortaz E. Dendritic cells in pathogenesis of COPD. *Curr Pharm Des.* (2012) 18:2329–35. doi: 10.2174/138161212800166068
81. Barnes PJ. Immunology of asthma and chronic obstructive pulmonary disease. *Nat Rev Immunol.* (2008) 8:183–92. doi: 10.1038/nri2254
82. Brusselle GG, Joos GF, Bracke KR. New insights into the immunology of chronic obstructive pulmonary disease. *Lancet* (2011) 378:1015–26. doi: 10.1016/S0140-6736(11)60988-4
83. Bhat TA, Panzica L, Kalathil SG, Thanavala Y. Immune dysfunction in patients with chronic obstructive pulmonary disease. *Ann Am Thorac Soc.* (2015) 12(Suppl. 2):S169–75. doi: 10.1513/AnnalsATS.201503-126AW
84. Maes T, Bracke KR, Vermaelen KY, Demedts IK, Joos GF, Pauwels RA, et al. Murine TLR4 is implicated in cigarette smoke-induced pulmonary inflammation. *Int Arch Allergy Immunol.* (2006) 141:354–68. doi: 10.1159/000095462
85. Mukherjee S, Karmakar S, Babu SP. TLR2 and TLR4 mediated host immune responses in major infectious diseases: a review. *Braz J Infect Dis.* (2016) 20:193–204. doi: 10.1016/j.bjid.2015.10.011
86. Hammad H, Lambrecht BN. Barrier epithelial cells and the control of type 2 immunity. *Immunity* (2015) 43:29–40. doi: 10.1016/j.immuni.2015.07.007
87. Lee J, Taneja V, Vassallo R. Cigarette smoking and inflammation: cellular and molecular mechanisms. *J Dent Res.* (2012) 91:142–9. doi: 10.1177/0022034511421200
88. Mortaz E, Henricks PA, Kraneveld AD, Givi ME, Garssen J, Folkerts G. Cigarette smoke induces the release of CXCL-8 from human bronchial epithelial cells via TLRs and induction of the inflammasome. *Biochim Biophys Acta* (2011) 1812:1104–10. doi: 10.1016/j.bbadis.2011.06.002
89. Byers DE, Alexander-Brett J, Patel AC, Agapov E, Dang-Vu G, Jin X, et al. Long-term IL-33-producing epithelial progenitor cells in chronic obstructive lung disease. *J Clin Invest.* (2013) 123:3967–82. doi: 10.1172/JCI65570
90. Barnes PJ. Mediators of chronic obstructive pulmonary disease. *Pharmacol Rev.* (2004) 56:515–48. doi: 10.1124/pr.56.4.2
91. Russell RE, Thorley A, Culpitt SV, Dodd S, Donnelly LE, Demattos C, et al. Alveolar macrophage-mediated elastolysis: roles of matrix metalloproteinases, cysteine, and serine proteases. *Am J Physiol Lung Cell Mol Physiol.* (2002) 283:L867–73. doi: 10.1152/ajplung.00020.2002
92. Culpitt SV, Rogers DF, Shah P, De Matos C, Russell RE, Donnelly LE, et al. Impaired inhibition by dexamethasone of cytokine release by alveolar macrophages from patients with chronic obstructive pulmonary disease. *Am J Respir Crit Care Med.* (2003) 167:24–31. doi: 10.1164/rccm.200204-298OC
93. Traves SL, Culpitt SV, Russell RE, Barnes PJ, Donnelly LE. Increased levels of the chemokines GROalpha and MCP-1 in sputum samples from patients with COPD. *Thorax* (2002) 57:590–5. doi: 10.1136/thorax.57.7.590
94. Hogg JC, Chu F, Utokaparch S, Woods R, Elliott WM, Buzatu L, et al. The nature of small-airway obstruction in chronic obstructive pulmonary disease. *N Engl J Med.* (2004) 350:2645–53. doi: 10.1056/NEJMoa032158
95. Di Stefano A, Capelli A, Lusuardi M, Balbo P, Vecchio C, Maestrelli P, et al. Severity of airflow limitation is associated with severity of airway inflammation in smokers. *Am J Respir Crit Care Med.* (1998) 158:1277–85. doi: 10.1164/ajrccm.158.4.9802078
96. Liu J, Pang Z, Wang G, Guan X, Fang K, Wang Z, et al. Advanced role of neutrophils in common respiratory diseases. *J Immunol Res.* (2017) 2017:6710278. doi: 10.1155/2017/6710278
97. Di Stefano A, Maestrelli P, Roggeri A, Turato G, Calabro S, Potena A, et al. Upregulation of adhesion molecules in the bronchial mucosa of subjects with chronic obstructive bronchitis. *Am J Respir Crit Care Med.* (1994) 149(3 Pt 1):803–10. doi: 10.1164/ajrccm.149.3.7509705
98. Quint JK, Wedzicha JA. The neutrophil in chronic obstructive pulmonary disease. *J Allergy Clin Immunol.* (2007) 119:1065–71. doi: 10.1016/j.jaci.2006.12.640
99. Vaidyanathan A, Damodar KS. Increased metabolic activity of neutrophils in patients with chronic obstructive pulmonary disease. *Lung India* (2015) 32:589–92. doi: 10.4103/0970-2113.168134
100. Keatings VM, Barnes PJ. Granulocyte activation markers in induced sputum: comparison between chronic obstructive pulmonary disease, asthma, and normal subjects. *Am J Respir Crit Care Med.* (1997) 155:449–53. doi: 10.1164/ajrccm.155.2.9032177
101. Fahy JV, Dickey BF. Airway mucus function and dysfunction. *N Engl J Med.* (2010) 363:2233–47. doi: 10.1056/NEJMra0910061
102. Jo EK, Kim JK, Shin DM, Sasakawa C. Molecular mechanisms regulating NLRP3 inflammasome activation. *Cell Mol Immunol.* (2016) 13:148–59. doi: 10.1038/cmi.2015.95
103. Colarusso C, Terlizzi M, Molino A, Pinto A, Sorrentino R. Role of the inflammasome in chronic obstructive pulmonary disease (COPD). *Oncotarget* (2017) 8:81813–24. doi: 10.18632/oncotarget.17850
104. Wang H, Lv C, Wang S, Ying H, Weng Y, Yu W. NLRP3 inflammasome involves in the acute exacerbation of patients with chronic obstructive pulmonary disease. *Inflammation* (2018) 41:1321–33. doi: 10.1007/s10753-018-0780-0
105. Kim K, Kim HJ, Binas B, Kang JH, Chung IY. Inflammatory mediators ATP and S100A12 activate the NLRP3 inflammasome to induce MUC5AC production in airway epithelial cells. *Biochem Biophys Res Commun.* (2018). doi: 10.1016/j.bbrc.2018.06.057
106. Uh ST, Koo SM, Kim Y, Kim K, Park S, Jang AS, et al. The activation of NLRP3-inflammsome by stimulation of diesel exhaust particles in lung tissues from emphysema model and RAW 264.7 cell line. *Korean J Intern Med.* (2017) 32:865–74. doi: 10.3904/kjim.2016.033
107. Demedts IK, Bracke KR, Van Pottelberge G, Testelmans D, Verleden GM, Vermassen FE, et al. Accumulation of dendritic cells and increased CCL20 levels in the airways of patients with chronic obstructive pulmonary disease. *Am J Respir Crit Care Med.* (2007) 175:998–1005. doi: 10.1164/rccm.200608-1113OC

108. D'Hulst A I, Maes T, Bracke KR, Demedts IK, Tournoy KG, Joos GF, et al. Cigarette smoke-induced pulmonary emphysema in scid-mice. Is the acquired immune system required? *Respir Res.* (2005) 6:147. doi: 10.1186/1465-9921-6-147
109. Upham JW, Xi Y. Dendritic cells in human lung disease: recent advances. *Chest* (2017) 151:668–73. doi: 10.1016/j.chest.2016.09.030
110. Saetta M, Mariani M, Panina-Bordignon P, Turato G, Buonsanti C, Baraldo S, et al. Increased expression of the chemokine receptor CXCR3 and its ligand CXCL10 in peripheral airways of smokers with chronic obstructive pulmonary disease. *Am J Respir Crit Care Med.* (2002) 165:1404–9. doi: 10.1164/rccm.2107139
111. Costa C, Rufino R, Traves SL, Lapa ESJR, Barnes PJ, Donnelly LE. CXCR3 and CCR5 chemokines in induced sputum from patients with COPD. *Chest* (2008) 133:26–33. doi: 10.1378/chest.07-0393
112. Majo J, Ghezzo H, Cosio MG. Lymphocyte population and apoptosis in the lungs of smokers and their relation to emphysema. *Eur Respir J.* (2001) 17:946–53. doi: 10.1183/09031936.01.17509460
113. Di Stefano A, Caramori G, Gnemmi I, Contoli M, Vicari C, Capelli A, et al. T helper type 17-related cytokine expression is increased in the bronchial mucosa of stable chronic obstructive pulmonary disease patients. *Clin Exp Immunol.* (2009) 157:316–24. doi: 10.1111/j.1365-2249.2009.03965.x
114. Pridgeon C, Bugeon L, Donnelly L, Straschil U, Tudhope SJ, Fenwick P, et al. Regulation of IL-17 in chronic inflammation in the human lung. *Clin Sci (Lond.)* (2011) 120:515–24. doi: 10.1042/CS20100417
115. De Grove KC, Provoost S, Verhamme FM, Bracke KR, Joos GF, Maes T, et al. Characterization and quantification of innate lymphoid cell subsets in human lung. *PLoS ONE* (2016) 11:e0145961. doi: 10.1371/journal.pone.0145961
116. Xia J, Zhao J, Shang J, Li M, Zeng Z, Zhao J, et al. Increased IL-33 expression in chronic obstructive pulmonary disease. *Am J Physiol Lung Cell Mol Physiol.* (2015) 308:L619–27. doi: 10.1152/ajplung.00305.2014
117. Ying S, O'Connor B, Ratoff J, Meng Q, Fang C, Cousins D, et al. Expression and cellular provenance of thymic stromal lymphopoietin and chemokines in patients with severe asthma and chronic obstructive pulmonary disease. *J Immunol.* (2008) 181:2790–8. doi: 10.1016/j.jaci.2004.12.051
118. van der Strate BW, Postma DS, Brandsma CA, Melgert BN, Luinge MA, Geerlings M, et al. Cigarette smoke-induced emphysema: a role for the B cell? *Am J Respir Crit Care Med.* (2006) 173:751–8. doi: 10.1164/rccm.200504-594OC
119. Lee SH, Goswami S, Grudo A, Song LZ, Bandi V, Goodnight-White S, et al. Antielastin autoimmunity in tobacco smoking-induced emphysema. *Nat Med.* (2007) 13:567–9. doi: 10.1038/nm1583
120. Karayama M, Inui N, Suda T, Nakamura Y, Nakamura H, Chida K. Antiendothelial cell antibodies in patients with COPD. *Chest* (2010) 138:1303–8. doi: 10.1378/chest.10-0863
121. Feghali-Bostwick CA, Gadgil AS, Otterbein LE, Pilewski JM, Stoner MW, Csizmadia E, et al. Autoantibodies in patients with chronic obstructive pulmonary disease. *Am J Respir Crit Care Med.* (2008) 177:156–63. doi: 10.1164/rccm.200701-014OC
122. Koethe SM, Kuhnmuench JR, Becker CG. Neutrophil priming by cigarette smoke condensate and a tobacco anti-idiotypic antibody. *Am J Pathol.* (2000) 157:1735–43. doi: 10.1016/S0002-9440(10)64810-9
123. Nahm DH, Lee YE, Yim EJ, Park HS, Yim H, Kang Y, et al. Identification of cytokeratin 18 as a bronchial epithelial autoantigen associated with nonallergic asthma. *Am J Respir Crit Care Med.* (2002) 165:1536–9. doi: 10.1164/rccm.200201-009OC
124. Caramori G, Ruggeri P, Di Stefano A, Mumby S, Girbino G, Adcock IM, et al. Autoimmunity and COPD: clinical implications. *Chest* (2018) 153:1424–31. doi: 10.1016/j.chest.2017.10.033
125. Cosio MG. Autoimmunity, T-cells and STAT-4 in the pathogenesis of chronic obstructive pulmonary disease. *Eur Respir J.* (2004) 24:3–5. doi: 10.1183/09031936.04.00043104
126. Agusti A, MacNee W, Donaldson K, Cosio M. Hypothesis: does COPD have an autoimmune component? *Thorax* (2003) 58:832–4. doi: 10.1136/thorax.58.10.832
127. Kirkham PA, Caramori G, Casolari P, Papi AA, Edwards M, Shamji B, et al. Oxidative stress-induced antibodies to carbonyl-modified protein correlate with severity of chronic obstructive pulmonary disease. *Am J Respir Crit Care Med.* (2011) 184:796–802. doi: 10.1164/rccm.201010-1605OC
128. Hurst JR, Wedzicha JA. What is (and what is not) a COPD exacerbation: thoughts from the new GOLD guidelines. *Thorax* (2007) 62:198–9. doi: 10.1136/thx.2007.077883
129. Wedzicha JA, Seemungal TA. COPD exacerbations: defining their cause and prevention. *Lancet* (2007) 370:786–96. doi: 10.1016/S0140-6736(07)61382-8
130. Pavord ID, Jones PW, Burgel PR, Rabe KF. Exacerbations of COPD. *Int J Chron Obstruct Pulmon Dis.* (2016) 11:21–30. doi: 10.2147/COPD.S85978
131. Seemungal TA, Donaldson GC, Bhowmik A, Jeffries DJ, Wedzicha JA. Time course and recovery of exacerbations in patients with chronic obstructive pulmonary disease. *Am J Respir Crit Care Med.* (2000) 161:1608–13. doi: 10.1164/ajrccm.161.5.9908022
132. Sapey E, Stockley RA. COPD exacerbations. 2: aetiology. *Thorax* (2006) 61:250–8. doi: 10.1136/thx.2005.041822
133. Ko FW, Chan KP, Hui DS, Goddard JR, Shaw JG, Reid DW, et al. Acute exacerbation of COPD. *Respirology* (2016) 21:1152–65. doi: 10.1111/resp.12780
134. Eldika N, Sethi S. Role of nontypeable *Haemophilus influenzae* in exacerbations and progression of chronic obstructive pulmonary disease. *Curr Opin Pulm Med.* (2006) 12:118–24. doi: 10.1097/01.mcp.0000208451.50231.8f
135. Celli BR, Barnes PJ. Exacerbations of chronic obstructive pulmonary disease. *Eur Respir J.* (2007) 29:1224–38. doi: 10.1183/09031936.00109906
136. Wilkinson TMA, Aris E, Bourne S, Clarke SC, Peeters M, Pascal TG, et al. A prospective, observational cohort study of the seasonal dynamics of airway pathogens in the aetiology of exacerbations in COPD. *Thorax* (2017) 72:919–27. doi: 10.1136/thoraxjnl-2016-209023
137. Seemungal T, Harper-Owen R, Bhowmik A, Moric I, Sanderson G, Message S, et al. Respiratory viruses, symptoms, and inflammatory markers in acute exacerbations and stable chronic obstructive pulmonary disease. *Am J Respir Crit Care Med.* (2001) 164:1618–23. doi: 10.1164/ajrccm.164.9.2105011
138. Kurai D, Saraya T, Ishii H, Takizawa H. Virus-induced exacerbations in asthma and COPD. *Front Microbiol.* (2013) 4:293. doi: 10.3389/fmicb.2013.00293
139. Mohan A, Chandra S, Agarwal D, Guleria R, Broor S, Gaur B, et al. Prevalence of viral infection detected by PCR and RT-PCR in patients with acute exacerbation of COPD: a systematic review. *Respirology* (2010) 15:536–42. doi: 10.1111/j.1440-1843.2010.01722.x
140. Biancardi E, Fennell M, Rawlinson W, Thomas PS. Viruses are frequently present as the infecting agent in acute exacerbations of chronic obstructive pulmonary disease in patients presenting to hospital. *Intern Med J.* (2016) 46:1160–5. doi: 10.1111/imj.13213
141. Hewitt R, Farne H, Ritchie A, Luke E, Johnston SL, Mallia P. The role of viral infections in exacerbations of chronic obstructive pulmonary disease and asthma. *Ther Adv Respir Dis.* (2016) 10:158–74. doi: 10.1177/1753465815618113
142. Koul PA, Mir H, Akram S, Potdar V, Chadha MS. Respiratory viruses in acute exacerbations of chronic obstructive pulmonary disease. *Lung India* (2017) 34:29–33. doi: 10.4103/0970-2113.197099
143. Jafarinejad H, Moghoofei M, Mostafaei S, Salimian J, Azimzadeh Jamalkandi S, Ahmadi A. Worldwide prevalence of viral infection in AECOPD patients: a meta-analysis. *Microb Pathog.* (2017) 113:190–6. doi: 10.1016/j.micpath.2017.10.021
144. Britto CJ, Brady V, Lee S, Dela Cruz CS. Respiratory viral infections in chronic lung diseases. *Clin Chest Med.* (2017) 38:87–96. doi: 10.1016/j.ccm.2016.11.014
145. Yin T, Zhu Z, Mei Z, Feng J, Zhang W, He Y, et al. Analysis of viral infection and biomarkers in patients with acute exacerbation of chronic obstructive pulmonary disease. *Clin Respir J.* (2018) 12:1228–39. doi: 10.1111/crj.12656
146. Chang CL, Sullivan GD, Karalus NC, Mills GD, McLachlan JD, Hancox RJ. Predicting early mortality in acute exacerbation of chronic obstructive pulmonary disease using the CURB65 score. *Respirology* (2011) 16:146–51. doi: 10.1111/j.1440-1843.2010.01866.x
147. Lou P, Zhu Y, Chen P, Zhang P, Yu J, Zhang N, et al. Vulnerability, beliefs, treatments and economic burden of chronic obstructive pulmonary disease in rural areas in China: a cross-sectional study. *BMC Public Health* (2012) 12:287. doi: 10.1186/1471-2458-12-287

148. Rosell A, Monso E, Soler N, Torres F, Angrill J, Riise G, et al. Microbiologic determinants of exacerbation in chronic obstructive pulmonary disease. *Arch Intern Med.* (2005) 165:891–7. doi: 10.1001/archinte.165.8.891
149. Wang Z, Bafadhel M, Haldar K, Spivak A, Mayhew D, Miller BE, et al. Lung microbiome dynamics in COPD exacerbations. *Eur Respir J.* (2016) 47:1082–92. doi: 10.1183/13993003.01406-2015
150. Polverino E, Rosales-Mayor E, Benegas M, Menendez R, Alcaraz-Serrano V, Ansotegui E, et al. Pneumonic and non-pneumonic exacerbations in bronchiectasis: clinical and microbiological differences. *J Infect.* (2018) 77:99–106. doi: 10.1016/j.jinf.2018.04.006
151. Mayhew D, Devos N, Lambert C, Brown JR, Clarke SC, Kim VL, et al. Longitudinal profiling of the lung microbiome in the AERIS study demonstrates repeatability of bacterial and eosinophilic COPD exacerbations. *Thorax* (2018) 73:422–30. doi: 10.1136/thoraxjnl-2017-210408
152. Simpson JL, Baines KJ, Horvat JC, Essilfie AT, Brown AC, Tooze M, et al. COPD is characterized by increased detection of *Haemophilus influenzae, Streptococcus pneumoniae* and a deficiency of *Bacillus* species. *Respirology* (2016) 21:697–704. doi: 10.1111/resp.12734
153. Sethi S, Evans N, Grant BJ, Murphy TF. New strains of bacteria and exacerbations of chronic obstructive pulmonary disease. *N Engl J Med.* (2002) 347:465–71. doi: 10.1056/NEJMoa012561
154. Rangelov K, Sethi S. Role of infections. *Clin Chest Med.* (2014) 35:87–100. doi: 10.1016/j.ccm.2013.09.012
155. Bafadhel M, McKenna S, Terry S, Mistry V, Reid C, Haldar P, et al. Acute exacerbations of chronic obstructive pulmonary disease: identification of biologic clusters and their biomarkers. *Am J Respir Crit Care Med.* (2011) 184:662–71. doi: 10.1164/rccm.201104-0597OC
156. George SN, Garcha DS, Mackay AJ, Patel AR, Singh R, Sapsford RJ, et al. Human rhinovirus infection during naturally occurring COPD exacerbations. *Eur Respir J.* (2014) 44:87–96. doi: 10.1183/09031936.00223113
157. Utokaparch S, Sze MA, Gosselink JV, McDonough JE, Elliott WM, Hogg JC, et al. Respiratory viral detection and small airway inflammation in lung tissue of patients with stable, mild COPD. *COPD* (2014) 11:197–203. doi: 10.3109/15412555.2013.836166
158. D'Anna SE, Balbi B, Cappello F, Carone M, Di Stefano A. Bacterial-viral load and the immune response in stable and exacerbated COPD: significance and therapeutic prospects. *Int J Chron Obstruct Pulmon Dis.* (2016) 11:445–53. doi: 10.2147/COPD.S93398
159. Unger BL, Faris AN, Ganesan S, Comstock AT, Hershenson MB, Sajjan US. Rhinovirus attenuates non-typeable *Haemophilus influenzae*-stimulated IL-8 responses via TLR2-dependent degradation of IRAK-1. *PLoS Pathog.* (2012) 8:e1002969. doi: 10.1371/journal.ppat.1002969
160. Gulraiz F, Bellinghausen C, Bruggeman CA, Stassen FR. *Haemophilus influenzae* increases the susceptibility and inflammatory response of airway epithelial cells to viral infections. *FASEB J.* (2015) 29:849–58. doi: 10.1096/fj.14-254359
161. Bellinghausen C, Gulraiz F, Heinzmann AC, Dentener MA, Savelkoul PH, Wouters EF, et al. Exposure to common respiratory bacteria alters the airway epithelial response to subsequent viral infection. *Respir Res.* (2016) 17:68. doi: 10.1186/s12931-016-0382-z
162. Sajjan U, Wang Q, Zhao Y, Gruenert DC, Hershenson MB. Rhinovirus disrupts the barrier function of polarized airway epithelial cells. *Am J Respir Crit Care Med.* (2008) 178:1271–81. doi: 10.1164/rccm.200801-136OC
163. Wang JH, Kwon HJ, Jang YJ. Rhinovirus enhances various bacterial adhesions to nasal epithelial cells simultaneously. *Laryngoscope* (2009) 119:1406–11. doi: 10.1002/lary.20498
164. Jia L, Xie J, Zhao J, Cao D, Liang Y, Hou X, et al. Mechanisms of severe mortality-associated bacterial co-infections following influenza virus infection. *Front Cell Infect Microbiol.* (2017) 7:338. doi: 10.3389/fcimb.2017.00338
165. Oliver BG, Lim S, Wark P, Laza-Stanca V, King N, Black JL, et al. Rhinovirus exposure impairs immune responses to bacterial products in human alveolar macrophages. *Thorax* (2008) 63:519–25. doi: 10.1136/thx.2007.0 81752
166. Arnason JW, Murphy JC, Kooi C, Wiehler S, Traves SL, Shelfoon C, et al. Human β-defensin-2 production upon viral and bacterial co-infection is attenuated in COPD. *PLoS ONE* (2017) 12:e0175963. doi: 10.1371/journal.pone.0175963
167. McCullers JA. The co-pathogenesis of influenza viruses with bacteria in the lung. *Nat Rev Microbiol.* (2014) 12:252–62. doi: 10.1038/nrmicro3231
168. Bellinghausen C, Rohde GGU, Savelkoul PHM, Wouters EFM, Stassen FRM. Viral-bacterial interactions in the respiratory tract. *J Gen Virol.* (2016) 97:3089–102. doi: 10.1099/jgv.0.000627
169. Welte T, Miravitlles M. Viral, bacterial or both? Regardless, we need to treat infection in COPD. *Eur Respir J.* (2014) 44:11–3. doi: 10.1183/09031936.00041914
170. Wark PA, Tooze M, Powell H, Parsons K. Viral and bacterial infection in acute asthma and chronic obstructive pulmonary disease increases the risk of readmission. *Respirology* (2013) 18:996–1002. doi: 10.1111/resp.12099
171. Papi A, Bellettato CM, Braccioni F, Romagnoli M, Casolari P, Caramori G, et al. Infections and airway inflammation in chronic obstructive pulmonary disease severe exacerbations. *Am J Respir Crit Care Med.* (2006) 173:1114–21. doi: 10.1164/rccm.200506-859OC
172. Wilkinson TM, Hurst JR, Perera WR, Wilks M, Donaldson GC, Wedzicha JA. Effect of interactions between lower airway bacterial and rhinoviral infection in exacerbations of COPD. *Chest* (2006) 129:317–24. doi: 10.1378/chest.129.2.317
173. Perotin JM, Dury S, Renois F, Deslee G, Wolak A, Duval V, et al. Detection of multiple viral and bacterial infections in acute exacerbation of chronic obstructive pulmonary disease: a pilot prospective study. *J Med Virol.* (2013) 85:866–73. doi: 10.1002/jmv.23495
174. Kawamatawong T, Apiwattanaporn A, Siricharoonwong W. Serum inflammatory biomarkers and clinical outcomes of COPD exacerbation caused by different pathogens. *Int J Chron Obstruct Pulmon Dis.* (2017) 12:1625–30. doi: 10.2147/COPD.S132132
175. Amatngalim GD, Schrumpf JA, Henic A, Dronkers E, Verhoosel RM, Ordonez SR, et al. Antibacterial defense of human airway epithelial cells from chronic obstructive pulmonary disease patients induced by acute exposure to nontypeable *Haemophilus influenzae*: modulation by cigarette smoke. *J Innate Immun.* (2017) 9:359–74. doi: 10.1159/000455193
176. Parameswaran GI, Sethi S, Murphy TF. Effects of bacterial infection on airway antimicrobial peptides and proteins in COPD. *Chest* (2011) 140:611–7. doi: 10.1378/chest.10-2760
177. Berenson CS, Kruzel RL, Eberhardt E, Sethi S. Phagocytic dysfunction of human alveolar macrophages and severity of chronic obstructive pulmonary disease. *J Infect Dis.* (2013) 208:2036–45. doi: 10.1093/infdis/jit400
178. Taylor AE, Finney-Hayward TK, Quint JK, Thomas CM, Tudhope SJ, Wedzicha JA, et al. Defective macrophage phagocytosis of bacteria in COPD. *Eur Respir J.* (2010) 35:1039–47. doi: 10.1183/09031936.00036709
179. Sapey E, Stockley JA, Greenwood H, Ahmad A, Bayley D, Lord JM, et al. Behavioral and structural differences in migrating peripheral neutrophils from patients with chronic obstructive pulmonary disease. *Am J Respir Crit Care Med.* (2011) 183:1176–86. doi: 10.1164/rccm.201008-1285OC
180. Sze MA, Hogg JC, Sin DD. Bacterial microbiome of lungs in COPD. *Int J Chron Obstruct Pulmon Dis.* (2014) 9:229–38. doi: 10.2147/COPD.S38932
181. Cookson W, Cox MJ, Moffatt MF. New opportunities for managing acute and chronic lung infections. *Nat Rev Microbiol.* (2018) 16:111–20. doi: 10.1038/nrmicro.2017.122
182. Mammen MJ, Sethi S. COPD and the microbiome. *Respirology* (2016) 21:590–9. doi: 10.1111/resp.12732
183. Wang L, Hao K, Yang T, Wang C. Role of the lung microbiome in the pathogenesis of chronic obstructive pulmonary disease. *Chin Med J. (Engl.)* (2017) 130:2107–11. doi: 10.4103/0366-6999.211452
184. Pienkowska K, Wiehlmann L, Tummler B. Airway microbial metagenomics. *Microbes Infect.* (2017) 2017:S1286-4579(17)30224-1. doi: 10.1016/j.micinf.2017.12.002
185. Hussell T, Lui S, Jagger C, Morgan D, Brand O. The consequence of matrix dysfunction on lung immunity and the microbiome in COPD. *Eur Respir Rev.* (2018) 27:180032. doi: 10.1183/16000617.0032-2018
186. O'Dwyer DN, Dickson RP, Moore BB. The lung microbiome, immunity, and the pathogenesis of chronic lung disease. *J Immunol.* (2016) 196:4839–47. doi: 10.4049/jimmunol.1600279
187. Monso E. Microbiome in chronic obstructive pulmonary disease. *Ann Transl Med.* (2017) 5:251. doi: 10.21037/atm.2017.04.20

188. Ghebre MA, Pang PH, Diver S, Desai D, Bafadhel M, Haldar K, et al. Biological exacerbation clusters demonstrate asthma and chronic obstructive pulmonary disease overlap with distinct mediator and microbiome profiles. *J Allergy Clin Immunol.* (2018) 141:2027.e12–36.e12. doi: 10.1016/j.jaci.2018.04.013
189. Saeedi P, Salimian J, Ahmadi A, Imani Fooladi AA. The transient but not resident (TBNR) microbiome: a Yin Yang model for lung immune system. *Inhal Toxicol.* (2015) 27:451–61. doi: 10.3109/08958378.2015.1070220
190. Molyneaux PL, Mallia P, Cox MJ, Footitt J, Willis-Owen SA, Homola D, et al. Outgrowth of the bacterial airway microbiome after rhinovirus exacerbation of chronic obstructive pulmonary disease. *Am J Respir Crit Care Med.* (2013) 188:1224–31. doi: 10.1164/rccm.201302-0341OC
191. Engel M, Endesfelder D, Schloter-Hai B, Kublik S, Granitsiotis MS, Boschetto P, et al. Influence of lung CT changes in chronic obstructive pulmonary disease (COPD) on the human lung microbiome. *PLoS ONE* (2017) 12:e0180859. doi: 10.1371/journal.pone.0180859
192. Tangedal S, Aanerud M, Gronseth R, Drengenes C, Wiker HG, Bakke PS, et al. Comparing microbiota profiles in induced and spontaneous sputum samples in COPD patients. *Respir Res.* (2017) 18:164. doi: 10.1186/s12931-017-0645-3
193. Diao W, Shen N, Du Y, Qian K, He B. Characterization of throat microbial flora in smokers with or without COPD. *Int J Chron Obstruct Pulmon Dis.* (2017) 12:1933–46. doi: 10.2147/COPD.S140243
194. Garcia-Nunez M, Millares L, Pomares X, Ferrari R, Perez-Brocal V, Gallego M, et al. Severity-related changes of bronchial microbiome in chronic obstructive pulmonary disease. *J Clin Microbiol.* (2014) 52:4217–23. doi: 10.1128/JCM.01967-14
195. Huang YJ, Sethi S, Murphy T, Nariya S, Boushey HA, Lynch SV. Airway microbiome dynamics in exacerbations of chronic obstructive pulmonary disease. *J Clin Microbiol.* (2014) 52:2813–23. doi: 10.1128/JCM.00035-14
196. Jubinville E, Veillette M, Milot J, Maltais F, Comeau AM, Levesque RC, et al. Exacerbation induces a microbiota shift in sputa of COPD patients. *PLoS ONE* (2018) 13:e0194355. doi: 10.1371/journal.pone.0194355
197. Shukla SD, Budden KF, Neal R, Hansbro PM. Microbiome effects on immunity, health and disease in the lung. *Clin Transl Immunol.* (2017) 6:e133. doi: 10.1038/cti.2017.6
198. Dicker AJ, Crichton ML, Pumphrey EG, Cassidy AJ, Suarez-Cuartin G, Sibila O, et al. Neutrophil extracellular traps are associated with disease severity and microbiota diversity in patients with chronic obstructive pulmonary disease. *J Allergy Clin Immunol.* (2018) 141:117–27. doi: 10.1016/j.jaci.2017.04.022
199. Yadava K, Pattaroni C, Sichelstiel AK, Trompette A, Gollwitzer ES, Salami O, et al. Microbiota promotes chronic pulmonary inflammation by enhancing IL-17A and autoantibodies. *Am J Respir Crit Care Med.* (2016) 193:975–87. doi: 10.1164/rccm.201504-0779OC
200. Sze MA, Dimitriu PA, Hayashi S, Elliott WM, McDonough JE, Gosselink JV, et al. The lung tissue microbiome in chronic obstructive pulmonary disease. *Am J Respir Crit Care Med.* (2012) 185:1073–80. doi: 10.1164/rccm.201111-2075OC
201. Sze MA, Dimitriu PA, Suzuki M, McDonough JE, Campbell JD, Brothers JF, et al. Host response to the lung microbiome in chronic obstructive pulmonary disease. *Am J Respir Crit Care Med.* (2015) 192:438–45. doi: 10.1164/rccm.201502-0223OC
202. Chalmers JD, McHugh BJ, Doherty C, Smith MP, Govan JR, Kilpatrick DC, et al. Mannose-binding lectin deficiency and disease severity in non-cystic fibrosis bronchiectasis: a prospective study. *Lancet Respir Med.* (2013) 1:224–32. doi: 10.1016/S2213-2600(13)70001-8
203. Dicker AJ, Crichton ML, Cassidy AJ, Brady G, Hapca A, Tavendale R, et al. Genetic mannose binding lectin deficiency is associated with airway microbiota diversity and reduced exacerbation frequency in COPD. *Thorax* (2018) 73:510–8. doi: 10.1136/thoraxjnl-2016-209931
204. Chambers DC, Gellatly SL, Hugenholtz P, Hansbro PM. JTD special edition 'Hot topics in COPD'-the microbiome in COPD. *J Thorac Dis.* (2014) 6:1525–31. doi: 10.3978/j.issn.2072-1439.2014.11.08
205. Erb-Downward JR, Thompson DL, Han MK, Freeman CM, McCloskey L, Schmidt LA, et al. Analysis of the lung microbiome in the "healthy" smoker and in COPD. *PLoS ONE* (2011) 6:e16384. doi: 10.1371/journal.pone.0016384
206. Hilty M, Burke C, Pedro H, Cardenas P, Bush A, Bossley C, et al. Disordered microbial communities in asthmatic airways. *PLoS ONE* (2010) 5:e8578. doi: 10.1371/journal.pone.0008578
207. Ahearn CP, Gallo MC, Murphy TF. Insights on persistent airway infection by non-typeable *Haemophilus influenzae* in chronic obstructive pulmonary disease. *Pathog Dis.* (2017) 75:ftx042. doi: 10.1093/femspd/ftx042
208. Van Eldere J, Slack MP, Ladhani S, Cripps AW. Non-typeable *Haemophilus influenzae*, an under-recognised pathogen. *Lancet Infect Dis.* (2014) 14:1281–92. doi: 10.1016/S1473-3099(14)70734-0
209. Puig C, Grau I, Marti S, Tubau F, Calatayud L, Pallares R, et al. Clinical and molecular epidemiology of *Haemophilus influenzae* causing invasive disease in adult patients. *PLoS ONE* (2014) 9:e112711. doi: 10.1371/journal.pone.0112711
210. Resman F, Ristovski M, Ahl J, Forsgren A, Gilsdorf JR, Jasir A, et al. Invasive disease caused by *Haemophilus influenzae* in Sweden 1997-2009; evidence of increasing incidence and clinical burden of non-type b strains. *Clin Microbiol Infect.* (2011) 17:1638–45. doi: 10.1111/j.1469-0691.2010.03417.x
211. Langereis JD, de Jonge MI. Invasive disease caused by Nontypeable *Haemophilus influenzae. Emerg Infect Dis.* (2015) 21:1711–8. doi: 10.3201/eid2110.150004
212. Sriram KB, Cox AJ, Clancy RL, Slack MPE, Cripps AW. Nontypeable *Haemophilus influenzae* and chronic obstructive pulmonary disease: a review for clinicians. *Crit Rev Microbiol.* (2018) 44:125–42. doi: 10.1080/1040841X.2017.1329274
213. Loens K, Van Heirstraeten L, Malhotra-Kumar S, Goossens H, Ieven M. Optimal sampling sites and methods for detection of pathogens possibly causing community-acquired lower respiratory tract infections. *J Clin Microbiol.* (2009) 47:21–31. doi: 10.1128/JCM.02037-08
214. Dickson RP, Martinez FJ, Huffnagle GB. The role of the microbiome in exacerbations of chronic lung diseases. *Lancet* (2014) 384:691–702. doi: 10.1016/S0140-6736(14)61136-3
215. Beasley V, Joshi PV, Singanayagam A, Molyneaux PL, Johnston SL, Mallia P. Lung microbiology and exacerbations in COPD. *Int J Chron Obstruct Pulmon Dis.* (2012) 7:555–69. doi: 10.2147/COPD.S28286
216. Sethi S, Maloney J, Grove L, Wrona C, Berenson CS. Airway inflammation and bronchial bacterial colonization in chronic obstructive pulmonary disease. *Am J Respir Crit Care Med.* (2006) 173:991–8. doi: 10.1164/rccm.200509-1525OC
217. Bandi V, Apicella MA, Mason E, Murphy TF, Siddiqi A, Atmar RL, et al. Nontypeable *Haemophilus influenzae* in the lower respiratory tract of patients with chronic bronchitis. *Am J Respir Crit Care Med.* (2001) 164:2114–9. doi: 10.1164/ajrccm.164.11.2104093
218. Millares L, Ferrari R, Gallego M, Garcia-Nunez M, Perez-Brocal V, Espasa M, et al. Bronchial microbiome of severe COPD patients colonised by *Pseudomonas aeruginosa. Eur J Clin Microbiol Infect Dis.* (2014) 33:1101–11. doi: 10.1007/s10096-013-2044-0
219. Finney LJ, Ritchie A, Pollard E, Johnston SL, Mallia P. Lower airway colonization and inflammatory response in COPD: a focus on *Haemophilus influenzae. Int J Chron Obstruct Pulmon Dis.* (2014) 9:1119–32. doi: 10.2147/COPD.S54477
220. Doring G, Parameswaran IG, Murphy TF. Differential adaptation of microbial pathogens to airways of patients with cystic fibrosis and chronic obstructive pulmonary disease. *FEMS Microbiol Rev.* (2011) 35:124–46. doi: 10.1111/j.1574-6976.2010.00237.x
221. Cullen L, McClean S. Bacterial adaptation during chronic respiratory infections. *Pathogens* (2015) 4:66–89. doi: 10.3390/pathogens4010066
222. Zhang L, Xie J, Patel M, Bakhtyar A, Ehrlich GD, Ahmed A, et al. Nontypeable *Haemophilus influenzae* genetic islands associated with chronic pulmonary infection. *PLoS ONE* (2012) 7:e44730. doi: 10.1371/journal.pone.0044730
223. Qu J, Lesse AJ, Brauer AL, Cao J, Gill SR, Murphy TF. Proteomic expression profiling of *Haemophilus influenzae* grown in pooled human sputum from adults with chronic obstructive pulmonary disease reveal antioxidant and stress responses. *BMC Microbiol.* (2010) 10:162. doi: 10.1186/1471-2180-10-162
224. Wong SM, Bernui M, Shen H, Akerley BJ. Genome-wide fitness profiling reveals adaptations required by *Haemophilus* in coinfection with influenza

A virus in the murine lung. *Proc Natl Acad Sci USA.* (2013) 110:15413–8. doi: 10.1073/pnas.1311217110

225. Pettigrew MM, Ahearn CP, Gent JF, Kong Y, Gallo MC, Munro JB, et al. *Haemophilus influenzae* genome evolution during persistence in the human airways in chronic obstructive pulmonary disease. *Proc Natl Acad Sci USA.* (2018) 115:E3256–E65. doi: 10.1073/pnas.1719654115
226. Murphy TF, Kirkham C, Jones MM, Sethi S, Kong Y, Pettigrew MM. Expression of IgA proteases by *Haemophilus influenzae* in the respiratory tract of adults with chronic obstructive pulmonary disease. *J Infect Dis.* (2015) 212:1798–805. doi: 10.1093/infdis/jiv299
227. Murphy TF, Kirkham C, Gallo MC, Yang Y, Wilding GE, Pettigrew MM. Immunoglobulin A protease variants facilitate intracellular survival in epithelial cells by nontypeable *Haemophilus influenzae* that persist in the human respiratory tract in chronic obstructive pulmonary disease. *J Infect Dis.* (2017) 216:1295–302. doi: 10.1093/infdis/jix471
228. Gallo MC, Kirkham C, Eng S, Bebawee RS, Kong Y, Pettigrew MM, et al. Changes in IgA protease expression are conferred by changes in genomes during persistent infection by nontypeable *Haemophilus influenzae* in chronic obstructive pulmonary disease. *Infect Immun.* (2018) 86(8). doi: 10.1128/IAI.00313-18
229. Puig C, Domenech A, Garmendia J, Langereis JD, Mayer P, Calatayud L, et al. Increased biofilm formation by nontypeable *Haemophilus influenzae* isolates from patients with invasive disease or otitis media versus strains recovered from cases of respiratory infections. *Appl Environ Microbiol.* (2014) 80:7088–95. doi: 10.1128/AEM.02544-14
230. Swords WE. Nontypeable *Haemophilus influenzae* biofilms: role in chronic airway infections. *Front Cell Infect Microbiol.* (2012) 2:97. doi: 10.3389/fcimb.2012.00097
231. Kaufhold I, Osbahr S, Shima K, Marwitz S, Rohmann K, Dromann D, et al. Nontypeable *Haemophilus influenzae* (NTHi) directly interfere with the regulation of E-cadherin in lung epithelial cells. *Microbes Infect.* (2017) 19:560–6. doi: 10.1016/j.micinf.2017.07.002
232. Singh B, Fleury C, Jalalvand F, Riesbeck K. Human pathogens utilize host extracellular matrix proteins laminin and collagen for adhesion and invasion of the host. *FEMS Microbiol Rev.* (2012) 36:1122–80. doi: 10.1111/j.1574-6976.2012.00340.x
233. Singh R, Mackay AJ, Patel AR, Garcha DS, Kowlessar BS, Brill SE, et al. Inflammatory thresholds and the species-specific effects of colonising bacteria in stable chronic obstructive pulmonary disease. *Respir Res.* (2014) 15:114. doi: 10.1186/s12931-014-0114-1
234. Liu T, Zhang L, Joo D, Sun SC. NF-κB signaling in inflammation. *Signal Transduct Target Ther.* (2017) 2:e17023. doi: 10.1038/sigtrans.2017.23
235. Moghaddam SJ, Clement CG, De la Garza MM, Zou X, Travis EL, Young HW, et al. *Haemophilus influenzae* lysate induces aspects of the chronic obstructive pulmonary disease phenotype. *Am J Respir Cell Mol Biol.* (2008) 38:629–38. doi: 10.1165/rcmb.2007-0366OC
236. Ganesan S, Comstock AT, Kinker B, Mancuso P, Beck JM, Sajjan US. Combined exposure to cigarette smoke and nontypeable *Haemophilus influenzae* drives development of a COPD phenotype in mice. *Respir Res.* (2014) 15:11. doi: 10.1186/1465-9921-15-11
237. Tan WS, Peh HY, Liao W, Pang CH, Chan TK, Lau SH, et al. Cigarette smoke-induced lung disease predisposes to more severe infection with nontypeable *Haemophilus influenzae*: protective effects of andrographolide. *J Nat Prod.* (2016) 79:1308–15. doi: 10.1021/acs.jnatprod.5b01006
238. Oliveira-Nascimento L, Massari P, Wetzler LM. The Role of TLR2 in infection and immunity. *Front Immunol.* (2012) 3:79. doi: 10.3389/fimmu.2012.00079
239. Kawasaki T, Kawai T. Toll-like receptor signaling pathways. *Front Immunol.* (2014) 5:461. doi: 10.3389/fimmu.2014.00461
240. Vaure C, Liu Y. A comparative review of toll-like receptor 4 expression and functionality in different animal species. *Front Immunol.* (2014) 5:316. doi: 10.3389/fimmu.2014.00316
241. Berenson CS, Murphy TF, Wrona CT, Sethi S. Outer membrane protein P6 of nontypeable *Haemophilus influenzae* is a potent and selective inducer of human macrophage proinflammatory cytokines. *Infect Immun.* (2005) 73:2728–35. doi: 10.1128/IAI.73.5.2728-2735.2005
242. Shuto T, Xu H, Wang B, Han J, Kai H, Gu XX, et al. Activation of NF-kappa B by nontypeable *Hemophilus influenzae* is mediated by toll-like receptor 2-TAK1-dependent NIK-IKK alpha /beta-I kappa B alpha and MKK3/6-p38 MAP kinase signaling pathways in epithelial cells. *Proc Natl Acad Sci USA.* (2001) 98:8774–9. doi: 10.1073/pnas.151236098
243. Wang X, Moser C, Louboutin JP, Lysenko ES, Weiner DJ, Weiser JN, et al. Toll-like receptor 4 mediates innate immune responses to *Haemophilus influenzae* infection in mouse lung. *J Immunol.* (2002) 168:810–5. doi: 10.4049/jimmunol.168.2.810
244. Wieland CW, Florquin S, Maris NA, Hoebe K, Beutler B, Takeda K, et al. The MyD88-dependent, but not the MyD88-independent, pathway of TLR4 signaling is important in clearing nontypeable *Haemophilus influenzae* from the mouse lung. *J Immunol.* (2005) 175:6042–9. doi: 10.4049/jimmunol.175.9.6042
245. Xu F, Xu Z, Zhang R, Wu Z, Lim JH, Koga T, et al. Nontypeable *Haemophilus influenzae* induces COX-2 and PGE2 expression in lung epithelial cells via activation of p38 MAPK and NF-kappa B. *Respir Res.* (2008) 9:16. doi: 10.1186/1465-9921-9-16
246. Piras V, Selvarajoo K. Beyond MyD88 and TRIF Pathways in Toll-Like Receptor Signaling. *Front Immunol.* (2014) 5:70. doi: 10.3389/fimmu.2014.00070
247. Jungnickel C, Schnabel PA, Bohle R, Wiewrodt R, Herr C, Bals R, et al. Nontypeable *Haemophilus influenzae*-promoted proliferation of Kras-induced early adenomatous lesions is completely dependent on Toll-like receptor signaling. *Am J Pathol.* (2017) 187:973–9. doi: 10.1016/j.ajpath.2017.01.003
248. Heyl KA, Klassert TE, Heinrich A, Muller MM, Klaile E, Dienemann H, et al. Dectin-1 is expressed in human lung and mediates the proinflammatory immune response to nontypeable *Haemophilus influenza. MBio* (2014) 5:e01492-14. doi: 10.1128/mBio.01492-14
249. Xu X, Steere RR, Fedorchuk CA, Pang J, Lee JY, Lim JH, et al. Activation of epidermal growth factor receptor is required for NTHi-induced NF-kappaB-dependent inflammation. *PLoS ONE* (2011) 6:e28216. doi: 10.1371/journal.pone.0028216
250. Mikami F, Gu H, Jono H, Andalibi A, Kai H, Li JD. Epidermal growth factor receptor acts as a negative regulator for bacterium nontypeable *Haemophilus influenzae*-induced Toll-like receptor 2 expression via an Src-dependent p38 mitogen-activated protein kinase signaling pathway. *J Biol Chem.* (2005) 280:36185–94. doi: 10.1074/jbc.M503941200
251. Koff JL, Shao MX, Ueki IF, Nadel JA. Multiple TLRs activate EGFR via a signaling cascade to produce innate immune responses in airway epithelium. *Am J Physiol Lung Cell Mol Physiol.* (2008) 294:L1068–75. doi: 10.1152/ajplung.00025.2008
252. Rotta Detto Loria J, Rohmann K, Droemann D, Kujath P, Rupp J, Goldmann T, et al. Nontypeable *Haemophilus influenzae* infection upregulates the NLRP3 inflammasome and leads to caspase-1-dependent secretion of interleukin-1β - a possible pathway of exacerbations in COPD. *PLoS ONE* (2013) 8:e66818. doi: 10.1371/journal.pone.0066818
253. Watanabe T, Jono H, Han J, Lim DJ, Li JD. Synergistic activation of NF-kappaB by nontypeable *Haemophilus influenzae* and tumor necrosis factor alpha. *Proc Natl Acad Sci USA.* (2004) 101:3563–8. doi: 10.1073/pnas.0400557101
254. Ishinaga H, Jono H, Lim JH, Kweon SM, Xu H, Ha UH, et al. TGF-beta induces p65 acetylation to enhance bacteria-induced NF-kappaB activation. *EMBO J.* (2007) 26:1150–62. doi: 10.1038/sj.emboj.7601546
255. Maciejewski BA, Jamieson KC, Arnason JW, Kooi C, Wiehler S, Traves SL, et al. Rhinovirus-bacteria coexposure synergistically induces CCL20 production from human bronchial epithelial cells. *Am J Physiol Lung Cell Mol Physiol.* (2017) 312:L731–40. doi: 10.1152/ajplung.00362.2016
256. Marti-Lliteras P, Regueiro V, Morey P, Hood DW, Saus C, Sauleda J, et al. Nontypeable *Haemophilus influenzae* clearance by alveolar macrophages is impaired by exposure to cigarette smoke. *Infect Immun.* (2009) 77:4232–42. doi: 10.1128/IAI.00305-09
257. Moon SK, Lee HY, Pan H, Takeshita T, Park R, Cha K, et al. Synergistic effect of interleukin 1 alpha on nontypeable *Haemophilus influenzae*-induced up-regulation of human beta-defensin 2 in middle ear epithelial cells. *BMC Infect Dis.* (2006) 6:12. doi: 10.1186/1471-2334-6-12

258. Moon SK, Lee HY, Li JD, Nagura M, Kang SH, Chun YM, et al. Activation of a Src-dependent Raf-MEK1/2-ERK signaling pathway is required for IL-1alpha-induced upregulation of beta-defensin 2 in human middle ear epithelial cells. *Biochim Biophys Acta* (2002) 1590:41–51. doi: 10.1016/S0167-4889(02)00196-9
259. Sibille Y, Reynolds HY. Macrophages and polymorphonuclear neutrophils in lung defense and injury. *Am Rev Respir Dis.* (1990) 141:471–501. doi: 10.1164/ajrccm/141.2.471
260. Yamasaki K, Eeden SFV. Lung macrophage phenotypes and functional responses: Role in the pathogenesis of COPD. *Int J Mol Sci.* (2018) 19(2). doi: 10.3390/ijms19020582
261. Kruger P, Saffarzadeh M, Weber AN, Rieber N, Radsak M, von Bernuth H, et al. Neutrophils: between host defence, immune modulation, and tissue injury. *PLoS Pathog.* (2015) 11:e1004651. doi: 10.1371/journal.ppat.1004651
262. Segal AW. How neutrophils kill microbes. *Annu Rev Immunol.* (2005) 23:197–223. doi: 10.1146/annurev.immunol.23.021704.115653
263. King PT, Sharma R, O'Sullivan K, Selemidis S, Lim S, Radhakrishna N, et al. Nontypeable *Haemophilus influenzae* induces sustained lung oxidative stress and protease expression. *PLoS ONE* (2015) 10:e0120371. doi: 10.1371/journal.pone.0120371
264. Juneau RA, Pang B, Weimer KE, Armbruster CE, Swords WE. Nontypeable *Haemophilus influenzae* initiates formation of neutrophil extracellular traps. *Infect Immun.* (2011) 79:431–8. doi: 10.1128/IAI.00660-10
265. Houghton AM. Matrix metalloproteinases in destructive lung disease. *Matrix Biol.* (2015) 44–46:167–74. doi: 10.1016/j.matbio.2015.02.002
266. McGuinness AJ, Sapey E. Oxidative stress in COPD: sources, markers, and potential mechanisms. *J Clin Med.* (2017) 6:E21. doi: 10.3390/jcm6020021
267. Rogers LK, Cismowski MJ. Oxidative stress in the lung - the essential paradox. *Curr Opin Toxicol.* (2018) 7:37–43. doi: 10.1016/j.cotox.2017.09.001
268. King PT, Hutchinson PE, Johnson PD, Holmes PW, Freezer NJ, Holdsworth SR. Adaptive immunity to nontypeable *Haemophilus influenzae*. *Am J Respir Crit Care Med.* (2003) 167:587–92. doi: 10.1164/rccm.200207-728OC
269. King P, Ngui J, Oppedisano F, Robins-Browne R, Holmes P, Holdsworth S. Effect of interferon gamma and CD40 ligation on intracellular monocyte survival of nontypeable *Haemophilus influenzae*. *APMIS* (2008) 116:1043–9. doi: 10.1111/j.1600-0463.2008.01078.x
270. King PT, Lim S, Pick A, Ngui J, Prodanovic Z, Downey W, et al. Lung T-cell responses to nontypeable *Haemophilus influenzae* in patients with chronic obstructive pulmonary disease. *J Allergy Clin Immunol.* (2013) 131:1314.e14–21.e14. doi: 10.1016/j.jaci.2012.09.030
271. Lu C, Zhang X, Ma C, Xu W, Gan L, Cui J, et al. Nontypeable *Haemophilus influenzae* DNA stimulates type I interferon expression via STING signaling pathway. *Biochim Biophys Acta* (2018) 1865:665–73. doi: 10.1016/j.bbamcr.2018.01.011
272. Kalathil SG, Lugade AA, Pradhan V, Miller A, Parameswaran GI, Sethi S, et al. T-regulatory cells and programmed death 1+ T cells contribute to effector T-cell dysfunction in patients with chronic obstructive pulmonary disease. *Am J Respir Crit Care Med.* (2014) 190:40–50. doi: 10.1164/rccm.201312-2293OC
273. Guan X, Lu Y, Wang G, Gibson P, Chen F, Fang K, et al. The role of regulatory T cell in nontypeable *Haemophilus influenzae*-induced acute exacerbation of chronic obstructive pulmonary disease. *Mediators Inflamm.* (2018) 2018:8387150. doi: 10.1155/2018/8387150
274. McCann JR, Mason SN, Auten RL, St Geme JW, III, Seed PC. Early-life intranasal colonization with nontypeable *Haemophilus influenzae* exacerbates juvenile airway disease in mice. *Infect Immun.* (2016) 84:2022–30. doi: 10.1128/IAI.01539-15
275. Abe Y, Murphy TF, Sethi S, Faden HS, Dmochowski J, Harabuchi Y, et al. Lymphocyte proliferative response to P6 of *Haemophilus influenzae* is associated with relative protection from exacerbations of chronic obstructive pulmonary disease. *Am J Respir Crit Care Med.* (2002) 165:967–71. doi: 10.1164/ajrccm.165.7.2109009
276. Hinks TS, Wallington JC, Williams AP, Djukanovic R, Staples KJ, Wilkinson TM. Steroid-induced deficiency of mucosal-associated invariant T cells in the chronic obstructive pulmonary disease lung. Implications for nontypeable *Haemophilus influenzae* Infection. *Am J Respir Crit Care Med.* (2016) 194:1208–18. doi: 10.1164/rccm.201601-0002OC
277. Riesbeck K. Inhaled corticosteroids in chronic obstructive pulmonary disease. A two-edged sword. *Am J Respir Crit Care Med.* (2016) 194:1177–8. doi: 10.1164/rccm.201605-0942ED
278. Li W, Zhang X, Yang Y, Yin Q, Wang Y, Li Y, et al. Recognition of conserved antigens by Th17 cells provides broad protection against pulmonary *Haemophilus influenzae* infection. *Proc Natl Acad Sci USA.* (2018) 115:E7149–57. doi: 10.1073/pnas.1802261115
279. Miller RD, Gleich GJ, Offord KP, Dunnette SL. Immunoglobulin concentrations in serum and nasal secretions in chronic obstructive pulmonary disease. A matched-pair study. *Am Rev Respir Dis.* (1979) 119:229–38. doi: 10.1164/arrd.1979.119.2.229
280. Groeneveld K, Eijk PP, van Alphen L, Jansen HM, Zanen HC. *Haemophilus influenzae* infections in patients with chronic obstructive pulmonary disease despite specific antibodies in serum and sputum. *Am Rev Respir Dis.* (1990) 141(5 Pt 1):1316–21. doi: 10.1164/ajrccm/141.5_Pt_1.1316
281. Otczyk DC, Cripps AW. Mucosal immunization: a realistic alternative. *Hum Vaccin.* (2010) 6:978–1006. doi: 10.4161/hv.6.12.13142
282. Yi K, Murphy TF. Mapping of a strain-specific bactericidal epitope to the surface-exposed loop 5 on the P2 porin protein of non-typeable *Haemophilus influenzae*. *Microb Pathog.* (1994) 17:277–82. doi: 10.1006/mpat.1994.1073
283. Staples KJ, Taylor S, Thomas S, Leung S, Cox K, Pascal TG, et al. Relationships between mucosal antibodies, non-typeable *Haemophilus influenzae* (NTHi) infection and airway inflammation in COPD. *PLoS ONE* (2016) 11:e0167250. doi: 10.1371/journal.pone.0167250
284. Polosukhin VV, Cates JM, Lawson WE, Zaynagetdinov R, Milstone AP, Massion PP, et al. Bronchial secretory immunoglobulin a deficiency correlates with airway inflammation and progression of chronic obstructive pulmonary disease. *Am J Respir Crit Care Med.* (2011) 184:317–27. doi: 10.1164/rccm.201010-1629OC
285. Millares L, Marin A, Garcia-Aymerich J, Sauleda J, Belda J, Monso E, et al. Specific IgA and metalloproteinase activity in bronchial secretions from stable chronic obstructive pulmonary disease patients colonized by *Haemophilus influenzae*. *Respir Res.* (2012) 13:113. doi: 10.1186/1465-9921-13-113
286. Meshi B, Vitalis TZ, Ionescu D, Elliott WM, Liu C, Wang XD, et al. Emphysematous lung destruction by cigarette smoke. The effects of latent adenoviral infection on the lung inflammatory response. *Am J Respir Cell Mol Biol.* (2002) 26:52–7. doi: 10.1165/ajrcmb.26.1.4253
287. Gohy ST, Detry BR, Lecocq M, Bouzin C, Weynand BA, Amatngalim GD, et al. Polymeric immunoglobulin receptor down-regulation in chronic obstructive pulmonary disease. Persistence in the cultured epithelium and role of transforming growth factor-β. *Am J Respir Crit Care Med.* (2014) 190:509–21. doi: 10.1164/rccm.201311-1971OC
288. Richmond BW, Brucker RM, Han W, Du RH, Zhang Y, Cheng DS, et al. Airway bacteria drive a progressive COPD-like phenotype in mice with polymeric immunoglobulin receptor deficiency. *Nat Commun.* (2016) 7:11240. doi: 10.1038/ncomms11240
289. Van der Hilst JC, Smits BW, van der Meer JW. Hypogammaglobulinaemia: cumulative experience in 49 patients in a tertiary care institution. *Neth J Med.* (2002) 60:140–7.
290. Storisteanu DM, Pocock JM, Cowburn AS, Juss JK, Nadesalingam A, Nizet V, et al. Evasion of neutrophil extracellular traps by respiratory pathogens. *Am J Respir Cell Mol Biol.* (2017) 56:423–31. doi: 10.1165/rcmb.2016-0193PS
291. Berenson CS, Garlipp MA, Grove LJ, Maloney J, Sethi S. Impaired phagocytosis of nontypeable *Haemophilus influenzae* by human alveolar macrophages in chronic obstructive pulmonary disease. *J Infect Dis.* (2006) 194:1375–84. doi: 10.1086/508428
292. Berenson CS, Kruzel RL, Eberhardt E, Dolnick R, Minderman H, Wallace PK, et al. Impaired innate immune alveolar macrophage response and the predilection for COPD exacerbations. *Thorax* (2014) 69:811–8. doi: 10.1136/thoraxjnl-2013-203669
293. Berenson CS, Wrona CT, Grove LJ, Maloney J, Garlipp MA, Wallace PK, et al. Impaired alveolar macrophage response to *Haemophilus* antigens in chronic obstructive lung disease. *Am J Respir Crit Care Med.* (2006) 174:31–40. doi: 10.1164/rccm.200509-1461OC
294. Lea SR, Reynolds SL, Kaur M, Simpson KD, Hall SR, Hessel EM, et al. The effects of repeated Toll-like receptors 2 and 4 stimulation in COPD

alveolar macrophages. *Int J Chron Obstruct Pulmon Dis.* (2018) 13:771–80. doi: 10.2147/COPD.S97071

295. Knobloch J, Schild K, Jungck D, Urban K, Muller K, Schweda EK, et al. The T-helper cell type 1 immune response to gram-negative bacterial infections is impaired in COPD. *Am J Respir Crit Care Med.* (2011) 183:204–14. doi: 10.1164/rccm.201002-0199OC
296. MacRedmond RE, Greene CM, Dorscheid DR, McElvaney NG, O'Neill SJ. Epithelial expression of TLR4 is modulated in COPD and by steroids, salmeterol and cigarette smoke. *Respir Res.* (2007) 8:84. doi: 10.1186/1465-9921-8-84
297. von Scheele I, Larsson K, Dahlen B, Billing B, Skedinger M, Lantz AS, et al. Toll-like receptor expression in smokers with and without COPD. *Respir Med.* (2011) 105:1222–30. doi: 10.1016/j.rmed.2011.02.012
298. Tripathi PM, Kant S, Yadav RS, Kushwaha RAS, Prakash V, Rizvi SHM, et al. Expression of Toll-like receptor 2 and 4 in peripheral blood neutrophil cells from patients with chronic obstructive pulmonary disease. *Oman Med J.* (2017) 32:477–85. doi: 10.5001/omj.2017.92
299. Freeman CM, Martinez FJ, Han MK, Washko GR, Jr., McCubbrey AL, Chensue SW, et al. Lung CD8+ T cells in COPD have increased expression of bacterial TLRs. *Respir Res.* (2013) 14:13. doi: 10.1186/1465-9921-14-13
300. Pouwels SD, van Geffen WH, Jonker MR, Kerstjens HA, Nawijn MC, Heijink IH. Increased neutrophil expression of pattern recognition receptors during COPD exacerbations. *Respirology* (2017) 22:401–4. doi: 10.1111/resp.12912
301. Budulac SE, Boezen HM, Hiemstra PS, Lapperre TS, Vonk JM, Timens W, et al. Toll-like receptor (TLR2 and TLR4) polymorphisms and chronic obstructive pulmonary disease. *PLoS ONE* (2012) 7:e43124. doi: 10.1371/journal.pone.0043124
302. Berenson CS, Kruzel RL, Wrona CT, Mammen MJ, Sethi S. Impaired innate COPD alveolar macrophage responses and Toll-like receptor-9 polymorphisms. *PLoS ONE* (2015) 10:e0134209. doi: 10.1371/journal.pone.0134209
303. Kumagai Y, Takeuchi O, Akira S. TLR9 as a key receptor for the recognition of DNA. *Adv Drug Deliv Rev.* (2008) 60:795–804. doi: 10.1016/j.addr.2007.12.004
304. Drannik AG, Pouladi MA, Robbins CS, Goncharova SI, Kianpour S, Stampfli MR. Impact of cigarette smoke on clearance and inflammation after *Pseudomonas aeruginosa* infection. *Am J Respir Crit Care Med.* (2004) 170:1164–71. doi: 10.1164/rccm.200311-1521OC
305. Metcalfe HJ, Lea S, Hughes D, Khalaf R, Abbott-Banner K, Singh D. Effects of cigarette smoke on Toll-like receptor (TLR) activation of chronic obstructive pulmonary disease (COPD) macrophages. *Clin Exp Immunol.* (2014) 176:461–72. doi: 10.1111/cei.12289
306. Berenson CS, Kruzel RL, Sethi S. The impact of exogenous factors on respiratory pathogen-induced innate alveolar macrophage responses in COPD. *Immunol Invest.* (2016) 45:130–47. doi: 10.3109/08820139.2015.1113427
307. Harvey CJ, Thimmulappa RK, Sethi S, Kong X, Yarmus L, Brown RH, et al. Targeting Nrf2 signaling improves bacterial clearance by alveolar macrophages in patients with COPD and in a mouse model. *Sci Transl Med.* (2011) 3:78ra32. doi: 10.1126/scitranslmed.3002042
308. Tay HL, Kaiko GE, Plank M, Li J, Maltby S, Essilfie AT, et al. Antagonism of miR-328 increases the antimicrobial function of macrophages and neutrophils and rapid clearance of non-typeable *Haemophilus influenzae* (NTHi) from infected lung. *PLoS Pathog.* (2015) 11:e1004549. doi: 10.1371/journal.ppat.1004549
309. Gaschler GJ, Skrtic M, Zavitz CC, Lindahl M, Onnervik PO, Murphy TF, et al. Bacteria challenge in smoke-exposed mice exacerbates inflammation and skews the inflammatory profile. *Am J Respir Crit Care Med.* (2009) 179:666–75. doi: 10.1164/rccm.200808-1306OC
310. Gaschler GJ, Zavitz CC, Bauer CM, Stampfli MR. Mechanisms of clearance of nontypeable *Haemophilus influenzae* from cigarette smoke-exposed mouse lungs. *Eur Respir J.* (2010) 36:1131–42. doi: 10.1183/09031936.00113909
311. Lugade AA, Bogner PN, Thatcher TH, Sime PJ, Phipps RP, Thanavala Y. Cigarette smoke exposure exacerbates lung inflammation and compromises immunity to bacterial infection. *J Immunol.* (2014) 192:5226–35. doi: 10.4049/jimmunol.1302584
312. Bhat TA, Kalathil SG, Bogner PN, Miller A, Lehmann PV, Thatcher TH, et al. Secondhand smoke induces inflammation and impairs immunity to respiratory infections. *J Immunol.* (2018) 200:2927–40. doi: 10.4049/jimmunol.1701417
313. Sharan R, Perez-Cruz M, Kervoaze G, Gosset P, Weynants V, Godfroid F, et al. Interleukin-22 protects against non-typeable *Haemophilus influenzae* infection: alteration during chronic obstructive pulmonary disease. *Mucosal Immunol.* (2017) 10:139–49. doi: 10.1038/mi.2016.40
314. Roos AB, Sethi S, Nikota J, Wrona CT, Dorrington MG, Sanden C, et al. IL-17A and the promotion of neutrophilia in acute exacerbation of chronic obstructive pulmonary disease. *Am J Respir Crit Care Med.* (2015) 192:428–37. doi: 10.1164/rccm.201409-1689OC
315. Singh D. Chronic obstructive pulmonary disease, neutrophils and bacterial infection: a complex web involving IL-17 and IL-22 unravels. *EBioMed.* (2015) 2:1580–1. doi: 10.1016/j.ebiom.2015.10.021
316. Persson LJ, Aanerud M, Hardie JA, Miodini Nilsen R, Bakke PS, Eagan TM, et al. Antimicrobial peptide levels are linked to airway inflammation, bacterial colonisation and exacerbations in chronic obstructive pulmonary disease. *Eur Respir J.* (2017) 49:1601328. doi: 10.1183/13993003.01328-2016
317. Hiemstra PS, Amatngalim GD, van der Does AM, Taube C. Antimicrobial peptides and innate lung defenses: role in infectious and noninfectious lung diseases and therapeutic applications. *Chest* (2016) 149:545–51. doi: 10.1378/chest.15-1353
318. Sallenave JM. Secretory leukocyte protease inhibitor and elafin/trappin-2: versatile mucosal antimicrobials and regulators of immunity. *Am J Respir Cell Mol Biol.* (2010) 42:635–43. doi: 10.1165/rcmb.2010-0095RT
319. Seiler F, Lepper PM, Bals R, Beisswenger C. Regulation and function of antimicrobial peptides in immunity and diseases of the lung. *Protein Pept Lett.* (2014) 21:341–51. doi: 10.2174/09298665113206660100
320. Marsland BJ, Gollwitzer ES. Host-microorganism interactions in lung diseases. *Nat Rev Immunol.* (2014) 14:827–35. doi: 10.1038/nri3769
321. Abou Alaiwa MH, Reznikov LR, Gansemer ND, Sheets KA, Horswill AR, Stoltz DA, et al. pH modulates the activity and synergism of the airway surface liquid antimicrobials beta-defensin-3 and LL-37. *Proc Natl Acad Sci USA.* (2014) 111:18703–8. doi: 10.1073/pnas.1422091112
322. Kilsgard O, Andersson P, Malmsten M, Nordin SL, Linge HM, Eliasson M, et al. Peptidylarginine deiminases present in the airways during tobacco smoking and inflammation can citrullinate the host defense peptide LL-37, resulting in altered activities. *Am J Respir Cell Mol Biol.* (2012) 46:240–8. doi: 10.1165/rcmb.2010-0500OC
323. Vollenweider DJ, Jarrett H, Steurer-Stey CA, Garcia-Aymerich J, Puhan MA. Antibiotics for exacerbations of chronic obstructive pulmonary disease. *Cochrane Database Syst Rev.* (2012) 12:CD010257. doi: 10.1002/14651858.CD010257
324. van Velzen P, Ter Riet G, Bresser P, Baars JJ, van den Berg BTJ, van den Berg JWK, et al. Doxycycline for outpatient-treated acute exacerbations of COPD: a randomised double-blind placebo-controlled trial. *Lancet Respir Med.* (2017) 5:492–9. doi: 10.1016/S2213-2600(17)30165-0
325. Clinical and Laboratory Standards Institute (CLSI). *Performance Standards for Antimicrobial Susceptibility Testing, 28th ed.* CLSI supplement M100. Wayne, PA: Clinical and Laboratory Standards Institute (2018). p. 296.
326. The European Committee on Antimicrobial Susceptibility Testing. *Breakpoint Tables for Interpretation of MICs and Zone Diameters. Version 8.1* (2018). Available online at: http://www.eucast.org/
327. Pettigrew MM, Tsuji BT, Gent JF, Kong Y, Holden PN, Sethi S, et al. Effect of fluoroquinolones and macrolides on eradication and resistance of *Haemophilus influenzae* in chronic obstructive pulmonary disease. *Antimicrob Agents Chemother.* (2016) 60:4151–8. doi: 10.1128/AAC.00301-16
328. Skaare D, Anthonisen IL, Caugant DA, Jenkins A, Steinbakk M, Strand L, et al. Multilocus sequence typing and *ftsI* sequencing: a powerful tool for surveillance of penicillin-binding protein 3-mediated beta-lactam resistance in nontypeable *Haemophilus influenzae. BMC Microbiol.* (2014) 14:131. doi: 10.1186/1471-2180-14-131
329. Tristram S, Jacobs MR, Appelbaum PC. Antimicrobial resistance in *Haemophilus influenzae. Clin Microbiol Rev.* (2007) 20:368–89. doi: 10.1128/CMR.00040-06
330. Resman F, Ristovski M, Forsgren A, Kaijser B, Kronvall G, Medstrand P, et al. Increase of β-lactam-resistant invasive *Haemophilus influenzae* in

Sweden, 1997 to 2010. *Antimicrob Agents Chemother.* (2012) 56:4408–15. doi: 10.1128/AAC.00415-12

331. Skaare D, Anthonisen IL, Kahlmeter G, Matuschek E, Natas OB, Steinbakk M, et al. Emergence of clonally related multidrug resistant *Haemophilus influenzae* with penicillin-binding protein 3-mediated resistance to extended-spectrum cephalosporins, Norway, 2006 to 2013. *Euro Surveill.* (2014) 19:20986. doi: 10.2807/1560-7917.es2014.19.49.20986
332. Garcia-Cobos S, Campos J, Lazaro E, Roman F, Cercenado E, Garcia-Rey C, et al. Ampicillin-resistant non-beta-lactamase-producing *Haemophilus influenzae* in Spain: recent emergence of clonal isolates with increased resistance to cefotaxime and cefixime. *Antimicrob Agents Chemother.* (2007) 51:2564–73. doi: 10.1128/AAC.00354-07
333. Okabe T, Yamazaki Y, Shiotani M, Suzuki T, Shiohara M, Kasuga E, et al. An amino acid substitution in PBP-3 in *Haemophilus influenzae* associate with the invasion to bronchial epithelial cells. *Microbiol Res.* (2010) 165:11–20. doi: 10.1016/j.micres.2008.03.003
334. Atkins NA, Kunde DA, Zosky G, Tristram SG. Genotypically defined beta-lactamase-negative ampicillin-resistant isolates of non-typable *Haemophilus influenzae* are associated with increased invasion of bronchial epithelial cells *in vitro*. *J Med Microbiol.* (2014) 63(Pt 10):1400–3. doi: 10.1099/jmm.0.077966-0
335. Herath SC, Poole P. Prophylactic antibiotic therapy for chronic obstructive pulmonary disease (COPD). *Cochrane Database Syst Rev.* (2013) CD009764. doi: 10.1002/14651858.CD009764.pub2
336. Pomares X, Monton C, Bullich M, Cuevas O, Oliva JC, Gallego M, et al. Clinical and safety outcomes of long-term azithromycin therapy in severe COPD beyond the first year of treatment. *Chest* (2018) 153:1125–33. doi: 10.1016/j.chest.2018.01.044
337. Shimizu T, Shimizu S. Azithromycin inhibits mucus hypersecretion from airway epithelial cells. *Mediators Inflamm.* (2012) 2012:265714. doi: 10.1155/2012/265714
338. Araki N, Yanagihara K, Morinaga Y, Yamada K, Nakamura S, Yamada Y, et al. Azithromycin inhibits nontypeable *Haemophilus influenzae*-induced MUC5AC expression and secretion via inhibition of activator protein-1 in human airway epithelial cells. *Eur J Pharmacol.* (2010) 644:209–14. doi: 10.1016/j.ejphar.2010.06.056
339. Hodge S, Reynolds PN. Low-dose azithromycin improves phagocytosis of bacteria by both alveolar and monocyte-derived macrophages in chronic obstructive pulmonary disease subjects. *Respirology* (2012) 17:802–7. doi: 10.1111/j.1440-1843.2012.02135.x
340. Euba B, Moleres J, Viadas C, Barberan M, Caballero L, Grillo MJ, et al. Relationship between azithromycin susceptibility and administration efficacy for nontypeable *Haemophilus influenzae* respiratory infection. *Antimicrob Agents Chemother.* (2015) 59:2700–12. doi: 10.1128/AAC.04447-14
341. Hodge S, Tran HB, Hamon R, Roscioli E, Hodge G, Jersmann H, et al. Nonantibiotic macrolides restore airway macrophage phagocytic function with potential anti-inflammatory effects in chronic lung diseases. *Am J Physiol Lung Cell Mol Physiol.* (2017) 312:L678–L87. doi: 10.1152/ajplung.00518.2016
342. Murphy TF. Vaccines for nontypeable *Haemophilus influenzae*: the future is now. *Clin Vaccine Immunol.* (2015) 22:459–66. doi: 10.1128/CVI.00089-15

7

Limited Innovations After More than 65 Years of Immunoglobulin Replacement Therapy: Potential of IgA- and IgM-Enriched Formulations to Prevent Bacterial Respiratory Tract Infections

Jeroen D. Langereis[1,2]**, *Michiel van der Flier*[1,2,3,4] *and Marien I. de Jonge*[1,2]

[1] Section Pediatric Infectious Diseases, Laboratory of Medical Immunology, Radboud Institute for Molecular Life Sciences, Nijmegen, Netherlands, [2] Radboud Center for Infectious Diseases, Nijmegen, Netherlands, [3] Pediatric Infectious Diseases and Immunology, Amalia Children's Hospital, Nijmegen, Netherlands, [4] Expertise Center for Immunodeficiency and Autoinflammation (REIA), Radboudumc, Nijmegen, Netherlands

Correspondence:
Jeroen D. Langereis
Jeroen.Langereis@radboudumc.nl

Patients with primary immunoglobulin deficiency have lower immunoglobulin levels or decreased immunoglobulin function, which makes these patients more susceptible to bacterial infection. Most prevalent are the selective IgA deficiencies (∼1:3,000), followed by common variable immune deficiency (∼1:25,000). Agammaglobulinemia is less common (∼1:400,000) and is characterized by very low or no immunoglobulin production resulting in a more severe disease phenotype. Therapy for patients with agammaglobulinemia mainly relies on prophylactic antibiotics and the use of IgG replacement therapy, which successfully reduces the frequency of invasive bacterial infections. Currently used immunoglobulin preparations contain only IgG. As a result, concurrent IgA and IgM deficiency persist in a large proportion of agammaglobulinemia patients. Especially patients with IgM deficiency remain at risk for recurrent infections at mucosal surfaces, which includes the respiratory tract. IgA and IgM have multiple functions in the protection against bacterial infections at the mucosal surface. Because of their multimeric structure, both IgA and IgM are able to agglutinate bacteria efficiently. Agglutination allows for entrapment of bacteria in mucus that increases clearance from the respiratory tract. IgA is also important for blocking bacterial adhesion by interfering with bacterial adhesion receptors. IgM in its place is very well capable of activating complement, therefore, it is thought to be important in complement-mediated protection at the mucosal surface. The purpose of this Mini Review is to highlight the latest advances regarding IgA- and IgM-enriched immunoglobulin replacement therapy. We describe the different IgA- and IgM-enriched IgG formulations, their possible modes of action and potential to protect against respiratory tract infections in patients with primary immunoglobulin deficiencies.

Keywords: IgM, IgA, IgG, immunoglobulin replacement therapy, respiratory tract infections, primary immunodeficiencies, complement system proteins, bacterial infections

ROLE FOR IMMUNOGLOBULIN SUBCLASSES IN PROTECTION AGAINST BACTERIAL INFECTIONS

Immunoglobulin production by B-lymphocytes is a sophisticated adaptive immune defense mechanisms evolved in jawed vertebrates (1). The absolute importance for immunoglobulins in protection against infections is illustrated in patients that completely lack immunoglobulin production, which is a lethal condition due to increased susceptibility for invasive infection (2). There are 5 main classes of immunoglobulins; IgG, IgM, IgA, IgD and IgE, all having different properties and functions (3). For this Mini Review, we will focus on IgG, IgM, and IgA and their role in protection against bacterial respiratory tract infections.

Immunoglobulins are with 10–22 g/L a major serum constituent. The majority of serum immunoglobulins are IgG (~75%), followed by IgA (~15%) and IgM (~10%) (4). IgG can be subdivided into IgG1, IgG2, IgG3 and IgG4 and IgA can be subdivided into IgA1 and IgA2. The half-life of immunoglobulins vary, with 3 to 4 weeks for IgG1, IgG2 and IgG4, whereas this is around 2 weeks for IgG3 (5, 6). Half-life for IgA and IgM is with 5 to 6 days much shorter compared to IgG (6, 7).

The different immunoglobulins have specific functions in immunity. Upon binding to their targets, both IgG and IgM are capable of activating complement through binding of C1q. The ability to activate complement for IgG subclasses varies due to differences in C1q binding, which is highest for IgG3, followed by IgG1, IgG2 and is absent for IgG4 (8, 9). Recent data indicate that IgG oligomerizes into hexamers, forming an optimal configuration for C1q binding (10). This oligomerization might explain the more efficient activation of complement by IgM, (11–13) because it is present as polymeric structures (pIgM) (14).

IgA is not able to activate complement directly. There are two subclasses of IgA, IgA1 and IgA2, characterized by differences in their hinge region (15). Whereas IgA1 is the predominant subclass in serum, both IgA1 and IgA2 are present on the mucosal surface (16). The majority of IgA at the mucosal surface is dimeric (dIgA) (16), whereas the majority in serum is monomeric (17). IgA is most abundant at mucosal surfaces where it has a role in protection against toxins, viruses and bacteria by means of direct neutralization, or by preventing attachment to the mucosal epithelium (18, 19).

IgA and IgM can be transported to mucosal surfaces through the polymeric immunoglobulin receptor (pIgR) (20). Only polymeric immunoglobulins containing a J-chain can be transported by this receptor (21). The pIgR present on the basolateral side of epithelial cells binds dIgA and pIgM, which facilitates transcytosis to the apical side, where it is cleaved off and leaving the secretory components attached, resulting in the formation of secretory IgA (sIgA) or sIgM (22, 23). Association of the secretory component enhances resistance to proteolysis (24), but does not affect the ability to activate complement (25).

IgG is not transported by the pIgR, but through the neonatal Fc receptor (FcRn) (26). FcRn is able to transport IgG from the basolateral to the apical side, and vice versa (27). This FcRn-mediated retrograde transport and recycling of IgG is thought to contribute to the prolonged half-life in serum (28, 29).

A successful strategy to protect healthy individuals from respiratory tract infections is the use of vaccination. In the early 1990s, the *Haemophilus influenzae* serotype B (Hib) conjugate vaccine entered the market, which decreased invasive Hib disease cases substantially in many countries (30–33). This Hib conjugate vaccine is highly immunogenic and increases capsule-specific antibody levels that not only protects against disease such as pneumonia and meningitis, but also against nasopharyngeal colonization (34). Hib vaccination elicits a combination of serum immunoglobulin subclasses, mainly IgG, but also IgM and IgA (35). Vaccination of children with the *Streptococcus pneumoniae* polysaccharide conjugate vaccines (PCV) has shown to increase capsule-specific IgG antibody levels (36) and confer protection against nasopharyngeal colonization, otitis media, pneumoniae and bacteremia (37–39). Vaccine-induced polysaccharide capsule-specific antibodies initiate complement deposition on the bacterial surface, which is essential for opsonophagocytic killing of *S. pneumoniae* and *H. influenzae* in whole blood (40).

IMMUNOGLOBULIN DEFICIENCIES

The diverse roles of the different immunoglobulin subclasses in protection against infections is illustrated in patients with primary immune deficiencies (PID), as described in more detail below.

Selective IgA Deficiency

Selective IgA deficiency (sIgAD) is characterized by serum IgA level of <7 mg/dL, with normal levels of both IgG and IgM in individuals more than 4 years of age (41). Most patients are clinically asymptomatic, but others show recurrent infections, allergies and autoimmunity (2). Although rather prevalent, the exact pathogenesis is unknown. Since sIgAD is heterogeneous in presentation of disease symptoms, it is likely that different aetiologies might be involved in the cause of this disease. There is evidence for genetic predisposition based on familial clustering, and mutations in many genes involved in cellular and humoral immunity have been associated with sIgAD (42).

Recurrent respiratory tract infections are the most common disease associated with sIgAD (43–45). When divided into complete and partial IgA deficiency, a history of chronic or recurrent infections is more often found in patients with complete IgA deficiency (77%), compared to partial IgA deficiency (20%) (44), suggesting that a lower IgA is associated with frequent infections. Elevated levels of IgG or IgM are found in a proportion of sIgAD patients (44–47), which might compensate the IgA deficiency. Patients with sIgAD who had

Abbreviations: Btk, Bruton tyrosine kinase; CVID, Common variable immune deficiency; dIgA, Dimeric IgA; FcRN, Neonatal Fc receptor; FFP, Fresh frozen plasma; IgGRT, IgG replacement therapy; IgRT, Immunoglobulin replacement therapy=; IM-IgGRT, Intramuscular IgG replacement therapy; IV-IgGRT, Intravenous IgG replacement therapy; PID, Primary immune deficiencies; pIgM, Polymeric IgM; SC-IgGRT, Subcutaneously IgG replacement therapy; sIgA, Secretory IgA; sIgAD, Selective IgA deficienciy; sIgM, Secretory IgM; sIgMD, Selective IgM deficienciy; XLA, X-lined agammaglobulinemia.

higher saliva IgM levels showed a lower infection incidence (47), although this was not found in a later study (46). Patients with sIgAD are usually not treated with IgG replacement therapy (IgGRT), but it is recommended for individuals with IgA deficiency and concomitant IgG2 subclass deficiency (48).

Selective IgM Deficiency

The European Society for Immunodeficiencies (ESID) Registry defines selective IgM deficiency (sIgMD) as a serum IgM concentration of 2 standard deviations below the normal level, with normal levels of serum IgA and IgG, normal vaccination responses and absence of T cell defects (41). The immunological and clinical phenotype of sIgMD is very heterogeneous and patients can remain asymptomatic (49). Similar to sIgAD, patients with sIgMD often present with recurrent respiratory problems (49, 50). In a cohort of 17 sIgMD patients, recurrent upper respiratory tract infections were observed in 5 out of 6 patients with undetectable IgM levels (<0.05 g/L) (49). Although for most sIgMD patients IgGRT was not required (49), it is recommended for patients with recurrent or severe infections (51).

Common Variable Immune Deficiencies

Patients with common variable immune deficiencies (CVID) are characterized by a marked decrease of IgG or IgA with or without low IgM levels, poor specific immunoglobulin responses to vaccination and no profound T-cell deficiency (41). A monogenic cause has been identified in 2–10% of CVID patients, but most patients appear to be polygenic or multifactorial disorders (52). Most CVID patients present with infectious manifestations, commonly of the upper and lower respiratory tract (53). The majority (70%) of CVID patients develop chronic pulmonary complications including bronchiectasis and bronchial wall thickening (54). To prevent especially respiratory tract infections, IgGRT is the mainstay treatment for CVID patients (55).

Agammaglobulinemia

Patients with agammaglobulinemia have very low or no serum immunoglobulin levels, making these patients highly susceptible to infections (2). The largest group of patients have X-linked agammaglobulinemia (XLA), which is a caused by a defect in the *Btk* gene encoding Bruton Tyrosine Kinsase (Btk), which accounts for 85% of agammaglobulinemia patients. IgGRT is recommended for all agammaglobulinemia patients to reduce infections (56). Bacterial infections of the respiratory tract are often seen in patients with agammaglobulinemia, prior to diagnosis, but also after initiation of IgGRT (57–60), likely due to the absence of IgA and IgM antibodies in IgGRT. As a results, a large proportion of agammaglobulinemia patients develop chronic lung diseases (57, 59).

PAST, PRESENT AND FUTURE OF IMMUNOGLOBULIN REPLACEMENT THERAPY

IgG for IgGRT is traditionally collected from the Cohn fraction II after cold methanol precipitation (61, 62) and used to prevent infections in patients with PID. Despite IgGRT, recurrent infections, mainly of the respiratory tract, are reported (57–60), and is associated with a lowered life-expectancy of CVID and agammaglobulinemia patients (63, 64). Currently used immunoglobulin preparations contain only IgG. As a result, concurrent IgA and IgM deficiency persists in a large proportion of immunoglobulin deficient patients, which results in recurrent infections and development of chronic lung diseases such as bronchiectasis (65, 66). Here, we summarize the current and novel immunoglobulin replacement therapies possibly effective in preventing bacterial respiratory tract infections.

In the Beginning; 1952

IgGRT was first introduced in 1952 by Colonel Ogden Bruton and applied to the first patient with agammaglobulinemia (67). This patient had an extensive history of infections, including osteomyelitis, gastrointestinal infection, and multiple episodes of epidemic parotitis, otitis media, pneumonia and sepsis for 4.5 years. After the third episode of epidemic parotitis, it was found that the serum of this patient was deficient for immunoglobulins. The patient was given subcutaneous IgGRT (SC-IgGRT) and was free of invasive infections (67, 68). After this first success, more individuals with agammaglobulinemia and other PID were treated with IgGRT. Most patients received intramuscular IgGRT (IM-IgGRT) (60) because uptake and bioavailability of IgG from the muscle is better as compared to fatty tissue where it is deposited by SC-IgGRT (69). However, injections were painful and the volume that can be given is limited, therefore, alternative administration methods were explored.

An advantage for SC-IgGRT is the ability for home treatment, which was shown to be feasible and safe (70). Home treatment is more convenient, and prevents loss of school or workdays and hospital costs (70). Although SC-IgGRT was initially limited by a slow infusion, this improved considerably over the past years (71). Recently, a new SC-IgGRT formulation containing recombinant hyaluronidase, which is an enzyme that cleaves the extracellular matrix and increases tissue permeability. Therefore, the use of recombinant hyaluronidase enables administration of larger volumes of IgG and thereby decreases dosing frequency to once in the 3–4 weeks, is in clinical trial (72).

Next Step, Intravenous IgG Replacement Therapy

The largest disadvantage of both SC-IgGRT and IM-IgGRT is the limited volume that can be administered per dose. As a result, the patient requires frequent dosing, typically every week. With intravenous IgGRT (IV-IgGRT), larger volumes can be giving, which decreases the frequency of dosing to once in the 3–4 weeks. However, it requires venous access and the incidence of systemic adverse reactions were high in the early years, mainly due to vasomotor and cardiovascular manifestations, which was most likely due to immunoglobulin aggregation and complement activation (56, 73, 74). Later, modification of IV-IgGRT by for instance ß-propiolactone, which prevents aggregation (75), reduced the number of side-effects considerably (76) and soon became the routine treatment regimen (77, 78). In a head-to-head comparison, IV-IgGRT was given once every 4 weeks and SC-IgGRT every week. Significant improvement in clinical parameters such as a lower number of days with acute respiratory infections and IgG trough levels were found for IV-IgGRT (74). This even improved further when IV-IgGRT was given once every 3 weeks (74). Important for protection against respiratory infections, serum opsonic capacity of *H. influenzae* and *S. pneumoniae* increased when IV-IgGRT was administered once every 3 weeks as compared to once every 4 weeks (74).

POSSIBLE IMPROVEMENTS; IgA- AND/OR IgM-ENRICHED IMMUNOGLOBULIN REPLACEMENT THERAPY

Nowadays, both SC-IgGRT and IV-IgGRT are used to prevent infections in patients with PID and are proven to be safe (79). The choice of therapy is mainly based on the clinical condition of the patient, side effects and patient's preference, as SC-IgGRT therapy can be administered by the patient at home independent of help from health care professionals. However, as mentioned above, the current IgGRT has an important limitation; it contains only IgG, resulting in the absence or low levels of IgA and/or IgM in patients with PID. Despite IgGRT, many patients with PID develop chronic lung disease (57, 59, 66). Therefore, improvements in therapy are needed, which might be the addition of IgA and/or IgM.

There are a limited number of IgA- and/or IgM-enriched immunoglobulin preparations used in clinical practice. Here, we summarize studies that have used IgA- and/or IgM-enriched immunoglobulin products, mainly in treatment of acute bacterial infections in general and highlight the studies focused on infections in immunoglobulin deficient patients.

Fresh Frozen Plasma

Fresh frozen plasma (FFP) was advocated over IM-IgGRT by Richard Stiehm in 1975 (80) and was next to IM-IgGRT used in the early days (81). The IgG levels achieved with FFP treatment were significantly higher as compared to IM-IgGRT, while IgM and IgA levels were only slightly increased (80). The use of FFP has limited or no side effects, but to reach a normal level of IgA and IgM, it should be given at a high frequency (~ twice a week), which is inconvenient for the patient. FFP was also given to PID patients with chronic gastro-intestinal infections as add-on therapy to their normal IgGRT. Two patients with relapsing *Campylobacter jejuni* infection were given FFP for 2 or 4 weeks (500 mL twice weekly), which resulted in complete recovery of both patients (82). Plasma infusion resulted in detectable serum IgA levels in two patients and detectable serum IgM levels in 1 patients (82). Although we have not found direct evidence, FFP might be beneficial as an treatment, next to normal IgGRT, to eliminate chronic bacterial respiratory tract infections.

Pentaglobin

Pentaglobin is an IgA- and IgM-containing immunoglobulin preparation collected from Cohn fraction III, consisting of 72% IgG, 12% IgM, and 16% IgA for intravenous use (83). Pentaglobin is treated with ß-propiolactone, which decreases immunoglobulin aggregation, but also affects complement fixation and Fc-binding capacity (84, 85). A clear beneficial effect of Pentoglobin in comparison to conventional intravenous IgG is its effective reduction of endotoxin (86, 87). Direct effects on bacterial killing has also been observed by *in vitro* experiments. For instance, Pentaglobin had a greater opsonic activity against *Pseudomonas aeruginosa*, *Staphylococcus aureus* and *Escherichia coli*, in comparison to IV-IgGRT (88, 89). In a *S. aureus* mouse sepsis model, the number of bacteria in liver and kidney were significantly lower for animals receiving Pentaglobin in comparison to animals receiving IV-IgGRT Intratect (89). Pentaglobin has to our knowledge not been used as replacement for conventional IgGRT, but, it has successfully been applied to treat two hypogammaglobulinemia patients with persistent gastroenteric *C. jejuni* infections (90). In these two patients, six dosages of Pentaglobin at 3-week intervals were well tolerated (90). After the first dose, an increased serum bactericidal antibody activity against *C. jejuni* was measured and treatment resulted in the elimination of the *C. jejuni* infections (90). This result is in line with the use of IgA- and IgM-containing FFP, which was also successfully used to treat chronic *C. jejuni* infections (82). We have found a remarkable increase in complement-mediated killing of *C. jejuni* (31) by supplementing purified serum IgM to serum of a patients with agammaglobulinemia, supporting an important role for IgM in complement-mediated protection against bacterial pathogens.

Trimodulin

Trimodulin (BT-588, predecessor BT-086) contains twice the amount of IgA (21%) and IgM (23%) in comparison to Pentaglobin. Trimodulin is not treated with ß-propiolactone and showed approximately 10-fold increase in opsonization of *E. coli* compared to Pentaglobin (91). In a rabbit model for endotoxemia, Trimodulin showed an increased elimination of *E. coli* from the bloodstream (92). Recently, the results of a phase II trial, which included 160 patients with severe community-acquired pneumonia, were published (93). Although no difference was observed for ventilator-free days between the placebo and Trimodulin groups, *post-hoc* analyses supported improved outcome in patients with elevated CRP, reduced IgM, or both. In addition, Trimodulin seemed to prevent secondary bacterial infections because infection-related treatment-emergent adverse events were significantly decreased from 57% in the placebo group to 33% in the Trimodulin-treated patients (93). Since IgA and IgM concentrations present in Trimodulin are higher compared to Pentaglobin, we would expect an additive effect on preventing bacterial infections of the respiratory tract, although this has not been determined to date.

IgAbulin

IgAbulin is an IgA-enriched IgG preparation, which was shown to prevent necrotizing enterocolitis when administered orally to babies with low birth weight (94) and has successfully been used to treat children with chronic diarrhea (95). Oral administration of IgAbulin daily for 3 weeks decreased the number of stools per day and improved the consistency of the stools (95). So far, IgA-enriched IgGRT has not been used to prevent or treat bacterial respiratory tract infections. Since IgA is the most abundant immunoglobulin isotype on the respiratory tract mucosal surface, with divers functions in preventing bacterial infections, it might help in preventing and clearing bacterial infections. A possible limitation of the current IgA-enriched immunoglobulin preparations is that they are isolated from plasma, and plasma-derived IgA is mainly IgA1, which is more sensitive to bacterial IgA proteases (96), in comparison to IgA2, which is most abundant on the mucosal surface (16). In addition, the majority of serum-derived IgA is monomeric (17), in contrast to locally produced IgA, which is mainly dimeric (16). But, administration of sufficient IgA might potentially be effective in preventing bacterial respiratory tract infections, especially in PID patients with concurrent IgA deficiency.

Purified Serum IgA and IgM Linked to Recombinant Secretory Component

Although not in clinical trials, plasma-derived IgA and IgM containing recombinant secretory component have been tested in animal studies with promising results. It has been shown that plasma-derived IgA and IgM can bind recombinant secretory component to form sIgA and sIgM (97). Addition of the secretory component increased resistance to protease activity and showed to prevent *Shigella flexneri*-induced intestine epithelial cell damage in an *in vitro* cell model (98). sIgA and sIgM preparations were found to bind and agglutinate *Salmonella enterica* Typhimurium (99). Oral administration of sIgA and sIgM preparations effectively limited *S. Typhimurium* infection and systemic dissemination in mice (99). No results were published regarding the effects on protection of bacterial respiratory pathogens, but since these sIgA and sIgM preparations are able to block bacterial adhesion, it is expected to prevent acquisition of bacteria in the respiratory tract when applied to the airways. In addition, these sIgA and sIgM preparations are not treated with ß-propiolactone, preserving natural complement fixating activity. Future experiments are required to address the efficacy to prevent bacterial respiratory tract infections.

CONCLUDING REMARKS

Current IgGRT treatment has not shown to prevent bacterial respiratory tract infections in a selection of PID patients. Based on the clinical presentation of patients with IgA and IgM deficiencies, who mainly present with respiratory tract infections, it is conceivable that IgA- and/or IgM-enriched immunoglobulin replacement therapy with biologically active IgA and/or IgM have the potential to prevent these type of infections. In the near future, pre-clinical *in vitro* assays, animal experiments and clinical trials have to be conducted to determine whether IgA and/or IgM-enriched immunoglobulin replacement therapy would prevent bacterial respiratory tract infections in patients with PID.

AUTHOR CONTRIBUTIONS

JL wrote the initial manuscript. MvdF and MdJ edited and approved the final manuscript.

REFERENCES

1. Hsu E, Pulham N, Rumfelt LL, Flajnik MF. The plasticity of immunoglobulin gene systems in evolution. *Immunol Rev.* (2006) 210:8–26. doi: 10.1111/j.0105-2896.2006.00366.x
2. Sullivan KE, Stiehm ER. *Stiehm's Immune Deficiencies.* London; San Diego, CA: Elsevier/AP (2014).
3. Janeway C. Immunobiology: the immune system in health and disease. New York, NY: Garland Science (2005).
4. Schroeder HW Jr, Cavacini L. Structure and function of immunoglobulins. *J Allergy Clin Immunol.* (2010) 125(2 Suppl. 2):S41–52. doi: 10.1016/j.jaci.2009.09.046
5. Mankarious S, Lee M, Fischer S, Pyun KH, Ochs HD, Oxelius VA, et al. The half-lives of IgG subclasses and specific antibodies in patients with primary immunodeficiency who are receiving intravenously administered immunoglobulin. *J Lab Clin Med.* (1988) 112:634–40.
6. Waldmann TA, Strober W. Metabolism of immunoglobulins. *Prog Allergy* (1969) 13:1–110.
7. Barth WF, Wochner RD, Waldmann TA, Fahey JL. Metabolism of human gamma macroglobulins. *J Clin Invest.* (1964) 43:1036–48. doi: 10.1172/JCI104987
8. Bindon CI, Hale G, Bruggemann M, Waldmann H. Human monoclonal IgG isotypes differ in complement activating function at the level of C4 as well as C1q. *J Exp Med.* (1988) 168:127–42.
9. Tao MH, Smith RI, Morrison SL. Structural features of human immunoglobulin G that determine isotype-specific differences in complement activation. *J Exp Med.* (1993) 178:661–7.
10. Diebolder CA, Beurskens FJ, de Jong RN, Koning RI, Strumane K, Lindorfer MA, et al. Complement is activated by IgG hexamers assembled at the cell surface. *Science* (2014) 343:1260–3. doi: 10.1126/science.1248943
11. Pluschke G, Bordmann G, Daoudaki ME, Lambris JD, Achtman M, Neibert M. Isolation of rat IgM to IgG hybridoma isotype switch variants and analysis of the efficiency of rat Ig in complement activation. *Eur J Immunol.* (1989) 19:131–5. doi: 10.1002/eji.1830190121
12. Raff HV, Bradley C, Brady W, Donaldson K, Lipsich L, Maloney G, et al. Comparison of functional activities between IgG1 and IgM class-switched human monoclonal antibodies reactive with group B streptococci or Escherichia coli K1. *J Infect Dis.* (1991) 163:346–54.
13. Sabharwal UK, Vaughan JH, Fong S, Bennett PH, Carson DA, Curd JG. Activation of the classical pathway of complement by rheumatoid factors. Assessment by radioimmunoassay for C4. *Arthritis Rheum.* (1982) 25:161–7.
14. Davis AC, Roux KH, Shulman MJ. On the structure of polymeric IgM. *Eur J Immunol.* (1988) 18:1001–8. doi: 10.1002/eji.1830180705
15. Frangione B, Wolfenstein MJ. Todel: partial duplication in the "hinge" region of IgA 1 myeloma proteins. *Proc Natl Acad Sci USA.* (1972) 69:3673–6.
16. Delacroix DL, Dive C, Rambaud JC, Vaerman JP. IgA subclasses in various secretions and in serum. *Immunology* (1982) 47:383–5.
17. Delacroix DL, Elkom KB, Geubel AP, Hodgson HF, Dive C, Vaerman JP. Changes in size, subclass, and metabolic properties of serum immunoglobulin A in liver diseases and in other diseases with high serum immunoglobulin A. *J Clin Invest.* (1983) 71:358–67.
18. Woof JM, Mestecky J. Mucosal immunoglobulins. *Immunol Rev.* (2005) 206:64–82. doi: 10.1111/j.0105-2896.2005.00290.x
19. Johnson S, Sypura WD, Gerding DN, Ewing SL, Janoff EN. Selective neutralization of a bacterial enterotoxin by serum immunoglobulin A in response to mucosal disease. *Infect Immun.* (1995) 63:3166–73.
20. Crago SS, Kulhavy R, Prince SJ, Mestecky J. Secretory component of epithelial cells is a surface receptor for polymeric immunoglobulins. *J Exp Med.* (1978) 147:1832–7.

21. Brandtzaeg P, Prydz H. Direct evidence for an integrated function of J chain and secretory component in epithelial transport of immunoglobulins. *Nature* (1984) 311:71–3.
22. Mostov KE, Kraehenbuhl JP, Blobel G. Receptor-mediated transcellular transport of immunoglobulin: synthesis of secretory component as multiple and larger transmembrane forms. *Proc Natl Acad Sci USA.* (1980) 77:7 257–61.
23. Mostov KE, Blobel G. A transmembrane precursor of secretory component. The receptor for transcellular transport of polymeric immunoglobulins. *J Biol Chem.* (1982) 257:11816–21.
24. Underdown BJ, Dorrington KJ. Studies on the structural and conformational basis for the relative resistance of serum and secretory immunoglobulin A to proteolysis. *J Immunol.* (1974) 112:949–59.
25. Michaelsen TE, Emilsen S, Sandin RH, Granerud BK, Bratlie D, Ihle O, et al. Human secretory IgM antibodies activate human complement and offer protection at mucosal surface. *Scand J Immunol.* (2017) 85:43–50. doi: 10.1111/sji.12508
26. Simister NE, Rees AR. Isolation and characterization of an Fc receptor from neonatal rat small intestine. *Eur J Immunol.* (1985) 15:733–8. doi: 10.1002/eji.1830150718
27. Dickinson BL, Badizadegan K, Wu Z, Ahouse JC, Zhu X, Simister NE, et al. Bidirectional FcRn-dependent IgG transport in a polarized human intestinal epithelial cell line. *J Clin Invest.* (1999) 104:903–11. doi: 10.1172/JCI6968
28. Ghetie V, Hubbard JG, Kim JK, Tsen MF, Lee Y, Ward ES. Abnormally short serum half-lives of IgG in beta 2-microglobulin-deficient mice. *Eur J Immunol.* (1996) 26:690–6. doi: 10.1002/eji.1830260327
29. Junghans RP, Anderson CL. The protection receptor for IgG catabolism is the beta2-microglobulin-containing neonatal intestinal transport receptor. *Proc Natl Acad Sci USA.* (1996) 93:5512–6.
30. Bisgard KM, Kao A, Leake J, Strebel PM, Perkins BA, Wharton M. Haemophilus influenzae invasive disease in the United States, 1994-1995: near disappearance of a vaccine-preventable childhood disease. *Emerg Infect Dis.* (1998) 4:229–37. doi: 10.3201/eid0402.980210
31. Langereis JD, Henriet SS, Kuipers S, Weemaes CMR, van der Burg M, de Jonge MI, et al. IgM augments complement bactericidal activity with serum from a patient with a novel CD79a mutation. *J Clin Immunol.* (2018) 38:185–92. doi: 10.1007/s10875-017-0474-7
32. Peltola H, Kilpi T, Anttila M. Rapid disappearance of Haemophilus influenzae type b meningitis after routine childhood immunisation with conjugate vaccines. *Lancet* (1992) 340:592–4.
33. van Alphen L, Spanjaard L, van der Ende A, Schuurman I, Dankert J. Effect of nationwide vaccination of 3-month-old infants in the Netherlands with conjugate *Haemophilus influenzae* type b vaccine: high efficacy and lack of herd immunity. *J Pediatr.* (1997) 131:869–73.
34. Ladhani SN. Two decades of experience with the haemophilus influenzae serotype b conjugate vaccine in the United Kingdom. *Clin Ther.* (2012) 34:385–99. doi: 10.1016/j.clinthera.2011.11.027
35. Barra A, Dagan R, Preud'homme JL, Bajart A, Danve B, Fritzell B. Characterization of the serum antibody response induced by Haemophilus influenzae type b tetanus protein-conjugate vaccine in infants receiving a DTP-combined vaccine from 2 months of age. *Vaccine* (1993) 11:1 003–6.
36. Bryant KA, Block SL, Baker SA, Gruber WC, Scott DA, PCVIS Group. Safety and immunogenicity of a 13-valent pneumococcal conjugate vaccine. *Pediatrics* (2010) 125:866–75. doi: 10.1542/peds.2009-1405
37. Black S, Shinefield H, Fireman B, Lewis E, Ray P, Hansen JR, et al. Efficacy, safety, and immunogenicity of heptavalent pneumococcal conjugate vaccine in children. *Am J Manag Care* (2000) 6:S536–49. doi: 10.1097/00006454-200003000-00003
38. Eskola J, Kilpi T, Palmu A, Jokinen J, Haapakoski J, Herva E, et al. Efficacy of a pneumococcal conjugate vaccine against acute otitis media. *New Eng J Med.* (2001) 344:403–9. doi: 10.1056/Nejm200102083440602
39. Shinefield H, Black S, Ray P, Fireman B, Schwalbe J, Lewis E. Efficacy, immunogenicity and safety of heptavalent pneumococcal conjugate vaccine in low birth weight and preterm infants. *Pediatr Infect Dis J.* (2002) 21:182–6. doi: 10.1097/00006454-200203000-00003
40. van der Maten E, de Jonge MI, de Groot R, van der Flier M, Langereis JD. A versatile assay to determine bacterial and host factors contributing to opsonophagocytotic killing in hirudin-anticoagulated whole blood. *Sci Rep.* (2017) 7:42137. doi: 10.1038/srep42137
41. European Society for Immunodeficiencies. *Registry-Diagnosis criteria*, April 19th 2018. Available online at https://esid.org/Working-Parties/Registry/Diagnosis-criteria
42. Abolhassani H, Aghamohammadi A, Hammarstrom L. Monogenic mutations associated with IgA deficiency. *Expert Rev Clin Immunol.* (2016) 12:1321–35. doi: 10.1080/1744666X.2016.1198696
43. Aghamohammadi A, Cheraghi T, Gharagozlou M, Movahedi M, Rezaei N, Yeganeh M, et al. IgA deficiency: correlation between clinical and immunological phenotypes. *J Clin Immunol.* (2009) 29:130–6. doi: 10.1007/s10875-008-9229-9
44. Burgio GR, Duse M, Monafo V, Ascione A, Nespoli L. Selective IgA deficiency: clinical and immunological evaluation of 50 pediatric patients. *Eur J Pediatr.* (1980) 133:101–6.
45. Aytekin C, Tuygun N, Gokce S, Dogu F, Ikinciogullari A. Selective IgA deficiency: clinical and laboratory features of 118 children in Turkey. *J Clin Immunol.* (2012) 32:961–6. doi: 10.1007/s10875-012-9702-3
46. Norhagen G, Engstrom PE, Hammarstrom L, Soder PO, Smith CI. Immunoglobulin levels in saliva in individuals with selective IgA deficiency: compensatory IgM secretion and its correlation with HLA and susceptibility to infections. *J Clin Immunol.* (1989) 9:279–86.
47. Mellander L, Bjorkander J, Carlsson B, Hanson LA. Secretory antibodies in IgA-deficient and immunosuppressed individuals. *J Clin Immunol.* (1986) 6:284–91.
48. Orange JS, Hossny EM, Weiler CR, Ballow M, Berger M, Bonilla FA, et al. Use of intravenous immunoglobulin in human disease: a review of evidence by members of the primary immunodeficiency committee of the american academy of allergy, asthma and immunology. *J Allergy Clin Immunol.* (2006) 117(4 Suppl):S525–53. doi: 10.1016/j.jaci.2006.01.015
49. Chovancova Z, Kralickova P, Pejchalova A, Bloomfield M, Nechvatalova J, Vlkova M, et al. Selective IgM deficiency: clinical and laboratory features of 17 patients and a review of the literature. *J Clin Immunol.* (2017) 37:559–74. doi: 10.1007/s10875-017-0420-8
50. Janssen LMA, Macken T, Creemers MCW, Pruijt JFM, Eijk JJJ, de Vries E. Truly selective primary IgM deficiency is probably very rare. *Clin Exp Immunol.* (2018) 191:203–11. doi: 10.1111/cei.13065
51. Gupta S, Gupta A. Selective IgM deficiency-an underestimated primary immunodeficiency. *Front Immunol.* (2017) 8:1056. doi: 10.3389/fimmu.2017.01056
52. Bogaert DJ, Dullaers M, Lambrecht BN, Vermaelen KY, De Baere E, Haerynck F. Genes associated with common variable immunodeficiency: one diagnosis to rule them all? *J Med Genet.* (2016) 53:575–90. doi: 10.1136/jmedgenet-2015-103690
53. Oksenhendler E, Gerard L, Fieschi C, Malphettes M, Mouillot G, Jaussaud R, et al. Infections in 252 patients with common variable immunodeficiency. *Clin Infect Dis.* (2008) 46:1547–54. doi: 10.1086/587669
54. Touw CM, van de Ven AA, de Jong PA, Terheggen-Lagro S, Beek E, Sanders EA, et al. Detection of pulmonary complications in common variable immunodeficiency. *Pediatr Allergy Immunol.* (2010) 21:793–805. doi: 10.1111/j.1399-3038.2009.00963.x
55. Busse PJ, Razvi S, Cunningham-Rundles C. Efficacy of intravenous immunoglobulin in the prevention of pneumonia in patients with common variable immunodeficiency. *J Allergy Clin Immunol.* (2002) 109:1001–4. doi: 10.1067/mai.2002.124999
56. Ammann AJ, Ashman RF, Buckley RH, Hardie WR, Krantmann HJ, Nelson J, et al. Use of intravenous gamma-globulin in antibody immunodeficiency: results of a multicenter controlled trial. *Clin Immunol Immunopathol.* (1982) 22:60–7.
57. Plebani A, Soresina A, Rondelli R, Amato GM, Azzari C, Cardinale F, et al. Clinical, immunological, and molecular analysis in a large cohort of patients with X-linked agammaglobulinemia: an Italian multicenter study. *Clin Immunol.* (2002) 104:221–30. doi: 10.1006/clim.2002.5241

58. Winkelstein JA, Marino MC, Lederman HM, Jones SM, Sullivan K, Burks AW, et al. X-linked agammaglobulinemia: report on a United States registry of 201 patients. *Medicine* (2006) 85:193–202. doi: 10.1097/01.md.0000229482.27398.ad
59. Basile N, Danielian S, Oleastro M, Rosenzweig S, Prieto E, Rossi J, et al. Clinical and molecular analysis of 49 patients with X-linked agammaglobulinemia from a single center in Argentina. *J Clin Immunol.* (2009) 29:123–9. doi: 10.1007/s10875-008-9227-y
60. Lederman HM, Winkelstein JA. X-linked agammaglobulinemia: an analysis of 96 patients. *Medicine* (1985) 64:145–56.
61. Cohn EJ, Strong LE, Hughes WL, Mulford DJ, Ashworth JN, Melin M, et al. Preparation and properties of serum and plasma proteins; a system for the separation into fractions of the protein and lipoprotein components of biological tissues and fluids. *J Am Chem Soc.* (1946) 68:459–75.
62. Oncley JL, Melin M, Richert DA, Cameron JW, Gross PM. The separation of the antibodies, isoagglutinins, prothrombin, plasminogen and beta1-lipoprotein into subfractions of human plasma. *J Am Chem Soc.* (1949) 71:541–50.
63. Shillitoe B, Gennery A. X-Linked Agammaglobulinaemia: outcomes in the modern era. *Clin Immunol.* (2017) 183:54–62. doi: 10.1016/j.clim.2017.07.008
64. Cunningham-Rundles C, Bodian C. Common variable immunodeficiency: clinical and immunological features of 248 patients. *Clin Immunol.* (1999) 92:34–48. doi: 10.1006/clim.1999.4725
65. Quinti I, Soresina A, Guerra A, Rondelli R, Spadaro G, Agostini C, et al. Effectiveness of immunoglobulin replacement therapy on clinical outcome in patients with primary antibody deficiencies: results from a multicenter prospective cohort study. *J Clin Immunol.* (2011) 31:315–22. doi: 10.1007/s10875-011-9511-0
66. Hodkinson JP, Bangs C, Wartenberg-Demand A, Bauhofer A, Langohr P, Buckland MS, et al. Low IgA and IgM Is associated with a higher prevalence of bronchiectasis in primary antibody deficiency. *J Clin Immunol.* (2017) 37:329–31. doi: 10.1007/s10875-017-0381-y
67. Bruton OC. Agammaglobulinemia. *Pediatrics* (1952) 9:722–8.
68. Bruton OC. A decade with agammaglobulinemia. *J Pediatr.* (1962) 60:672–6.
69. Smith GN, Griffiths B, Mollison D, Mollison PL. Uptake of IgG after intramuscular and subcutaneous injection. *Lancet* (1972) 1:1208–12.
70. Ochs HD, Fischer SH, Lee ML, Delson ES, Kingdon HS, Wedgwood RJ. Intravenous immunoglobulin home treatment for patients with primary immunodeficiency diseases. *Lancet* (1986) 1:610–11.
71. Gardulf A, Hammarstrom L, Smith CI. Home treatment of hypogammaglobulinaemia with subcutaneous gammaglobulin by rapid infusion. *Lancet* (1991) 338:162–6.
72. Wasserman RL, Melamed I, Kobrynski L, Puck J, Gupta S, Doralt J, et al. Recombinant human hyaluronidase facilitated subcutaneous immunoglobulin treatment in pediatric patients with primary immunodeficiencies: long-term efficacy, safety and tolerability. *Immunotherapy* (2016) 8:1175–86. doi: 10.2217/imt-2016-0066
73. Barandun S, Kistler P, Jeunet F, Isliker H. Intravenous administration of human gamma-globulin. *Vox Sang.* (1962) 7:157–74.
74. Garbett ND, Currie DC, Cole PJ. Comparison of the clinical efficacy and safety of an intramuscular and an intravenous immunoglobulin preparation for replacement therapy in idiopathic adult onset panhypogammaglobulinaemia. *Clin Exp Immunol.* (1989) 76:1–7.
75. Stephan W. Undegraded human immunoglobulin for intravenous use. *Vox Sang.* (1975) 28:422–37.
76. Brennan VM, Salome-Bentley NJ, Chapel HMS. Immunology Nurses. Prospective audit of adverse reactions occurring in 459 primary antibody-deficient patients receiving intravenous immunoglobulin. Clin Exp Immunol. (2003) 133:247–51. doi: 10.1046/j.1365-2249.2003.02199.x
77. Nolte MT, Pirofsky B, Gerritz GA, Golding B. Intravenous immunoglobulin therapy for antibody deficiency. *Clin Exp Immunol.* (1979) 36:237–43.
78. Jager BV. Intravenous administration of modified gamma globulin. Several studies on a patient with agammaglobulinemia. *Arch Intern Med.* (1967) 119:60–4.
79. Gardulf A, Nicolay U, Asensio O, Bernatowska E, Bock A, Carvalho BC, et al. Rapid subcutaneous IgG replacement therapy is effective and safe in children and adults with primary immunodeficiencies–a prospective, multi-national study. *J Clin Immunol.* (2006) 26:177–85. doi: 10.1007/s10875-006-9002-x
80. Stiehm ER. Plasma therapy: an alternative to gamma globulin injections in immunodeficiency. *Birth Defects Orig Artic Ser.* (1975) 11:343–6.
81. Buckley RH. Plasma therapy in immunodeficiency diseases. *Am J Dis Child.* (1972) 124:376–81.
82. Kerstens PJ, Endtz HP, Meis JF, Oyen WJ, Koopman RJ, van den Broek PJ, van der Meer JW. Erysipelas-like skin lesions associated with *Campylobacter jejuni* septicemia in patients with hypogammaglobulinemia. *Eur J Clin Microbiol Infect Dis.* (1992) 11:842–7.
83. Stephan W, Dichtelmuller H, Schedel I. Properties and efficacy of a human immunoglobulin M preparation for intravenous administration. *Arzneimittelforschung* (1985) 35:933–6.
84. Stephan W. [Elimination of complement fixation of gamma-globulin by chemical modification with beta-propiolactone]. *Z Klin Chem Klin Biochem.* (1969) 7:282–6.
85. Jungi TW, Santer M, Lerch PG, Barandun S. Effect of various treatments of gamma-globulin (Igg) for achieving intravenous tolerance on the capacity to interact with human monocyte Fc-receptors - a comparative-study. *Vox Sang.* (1986) 51:18–26. doi: 10.1111/j.1423-0410.1986.tb00203.x
86. Wand S, Klages M, Kirbach C, Warszawska J, Meybohm P, Zacharowski K, et al. IgM-enriched immunoglobulin attenuates systemic endotoxin activity in early severe sepsis: a before-after cohort study. *PLoS ONE* (2016) 11:e0160907. doi: 10.1371/journal.pone.0160907
87. Behre G, Schedel I, Nentwig B, Wormann B, Essink M, Hiddemann W. Endotoxin concentration in neutropenic patients with suspected gram-negative sepsis: correlation with clinical outcome and determination of anti-endotoxin core antibodies during therapy with polyclonal immunoglobulin M-enriched immunoglobulins. *Antimicrob Agents Chemother.* (1992) 36:2139–46.
88. Garbett ND, Munro CS, Cole PJ. Opsonic activity of a new intravenous immunoglobulin preparation: pentaglobin compared with sandoglobulin. *Clin Exp Immunol.* (1989) 76:8–12.
89. Rossmann FS, Kropec A, Laverde D, Saaverda FR, Wobser D, Huebner J. *In vitro* and *in vivo* activity of hyperimmune globulin preparations against multiresistant nosocomial pathogens. *Infection* (2015) 43:169–75. doi: 10.1007/s15010-014-0706-1
90. Borleffs JC, Schellekens JF, Brouwer E, Rozenberg-Arska M. Use of an immunoglobulin M containing preparation for treatment of two hypogammaglobulinemic patients with persistent Campylobacter jejuni infection. *Eur J Clin Microbiol Infect Dis.* (1993) 12:772–5.
91. Langohr PL, Wartenberg-Demand, A, Ulrike W, Daelken, B. Treatment of severe community acquired pneumonia. In: *BIOTEST AG* (Dreieich) (2017). Available online at: http://www.freepatentsonline.com/WO2017157850.html
92. Shmygalev S, Damm M, Knels L, Strassburg A, Wunsche K, Dumke R, et al. IgM-enriched solution BT086 improves host defense capacity and energy store preservation in a rabbit model of endotoxemia. *Acta Anaesthesiol Scand.* (2016) 60:502–12. doi: 10.1111/aas.12652
93. Welte T, Dellinger RP, Ebelt H, Ferrer M, Opal SM, Singer M, et al. Efficacy and safety of trimodulin, a novel polyclonal antibody preparation, in patients with severe community-acquired pneumonia: a randomized, placebo-controlled, double-blind, multicenter, phase II trial (CIGMA study). *Intensive Care Med.* (2018) 44:438–48. doi: 10.1007/s00134-018-5143-7
94. Eibl MM, Wolf HM, Furnkranz H, Rosenkranz A. Prevention of necrotizing enterocolitis in low-birth-weight infants by IgA-IgG feeding. *N Engl J Med.* (1988) 319:1–7. doi: 10.1056/NEJM198807073190101
95. Casswall TH, Hammarstrom L, Veress B, Nord CE, Bogstedt A, Brockstedt U, et al. Oral IgA-IgG treatment of chronic non-specific diarrhoea in infants and children. *Acta Paediatr.* (1996) 85:1126–8.

96. Plaut AG, Wistar RJr, Capra JD. Differential susceptibility of human IgA immunoglobulins to streptococcal IgA protease. *J Clin Invest.* (1974) 54:1295–300. doi: 10.1172/JCI107875
97. Longet S, Miled S, Lotscher M, Miescher SM, Zuercher AW, Corthesy B. Human plasma-derived polymeric IgA and IgM antibodies associate with secretory component to yield biologically active secretory-like antibodies. *J Biol Chem.* (2013) 288:4085–94. doi: 10.1074/jbc.M112.410811
98. Longet S, Vonarburg C, Lotscher M, Miescher S, Zuercher A, Corthesy B. Reconstituted human polyclonal plasma-derived secretory-like IgM and IgA maintain the barrier function of epithelial cells infected with an enteropathogen. *J Biol Chem.* (2014) 289:21617–26. doi: 10.1074/jbc.M114.549139
99. Bioley G, Monnerat J, Lotscher M, Vonarburg C, Zuercher A, Corthesy B. Plasma-derived polyreactive secretory-like IgA and IgM opsonizing *Salmonella enterica* typhimurium reduces invasion and gut tissue inflammation through agglutination. *Front Immunol.* (2017) 8:1043. doi: 10.3389/fimmu.2017.01043

8

Mechanisms of Naturally Acquired Immunity to *Streptococcus pneumoniae*

Elisa Ramos-Sevillano, Giuseppe Ercoli and Jeremy S. Brown*

Centre for Inflammation and Tissue Repair, UCL Respiratory, London, United Kingdom

***Correspondence:**
Jeremy S. Brown
jeremy.brown@ucl.ac.uk

In this review we give an update on the mechanisms of naturally acquired immunity against *Streptococcus pneumoniae*, one of the major human bacterial pathogens that is a common cause of pneumonia, septicaemia, and meningitis. A clear understanding of the natural mechanisms of immunity to *S. pneumoniae* is necessary to help define why the very young and elderly are at high risk of disease, and for devising new prevention strategies. Recent data has shown that nasopharynx colonization by *S. pneumoniae* induces antibody responses to protein and capsular antigens in both mice and humans, and also induces Th17 CD4+ cellular immune responses in mice and increases pre-existing responses in humans. These responses are protective, demonstrating that colonization is an immunizing event. We discuss the data from animal models and humans on the relative importance of naturally acquired antibody and Th17 cells on immunity to *S. pneumoniae* at three different anatomical sites of infection, the nasopharynx (the site of natural asymptomatic carriage), the lung (site of pneumonia), and the blood (site of sepsis). Mouse data suggest that CD4+ Th17 cells prevent both primary and secondary nasopharyngeal carriage with no role for antibody induced by previous colonization. In contrast, antibody is necessary for prevention of sepsis but CD4+ cellular responses are not. Protection against pneumonia requires a combination of both antibody and Th17 cells, in both cases targeting protein rather than capsular antigen. Proof of which immune component prevents human infection is less easily available, but two recent papers demonstrate that human IgG targeting *S. pneumoniae* protein antigens is highly protective against septicaemia. The role of CD4+ responses to prior nasopharyngeal colonization for protective immunity in humans is unclear. The evidence that there is significant naturally-acquired immunity to *S. pneumoniae* independent of anti-capsular polysaccharide has clinical implications for the detection of subjects at risk of *S. pneumoniae* infections, and the data showing the importance of protein antigens as targets for antibody and Th17 mediated immunity should aid the development of new vaccine strategies.

Keywords: immunity, pneumococcus (*Streptococcus pneumoniae*), natural acquired immunity, pneumonia, protection

INTRODUCTION

Streptococcus pneumoniae is a major cause of acute otitis media, community-acquired pneumonia, bacterial sepsis, and meningitis and is estimated to be responsible for over 800,000 deaths annually in children (1). *S. pneumoniae* strains causing invasive infections are surrounded by a polysaccharide capsule layer that inhibits innate and adaptive immune responses to infection (2). The capsule has a varied biochemical composition and antigenic structure between *S. pneumoniae* strains, resulting in over 90 different capsular serotypes (3). Serotype specific *S. pneumoniae* vaccines have been developed using capsular antigen linked to carrier protein, termed pneumococcal conjugated vaccines (PCVs), and these are highly effective against the serotypes included in the vaccine (4–6). However, there is still a high level of mortality and morbidity due to *S. pneumoniae* infections due to the restricted serotype coverage of PCVs resulting in serotype-replacement disease, and their high cost leading to incomplete use of PCVs in low and middle-income countries. In addition, PCVs are less effective at preventing pneumonia compared to septicaemia and meningitis, despite pneumonia making the largest contribution to the burden of disease (1, 7, 8). Novel approaches are needed to overcome the limitations of the present PCV. One way of identifying new preventative strategies could be to define the mechanisms of natural adaptive immunity to *S. pneumoniae*, which could then be targeted to enhance immunity against infection in high-risk groups such as children and older adults. In this review we will discuss the evidence for naturally acquired adaptive immunity to *S. pneumoniae* and the mechanisms by which this maybe mediated.

CLINICAL AND EPIDEMIOLOGICAL EVIDENCE FOR ADAPTIVE IMMUNITY TO *S. PNEUMONIAE*

S. pneumoniae Nasopharyngeal Colonization

Unlike some major bacterial respiratory pathogens such as *Mycobacterium tuberculosis*, *S. pneumoniae* is also a ubiquitous human commensal of the upper respiratory tract, specifically of the nasopharynx. Colonization of the nasopharynx occurs in the first years of life and repeatedly thereafter (9–11). Successive episodes of colonization with different pneumococcal strains occur in children up to 2 years of age (9, 10), with the point prevalence of nasopharyngeal carriage estimated at 27–65% among infants. This colonization prevalence decreases with age to <10% during adult life (12–14), and even lower rates in the elderly (15). This decline in colonization seems to have a multifactorial nature, one element of could be maturation of the immune system with age. The main nasopharyngeal reservoir for the spread of *S. pneumoniae* is in children, and consequently vaccination of children with PCV (which prevents nasopharyngeal colonization) has resulted in significant herd immunity against adult *S. pneumoniae* pneumonia (12).

Epidemiological Evidence for Naturally Acquired Adaptive Immunity to *S. pneumoniae*

Subjects with defects of their adaptive immune response are more susceptible to *S. pneumoniae* infections. These groups include people with genetic or acquired defects in immunoglobulin production, and those who have severe defects of adaptive immunity due to stem cell transplantation or HIV infection (16–18). In addition, subjects with deficiencies in the classical pathway of complement activation have a massively increased incidence of pneumococcal septicaemia, meningitis, and bacterial pneumonia (19). Although this will reflect weakened complement-mediated innate immunity to *S. pneumoniae* (20), the classical complement pathway is also vital for antibody mediated killing of *S. pneumoniae* (2), and hence the susceptibility of subjects with classical pathway defects will partially reflect weakened antibody mediated immunity. Furthermore, the incidence of *S. pneumoniae* infection with age has a pronounced U shaped curve with the highest incidence in infants and the elderly (21), a pattern that suggests there is an adaptive immune response to *S. pneumoniae* that improves in children with maturity then perhaps wanes due to immunosenescence in the elderly. The frequency of *S. pneumoniae* septicaemia associated with pneumonia is also higher in infants than adults, indicating that in adults the immune system is able to prevent spread to the blood from the lungs. Overall, these epidemiological data indicate that there is significant naturally acquired adaptive immunity that helps prevent *S. pneumoniae* infections. Importantly, the incidence of infection with all serotypes falls at the same time (22), an epidemiological observation that suggests naturally acquired resistance to *S. pneumoniae* infections is mediated by serotype independent mechanisms rather than anticapsular antibody.

This evidence of naturally acquired adaptive immunity to *S. pneumoniae* leads to the question of how this has developed? Only a small proportion of humans have been exposed to *S. pneumoniae* during invasive diseases such as septicaemia and meningitis, and although many more humans will have had an episode of *S. pneumoniae* pneumonia this would have been with a single strain and capsular serotype. In contrast, almost all humans have been exposed to *S. pneumoniae* via nasopharyngeal colonization events on multiple occasions and by many different strains. Hence, if most (if not all) humans have a naturally acquired serotype-independent adaptive immunity to *S. pneumoniae* then this must have occurred because of colonization rather than active infectious disease.

Evidence That *S. pneumoniae* Nasopharyngeal Colonization Is an Immunizing Event

Data obtained during natural and experimental human infection and from mouse models have now shown conclusively that colonization of the nasopharynx by *S. pneumoniae* is indeed an immunizing event. Multiple longitudinal studies of serum antibody responses in infants show the development of antibody responses to *S. pneumoniae* capsular and protein antigens in serum and saliva after human colonization events (11, 14, 23, 24). In murine models, several authors have shown both antibody and T-cell mediated immune responses develop after a colonization event with *S. pneumoniae* or exposure to *S. pneumoniae* antigens in the nasopharynx (25–32). In addition, after successful experimental human colonization with *S. pneumoniae* pre-existing antibody responses (33, 34) and *S. pneumoniae*-specific blood and lung IL-17 producing $CD4^+$ memory cells are increased (35), providing enhanced humoral and cellular immunity. These data confirm that colonization is an immunizing event, and this is supported by data from infants showing gradual increases in anti-protein antigen IgG responses with age and correlations between colonization events and increases in anti-capsular antibody for several serotypes (11).

Mechanisms of Naturally Acquired Adaptive Immune Protection Against *S. pneumoniae* Infection

The data discussed above demonstrate that humans do develop naturally acquired adaptive immune responses against *S. pneumoniae* in response to nasopharyngeal colonization and that these responses are likely to be protective. The adaptive response to nasopharyngeal colonization by *S. pneumoniae* includes acquisition of anti-capsular (14, 36, 37) and anti-protein antibodies (38–40), as well as $CD4^+$ cellular immune responses targeting protein antigens alone (39, 41). The observation of $CD4^+$ cellular immune responses is important, as Th17 $CD4^+$ responses are a common mechanism for pathogen clearance at mucosal surfaces via rapid recruitment of neutrophils to the site of infection, improved epithelial barrier function, and increased secretion of antibacterial peptides (42, 43). However, to effectively utilize these findings to design preventative strategies against *S. pneumoniae* it is necessary to go one step further and identify which of these responses actually protect against *S. pneumoniae* infections.

All currently licensed pneumococcal vaccines use polysaccharide capsular antigen, and capsular antibodies against the capsule are highly protective against infection caused by that serotype (5, 44, 45). As a consequence, historically the literature has also emphasized the role of anti-capsule antibodies as the mechanism for naturally acquired immunity against *S. pneumoniae* (46). This is supported by the early data showing that sera from survivors of severe *S. pneumoniae* provided serotype-specific protection when used as a passive antibody treatment (47–51). However, as mentioned above the epidemiological evidence suggests that naturally acquired immunity has a significant serotype-independent component. Analysis of datasets from several countries (e.g., USA, Finland and Israel), demonstrated a decrease in incidence of invasive disease with age independent of increases in serotype-specific antibody levels, suggesting a different mechanism of protection such as acquired immunity to non-capsular antigens or maturation of non-specific immune responses (22). Theoretical modeling also suggested that only 30–60% of the reduction in recolonization is led by anti-capsular immunity generated during previous colonization events (52). Animal model data has shown that antibody and more recently cell mediated immune responses targeting protein rather than capsular antigens can protect against *S. pneumoniae* infections, providing proof of principle that these capsular-antigen independent mechanisms could mediate naturally acquired immunity to *S. pneumoniae* in humans (25, 26, 38, 53). Which proteins dominant the human antibody response to *S. pneumoniae* protein antigens was recently defined by Croucher using a proteome microarray that displays more than 2,000 potential *S. pneumoniae* antigens. Of these, 208 had significant IgG responses in sera obtained from 35 healthy US adults. About half of these antigens were allelic variants of the highly variable surface proteins PspA, PspC, ZmpA, and ZmpB expressed by different *S. pneumoniae* strains (54). The remaining proteins recognized by human sera were more conserved between strains and were enriched in motifs for adhesion or degradation, cell wall metabolism, or solute binding for transport. These results are consistent with a previous screen reverse vaccinology approach that identified proteins recognized by antibody in human sera which identified the proteins PspC and PspA, along with PcsB and StkP (55). There are only limited data on the identification of *S. pneumoniae* antigens that induce Th17 $CD4^+$ cell responses as this is technically difficult. The available data was obtained in mice by screening of an expression library containing >96% of predicted pneumococcal protein and identified several proteins (including ABC transporter lipoproteins) that induce Th17 responses after exposure to whole pneumococci and as purified protein antigens, with little overlap between with antibody-inducing protein antigens (56).

Overall, the data from human and animal studies show colonization induces both anti-capsule and anti-protein antibody responses, and in addition cell mediated immunity to protein antigens. The anatomy, associated immunological tissues, and interactions with soluble immune effectors in mucosal lining fluid or in the plasma all vary between the common anatomical sites of *S. pneumoniae* infection, creating potential variations in the relative efficacy of different immune effectors for controlling *S. pneumoniae* infection between anatomical sites. Hence the following discussion of which mechanisms of naturally acquired adaptive immunity protect against *S. pneumoniae* is divided into three representative sites of infection; (i) the nasopharynx as a mucosal site colonized by *S. pneumoniae*; (ii) the blood as a site of systemic invasive infection; and (iii) the lungs as a deep site of mucosal infection intimately associated with the systemic circulation, and also the site responsible for the biggest burden of severe infections globally. In general, data from animal studies (mainly in mice) can clearly define protective mechanisms but is of more limited utility due to potential differences in immune function between species. However, after early childhood all humans have had multiple episodes of *S. pneumoniae* colonization each of which will stimulate some degree of immune response, and this background situation of considerable prior exposure to *S. pneumoniae* over many years is difficult to replicate in mouse models. Human data is directly relevant but it is usually only possible to provide potential correlations rather than direct proof between a specific immune effector and protection against disease.

Prevention of Subsequent Colonization

Mouse Data

Whether antibodies have an important role in controlling a primary episode of nasopharyngeal colonization by *S. pneumoniae* was investigated by McCool and Weiser using murine models of infection and mice knock out strains affecting specific aspects of antibody mediated immunity (38). They established a murine model of colonization in *xid* mice, which have a poor antibody response to polysaccharide capsule. *S. pneumoniae* clearance from the nasopharynx was similar in *xid* mice compared to wild-type mice. These results were corroborated using *uMT* mice, which lack B cell and antibody responses, which were also still able to clear *S. pneumoniae* nasopharyngeal colonization. These results demonstrate that antibody responses do not aid clearance of primary colonization events, and have been confirmed by other studies (57). Instead, protection against recolonization was lost in mice deficient in $CD4^+$ cells, highlighting the requirement of cellular immunity rather than antibody in protection against recolonization (58). Similar data were obtained using administration of the *S. pneumoniae* antigen cell wall polysaccharide intranasally, which inhibited subsequent colonization independent of antibody but dependent on $CD4^+$ cells (29). In addition, these authors confirmed for the first time an important role for IL-17 in preventing colonization, although the exact mechanism by which this cytokine provided protection was not determined. Vaccination with killed unencapsulated *S. pneumoniae* also induced Th17 $CD4^+$ immunity which prevented nasopharyngeal colonization with a heterologous *S. pneumoniae* serotype (27, 59).

The data obtained from these studies indicated an important role of $CD4^+$ cells rather than antibodies for prevention of a second episode of *S. pneumoniae* colonization, and this has been confirmed by more detailed investigation in mice. Zhang et al. demonstrated that the clearance of both the initial and second episode of *S. pneumoniae* colonization in adult mice was dependent on cellular responses rather than humoral immunity (58, 60). Clearance of the initial episode of colonization involved recruitment of monocytes/macrophages into the upper airway lumen via a TLR2-dependent mechanism which required an IL-17 secreting $CD4^+$ cell population (57, 60). Prevention of a second episode of colonization also required IL-17 and $CD4^+$ cells, and was mediated by rapid neutrophil recruitment to the nasopharynx. These findings are supported by other data showing $CD4^+$ cells and IL-17 are required for protection against colonization and mediate the protective effect of immunization with whole cell vaccines against colonization[28, 29, 31].

Overall, the murine data demonstrate that Th17 responses to protein antigens are critical for controlling *S. pneumoniae* colonization after a previous episode of colonization; subsequent work has identified several protein antigens that are able to induce Th17 mediated immunity but whether these antigens are the same for different *S. pneumoniae* strains is not known (56). These data do not preclude a potential role for vaccine induced antibody for prevention of colonization after vaccination, and in mice vaccination with protein antigens elicits protection against *S. pneumoniae* colonization (61, 62) and passive immunization with anticapsular antibodies prevents both colonization and transmission between littermates (63, 64).

Human Data

As discussed above longitudinal studies have demonstrated that antibodies to both protein and capsule antigens develop after episodes of *S. pneumoniae* colonization. As a consequence adult

		Anti-CPS antibody	Anti-protein antigen antibody	Protein antigen specific Th17 CD4 T cells
Carriage 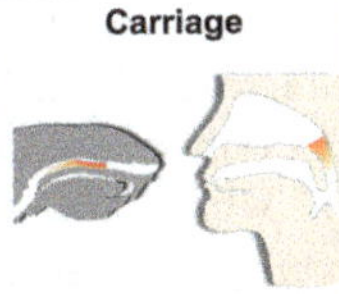	Mouse	Little effect[1] [32, 38, 53]	Little effect[2] [26, 32, 38, 53]	**Protective[2] (both 1er and 2er infection)** [32, 59, 60]
	Human	Not known[1]	Not known	Not known
Pneumonia 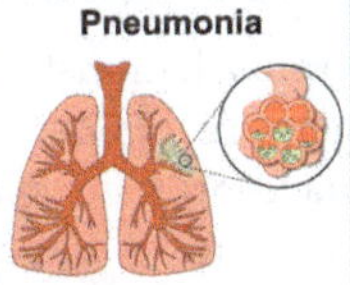	Mouse	Little effect[1]	**Protective[2]** [25, 26, 53, 71]	**Protective** [25, 78, 79]
	Human	Not known[1]	Not known	Not known
Septicaemia / IPD 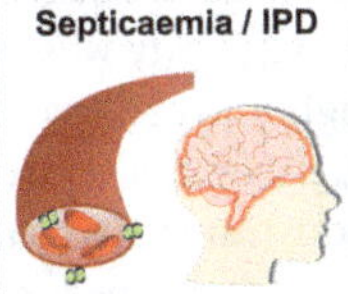	Mouse	Unclear[1] (strain dependent?)	**Protective[2]** [26, 70, 71]	Little effect [70]
	Human	**After IPD: protective[1]** After colonisation: unclear [44, 48, 50]	**Protective** [34, 75]	Not known

[1]Protection can be induced by vaccination with capsular antigen [2]Protection can be induced by vaccination with protein antigen

FIGURE 1 | Summary of what is known about the mechanisms of naturally acquired (as opposed to vaccine-induced) adaptive immunity to *S. pneumoniae* in mice and humans for three representative sites of infection, the nasopharynx, the lungs, and in the blood. The references relevant for each statement are as shown.

sera contains antibodies to multiple capsular *S. pneumoniae* serotypes and one hundred or so protein antigens (11, 54). In addition, different studies have identified Th17 CD4$^+$ responses to *S. pneumoniae* in adenoid tissue (65, 66), bronchoalveolar lavage (35), and blood (31, 35, 67). Evidence for which of these naturally acquired immune mechanisms can prevent colonization in humans is less readily obtained. The impressive reduction in *S. pneumoniae* vaccine serotype prevalence as nasopharyngeal commensals in populations vaccinated with PCV demonstrates that high levels of anti-capsular antibody do prevent colonization (5–7). Recent data obtained using the experimental human pneumococcal carriage model (EHPC) and murine models suggest anticapsular antibody inhibits the establishment of colonization by serotype-specific agglutination of *S. pneumoniae* (63, 68). Whether the lower levels of anti-capsular antibody induced by natural colonization rather than vaccination with a PCV is enough to prevent colonization is not clear.

The most important data on immune mechanisms that prevent colonization in humans has been obtained using the EHPC model. In this experimental human infection model, human volunteers are inoculated intranasally with a serotype 6B strain leading to successful nasopharyngeal colonization in approximately half of subjects (34). Previous colonization prevented recolonization with the same strain (34). In this model, all recruited subjects had detectable IgG levels to *S. pneumoniae* antigens prior to nasopharyngeal administration of *S. pneumoniae*, but anti-pneumococcal IgG levels did not correlate with whether colonization was successful or not (34). In contrast, a previous EHPC model suggested that antibodies to the *S. pneumoniae* surface protein PspA correlated with prevention of successful colonization, providing some evidence that anti-protein antibody may prevent colonization (33). Exposure to serotype 6B or 23F strains increased antibody responses to multiple *S. pneumoniae* proteins (e.g., PspA, PspC, PsaA, and PdB), with the highest increases in carriage positive subjects (33, 34, 69). Systemic anti-capsule antibodies were only detected in subjects that developed carriage after challenge (34). *S. pneumoniae* specific IL-17 secreting CD4$^+$ cells were found in the lung prior to exposure to the 6B strain but were increased in bronchoalveolar fluid 17-fold and in blood 8-fold in volunteers in which colonization was successful (35, 69). Overall these data confirm that pre-existing antibody and local CD4$^+$ cellular immunity to *S. pneumoniae* are significantly boosted by colonization events, and that this seems to prevent recolonization for at least a period of several months. However, the data are unable to define which of these immune mechanisms was important for the prevention of recolonization.

Prevention of *S. pneumoniae* Septicaemia and Meningitis

Mouse Data

Mouse data also clearly demonstrates that colonization of the nasopharynx promotes protection against invasive disease, but in contrast to prevention of colonization this is dependent on antibody mediated immunity, not CD4$^+$ cells. Cohen et al. showed that a previous episode of colonization with the *S. pneumoniae* D39 strain was highly protective against subsequent lethal invasive pneumonia, with the major effect being prevention of septicaemia (70). CD4$^+$ depleted mice were still protected against septicaemia, whereas no protection was seen in antibody deficient mice, and passive transfer of serum from colonized mice into immune naïve mice also protected against *S. pneumoniae* septicaemia. Similarly, Bou Ghanem *et al* found that previous colonization protected against *S. pneumoniae* pneumonia with septicaemia caused by the TIGR4 strain, with the most profound effect seen on blood colony forming units (CFU) (71). Repeated episodes of nasopharynx colonization in antibody deficient mice did not induced any protection whereas protection persisted after CD4$^+$ cell depletion, and the authors proposed long-lived antibody secreting CD138$^+$ cells were responsible for the protective effect of prior colonization. These data demonstrating the important role of antibody are perhaps not surprising as protection against septicaemia in mice is dependent on soluble mediators such as complement and naturally and induced antibody working in concert with the reticuloendothelial system, especially the spleen (72–74), rather than CD4$^+$ Th17 mediated mechanisms.

Human Data

It was commonly accepted for many years that the major mechanism of natural immunity against invasive pneumococcal disease (IPD) was anti-capsular antibodies generated by previous episodes of either colonization or infection (44, 48, 50). However, this assumption has been progressively threatened by epidemiological data as discussed above. More recently experimental data by Wilson et al. has demonstrated that antibody to protein rather than capsular antigen is a major mechanism of naturally acquired immunity to *S. pneumoniae* septicaemia and IPD (75). To do so the authors used Intravenous Immunoglobulin (IVIG) which is used to prevent infections in individuals with primary antibody deficiency (76, 77). IVIG contains the pooled IgG from the plasma of approximately a thousand donors who are unlikely to have been vaccinated against *S. pneumoniae* due to their lack of risk factors, and therefore contains the naturally acquired antibody repertoire for the population from which the donors are obtained. Antibodies to both *S. pneumoniae* capsule and multiple proteins were detected in IVIG. Immunoblots against lysates from different pneumococcal strains demonstrated a highly conserved pattern of protein targets recognized by IVIG, including major pneumococcal surface proteins such as choline binding proteins and lipoproteins. Importantly, opsonophagocytosis of *S. pneumoniae* was improved against unencapsulated bacteria but reduced when anticapsular antibody was depleted from the IVIG preparation. IVIG was highly protective against *S. pneumoniae* septicaemia in mouse models, even after depletion of anticapsular antibody. These data demonstrate there is a high level of naturally acquired antibody to *S. pneumoniae* protein antigens in adult sera that promotes bacterial clearance during sepsis. In addition, passive vaccination of mice with sera obtained from human EHPC subjects colonized with the serotype 6B strain conferred protection against the D39 serotype 2 strain in a pneumonia model in which lethality is driven by septicaemia (34). The data from these two studies provide direct proof that antiprotein antibody is an important mechanism of naturally acquired immunity to *S. pneumoniae* systemic infection.

Prevention of *S. pneumoniae* Pneumonia

The nasopharynx represents a mucosal site of infection, and septicaemia a systemic site, whereas the commonest site of serious infection, the lungs, represents a combination of the two. In the early stages of pneumonia infection is limited to interactions with the mucosal surface, which are similar to those found in the nasopharynx. As the infection develops there is a breakdown in the epithelial/endothelial barrier function and cellular recruitment to the alveoli, recruiting systemic soluble and white cell-mediated immune mechanisms to the alveoli. Hence, both mucosal and systemic mechanisms of adaptive immunity could potentially have roles in protection against *S. pneumoniae* pneumonia.

Mouse Data

Several studies have examined the role of colonization-induced immunity for protection against pneumonia in murine models. In a murine model of asymptomatic carriage with the D39 strain the number of CFU recovered from lung was reduced compared to control mice after a lethal pneumonia invasive challenge suggesting that colonization does improve local lung immunity against *S. pneumoniae* pneumonia (26). The authors also showed increased levels of IL-17A and $CD4^{+}$ cells in lungs of previously colonized mice, indicating a potential role for T cell mediated immunity for prevention of pneumonia. These data were developed by Wilson et al. using a non-invasive *S. pneumoniae* serotype 19F strain that only causes lung infection without sepsis to allow lung immunity to be assessed separate to protection against systemic infection (25). Prior colonization protected against subsequent pneumonia, with a marked reduction in lung CFU. Additional experiments demonstrated that B cells, $CD4^{+}$ and IL-17 were each necessary for protection against *S. pneumoniae* pneumonia caused by the 19F strain. These results suggested that naturally acquired protective immunity to *S. pneumoniae* pneumonia required a combination of both humoral immunity and Th17 $CD4^{+}$ cells. Protection also required neutrophils, presumably as the main mechanism of bacterial killing, and previously colonized mice seemed to have a more rapid influx of neutrophils into the lungs during *S. pneumoniae* pneumonia compatible with improved local Th17 immunity (58). There was no detectable anti-capsular IgG responses after colonization. This suggested the humoral component of protection against pneumonia required anti-protein antibodies instead, and in agreement with previous mouse and human colonization models (28, 31, 69) the authors detected antibody responses to the important surface protein antigens PsaA, PhtD, and PpmA.

Two additional papers have also demonstrated an important role for Th17 $CD4^{+}$ cells induced by prior exposure to *S. pneumoniae* for protection against subsequent severe *S. pneumoniae* pneumonia (78, 79). In both these papers protection was seen against pneumonia caused by a different capsular serotype, demonstrating that it was dependent on recognition of protein antigens. Smith et al. used prior exposure to *S. pneumoniae* through self-limiting lung infection rather than colonization, and demonstrated that protection was specific to *S. pneumoniae* and required administration of live rather than dead bacteria, suggesting bacterial replication within the respiratory tract was necessary. Importantly, they identified a population of tissue resident memory T cells within the lungs that mediated the antigen specific Th17 immunity to *S. pneumoniae* and that was restricted to the lobe that had been previously exposed to *S. pneumoniae*. It remains to be seen whether the low quantities of bacteria that reach the lung due to microaspiration from "pure" nasopharyngeal colonization are also sufficient to induce this population of lung tissue resident memory T cells.

Human Data

The increased incidence of lung infection in patients with immunoglobulin deficiencies (16, 80), HIV infection (81), or inherited disorders affecting IL-17 pathways [e.g., hyperIgE syndrome (82)], do indicate roles for both antibody and Th17 $CD4^{+}$ cells for protection against *S. pneumoniae* pneumonia in humans as well as mice. However, these data are confounded by the presence of additional immune effects for each condition, with even immunoglobulin deficiencies resulting in functional impairment of *S. pneumoniae*-specific $CD4^{+}$ cells (83). As previously mentioned, data obtained using bronchoalveolar lavage fluid has confirmed there are pre-existing $CD4^{+}$ cells present in the human lung that produce IL-17 (and often TNFalpha) when stimulated with *S. pneumoniae* (36). The authors demonstrated that IL-17 improved *S. pneumoniae* killing mediated by either macrophages or neutrophils (31), providing an additional mechanism by which IL-17 can assist immunity to extracellular bacteria. BALF also contains antibody to *S. pneumoniae* protein and capsular antigens (33, 34, 69). Hence the human data has identified local pulmonary Th17 $CD4^{+}$ and antibody specific for *S. pneumoniae* that are boosted by nasopharyngeal colonization which could potentially assist lung immunity to pneumonia as has been described in mouse models. However, the additional step of identifying which of these immune responses is actually protective against *S. pneumoniae* lung infection in humans is not easily achieved.

Implications of Data on Naturally Acquired Immunity to *S. pneumoniae*

As described above murine studies have defined how naturally acquired immunity due to prior colonization can protect against *S. pneumoniae* infections, and much of the data has been reinforced by epidemiological and experimental data obtained from humans. These mechanisms are summarized in **Figure 1**. In this last section, we will discuss how the data on naturally acquired infection may effect vaccination strategies and our understanding of the mechanisms underpinning susceptibility to *S. pneumoniae* in high risk groups.

In children, pneumococcal colonization events occur frequently and as discussed above this is necessary for the development of immunity against *S. pneumoniae*. During adulthood, colonization rates hugely decrease (15, 36, 84), but the data from the EHPC model clearly show that a colonization event still stimulates a boost to the pre-existing immune responses (34, 35, 69). Hence colonization has significant immune benefits to the host that could be affected if the ecology of *S. pneumoniae* colonization is altered. Multiple studies have indeed shown that routine PCV vaccination in children has profound effects on *S. pneumoniae* colonization, with hugely decreased carriage rates of the serotypes present in the vaccine (5, 6). However, there has been a parallel increase in colonization with non-vaccine serotypes reported to have a lower invasive disease potential (85, 86), and this alteration of carriage serotype ecology in favor or less invasive serotypes should also maintain the beneficial effects of colonization on natural mechanisms of immunity. If more aggressive preventative strategies reduce overall *S. pneumoniae* carriage rates then there might be a reduction in the strength of naturally immunity, and potentially a paradoxical increase risk of infection in adults.

The data on naturally acquired immunity should also help identify why certain risk groups such as the elderly, patients with chronic lung disease, or HIV infection are highly susceptible to *S. pneumoniae* infections. Studies performed both in mice and patients have highlighted the phenomenon of immunosenescence (87, 88), including an increase in baseline inflammation that seems to impair the development of immunity against *S. pneumoniae* after colonization (88, 89). In the elderly the reduced frequency of colonization events (15, 90) and the decreased levels and activity of IgM memory B cells (91) could also have an impact on colonization-induced immunity to *S. pneumoniae. Streptococcus pneumoniae* specific CD4 responses are dysregulated by HIV infection (92), and these may underpin the greatly increased susceptibility of HIV positive subjects to *S. pneumoniae* infections. How age and comorbidity affects naturally acquired adaptive responses needs to be clearly defined so that there is a much clearer understanding why these groups are highly susceptible to *S. pneumoniae*. Effective methods of measuring the strength of antiprotein and $CD4^+$ cellular immune response to *S. pneumoniae* could also considerable improve our ability to measure susceptibility to this pathogen, which at present depends on measuring anticapsular antibody levels alone.

The recognition that there is a significant element on natural adaptive immunity to *S. pneumoniae* should also provide opportunities for new strategies of vaccination for prevention of *S. pneumoniae* infections. Firstly, strategies could be developed that boost existing naturally acquired immunity, especially in high risk subjects. Secondly, by knowing the mechanisms required for preventing specific diseases such as pneumonia these could be targeted by novel vaccines, for example by aiming to induce $CD4^+$ cellular (mainly Th17) mediated immunity. Furthermore, the recognition that protein antigens in humans can provide significant immunity should boost research into vaccines that induce immune responses to protein antigen.

SUMMARY

This review has discussed the induction and mechanisms of the naturally acquired immune response to *S. pneumoniae*. Multiple lines of evidence from animal experiments and in humans have convincingly demonstrated that nasopharyngeal colonization stimulates significant levels of naturally acquired immunity to *S. pneumoniae* that helps prevent subsequent colonization events as well as systemic and pulmonary infections. The mechanisms involved in preventing infection depends on anatomical site, with an emphasis on antibody during systemic infection and on Th17 $CD4^+$ cells for mucosal infection, with pneumonia seemingly a combination of the two. In contrast to previous assumptions, antibody to protein as well as capsular antigens has an important role. Future work is required to delineate which protein antigens are the most important for protective immunity and whether there are important roles for other cellular immune mechanisms [e.g., Tregs, which have been shown to be important for innate immunity (93)] as well as Th17 $CD4^+$ cells. Overall, these findings may lead to a much better understanding of why certain patient groups are at high risk of *S. pneumoniae* infection and should help improve future vaccine strategies.

AUTHOR CONTRIBUTIONS

ER-S, GE, and JB contributed to draft the manuscript. ER-S and JB contributed to revising it critically and wrote the final version.

REFERENCES

1. O'Brien KL, Wolfson LJ, Watt JP, Henkle E, Deloria-Knoll M, McCall N, et al. Burden of disease caused by *Streptococcus pneumoniae* in children younger than 5 years: global estimates. *Lancet.* (2009) 374:893–902. doi: 10.1016/S0140-6736(09)61204-6
2. Hyams C, Camberlein E, Cohen JM, Bax K, Brown JS.Hyams C, et al. The *Streptococcus pneumoniae* capsule inhibits complement activity and neutrophil phagocytosis by multiple mechanisms. *Infect Immun.* (2010) 78:704–15. doi: 10.1128/IAI.00881-09
3. Bentley SD, Aanensen DM, Mavroidi A, Saunders D, Rabbinowitsch E, Collins M, et al. Genetic analysis of the capsular biosynthetic locus from all 90 pneumococcal serotypes. *PLoS Genet.* (2006) 2:e31. doi: 10.1371/journal.pgen.0020031
4. Smit P, Oberholzer D, Hayden-Smith S, Koornhof HJ, Hilleman MR.Smit P, et al. Protective efficacy of pneumococcal polysaccharide vaccines. *JAMA.* (1977) 238:2613–6. doi: 10.1001/jama.1977.03280250039019
5. Shinefield HR, Black S. Efficacy of pneumococcal conjugate vaccines in large scale field trials. *Pediatr Infect Dis J.* (2000) 19:394–7. doi: 10.1097/00006454-200004000-00036
6. Whitney CG, Farley MM, Hadler J, Harrison LH, Bennett NM, Lynfield R, et al. Decline in invasive pneumococcal disease after the introduction of protein-polysaccharide conjugate vaccine. *N Engl J Med.* (2003) 348:1737–46. doi: 10.1056/NEJMoa022823
7. Bonten MJ, Huijts SM, Bolkenbaas M, Webber C, Patterson S, Gault S, et al. Polysaccharide conjugate vaccine against pneumococcal pneumonia in adults. *N Engl J Med.* (2015) 372:1114–25. doi: 10.1056/NEJMoa1408544
8. Jose RJ, Brown JS. Adult pneumococcal vaccination:advances, impact, and unmet needs. *Curr Opin Pulm Med.* (2017) 23:225–30. doi: 10.1097/MCP.0000000000000369
9. Hussain M, Melegaro A, Pebody RG, George R, Edmunds WJ, Talukdar R, et al. A longitudinal household study of *Streptococcus pneumoniae* nasopharyngeal carriage in a UK setting. *Epidemiol Infect.* (2005) 133:891–8. doi: 10.1017/S0950268805004012

10. Hill PC, Cheung YB, Akisanya A, Sankareh K, Lahai G, Greenwood BM, et al. Nasopharyngeal carriage of *Streptococcus pneumoniae* in Gambian infants:a longitudinal study. *Clin Infect Dis.* (2008) 46:807–14. doi: 10.1086/528688
11. Turner P, Turner C, Green N, Ashton L, Lwe E, Jankhot A, et al. Serum antibody responses to pneumococcal colonization in the first 2 years of life:results from an SE Asian longitudinal cohort study. *Clin Microbiol Infect.* (2013) 19:E551–8. doi: 10.1111/1469-0691.12431
12. Abdullahi O, Karani A, Tigoi CC, Mugo D, Kungu S, Wanjiru E, et al. The prevalence and risk factors for pneumococcal colonization of the nasopharynx among children in Kilifi District, Kenya. *PLoS ONE.* (2012) 7:e30787. doi: 10.1371/journal.pone.0030787
13. Yahiaoui RY, den Heijer CDj, van Bijnen EM, Paget WJ, Pringle M, Goossens H, et al. Prevalence and antibiotic resistance of commensal *Streptococcus pneumoniae* in nine European countries. *Future Microbiol.* (2016) 11:737–44. doi: 10.2217/fmb-2015-0011
14. Goldblatt D, Hussain M, Andrews N, Ashton L, Virta C, Melegaro A, et al. Antibody responses to nasopharyngeal carriage of *Streptococcus pneumoniae* in adults:a longitudinal household study. *J Infect Dis.* (2005) 192:387–93. doi: 10.1086/431524
15. Ridda I, Macintyre CR, Lindley R, McIntyre PB, Brown M, Oftadeh S, et al. Lack of pneumococcal carriage in the hospitalised elderly. *Vaccine.* (2010) 28:3902–4. doi: 10.1016/j.vaccine.2010.03.073
16. Oksenhendler E, Gérard L, Fieschi C, Malphettes M, Mouillot G, Jaussaud R, et al. Infections in 252 patients with common variable immunodeficiency. *Clin Infect Dis.* (2008) 46:1547–54. doi: 10.1086/587669
17. Kumar D, Humar A, Plevneshi A, Siegal D, Franke N, Green K, et al. Invasive pneumococcal disease in adult hematopoietic stem cell transplant recipients:a decade of prospective population-based surveillance. *Bone Marrow Transplant.* (2008) 41:743–7. doi: 10.1038/sj.bmt.1705964
18. Janoff EN, Breiman RF, Daley CL, Hopewell PC.Janoff EN, et al. Pneumococcal disease during HIV infection. Epidemiologic, clinical, and immunologic perspectives. *Ann Intern Med.* (1992) 117:314–24. doi: 10.7326/0003-4819-117-4-314
19. Jönsson G, Truedsson L, Sturfelt G, Oxelius VA, Braconier JH, Sjöholm AG.Jonsson G, et al. Hereditary C2 deficiency in Sweden:frequent occurrence of invasive infection, atherosclerosis, and rheumatic disease. *Medicine.* (2005) 84:23–34. doi: 10.1097/01.md.0000152371.22747.1e
20. Yuste J, Sen A, Truedsson L, Jönsson G, Tay LS, Hyams C, et al. Impaired opsonization with C3b and phagocytosis of *Streptococcus pneumoniae* in sera from subjects with defects in the classical complement pathway. *Infect Immun.* (2008) 76:3761–70. doi: 10.1128/IAI.00291-08
21. Melegaro A, Edmunds WJ, Pebody R, Miller E, George R.Melegaro A, et al. The current burden of pneumococcal disease in England and Wales. *J Infect.* (2006) 52:37–48. doi: 10.1016/j.jinf.2005.02.008
22. Lipsitch M, Whitney CG, Zell E, Kaijalainen T, Dagan R, Malley R. Are anticapsular antibodies the primary mechanism of protection against invasive pneumococcal disease? *PLoS Med.* (2005) 2:e15. doi: 10.1371/journal.pmed.0020015
23. Prevaes SM, van Wamel WJ, de Vogel CP, Veenhoven RH, van Gils EJ, van Belkum A, et al. Nasopharyngeal colonization elicits antibody responses to staphylococcal and pneumococcal proteins that are not associated with a reduced risk of subsequent carriage. *Infect Immun.* (2012) 80:2186–93. doi: 10.1128/IAI.00037-12
24. Simell B, Kilpi TM. Kayhty H. Pneumococcal carriage and otitis media induce salivary antibodies to pneumococcal capsular polysaccharides in children. *J Infect Dis.* (2002) 186:1106–14. doi: 10.1086/344235
25. Wilson R, Cohen JM, Jose RJ, de Vogel C, Baxendale H, Brown JS.Wilson R, et al. Protection against *Streptococcus pneumoniae* lung infection after nasopharyngeal colonization requires both humoral and cellular immune responses. *Mucosal Immunol.* (2015) 8:627–39. doi: 10.1038/mi.2014.95
26. Richards L, Ferreira DM, Miyaji EN, Andrew PW, Kadioglu A.Richards L, et al. The immunising effect of pneumococcal nasopharyngeal colonisation; protection against future colonisation and fatal invasive disease. *Immunobiology.* (2010) 215:251–63. doi: 10.1016/j.imbio.2009.12.004
27. Malley R, Lipsitch M, Stack A, Saladino R, Fleisher G, Pelton S, et al. Intranasal immunization with killed unencapsulated whole cells prevents colonization and invasive disease by capsulated pneumococci. *Infect Immun.* (2001) 69:4870–3. doi: 10.1128/IAI.69.8.4870-4873.2001
28. Malley R, Trzcinski K, Srivastava A, Thompson CM, Anderson PW, Lipsitch M.Malley R, et al. CD4+ T cells mediate antibody-independent acquired immunity to pneumococcal colonization. *Proc Natl Acad Sci USA.* (2005) 102:4848–53. doi: 10.1073/pnas.0501254102
29. Malley R, Srivastava A, Lipsitch M, Thompson CM, Watkins C, Tzianabos A, et al. Antibody-independent, interleukin−17A-mediated, cross-serotype immunity to pneumococci in mice immunized intranasally with the cell wall polysaccharide. *Infect Immun.* (2006) 74:2187–95. doi: 10.1128/IAI.74.4.2187-2195.2006
30. Basset A, Thompson CM, Hollingshead SK, Briles DE, Ades EW, Lipsitch M, et al. Antibody-independent, CD4+ T-cell-dependent protection against pneumococcal colonization elicited by intranasal immunization with purified pneumococcal proteins. *Infect Immun.* (2007) 75:5460–4. doi: 10.1128/IAI.00773-07
31. Lu YJ, Gross J, Bogaert D, Finn A, Bagrade L, Zhang Q, et al. Interleukin−17A mediates acquired immunity to pneumococcal colonization. *PLoS Pathog.* (2008) 4:e1000159. doi: 10.1371/journal.ppat.1000159
32. Bogaert D, Weinberger D, Thompson C, Lipsitch M, Malley R.Bogaert D, et al. Impaired innate and adaptive immunity to *Streptococcus pneumoniae* and its effect on colonization in an infant mouse model. *Infect Immun.* (2009) 77:1613–22. doi: 10.1128/IAI.00871-08
33. McCool TL, Cate TR, Moy G, Weiser JN.McCool TL, et al. The immune response to pneumococcal proteins during experimental human carriage. *J Exp Med.* (2002) 195:359–65. doi: 10.1084/jem.20011576
34. Ferreira DM, Neill DR, Bangert M, Gritzfeld JF, Green N, Wright AK, et al. Controlled human infection and rechallenge with *Streptococcus pneumoniae* reveals the protective efficacy of carriage in healthy adults. *Am J Respir Crit Care Med.* (2013) 187:855–64. doi: 10.1164/rccm.201212-2277OC
35. Wright AK, Bangert M, Gritzfeld JF, Ferreira DM, Jambo KC, Wright AD, et al. Experimental human pneumococcal carriage augments IL−17A-dependent T-cell defence of the lung. *PLoS Pathog.* (2013) 9:e1003274. doi: 10.1371/journal.ppat.1003274
36. Zhang Q, Bernatoniene J, Bagrade L, Pollard AJ, Mitchell TJ, Paton JC, et al. Serum and mucosal antibody responses to pneumococcal protein antigens in children:relationships with carriage status. *Eur J Immunol.* (2006) 36:46–57. doi: 10.1002/eji.200535101
37. Weinberger DM, Dagan R, Givon-Lavi N, Regev-Yochay G, Malley R, Lipsitch M.Weinberger DM, et al. Epidemiologic evidence for serotype-specific acquired immunity to pneumococcal carriage. *J Infect Dis.* (2008) 197:1511–8. doi: 10.1086/587941
38. McCool TL, Weiser JN. Limited role of antibody in clearance of *Streptococcus pneumoniae* in a murine model of colonization. *Infect Immun.* (2004) 72:5807–13. doi: 10.1128/IAI.72.10.5807-5813.2004
39. Zhang Q, Bernatoniene J, Bagrade L, Paton JC, Mitchell TJ, Hammerschmidt S, et al. Regulation of production of mucosal antibody to pneumococcal protein antigens by T-cell-derived gamma interferon and interleukin−10 in children. *Infect Immun.* (2006) 74:4735–43. doi: 10.1128/IAI.00165-06
40. Lebon A, Verkaik NJ, Labout JA, de Vogel CP, Hooijkaas H, Verbrugh HA, et al. Natural antibodies against several pneumococcal virulence proteins in children during the pre-pneumococcal-vaccine era:the generation R study. *Infect Immun.* (2011) 79:1680–7. doi: 10.1128/IAI.01379-10
41. Mureithi MW, Finn A, Ota MO, Zhang Q, Davenport V, Mitchell TJ, et al. T cell memory response to pneumococcal protein antigens in an area of high pneumococcal carriage and disease. *J Infect Dis.* (2009) 200:783–93. doi: 10.1086/605023
42. McAleer JP, Kolls JK. Directing traffic:IL−17 and IL−22 coordinate pulmonary immune defense. *Immunol Rev.* (2014) 260:129–44. doi: 10.1111/imr.12183
43. Curtis MM, Way SS. Interleukin−17 in host defence against bacterial, mycobacterial and fungal pathogens. *Immunology.* (2009) 126:177–85. doi: 10.1111/j.1365-2567.2008.03017.x
44. Macleod CM, Hodges RG. Prevention of pneumococcal pneumonia by immunization with specific capsular polysaccharides. *J Exp Med.* (1945) 82:445–65. doi: 10.1084/jem.82.6.445
45. Whitney CG. Preventing pneumococcal disease. ACIP recommends pneumococcal polysaccharide vaccine for all adults age > or = 65. *Geriatrics.* (2003) 58:20–2, 25.

46. Janoff EN, Musher DM. *Streptococcus pneumoniae, in Mandell, Douglas, and Bennett's Principles and Practice of Infectious Diseases.* Philadelphia: Saunders (2015).
47. Casadevall A. Antibody-based therapies for emerging infectious diseases. *Emerg Infect Dis.* (1996) 2:200–8. doi: 10.3201/eid0203.960306
48. Bull CG. The mechanism of the curative action of antipneumococcus serum. *J Exp Med.* (1915) 22:457–64. doi: 10.1084/jem.22.4.457
49. Casadevall A, Scharff MD. Serum therapy revisited:animal models of infection and development of passive antibody therapy. *Antimicrob Agents Chemother.* (1994) 38:1695–702. doi: 10.1128/AAC.38.8.1695
50. Bullowa JG, Wilcox C. Therapeutic serum for pneumococcus type V (Cooper) pneumonia. *J Clin Invest.* (1936) 15:711–4. doi: 10.1172/JCI100824
51. Bullowa JG. Pneumonias:their management. *Cal West Med.* (1937) 46:368–72.
52. Cobey S, Lipsitch M. Niche and neutral effects of acquired immunity permit coexistence of pneumococcal serotypes. *Science.* (2012) 335:1376–80. doi: 10.1126/science.1215947
53. Roche AM, King SJ. Weiser JN. Live attenuated *Streptococcus pneumoniae* strains induce serotype-independent mucosal and systemic protection in mice. *Infect Immun.* (2007) 75:2469–75. doi: 10.1128/IAI.01972-06
54. Croucher NJ, Campo JJ, Le TQ, Liang X, Bentley SD, Hanage WP, et al. Diverse evolutionary patterns of pneumococcal antigens identified by pangenome-wide immunological screening. *Proc Natl Acad Sci USA.* (2017) 114:E357–66. doi: 10.1073/pnas.1613937114
55. Giefing C, Meinke AL, Hanner M, Henics T, Bui MD, Gelbmann D, et al. Discovery of a novel class of highly conserved vaccine antigens using genomic scale antigenic fingerprinting of pneumococcus with human antibodies. *J Exp Med.* (2008) 205:117–31. doi: 10.1084/jem.20071168
56. Moffitt KL, Gierahn TM, Lu YJ, Gouveia P, Alderson M, Flechtner JB, et al. T(H)17-based vaccine design for prevention of *Streptococcus pneumoniae* colonization. *Cell Host Microbe.* (2011) 9:158–65. doi: 10.1016/j.chom.2011.01.007
57. Trzcinski K, Thompson C, Malley R, Lipsitch M. Antibodies to conserved pneumococcal antigens correlate with, but are not required for, protection against pneumococcal colonization induced by prior exposure in a mouse model. *Infect Immun.* (2005) 73:7043–6. doi: 10.1128/IAI.73.10.7043-7046.2005
58. Zhang Z, Clarke TB, Weiser JN. Cellular effectors mediating Th17-dependent clearance of pneumococcal colonization in mice. *J Clin Invest.* (2009) 119:1899–909. doi: 10.1172/JCI36731
59. Malley R, Morse SC, Leite LC, Areas AP, Ho PL, Kubrusly FS, et al. Multiserotype protection of mice against pneumococcal colonization of the nasopharynx and middle ear by killed nonencapsulated cells given intranasally with a nontoxic adjuvant. *Infect Immun.* (2004) 72:4290–2. doi: 10.1128/IAI.72.7.4290-4292.2004
60. van Rossum AM, Lysenko ES. Weiser JN. Host and bacterial factors contributing to the clearance of colonization by *Streptococcus pneumoniae* in a murine model. *Infect Immun.* (2005) 73:7718–26. doi: 10.1128/IAI.73.11.7718-7726.2005
61. Briles DE, Hollingshead SK, Paton JC, Ades EW, Novak L, van Ginkel FW, et al. Immunizations with pneumococcal surface protein A and pneumolysin are protective against pneumonia in a murine model of pulmonary infection with *Streptococcus pneumoniae. J Infect Dis.* (2003) 188:339–48. doi: 10.1086/376571
62. Balachandran P, Brooks-Walter A, Virolainen-Julkunen A, Hollingshead SK, Briles DE.Balachandran P, et al. Role of pneumococcal surface protein C in nasopharyngeal carriage and pneumonia and its ability to elicit protection against carriage of *Streptococcus pneumoniae. Infect Immun.* (2002) 70:2526–34. doi: 10.1128/IAI.70.5.2526-2534.2002
63. Roche AM, Richard AL, Rahkola JT, Janoff EN, Weiser JN.Roche AM, et al. Antibody blocks acquisition of bacterial colonization through agglutination. *Mucosal Immunol.* (2015) 8:176–85. doi: 10.1038/mi.2014.55
64. Zangari T, Wang Y, Weiser JN. *Streptococcus pneumoniae* Transmission is blocked by type-specific immunity in an infant mouse model. *MBio.* (2017) 8:e00188-17. doi: 10.1128/mBio.00188-17
65. Pido-Lopez J, Kwok WW, Mitchell TJ, Heyderman RS, Williams NA.Pido-Lopez J, et al. Acquisition of pneumococci specific effector and regulatory Cd4+ T cells localising within human upper respiratory-tract mucosal lymphoid tissue. *PLoS Pathog.* (2011) 7:e1002396. doi: 10.1371/journal.ppat.1002396
66. Zhang Q, Leong SC, McNamara PS, Mubarak A, Malley R, Finn A.Zhang Q, et al. Characterisation of regulatory T cells in nasal associated lymphoid tissue in children:relationships with pneumococcal colonization. *PLoS Pathog.* (2011) 7:e1002175. doi: 10.1371/journal.ppat.1002175
67. Lundgren A, Bhuiyan TR, Novak D, Kaim J, Reske A, Lu YJ, et al. Characterization of Th17 responses to *Streptococcus pneumoniae* in humans:comparisons between adults and children in a developed and a developing country. *Vaccine.* (2012) 30:3897–907. doi: 10.1016/j.vaccine.2012.03.082
68. Mitsi E, Roche AM, Reiné J, Zangari T, Owugha JT, Pennington SH, et al. Agglutination by anti-capsular polysaccharide antibody is associated with protection against experimental human pneumococcal carriage. *Mucosal Immunol.* (2017) 10:385–94. doi: 10.1038/mi.2016.71
69. Wright AK, Ferreira DM, Gritzfeld JF, Wright AD, Armitage K, Jambo KC, et al. Human nasal challenge with *Streptococcus pneumoniae* is immunising in the absence of carriage. *PLoS Pathog.* (2012) 8:e1002622. doi: 10.1371/journal.ppat.1002622
70. Cohen JM, Khandavilli S, Camberlein E, Hyams C, Baxendale HE, Brown JS.Cohen JM, et al. Protective contributions against invasive *Streptococcus pneumoniae* pneumonia of antibody and Th17-cell responses to nasopharyngeal colonisation. *PLoS ONE.* (2011) 6:e25558. doi: 10.1371/journal.pone.0025558
71. Bou Ghanem EN, Maung NHT, Siwapornchai N, Goodwin AE, Clark S, Muñoz-Elías EJ, et al. Nasopharyngeal exposure to *Streptococcus pneumoniae* induces extended age-dependent protection against pulmonary infection mediated by antibodies and CD138(+) cells. *J Immunol.* (2018) 200:3739–51. doi: 10.4049/jimmunol.1701065
72. Brown JS, Hussell T, Gilliland SM, Holden DW, Paton JC, Ehrenstein MR, et al. The classical pathway is the dominant complement pathway required for innate immunity to *Streptococcus pneumoniae* infection in mice. *Proc Natl Acad Sci USA.* (2002) 99:16969–74. doi: 10.1073/pnas.012669199
73. Kang YS, Do Y, Lee HK, Park SH, Cheong C, Lynch RM, et al. A dominant complement fixation pathway for pneumococcal polysaccharides initiated by SIGN-R1 interacting with C1q. *Cell.* (2006) 125:47–58. doi: 10.1016/j.cell.2006.01.046
74. Gerlini A, Colomba L, Furi L, Braccini T, Manso AS, Pammolli A, et al. The role of host and microbial factors in the pathogenesis of pneumococcal bacteraemia arising from a single bacterial cell bottleneck. *PLoS Pathog.* (2014) 10:e1004026. doi: 10.1371/journal.ppat.1004026
75. Wilson R, et al. Naturally acquired human immunity to pneumococcus is dependent on antibody to protein antigens. *PLoS Pathog.* (2017) 13:e1006137. doi: 10.1371/journal.ppat.1006137
76. Quinti I, Soresina A, Guerra A, Rondelli R, Spadaro G, Agostini C, et al. Effectiveness of immunoglobulin replacement therapy on clinical outcome in patients with primary antibody deficiencies:results from a multicenter prospective cohort study. *J Clin Immunol.* (2011) 31:315–22. doi: 10.1007/s10875-011-9511-0
77. Pourpak Z, Aghamohammadi A, Sedighipour L, Farhoudi A, Movahedi M, Gharagozlou M, et al. Effect of regular intravenous immunoglobulin therapy on prevention of pneumonia in patients with common variable immunodeficiency. *J Microbiol Immunol Infect.* (2006) 39:114–20.
78. Wang Y, Jiang B, Guo Y, Li W, Tian Y, Sonnenberg GF, et al. Cross-protective mucosal immunity mediated by memory Th17 cells against *Streptococcus pneumoniae* lung infection. *Mucosal Immunol.* (2017) 10:250–9. doi: 10.1038/mi.2016.41
79. Smith NM, Wasserman GA, Coleman FT, Hilliard KL, Yamamoto K, Lipsitz E, et al. Regionally compartmentalized resident memory T cells mediate naturally acquired protection against pneumococcal pneumonia. *Mucosal Immunol.* (2018) 11:220–35. doi: 10.1038/mi.2017.43
80. Rosen FS, Cooper MD, Wedgwood RJ. The primary immunodeficiencies. *N Engl J Med.* (1995) 333:431–40. doi: 10.1056/NEJM199508173330707
81. Dworkin MS, Ward JW, Hanson DL, Jones JL, Kaplan JE, .Dworkin MS, et al. Pneumococcal disease among human immunodeficiency virus-infected persons:incidence, risk factors, and impact of vaccination. *Clin Infect Dis.* (2001) 32:794–800. doi: 10.1086/319218

82. Milner JD, Brenchley JM, Laurence A, Freeman AF, Hill BJ, Elias KM, et al. Impaired T(H)17 cell differentiation in subjects with autosomal dominant hyper-IgE syndrome. *Nature.* (2008) 452:773–6. doi: 10.1038/nature06764
83. Perreau M, Vigano S, Bellanger F, Pellaton C, Buss G, Comte D, et al. Exhaustion of bacteria-specific CD4 T cells and microbial translocation in common variable immunodeficiency disorders. *J Exp Med.* (2014) 211:2033–45. doi: 10.1084/jem.20140039
84. Esposito S, Mari D, Bergamaschini L, Orenti A, Terranova L, Ruggiero L, et al. Pneumococcal colonization in older adults. *Immun Ageing.* (2016) 13:2. doi: 10.1186/s12979-016-0057-0
85. O'Brien KL, Millar EV, Zell ER, Bronsdon M, Weatherholtz R, Reid R, et al. Effect of pneumococcal conjugate vaccine on nasopharyngeal colonization among immunized and unimmunized children in a community-randomized trial. *J Infect Dis.* (2007) 196:1211–20. doi: 10.1086/521833
86. Lindstrand A, Galanis I, Darenberg J, Morfeldt E, Naucler P, Blennow M, et al. Unaltered pneumococcal carriage prevalence due to expansion of non-vaccine types of low invasive potential 8 years after vaccine introduction in Stockholm, Sweden. *Vaccine.* (2016) 34:4565–71. doi: 10.1016/j.vaccine.2016.07.031
87. Puchta A, Naidoo A, Verschoor CP, Loukov D, Thevaranjan N, Mandur TS, et al. TNF drives monocyte dysfunction with age and results in impaired anti-pneumococcal immunity. *PLoS Pathog.* (2016) 12:e1005368. doi: 10.1371/journal.ppat.1005368
88. Boyd AR, Orihuela CJ. Dysregulated inflammation as a risk factor for pneumonia in the elderly. *Aging Dis.* (2011) 2:487–500.
89. Krone CL, Trzcinski K, Zborowski T, Sanders EA, Bogaert D.Krone CL, et al. Impaired innate mucosal immunity in aged mice permits prolonged *Streptococcus pneumoniae* colonization. *Infect Immun.* (2013) 81:4615–25. doi: 10.1128/IAI.00618-13
90. Adler H, Ferreira DM, Gordon SB, Rylance J.Adler H, et al. Pneumococcal capsular polysaccharide immunity in the elderly. *Clin Vaccine Immunol.* (2017) 24: e00004–17. doi: 10.1128/CVI.00004-17
91. Shi Y, Yamazaki T, Okubo Y, Uehara Y, Sugane K, Agematsu K.Shi Y, et al. Regulation of aged humoral immune defense against pneumococcal bacteria by IgM memory B cell. *J Immunol.* (2005) 175:3262–7. doi: 10.4049/jimmunol.175.5.3262
92. Glennie SJ, Sepako E, Mzinza D, Harawa V, Miles DJ, Jambo KC, et al. Impaired CD4 T cell memory response to *Streptococcus pneumoniae* precedes CD4 T cell depletion in HIV-infected Malawian adults. *PLoS ONE.* (2011) 6:e25610. doi: 10.1371/journal.pone.0025610
93. Neill DR, Fernandes VE, Wisby L, Haynes AR, Ferreira DM, Laher A, et al. T regulatory cells control susceptibility to invasive pneumococcal pneumonia in mice. *PLoS Pathog.* (2012) 8:e1002660. doi: 10.1371/journal.ppat.1002660

9

Bordetella pertussis Whole Cell Immunization, Unlike Acellular Immunization, Mimics Naive Infection by Driving Hematopoietic Stem and Progenitor Cell Expansion in Mice

Melinda E. Varney[1,2], Dylan T. Boehm[1,2], Katherine DeRoos[1,2], Evan S. Nowak[1,2], Ting Y. Wong[1,2], Emel Sen-Kilic[1,2], Shebly D. Bradford[1,2], Cody Elkins[1,2], Matthew S. Epperly[1,2], William T. Witt[1,2], Mariette Barbier[1,2] and F. Heath Damron[1,2]*

[1] Department of Microbiology, Immunology, and Cell Biology, West Virginia University School of Medicine, Morgantown, WV, United States, [2] Vaccine Development Center at West Virginia University Health Sciences Center, Morgantown, WV, United States

***Correspondence:**
Melinda E. Varney
melinda.varney@hsc.wvu.edu

Hematopoietic stem and progenitor cell (HSPC) compartments are altered to direct immune responses to infection. Their roles during immunization are not well-described. To elucidate mechanisms for waning immunity following immunization with acellular vaccines (ACVs) against *Bordetella pertussis* (*Bp*), we tested the hypothesis that immunization with *Bp* ACVs and whole cell vaccines (WCVs) differ in directing the HSPC characteristics and immune cell development patterns that ultimately contribute to the types and quantities of cells produced to fight infection. Our data demonstrate that compared to control and ACV-immunized CD-1 mice, immunization with an efficacious WCV drives expansion of hematopoietic multipotent progenitor cells (MPPs), increases circulating white blood cells (WBCs), and alters the size and composition of lymphoid organs. In addition to MPPs, common lymphoid progenitor (CLP) proportions increase in the bone marrow of WCV-immunized mice, while B220$^+$ cell proportions decrease. Upon subsequent infection, increases in maturing B cell populations are striking in WCV-immunized mice. RNAseq analyses of HSPCs revealed that WCV and ACV-immunized mice vastly differ in developing VDJ gene segment diversity. Moreover, gene set enrichment analyses demonstrate WCV-immunized mice exhibit unique gene signatures that suggest roles for interferon (IFN) induced gene expression. Also observed in naïve infection, these IFN stimulated gene (ISG) signatures point toward roles in cell survival, cell cycle, autophagy, and antigen processing and presentation. Taken together, these findings underscore the impact of vaccine antigen and adjuvant content on skewing and/or priming HSPC populations for immune response.

Keywords: vaccination, *Bordetella pertussis*, respiratory pathogen, hematopoietic stem cell, immunobiology

INTRODUCTION

Innate and adaptive immune cells originate from hematopoietic stem cells (HSCs). Over an organism's lifetime, long-term HSCs (LT-HSCs) self-renew and generate short-term HSCs (ST-HSCs). ST-HSCs give rise to myeloid and lymphoid progenitors that differentiate into immune cells (1). Hematopoietic stem and progenitor cell (HSPC) renewal, expansion, and differentiation are tightly regulated to produce and maintain sufficient blood cells (2). Cell–cell interactions, microenvironment contributions, cytokines, and gene signature changes prompt HSPC expansion (1, 3). During infection, this results from: (1) direct pathogen interaction or signals that push differentiation and/or mobilization or (2) a pull to replenish leukocytes required for immune surveillance and clearing infection (4, 5). The immune system critically relies on these events to produce correct quantities and types of cells required for response to pathogens and stress (6). At sites of infection, innate and adaptive arms of the immune system work synergistically to clear infection and/or prevent recurrence. Long-term immunity is maintained by antigen-specific memory B and T cells. Recent evidence suggests that innate immune cells also provide long-term immunity independently (7–9).

While HSPCs direct immune responses to infections, little is known about their significance in immunization-induced immunity (10–17). Kaufmann et al. demonstrated that Bacillus Camette-Guerin (BCG) vaccination "educates" HSPCs to form components of innate immunity responsible for long-term immune protection from tuberculosis (9). Herein, we demonstrate that vaccine composition influences HSPC frequency by eliciting a unique transcriptional landscape that impacts both innate and adaptive immunity. Recent re-emergence of pertussis, a highly contagious respiratory infection caused by the Gram-negative bacterial pathogen *Bp*, prompted our use of a pertussis model to investigate the roles of HSPCs in vaccine efficacy. Immunization strategies were altered from the use of highly efficacious whole cell vaccines (WCVs), such as DTP, to acellular vaccines (ACV) (DTaP/tdap) in the 1990s. Evidence suggests that recent increases in pertussis cases are due in part to waning ACV protection (18–20). Epidemiological data indicate that when ACVs prevent disease, they may fail to completely prevent infection or transmission (18, 19). Without enhanced vaccines, pertussis incidence is expected to continue to rise, given that a greater proportion of the population over time will only be ACV-immunized. Because WCVs offer longer-lived protection (21), comparisons regarding how immune responses to ACV and WCV differ, including impact on HSPCs, may provide insight for next generation ACVs that are safe and efficacious.

To investigate the role of vaccine content on influencing HSPCs, it is essential to consider known components of each pertussis vaccine. Despite differences in overall antigenic content, WCVs, which are inactivated entire *Bp* organisms, and ACVs, which contain purified components of *Bp*, share some common antigens: pertussis toxin (PT), filamentous hemagglutinin (FHA), pertactin, and fimbriae. ACVs contain aluminum hydroxide, which contributes to a T helper (Th)2-polarized response. Conversely, lipo-oligosaccharide (LOS) in WCVs promotes Th1/Th17 responses (22) despite DTP combined vaccines' inclusion of alum. Little is known regarding the influence of the components of pertussis vaccines on HSPCs. Enzymatically active PT can induce HSC mobilization by blocking G protein function (23), but it is inactivated in ACVs and present only in low concentrations in WCVs (unpublished observations). Additionally, alum, which is present in ACVs and some WCVs, is known to induce granulopoiesis (24) while LOS, present only in WCVs, stimulates TLR4 signaling known to induce HSPC expansion in bone marrow (25).

In the present study, we tested the hypothesis that vaccine composition determines immune response by HSPCs. To do so, we assessed the impact ACVs and WCVs on HSPC expansion, differentiation, and downstream peripheral immune response. We demonstrate that WCVs (1) induce HSPC expansion, priming them for antigen processing and presentation, (2) increase extramedullary hematopoiesis providing stores of immature immune cells released by the spleen upon infection, and (3) prime HSPCs for rapid B cell maturation upon subsequent *Bp* challenge. We also show that ACVs have little impact on HSPCs. This knowledge provides insights into methods by which immune responses to ACVs and WCVs differ, thus introducing a novel area of study that may explain in part why waning immunity occurs with ACVs.

METHODS

Mouse Models

Phosphate buffered saline (PBS), 1/5th human dose of INFANRIX (GSK) human vaccine (DTap/ACV), or 1/5th human dose of National Institute for Biological Standards and WHO International Standard *Bp* vaccine (NIBSC 94-532) (WCV) were used to immunize 5-weeks-old female CD-1 mice (Charles River) by intraperitoneal injection (**Table S1**). Anesthetized mice were infected by intranasal administration of 2×10^7 colony forming units (CFU) of *Bp* strain UT25 (26) in 20 μl of PBS. *Bp* was handled using standard biosecurity and institutional procedures necessary for the use of a BSL-2 microorganism. These procedures were approved by the West Virginia University Institutional Biosafety Committee (protocol 17-11-01). Post-vaccination and challenge, organs/tissues were extracted in sterile conditions from mice euthanized by pentobarbital injection as recommended by the Panel on Euthanasia of the American Veterinary Medical Association. Cardiac puncture blood was collected. Serum was separated by centrifugation using Microtainer blood collection tubes (BD). Trachea and lungs were homogenized to determine bacterial burden. For *Bp* burden in the nares, 1 ml of PBS was flushed through the nares. Serial dilutions in PBS were plated on Bordet Gengou (BG) Agar containing 15% sheep's blood and streptomycin (100 μg/ml). Bone marrow extraction was performed by flushing RPMI media (ATCC) + 10% fetal bovine serum (FBS) (Sigma) through mouse femurs. Cells were pelleted by centrifugation (500 g) and red blood cell lysis was performed by incubating cells in 1 ml 1X BD PharmLyse™ (BD

Biosciences) for 2 min at 37°C. Cells were washed in 1X PBS containing 2% FBS and prepared for flow cytometry. Spleens were dissociated by being passed through a 70 μm mesh filter in 5 ml RPMI media (ATCC) + 10% FBS (Sigma) with the aid of a syringe plunger. Cells were pelleted by centrifugation (500 g) and red blood cell lysis was performed by incubating cells in 1 ml 1X BD PharmLyse™ (BD Biosciences) for 2 min at 37°C. Cells were washed in 1X PBS containing 2% FBS and prepared for flow cytometry. This study was reviewed and approved by the West Virginia University Institutional Animal Care and Use Committee (protocol Damron 14-1211).

Complete Blood Counts and Histology

Complete peripheral blood (PB) counts were analyzed using a Drew Scientific Hemavet 950. Briefly, a portion of PB from the cardiac puncture was collected using Microtainer blood collection tubes (BD) with a K2EDTA additive. After thorough mixing within the K2EDTA containing tube, blood was transferred to a 1.5 ml microcentrifuge tube and run on the Drew Scientific Hemavet 950. For tissue histology, tibias and spleens were fixed in formalin, embedded in paraffin blocks, sectioned, and stained with hematoxylin and eosin (H&E).

Flow Cytometry

Following Fc receptor blocking in PBS containing 2% FBS, 1×10^6 cells were incubated in antibody for 1 h at 4°C in the dark. Cells were then washed 2 times with PBS, and resuspended in fluorescence-activated cell sorting (FACS) buffer. Flow cytometry antibodies (listed in **Table S2**) were chosen to acquire a broad understanding of how different vaccine compositions influence the development of both innate and adaptive immune cells. FACS analyses were performed on BD LSRFortessa or FACSAria III cytometers. Data was analyzed using FlowJo_V10.

Cytokine Analysis

Spleen homogenates were pelleted by centrifugation (1,000 g for 5 min). Collected supernatant was stored at −80°C until analysis. Concentrations of cytokineswere determined by quantitative sandwich immunoassays, Meso Scale Discovery (Rockville, MD) V-PLEX Proinflammatory Panel (K15048G-1).

Isolation of RNA, Illumina Library Preparation, and Sequencing

RNA was prepared immediately using RNeasy purification kits (Qiagen) and quantified using Qubit 3.0 (ThermoFisher). RNA integrity was assessed using Agilent BioAnalyzer RNA Pico chip. Samples were submitted for Ribo-zero rRNA depletion (Illumina) and reassessed for RNA integrity. Samples were processed into libraries by the Ovation RNA-Seq System v2 (NuGEN) protocol. Quality control was performed on libraries using the KAPA qPCR QC assay (KAPA Biosystems). Libraries (36 total) were sequenced on an illumina HiSeq 1500 at the Marshall University Genomics Core facility, 2 × 50 bp resulting in ∼16 M reads per sample. Sequencing data was deposited to the Sequence Read Archive (reference number SRP130256, BioProject number PRJNA430726).

RNAseq Bioinformatic Analyses

Reads were analyzed using CLC Genomics Workbench 9.5. Default settings were used for mapping reads against the GRCm38 *mus musculus* genome. Fold changes in gene expression and statistical analyses were performed using Extraction of Differential Gene Expression (EDGE) test on *p*-values. Venn diagrams and gene set enrichment were established using Venny 2.1 (27) and PANTHER, respectively. Significant data was determined by FDR (<0.05). In Ingenuity Pathway Analysis (IPA), significant genes ($p < 0.05$) were uploaded into software and datasets were compared across immunization and challenge conditions. IPA's Upstream Regulator analytic was utilized to identify upstream transcriptional regulators.

Immunoglobulin and B- and T-Cell Receptor Profiling

B cell clones were identified using MiXCR software (MiLabratory) (28), capable of generating quantitated clonotypes of immunoglobulins. Reads were merged using concatenation and imported into MiXCR software and aligned to each other to generate clonotypes based on Variable (V), Diversity (D), and Joining (J) (VDJ) segment regions of unique immunoglobulins specific to each sample. Clone data was grouped based on vaccine received and time point. Clonotypes were separated into T and B cells based on T-cell receptor or B-cell receptor specific sequences. Prepared data files were imported into VDJtools (MiLabratory) for data representation as previously described (29).

Statistical Analysis

Results are depicted as mean ± SEM. Excluding RNAseq statistics described above, all other statistical analyses were performed using two way ANOVAs and Tukey's multiple comparisons. GraphPad Prism software was used for statistical analysis.

RESULTS

Vaccine Content Determines Peripheral Immune Response to *Bp* Challenge

To investigate how vaccine impact on HSPCs contributes to immunity to pertussis in CD-1 outbred mice, we utilized a vaccination and challenge workflow (**Figure 1A**) for profiling immune responses after primary and boost immunizations as well *Bp* challenge. Five-weeks-old mice were immunized with PBS (vehicle control), ACV, or WCV (**Table S1**), boosted, and subsequently challenged with *Bp*. Although ACVs wane in immune protection over time in humans (18–20), short-term experiments in mice show similar initial clearance of bacterial burden in sites of respiratory infection (lung, nasal wash, and trachea) in both groups (**Figure 1B**) with 1/5th human doses. Serological analysis of Ig(A+G+M) indicates that only the ACV induces detectable anti-PT, whereas both the ACV and WCV induce anti-FHA. As expected, the LOS-containing WCV induces production of anti-LOS (serology data not shown).

To demonstrate consistency of our model with other groups, we assessed PB cell counts. Pertussis causes leukocytosis in humans, rodents, and baboons (30–32), and WCV immunization

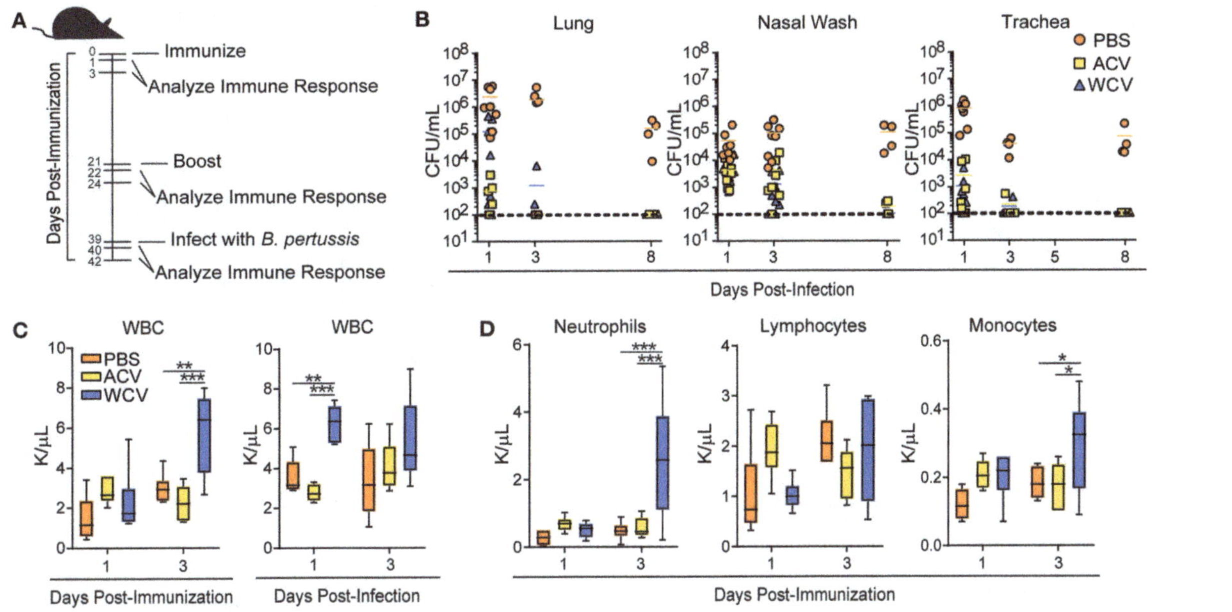

FIGURE 1 | Vaccine content determines PB immune response to *Bp* challenge. **(A)** The workflow for immunization and infection schedules of 5-weeks-old female CD-1 mice is represented. Mice were immunized with phosphate buffered saline (PBS), *Bp* acellular vaccine (ACV), or *Bp* whole cell vaccine (WCV) and infected with 2 × 10^7 CFU UT25 *Bp*. Immune responses in mice were evaluated at 1 and 3 days after immunization, boost, and infection. **(B)** *Bp* bacterial burden was measured in lung, nasal wash, and trachea of mice ($n = 4$–8/group for each time point) by counting CFUs produced 3 days after plating and incubating serial dilutions of homogenates on BG containing streptomycin (100 μg/ml) at 37°C. **(C)** White blood cell counts were measured ($n = 5$–6/group for each time point) on a Drew Scientific Hemavet 950 at days 1 and 3 post-immunization and days 1 and 3 post-infection $^{**}p < 0.01$; $^{***}p < 0.001$. **(D)** Differential white blood cell counts measured on days 1 and 3 post-immunization are represented. $^{*}p < 0.05$; 2-way ANOVAs with Tukey's multiple comparisons. Bars extend to represent minimum to maximum values, while the line represents the mean.

has been shown to also result in leukocytosis (33). Our WCV-immunized mice exhibit increases in white blood cells at day 3 post-immunization when compared to PBS and ACV-immunized mice. WBCs increase again following subsequent infection (day 1) (**Figure 1C**) in WCV-immunized mice. Increases in WBCs are attributed to increased myeloid cells, particularly neutrophils and monocytes (**Figure 1D**). Mimicking *Bp* infection, our WCV immunization model induces leukocytosis in response to immunization. These data directed our attention to upstream events leading to WBC responses.

WCV Content Alters the Size and Composition of Peripheral Lymphoid Organs

To determine how each vaccination further effects the periphery, evaluations of lymphoid organs were performed. Two major lymphoid organs, which defend the body against invading pathogens include the thymus and the spleen. Thymus and spleen weights were recorded throughout our experimental schedule. Though only minor differences occur between vaccination groups in thymus weight and cell population proportions (data not shown), spleen sizes (**Figure S1A**), and weights (**Figure 2A**) increase progressively post-immunization with the WCV when compared to other groups. Cell counts following RBC lysis confirm increased spleen cellularity in WCV-immunized mice (data not shown). Spleens then decrease dramatically and rapidly in size and weight (2.45-fold) upon *Bp* infection (**Figure S1A** and **Figure 2A**), suggesting that cells migrate from the spleen to sites of infection. Similarly, naïve infected mice also exhibit decreases in spleen weight (1.94-fold) upon infection, but this occurrence is delayed when compared to WCV-immunized mice. Naïve mice exhibit a reduction in spleen weight 3 days post-infection, whereas WCV-immunized mice exhibit reduced spleen weight at 1 day post-infection. By day 3 post-infection spleen sizes are beginning to increase again in WCV-immunized mice. Flow cytometric analysis of splenocytes revealed that CD11b$^+$GR-1$^+$ myeloid cell proportions (**Figure S1B** and **Figure 2B**) are significantly increased in WCV-immunized mice, suggesting that they contribute to increased spleen size. CD11b$^+$GR-1$^+$ cells comprise a heterogeneous population of myeloid cells including myeloid progenitors, immature macrophages, immature granulocytes, and immature dendritic cells (34).

WCV-immunized mice display proportional decreases in splenic CD3e$^+$ T cells (post-immunization day 3, post-boost day 3, and post-infection day 3 and B220$^+$ B cells (post-boost days 3 and 12) (**Figures 2C,D**). To determine if proportional decreases were due only to reflect the increased myeloid cells in the spleen, total B and T cells were assessed in the spleen at days 1 and 3 post-immunization and post-infection (**Figures S1C,D**). Total B cells do not differ between groups post-immunization. T cell proportional decreases in WCV-immunized mice, however,

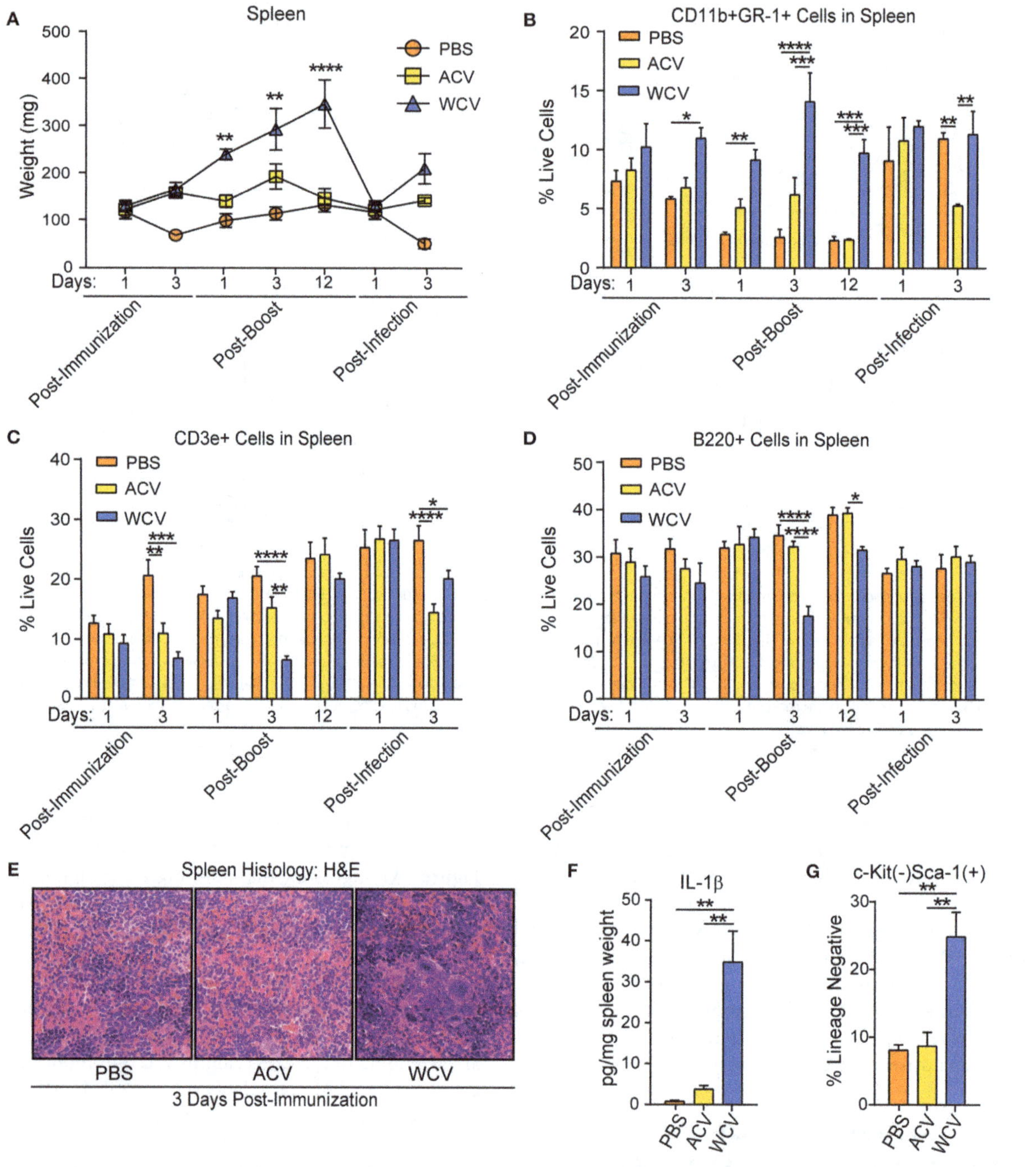

FIGURE 2 | WCV content induces alterations in the size and composition of peripheral lymphoid organs suggesting extramedullary hematopoiesis may occur. **(A)** Spleen weights from CD-1 mice ($n = 4$/group for each time point) immunized with phosphate buffered saline (PBS), *Bp* acellular vaccine (ACV), or *Bp* whole cell vaccine (WCV) were recorded at the indicated time points across the immunization and infection schedule. **(B)** CD11b$^+$Gr-1$^+$ cell proportions in the spleen ($n = 4$/group for each time point) were measured by flow cytometric analysis. **(C)** CD3e$^+$ cell proportions in the spleen ($n = 4$/group for each time point) were measured by flow cytometric analysis. **(D)** B220$^+$ cell proportions in the spleen ($n = 4$/group for each time point) were measured by flow cytometric analysis. **(E)** Representative images were taken of H&E-stained spleen ($n = 4$/group) at 400X magnification. **(F)** IL-1β in spleen homogenate ($n = 4$/group) was measured by quantitative sandwich immunoassays. G. Proportions of lineage$^-$c-kit$^-$Sca-1$^+$ cells in the spleen ($n = 4$/group for each time point) were measured using flow cytometric analysis. $^*p < 0.05$; $^{**}p < 0.01$; $^{***}p < 0.001$; $^{****}p < 0.0001$; 2-way ANOVAs with Tukey's multiple comparisons. Error bars are mean ± SEM values.

are due in part to a decrease in total T cells at day 3 post-immunization. Upon subsequent infection (day 3), however, CD3e$^+$ T cells are present in higher proportions and total numbers in the spleen in PBS and WCV-immunized mice when compared to ACV-immunized mice (**Figure S1C** and **Figure 2C**). Interestingly, as myeloid cell proportions become similar to PBS and ACV-immunized mice following infection, both T and B cells are increased in total number in the spleen. To further elucidate to impact of immunization formulation on cell population dynamics and cellularity in the spleen, H&E staining of spleen cross sections (day 3 post-vaccination) were performed. This examination of histology confirms hypercellularity and increases in myeloid cells, including megakaryocytes, occurs in WCV-immunized mice when compared to other groups (**Figure 2E**).

Parallel to increases in myeloid cell proportions in the spleens of WCV-immunized mice, on post-immunization day 3, we observed a significant increase in splenic IL-1β production (**Figure 2F**). IL-1β, which is produced by myeloid cells, enhances lymphocyte processes such as antigen-primed CD4 and CD8 T-cell expansion, differentiation, and migration to the periphery as well as memory (35, 36). Additionally, on post-immunization day 3, when compared to PBS and ACV groups, WCV-immunized mice exhibit larger proportions of splenic Lineage$^-$Sca-1$^+$c-Kit$^-$ cells (**Figure 2G**), which have been described as lymphoid progenitor cells that expand in the spleen upon infection, preferentially maturing into B cells (37, 38). Taken together, these data suggest that extramedullary hematopoiesis, which can occur due to mobilization of bone marrow HSPCs to the spleen (39, 40), is expanded in WCV immunizations. Evidence gathered from kinetics of immature cell population changes in the spleen suggest that bone marrow HSPC compartment composition may play a role in splenic immune response to vaccination.

WCV Immunization Induces MPP Expansion in the Bone Marrow

All groups evaluated have a similar level of cellularity in the bone marrow following infection as evidenced by H&E staining of lengthwise cross-sections of tibia (**Figure 3A**) and total cell counts (data not shown). Flow cytometric analysis of bone marrow HSPCs demonstrates that Lineage-Sca-1$^+$c-Kit$^+$ (LSK) cell proportions increase in WCV-immunized mice when compared to PBS and ACV-immunized mice (**Figures 3B,C**). Interestingly, naïve mice elicit robust delayed LSK expansion upon *Bp* challenge (**Figure 3B**). Further analysis of LSK cells in WCV and naïve challenge indicate that the expanded LSK are CD48$^+$CD150$^-$ multipotent progenitor cells (MPPs) (**Figure 3D**). To gain insight into how proportions of these progenitors change among groups when compared to proportions of other populations, LT-HSC, ST-HSC, MPP, common lymphoid progenitor (CLP), common myeloid progenitor (CMP), granulocyte monocyte progenitor (GMP), and megakaryocyte erythrocyte progenitor (MEP) bone marrow populations were analyzed to be presented as parts of the whole HSPC compartment (**Figure 3E**). Major differences in HSPC proportions occur across vaccine groups. WCV-immunized mice exhibit large proportions of MPPs upon initial vaccination (day 1) and boost (day 1) that become reduced with time after each incidence (day 3 post immunization and boost), while ACV-immunized mice exhibit MPP proportions only slightly larger than those of PBS control (day 1 post-immunization, day 1 post-boost). It is evident that WCV-immunized mice post-vaccination (day 1) highly resemble naïve infection (PBS) post-challenge (day 3).

WCV Immunization Primes Bone Marrow HSPCs for Rapid Maturation of Developing B Cells Upon Subsequent Infection

In WCV-immunized mice, Lineage$^-$Sca-1$^-$c-kit$^+$ (LK) cell proportions are decreased upon boost and infection when compared to other groups (**Figure 4A**). Further analysis into the cell populations that comprise LK cells revealed a proportional decrease within WCV-immunized mice in MEP populations post-immunization (day 3) and post-infection (day 1) (**Figures 4C,D**). Regarding lymphoid progenitors, an increase in CLP proportions upon infection is observed in WCV-immunized mice (**Figure 4C**). Aside from B cells, no mature populations evaluated differed across groups (data not shown). B220$^+$ cell proportions, however, were reduced significantly in WCV mice post-immunization (day 3) and post-boost (day 3) (**Figure 4C**). Interestingly, post-infection (day 3), B220$^+$ cells in WCV-immunized mice showed signs of robust maturation processes (**Figure 4E**). Our data indicate that HSPC expansion in response to immunization and infection is a dynamic process, which prompted us to investigate the transcriptomic profiles of HSPCs to better understand the mechanisms and systems driving observed responses.

RNAseq Analysis of Developing VDJ Recombination in HSPCs

To characterize gene expression profiles of HPSCs in relation to immunization and challenge, HSPCs were isolated from the bone marrow of mice upon immunization and infection. Isolated RNA was converted into libraries for Illumina platform sequencing. We obtained expression data for ~60% of all encoded murine genes across all experimental groups (**Table S3**) indicating robust transcriptomic analysis. Since differential expansion of bone marrow B cell populations occurs in response to immunization (**Figure 4**), we hypothesized that B cell population dynamics coincide with differential VDJ recombination developing within HSPCs. VDJ recombination and somatic hypermutation during B cell development and affinity maturation are responsible for diversity of antigen-recognizing B cell receptors (BCRs). Highly variable complementarity determining region 3, which plays a critical role in antigen specificity and binding affinity, is located at the VDJ junction BCR heavy chains (41). Mapped reads were analyzed with MiTCRx and VJRtools to identify immunoglobulin sequences, building libraries of clonal types. **Figure 5A** shows resulting B cell repertoires for all immunization and infections conditions. Spectral plots show that both ACV and WCV immunization influence clonal populations compared to naïve (PBS) mice. Post-immunization (day 3), these clone repertoires return to a state more similar to naïve mice. Upon infection, the clone repertoires diversify and it becomes difficult to distinguish naïve infected or immunized groups. Investigation of per clone diversity revealed that only the WCV group exhibits enhanced amounts of any one clone. The IGKV15-103/IGKJ4

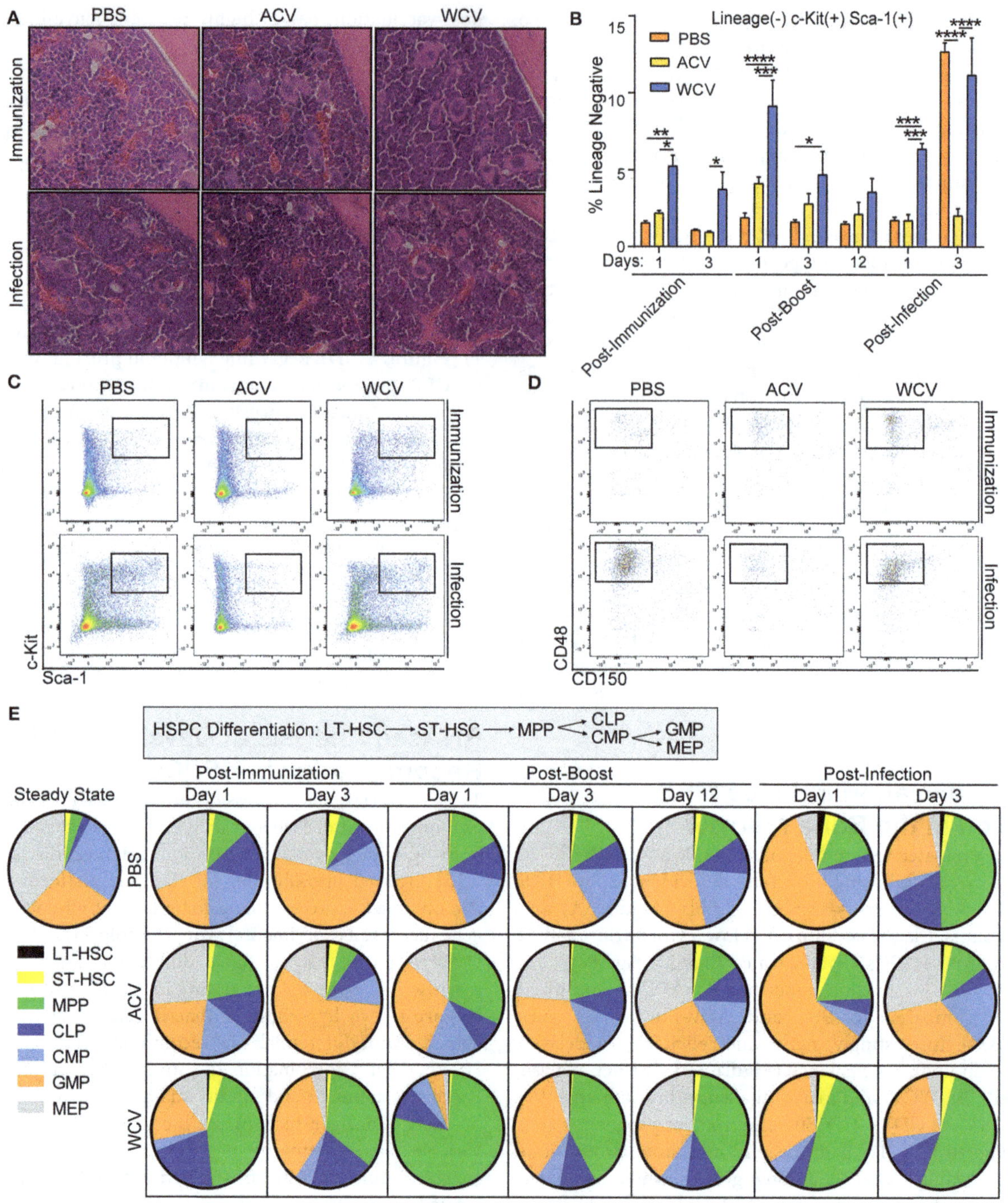

FIGURE 3 | WCV immunization induces MPP expansion in the bone marrow. **(A)** Representative images of cross sections of tibia from CD-1 mice ($n = 4$/group for each time point) immunized with phosphate buffered saline (PBS), *Bp* acellular vaccine (ACV), or *Bp* whole cell vaccine (WCV) and infected with 10^7 CFU *Bp* were taken at 400X magnification. **(B)** Proportions of lineage$^-$Sca-1$^+$ckit$^+$ (LSK) cells were evaluated in the bone marrow ($n = 4$/group for each time point) using flow cytometric analysis. **(C)** Representative dot plots of the flow cytometric analysis from 3B are shown. **(D)** Representative dot plots from further gating on LSK proportions to show CD48 and CD150 biexponential plot. **(E)** Hematopoietic stem and progenitor cell proportions were analyzed by flow cytometry and are represented as parts of the whole. $^*p < 0.05$; $^{**}p < 0.01$; $^{***}p < 0.001$; $^{****}p < 0.0001$; 2-way ANOVAs with Tukey's multiple comparisons. Error bars are mean ± SEM values.

clone was enriched in HSPCs from WCV-immunized mice and WCV-immunized mice that were subsequently infected. We speculate that this clone may be responsible for anti-LOS which is produced in high quantities in WCV-immunized mice. Enlarged spectral plots with labeled clones can be found in **Figures S2–S4**.

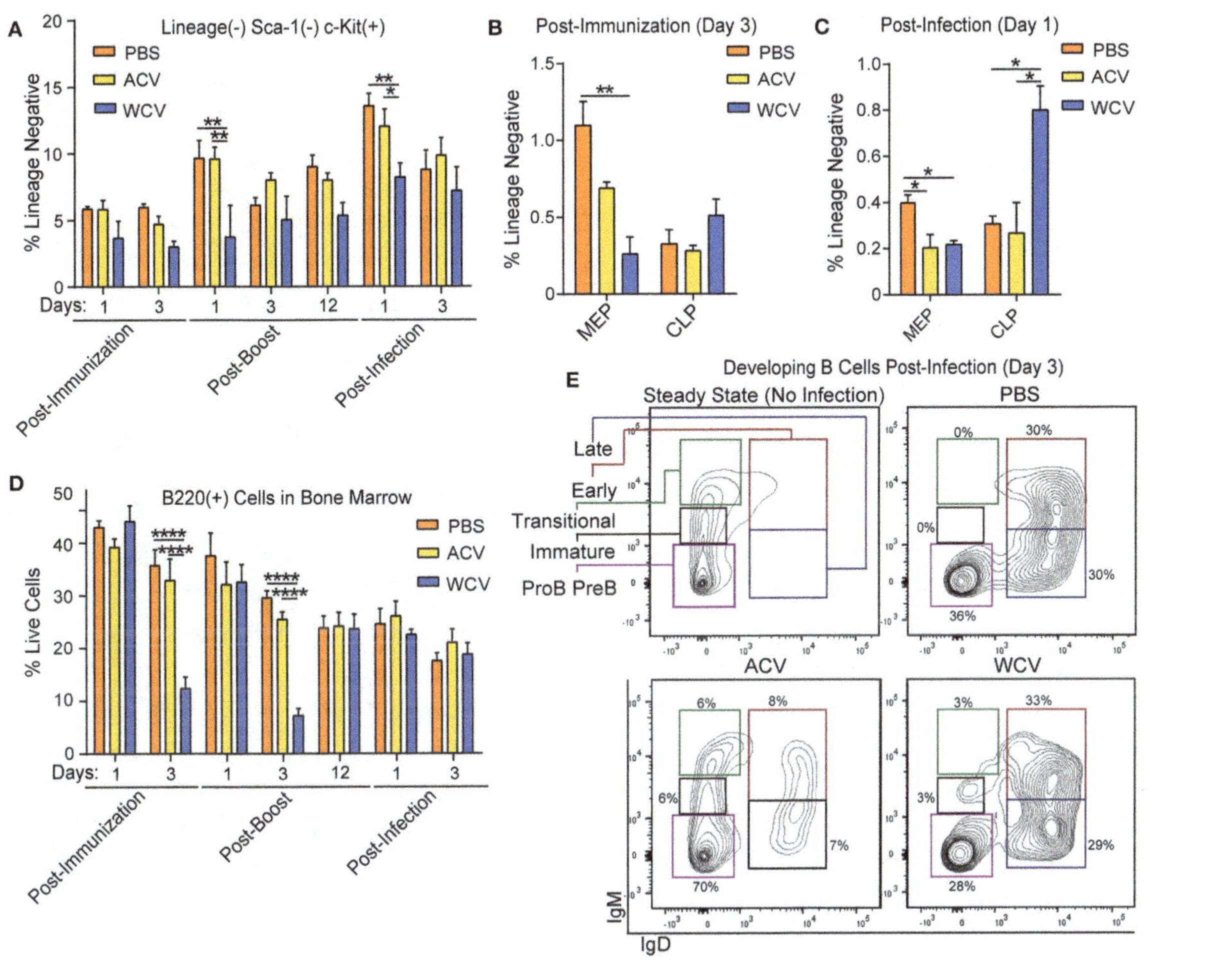

FIGURE 4 | WCV immunization prepares HSPCs for rapid maturation of developing B cells upon subsequent infection. **(A)** Proportions of lineage$^-$Sca-1$^+$ckit$^+$ (LK) cells were evaluated in the bone marrow of CD-1 mice ($n = 4$/group for each time point) immunized with phosphate buffered saline (PBS), *Bp* acellular vaccine (ACV), or *Bp* whole cell vaccine (WCV) and infected with 10^7 CFU *Bp* using flow cytometric analysis. **(B)** Proportions of megakaryocyte erythroid progenitors (MEPs) and common lymphoid progenitors (CLPs) were evaluated in mouse bone marrow ($n = 4$/group for each time point) post-immunization and **(C)** post-infection by flow cytometric analysis. **(D)** Proportions B220$^+$ cells were evaluated in mouse bone marrow ($n = 4$/group for each time point) using flow cytometric analysis. **(E)** Representative dot plots from further gating on cells from part D are shown. $^*p < 0.05$; $^{**}p < 0.01$; $^{****}p < 0.0001$; 2-way ANOVAs with Tukey's multiple comparisons. Error bars are mean ± SEM values.

Immunization and Infection Induces Unique Gene Expression Profiles of HSPCs

RNA sequencing (days 1 and 3 post-immunization, and days 1 and 3 post-infection) demonstrates that HSPCs respond to WCV-immunization by altering many immune response gene signatures. WCV-immunized mice exhibit >19-fold more differentially expressed genes when compared to ACV-immunized mice (**Figure S5A**). The most enriched of 18 significant gene signatures (fold change > 5) in this WCV HSPC gene set include protein folding, antigen processing and presentation, and response to interferons (IFNs) (**Figure S5B**). Genes differentially expressed only in HSPCs of ACV-immunized mice as well as genes differentially expressed in both immunization groups yielded no significantly enriched gene signatures.

Differential gene expression between vaccine groups upon challenge with *Bp* reveals that 35 genes overlap all groups, 88 genes exhibit unique overlap of naïve infection (PBS-immunized) and WCV, while 9 genes overlap ACV and naïve infected mice (**Figure S5C**). Enrichment of 123 genes differentially expressed in HSPCs from naïve infected mice that do not overlap with other groups resulted in signatures involving phagocytosis, complement, regulation of B cell activation, defense response to bacterium, and innate immune response (**Figure S5D**). Enrichment of genes uniquely overlapping naïve infection and WCV-immunized, *Bp*-infected mice produce similar defense response signatures (**Figure S5E**), but additionally include MHC class I and II processing and presentation and response to IFNs. No enriched pathways exist for differentially expressed genes that overlap naïve infection

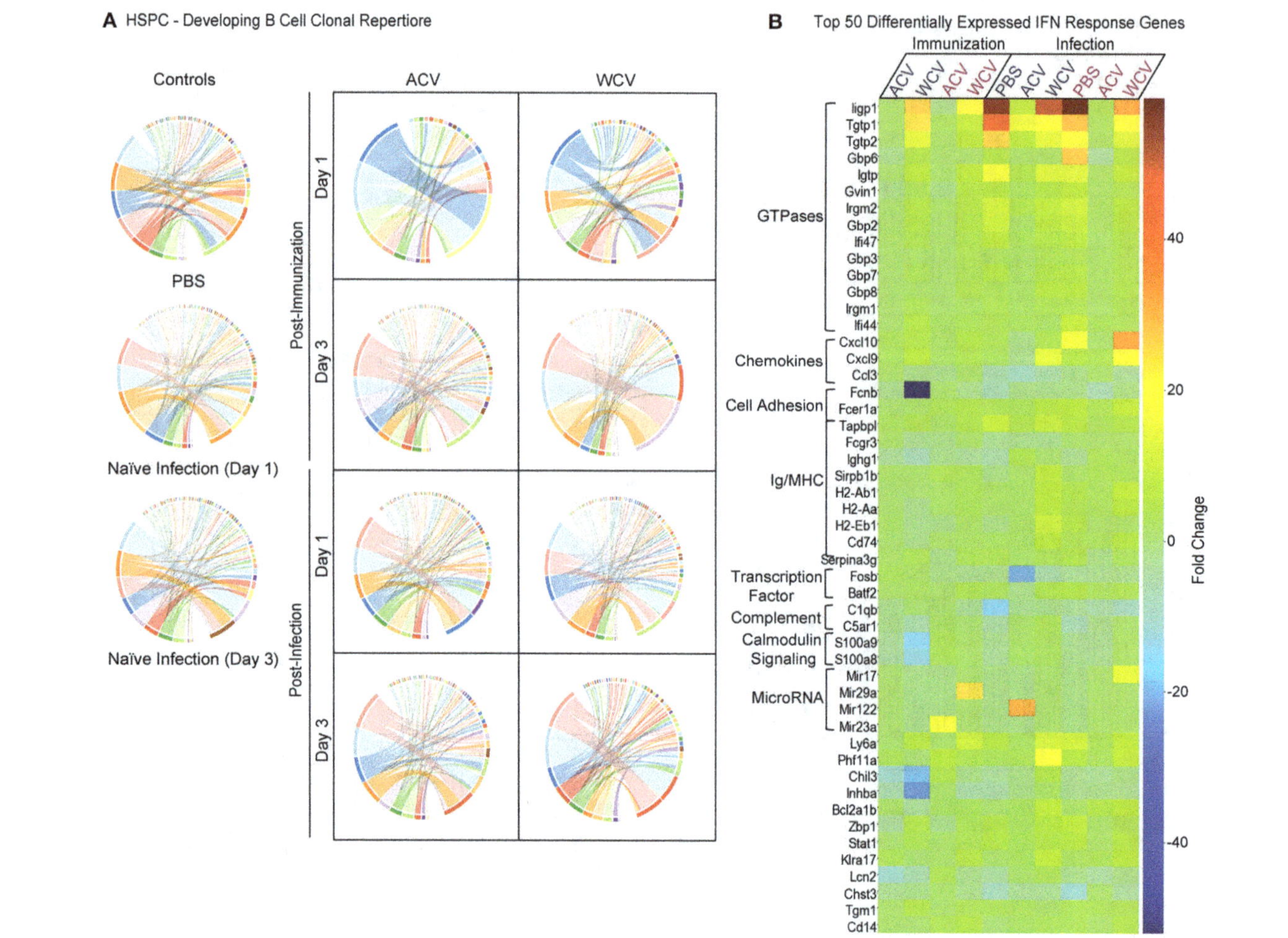

FIGURE 5 | Vaccine content drives the transcriptional landscape of HSPCs. **(A)** Pairwise overlap circos plots of HSPC B cell clonal repertoires (n = 6mice/group) were prepared using MiXCR software. Count, frequency and diversity panels correspond to the read count, frequency (both non-symmetric) and the total number of clonotypes that are shared between samples. Pairwise overlaps are stacked, i.e., segment arc length is not equal to sample size. **(B)** A heatmap was prepared to represent the top 50 differentially expressed genes downstream of IFNα, β, and/or γ across all immunization and infection groups. Day 1 for immunization and infection is shown below the dark blue text, while day 3 is shown below the magenta text. Gene sets for the heatmap were prepared using IPA's Upstream Regulator analytic tool. RNA was pooled from 2 mice for each sample n.

and ACV-immunized, *Bp*-infected mice. Additionally no enriched pathways exist for gene sets unique to WCV or ACV. Analysis of 35 genes overlapping all infection groups presents 8 significant gene signatures that resemble those observed in WCV immunization only (**Figure S5F**). Direct comparisons of initial immunization to naïve infection reveal that gene signature responses in HSPCs upon naïve infection resemble those of WCV-immunized, non-challenged mice as well. These include IFN response, MHC class I and II molecule production, chaperone folding, and immunoproteasome formation (data not shown), suggesting increased antigen processing and presentation.

Further highlighting mechanisms driving these immune responses, powerful algorithms and advanced analysis capabilities available through IPA allowed for the identification of transcriptional patterns that indicate a significant role for IFN stimulated gene (ISG) expression in HSPCs from WCV-immunized mice when compared to ACV-immunized mice. Z-scores, used to infer the activation state of predicted upstream transcriptional regulators, were increased in HSPCs from WCV-immunized mice for upstream IFNα, IFNβ, and IFNγ signaling when compared to ACV-immunized HSPCs. Similar to immunization, naïve infection and challenged WCV-immunized mice exhibited increased activation of these pathways compared to ACV-immunized mice. A heatmap displaying the top 50 differentially expressed IFN (α, β, and γ) stimulated genes is shown in **Figure 5B**.

Our proposed model for vaccine content influence on HSPCs through IFN signaling pathways is described in **Figure 6**. Briefly, we have propose that following vaccination with ACV, similar to PBS—immunized mice, cytokines in the PB impact the bone

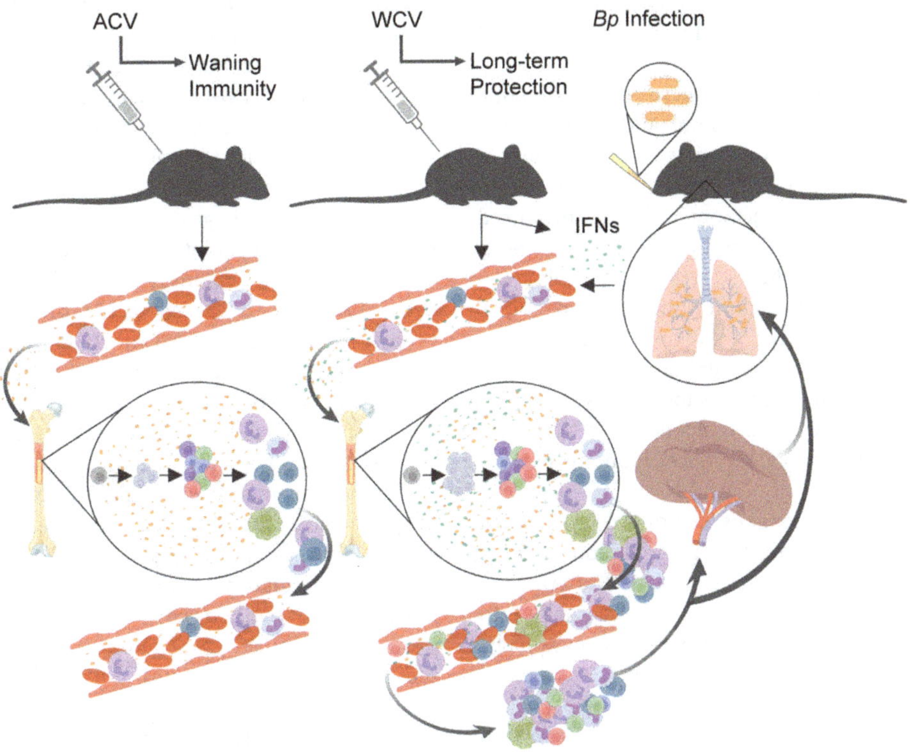

FIGURE 6 | Proposed model for vaccination and infection effects on HSPCs and downstream immune response. Following vaccination with ACV, similar to PBS (negative control) immunized mice, cytokines in the peripheral blood impact the bone marrow microenvironment to produce immune cells. Following vaccination with WCV, IFNs are produced and circulate in the blood, impacting the bone marrow microenvironment, thereby directing an expansion of HSPCs. In addition to HPSC proportional expansion, mature B cells decrease proportionally within in the bone marrow, while all other immune cells analyzed (T cells, macrophages, and granulocytes) do not significantly change. Given that bone marrow cellularity remains similar to PBS and ACV immunization groups, we hypothesize that upon production, select progenitors and differentiated cells move out of the marrow and into the peripheral blood where they migrate to the spleen. Upon subsequent infection, HSPCs undergo expansion again and cells in the peripheral blood and spleen migrate to sites of infection to clear *Bp*. During naïve infection, a similar process occurs. This model was created using BioRender.

marrow microenvironment to produce immune cells required for homeostasis. Following vaccination with WCV, however, we speculate that additional IFNs are produced and circulate in the blood, impacting the bone marrow microenvironment, thereby directing an expansion of HSPCs. In addition to HPSC proportional expansion, we observe that mature B cells decrease proportionally within in the bone marrow, while all other immune cells analyzed (T cells, macrophages, and granulocytes) do not significantly change. Given that bone marrow cellularity remains similar to PBS and ACV immunization groups, we hypothesize that upon production, select progenitors and differentiated cells move out of the marrow and into the PB where a subset of these cells migrate to the spleen. Upon subsequent infection, HSPCs undergo expansion again and cells in the PB and spleen migrate to sites of infection to clear *Bp*. During naïve infection, a similar process occurs. We propose that immune cell activation in the periphery results in IFN signaling that reaches HSPCs of the bone marrow, inducing ISG expression and influencing cell cycle, survival, autophagy, and innate immune signaling pathways among others.

DISCUSSION

Investigating the impact of altered HSPC populations following immunization is imperative to advancing knowledge that will inform the design of future vaccines. We have described how content of pertussis vaccines influences HSPC population kinetics and associated peripheral immune responses. While WCVs or ACVs allow mice to clear short-term infection, longevity of immune protection may reside in how HSPCs are influenced following immunization. This includes the propensity of these cells to undergo expansion and priming for future infection responses. Our data indicate that LSK cell populations are increased in the bone marrow following WCV immunization. This phenomenon mimics how LSK cells are impacted in response to naïve infection. HSPCs have the capacity to differentiate into all types of immune cells, and their expansion following immunization with an efficacious vaccine or naïve infection correlates with immune cell population changes in the PB and organs. Further investigation of the HSPC compartment revealed that LSK expansion is largely due to an increase in MPPs. Since MPPs support the generation of all types of mature blood cells, it is not surprising to find that cell populations of both myeloid and lymphoid lineages are altered in the bone marrow, blood, or spleen.

Lymphoid progenitor cell population increases in the bone marrow and spleen following WCV immunization suggest that greater proportions of B and T cells are undergoing early stages of development following WCV immunization when compared to PBS and ACV immunization. Furthermore, cytokines produced by the multitude of myeloid cells in the blood and spleen could impact the way in which these developing lymphocytes differentiate. Future studies will include kinetics of B and T cell development for several weeks following immunization. Regarding immature myeloid cell population increases in the spleen following immunization, these cells most likely produced by extramedullary hematopoiesis, seem to act as a reservoir, poised to move out to the respiratory tract upon subsequent infection.

In revealing molecular mechanisms responsible for HSPC alterations and downstream immune cell population changes observed, transcriptional signatures from HSPCs isolated from WCV immunization and naïve infection fall into interesting immune-related gene families. Involved in autophagy, immunoproteasome formation, molecular chaperone processes, and class I and class II MHC molecule components, these gene families suggest that HSPCs may be primed for antigen presentation. Taken together with the dynamics of B cell development and developing VDJ recombination within HSPCs, these data support a role for HSPC involvement in influencing long-term immune protection via impact on MHC class II antigen presenting B cell development.

The most striking gene expression change observed in infection and WCV immunization, but not acellular vaccination, involves IFN-inducible genes (**Figure 5B**). Type 1 and 2 IFNs are known for inducing HSC proliferation, which potentially explains bone marrow HSPC expansion (42–44). Essers et al. showed that in response to IFNα treatment, HSPCs exhibit increased Sca-1 and phosphorylation of STAT1 and PKB/Akt. Furthermore, they and others established that STAT1 and Sca-1 mediate IFNα-induced HSC proliferation. We speculate that signaling cascades downstream of IFNs, such as mTOR, PI3K, MAPK, and NFκB pathways, which are all affected in our datasets, influence HSPC frequency observed in our models. Beyond impacting cell survival, proliferation, and cell cycle, many IFN-regulated genes implicated in our data are involved in immune response. The immunity-related guanosine triphosphatase (IRG) family, for example, has well-documented roles in clearing infection (45, 46). Among other mechanisms, IRGs interfere with infectious pathogens by disrupting phagocytic vacuoles during infection (45, 46).

Of the IRG family, 47-kDa GTPases in mice include: Irgm1, Irgm2, Ifi47, Tgtp1, Tgtp2, Igtp1, and Igtp2, all of which are upregulated in naïve *Bp* infection and WCV immunization against *Bp*. Genetic deletion of 47-kDa GTPases severely impairs defense against many primarily intracellular pathogens: *Toxoplasma gondii, Trypanosoma cruzi, Leishmania major, Listeria monocytogenes, Mycobacterium* spp., including *Mycobacterium tuberculosis and Mycobacterium avium, Salmonella typhimurium,* and murine cytomegalovirus (46). Host immune clearance of intracellular pathogens is relies upon IFN-mediated cellular immunity(47). Though *Bp* is primarily considered an extracellular pathogen, it has also been shown to survive inside respiratory epithelial cells, human polymorphonuclear leukocytes, and human monocytes/macrophages (48–50). Moreover, Connelly et al. provided evidence that INFγ-induced GTPases play a role in PT-associated responses in the lungs during *Bp* infection (51). Though IFNγ is responsible for many immune responses (47), it has recently gained much attention in how it mediates GTPases to eliminate pathogens that survive inside of a cell. Mitchell et al. has reviewed the processes of immune clearance of intracellular microorganisms that particularly involve IFNγ GTPases (52). The two systems discussed (1) xenophagy and (2) interferon-regulated GTPase promotion of the rupture of pathogen-containing vacuoles and microbial degradation are thought to participate in cross-talk that balances the killing of pathogens within cells and inflammatory responses. Beyond this, methods by which GTPases are involved in protection against pathogens include: (1) trafficking from the endoplasmic reticulum and Golgi to phagosomes, (2) regulating survival of infected host cells, and (3) regulating pools of effector lymphocytes (45, 46). It has been proposed that when coupled with signals from Toll-like receptors, such as those recognizing LOS, the p47 GTPase family provides an enhanced sensory system for recognizing infectious agents as well (53).

Regarding HSPCs, genetic deletion of *Irgm1*, for which *IRGM* is a human ortholog, results in pancytopenia due to inadequate cell expansion when challenged with mycobacterium or *T. cruzi* (54, 55). Given that we observe high expression of IRG genes during HSPC expansion and robust enrichment of IFN- and STAT1-related genes in HSPCs of both naïve infection and WCV immunization, it can be argued that IFN influence on primitive hematopoietic cells is important in expanding bone marrow HSPCs for the promotion of leukocytosis. Feng et al. described an Irgm1 feedback mechanism in Th1 response that promotes antimicrobial function while limiting detrimental effects of IFNγ on effector T lymphocyte survival (56). Perhaps similarly, this and other GTPases upregulated in HSPCs following infection and WCV immunization are involved in peripheral expansion of immune effector cell populations during downstream Th1 responses to intracellular pathogens. Experts in the pertussis field often contribute WCV efficacy to preferential production of Th1 responses to *Bp* (57–60). We speculate that this is partly maintained by upregulated IRGs within HSPCs.

Relevant to our data, IRGs are also implicated in B cell maturation. IFNγ induces pre-B cells to exhibit surface immunoglobulin (61). Simultaneously, IFN-inducible GTPases increase in expression (61). We postulate that IFN signaling during efficacious vaccination mimics naïve infection, leading to various processes that impact HSPCs, including increased IFN-induced GTPase expression, increased priming of cells for antigen presentation, and skewed MPP and B cell maturation patterns. Similar to our studies, Kaufmann et al. found IFN signaling to be essential to LSK expansion following BCG vaccination. In their studies, it was needed to educate macrophages to provide long-term innate immune protection. Our work, together with additional studies in trained immunity (7–9), demonstrates that understanding the mechanisms by which IFN signaling may prime HSPCs to react to specific pathogens once cells have matured is underappreciated, offering a novel area of investigation regarding long-term immunity.

We expect this work highlighting the importance of vaccine content in influencing HSPC characteristics to provide new insights for the development of future pertussis vaccines as well as provide broad applicability to vaccine efficacy. Acellular pertussis vaccines protect mice against challenge in short term immunization/boost/challenge studies. Similarly, in humans, DTaP performed well in short-term clinical trials in Europe (62). However, with time it is clearly appreciated that DTaP/Tdap immunity wanes. We appreciate that there are substantial differences between murine models and human hosts. In the present study, however, we aimed to characterize HSPC expansion on the transcriptomic level. By identifying biomarkers that can be measured as a function of HSPC expansion, we may be able to develop protocols to better monitor early events in immunization for the purpose of developing vaccine formulations that induce longer term memory.

We hypothesize that the use of adjuvants that induce IFN responses and/or TLR4 signaling will enhance ACVs by influencing HSPC priming and expansion. Our future work with the use of rationally designed, functionally diverse lipid A adjuvants (63) will provide answers as to how induction of HSPC expansion in ACV-immunized mice may contribute to downstream immune responses. Once we have elucidated how these adjuvants may enhance vaccine-induced immunity in mice and other animal models, we expect that this knowledge will lead to improved ACV vaccines for use in humans. Furthermore, in future studies we expect to determine how pertussis immunization and subsequent infection impacts overall HSPC health and longevity.

AUTHOR CONTRIBUTIONS

MV, DB, KD, TW, ES, SB, CE, ME, WW, MB, and FD performed experiments. MV, EN, and FD analyzed results and composed figures. MV and FD designed experiments and composed the manuscript. All authors participated in the review of the manuscript.

ACKNOWLEDGMENTS

We thank Kathleen Brundage for assistance with cell sorting (West Virginia University Flow Cytometry Core). Instruments utilized in the WVU flow cytometry core are supported by the National Institutes of Health equipment grant number S10OD016165 and U51 GM104942 (WV CTSI) as well as the Institutional Development Awards (IDeA) from the National Institute of General Medical Sciences of the National Institutes of Health under grant numbers P30GM103488 (Cancer CoBRE) and P20GM103434 (INBRE). Additionally, we thank Ryan Percifield and Donald Primerano for assistance with library preparation and RNA sequencing (West Virginia University Genomics Core and Marshall University Genomics Core, respectively). We thank Deborah McLaughlin for assistance with preparation of pathology slides (West Virginia University Pathology Core).

SUPPLEMENTARY MATERIAL

Figure S1 | WCV induces alterations in spleen size and B and T cell population composition. **(A)**. Spleen sizes from CD-1 mice (n = 4/group for each time point) immunized with phosphate buffered saline (PBS), Bp acellular vaccine (ACV), or Bp whole cell vaccine (WCV) are shown in representative images for the indicated time points across the immunization and infection schedule. **(B)**. Representative dot plots from flow cytometric analysis described in **Figure 2B**. **(C)**. Total CD3e+ cells in the spleen (n = 4/group for each time point) were calculated by multiplying the percentage of CD3e+ live cells (**Figure 2C**) in the spleen by total number of live cells in the spleen. **(D)** Total B220+ cells in the spleen (n = 4/group for each time point) were calculated by multiplying the percentage of B220+ live cells in the spleen (**Figure 2D**) by total number of live cells in the spleen. $*p<0.05$; $**p<0.01$; $***p<0.001$; $****p<0.0001$; 2-way ANOVAs with Tukey's multiple comparisons. Error bars are mean ± SEM values.

Figure S2 | Enlargement of controls for the transcriptional landscape of HSPCs B cell clonal repertoires. Pairwise overlap circos plots of HSPC B cell clonal repertoires (n = 6mice/group) prepared using MiXCR software and shown in **Figure 5A** were enlarged for viewing individual clones. Count, frequency and diversity panels correspond to the read count, frequency (both non-symmetric) and the total number of clonotypes that are shared between samples. Pairwise overlaps are stacked, i.e., segment arc length is not equal to sample size.

Figure S3 | Enlargement of the post-immunization transcriptional landscape of HSPCs B cell clonal repertoires. Pairwise overlap circos plots of HSPC B cell clonal repertoires (n=6mice/group) prepared using MiXCR software and shown in **Figure 5A** were enlarged for viewing individual clones. Count, frequency and diversity panels correspond to the read count, frequency (both non-symmetric) and the total number of clonotypes that are shared between samples. Pairwise overlaps are stacked, i.e., segment arc length is not equal to sample size.

Figure S4 | Enlargement of the post-infection transcriptional landscape of HSPCs B cell clonal repertoires. Pairwise overlap circos plots of HSPC B cell clonal repertoires (n = 6mice/group) prepared using MiXCR software and shown in **Figure 5A** were enlarged for viewing individual clones. Count, frequency and diversity panels correspond to the read count, frequency (both non-symmetric) and the total number of clonotypes that are shared between samples. Pairwise overlaps are stacked, i.e., segment arc length is not equal to sample size.

Figure S5 | Vaccine content determines gene set enrichment of HSPCs. RNAseq was performed on HSPCs isolated from CD-1 mice on days 1 and 3 post immunization with PBS, ACV, or WCV and on days 1 and 3 post subsequent infection with Bp. **(A)** Venn diagram was prepared for significant differentially expressed genes in HSPCs of ACV- and WCV-immunized mice when compared to PBS control mice. **(B)** Gene signatures enriched (fold change>5) in the WCV-immunized HSPC gene set are shown. **(C)** A Venn diagram was prepared for significant differential gene expression in HSPCs from PBS-, ACV-, and WCV-immunized and subsequently Bp challenged mice when compared to PBS control mice. **(D)**. Gene signatures enriched (fold change>5) in the PBS vaccinated, Bp challenged HSPCs gene set are shown. **(E)** HSPC gene signatures enriched (fold change>5) that overlap PBS vaccinated, Bp challenged and WCV-immunized, Bp challenged mice are shown. **(F)**. HSPC gene signatures enriched (fold change > 5) that overlap all Bp challenged mice are shown. Venn diagrams and gene set enrichment were established using Venny 2.1 and PANTHER, respectively. Significant data was determined by FDR (<0.05).

Table S1 | Compositions of vaccines of this study.

Table S2 | Flow cytometry antibodies used in this study.

Table S3 | Summary of RNAseq performed in this study.

REFERENCES

1. Geissmann F, Manz MG, Jung S, Sieweke MH, Merad M, Ley K. Development of monocytes, macrophages, and dendritic cells. *Science* (2010) 327:656–61. doi: 10.1126/science.1178331
2. Takizawa H, Regoes RR, Boddupalli CS, Bonhoeffer S, Manz MG. Dynamic variation in cycling of hematopoietic stem cells in steady state and inflammation. *J Exp Med.* (2011) 208:273–84. doi: 10.1084/jem.20101643
3. Morrison SJ, Scadden DT. The bone marrow niche for haematopoietic stem cells. *Nature* (2014) 505:327–34. doi: 10.1038/nature12984
4. King KY, Goodell MA. Inflammatory modulation of HSCs: viewing the HSC as a foundation for the immune response. *Nat Rev Immunol.* (2011) 11:685–92. doi: 10.1038/nri3062
5. Baldridge MT, King KY, Goodell MA. Inflammatory signals regulate hematopoietic stem cells. *Trends Immunol.* (2011) 32:57–65. doi: 10.1016/j.it.2010.12.003
6. Glatman Zaretsky A, Engiles JB, Hunter CA. Infection-induced changes in hematopoiesis. *J Immunol.* (2014) 192:27–33. doi: 10.4049/jimmunol.1302061
7. Netea MG, Quintin J, van der Meer JW. Trained immunity: a memory for innate host defense. Cell Host Microbe. (2011) 9:355–61. doi: 10.1016/j.chom.2011.04.006
8. Netea MG, Joosten LA, Latz E, Mills KH, Natoli G, Stunnenberg HG, et al. Trained immunity: a program of innate immune memory in health and disease. *Science* (2016) 352:aaf1098. doi: 10.1126/science.aaf1098
9. Kaufmann E, Sanz J, Dunn JL, Khan N, Mendonca LE, Pacis A, et al. BCG educates hematopoietic stem cells to generate protective innate immunity against tuberculosis. *Cell* (2018) 172:176–90 e19. doi: 10.1016/j.cell.2017.12.031
10. Megias J, Yanez A, Moriano S, O'Connor JE, Gozalbo D, Gil ML. Direct Toll-like receptor-mediated stimulation of hematopoietic stem and progenitor cells occurs *in vivo* and promotes differentiation toward macrophages. *Stem Cells* (2012) 30:1486–95. doi: 10.1002/stem.1110
11. Yanez A, Flores A, Murciano C, O'Connor JE, Gozalbo D, Gil ML. Signalling through TLR2/MyD88 induces differentiation of murine bone marrow stem and progenitor cells to functional phagocytes in response to *Candida albicans*. *Cell Microbiol.* (2010) 12:114–28. doi: 10.1111/j.1462-5822.2009.01382.x
12. Yanez A, Murciano C, O'Connor JE, Gozalbo D, Gil ML. *Candida albicans* triggers proliferation and differentiation of hematopoietic stem and progenitor cells by a MyD88-dependent signaling. *Microbes Infect.* (2009) 11:531–5. doi: 10.1016/j.micinf.2009.01.011
13. Singh P, Yao Y, Weliver A, Broxmeyer HE, Hong SC, Chang CH. Vaccinia virus infection modulates the hematopoietic cell compartments in the bone marrow. *Stem Cells* (2008) 26:1009–16. doi: 10.1634/stemcells.2007-0461
14. Quinton LJ, Nelson S, Boe DM, Zhang P, Zhong Q, Kolls JK, et al. The granulocyte colony-stimulating factor response after intrapulmonary and systemic bacterial challenges. *J Infect Dis.* (2002) 185:1476–82. doi: 10.1086/340504
15. Zhang P, Nelson S, Bagby GJ, Siggins R II, Shellito JE, Welsh DA. The lineage-c-Kit+Sca-1+ cell response to *Escherichia coli* bacteremia in Balb/c mice. *Stem Cells* (2008) 26:1778–86. doi: 10.1634/stemcells.2007-1027
16. Kim JM, Oh YK, Kim YJ, Youn J, Ahn MJ. *Escherichia coli* up-regulates proinflammatory cytokine expression in granulocyte/macrophage lineages of CD34 stem cells via p50 homodimeric NF-kappaB. *Clin Exp Immunol.* (2004) 137:341–50. doi: 10.1111/j.1365-2249.2004.02542.x
17. Shahbazian LM, Quinton LJ, Bagby GJ, Nelson S, Wang G, Zhang P. *Escherichia coli* pneumonia enhances granulopoiesis and the mobilization of myeloid progenitor cells into the systemic circulation. *Crit Care Med.* (2004) 32:1740–6. doi: 10.1097/01.CCM.0000132900.84627.90
18. Klein NP, Bartlett J, Rowhani-Rahbar A, Fireman B, Baxter R. Waning protection after fifth dose of acellular pertussis vaccine in children. *N Eng J Med.* (2012) 367:1012–9. doi: 10.1056/NEJMoa1200850
19. Klein NP, Bartlett J, Fireman B, Aukes L, Buck PO, Krishnarajah G, et al. Waning protection following 5 doses of a 3-component diphtheria, tetanus, and acellular pertussis vaccine. *Vaccine* (2017) 35:3395–400. doi: 10.1016/j.vaccine.2017.05.008
20. Burdin N, Handy LK, Plotkin SA. What is wrong with pertussis vaccine immunity? the problem of waning effectiveness of pertussis vaccines. *Cold Spring Harb Perspect Biol.* (2017) 9:a029454. doi: 10.1101/cshperspect.a029454
21. Wendelboe AM, Van Rie A, Salmaso S, Englund JA. Duration of immunity against pertussis after natural infection or vaccination. *Pediatr Infect Dis J.* (2005) 24(Suppl. 5):S58–61. doi: 10.1097/01.inf.0000160914.59160.41
22. Ross PJ, Sutton CE, Higgins S, Allen AC, Walsh K, Misiak A, et al. Relative contribution of Th1 and Th17 cells in adaptive immunity to *Bordetella pertussis*: towards the rational design of an improved acellular pertussis vaccine. *PLoS Pathog.* (2013) 9:e1003264. doi: 10.1371/journal.ppat.1003264
23. Papayannopoulou T, Priestley GV, Bonig H, Nakamoto B. The role of G-protein signaling in hematopoietic stem/progenitor cell mobilization. *Blood* (2003) 101:4739–47. doi: 10.1182/blood-2002-09-2741
24. Cain DW, Snowden PB, Sempowski GD, Kelsoe G. Inflammation triggers emergency granulopoiesis through a density-dependent feedback mechanism. *PLoS ONE* (2011) 6:e19957. doi: 10.1371/journal.pone.0019957
25. Yanez A, Goodridge HS, Gozalbo D, Gil ML. TLRs control hematopoiesis during infection. *Eur J Immunol.* (2013) 43:2526–33. doi: 10.1002/eji.201343833
26. Brickman TJ, Armstrong SK. The ornithine decarboxylase gene odc is required for alcaligin siderophore biosynthesis in *Bordetella* spp.: putrescine is a precursor of alcaligin. *J Bacteriol.* (1996) 178:54–60.
27. Oliveros JC. *Venny. An Interactive Tool for Comparing Lists With Venn's Diagrams* (2007).
28. Bolotin DA, Poslavsky S, Mitrophanov I, Shugay M, Mamedov IZ, Putintseva EV, et al. MiXCR: software for comprehensive adaptive immunity profiling. *Nat Meth.* (2015) 12:380–1. doi: 10.1038/nmeth.3364
29. Shugay M, Bagaev DV, Turchaninova MA, Bolotin DA, Britanova OV, Putintseva EV, et al. VDJtools: unifying post-analysis of T cell receptor repertoires. *PLoS Comput Biol.* (2015) 11:e1004503. doi: 10.1371/journal.pcbi.1004503.
30. Carbonetti NH. Pertussis leukocytosis: mechanisms, clinical relevance and treatment. *Pathog Dis.* (2016) 74:ftw087. doi: 10.1093/femspd/ftw087
31. Morse SI, Morse JH. Isolation and properties of the leukocytosis- and lymphocytosis-promoting factor of *Bordetella pertussis*. *J Exp Med.* (1976) 143:1483–502.
32. Morse SI, Barron BA. Studies on the leukocytosis and lymphocytosis induced by *Bordetella pertussis*. 3. The distribution of transfused lymphocytes in pertussis-treated and normal mice. *J Exp Med.* (1970) 132:663–72.
33. Morse SI. Studies on the lymphocytosis induced in mice by *Bordetella pertussis*. *J Exp Med.* (1965) 121:49–68.

34. Gabrilovich DI, Nagaraj S. Myeloid-derived suppressor cells as regulators of the immune system. *Nat Rev Immunol.* (2009) 9:162–74. doi: 10.1038/nri 2506
35. Ben-Sasson SZ, Wang K, Cohen J, Paul WE. IL-1beta strikingly enhances antigen-driven CD4 and CD8 T-cell responses. *Cold Spring Harb Symp Quant Biol.* (2013) 78:117–24. doi: 10.1101/sqb.2013.78.0 21246
36. Ben-Sasson SZ, Hu-Li J, Quiel J, Cauchetaux S, Ratner M, Shapira I, et al. IL-1 acts directly on CD4 T cells to enhance their antigen-driven expansion and differentiation. *Proc Natl Acad Sci USA.* (2009) 106:7119–24. doi: 10.1073/pnas.0902745106
37. Ghosh D, Brown SL, Stumhofer JS. IL-17 promotes differentiation of splenic LSK- lymphoid progenitors into B cells following *Plasmodium yoelii* infection. *J Immunol.* (2017) 199:1783–95. doi: 10.4049/jimmunol.1601972
38. Ghosh D, Wikenheiser DJ, Kennedy B, McGovern KE, Stuart JD, Wilson EH, et al. An atypical splenic B cell progenitor population supports antibody production during plasmodium infection in mice. *J Immunol.* (2016) 197:1788–800. doi: 10.4049/jimmunol.1502199
39. Yamamoto K, Miwa Y, Abe-Suzuki S, Abe S, Kirimura S, Onishi I, et al. Extramedullary hematopoiesis: elucidating the function of the hematopoietic stem cell niche (Review). *Mol Med Rep.* (2016) 13:587–91. doi: 10.3892/mmr.2015.4621
40. Kim CH. Homeostatic and pathogenic extramedullary hematopoiesis. *J Blood Med.* (2010) 1:13–9. doi: 10.2147/JBM.S7224
41. Lee DW, Khavrutskii IV, Wallqvist A, Bavari S, Cooper CL, Chaudhury S. BRILIA: integrated tool for high-throughput annotation and lineage tree assembly of B-cell repertoires. *Front Immunol.* (2016) 7:681. doi: 10.3389/fimmu.2016.00681
42. Passegue E, Ernst P. IFN-alpha wakes up sleeping hematopoietic stem cells. *Nat Med.* (2009) 15:612–3. doi: 10.1038/nm0609-612
43. Baldridge MT, King KY, Boles NC, Weksberg DC, Goodell MA. Quiescent haematopoietic stem cells are activated by IFN-gamma in response to chronic infection. *Nature* (2010) 465:793–7. doi: 10.1038/nature09135
44. Essers MA, Offner S, Blanco-Bose WE, Waibler Z, Kalinke U, Duchosal MA, et al. IFNalpha activates dormant haematopoietic stem cells *in vivo*. *Nature* (2009) 458:904–8.
45. Kim BH, Shenoy AR, Kumar P, Bradfield CJ, MacMicking JD. IFN-inducible GTPases in host cell defense. *Cell Host Microbe.* (2012) 12:432–44. doi: 10.1016/j.chom.2012.09.00
46. Taylor GA, Feng CG, Sher A. p47 GTPases: regulators of immunity to intracellular pathogens. *Nat Rev Immunol.* (2004) 4:100–9. doi: 10.1038/nri1270
47. Schoenborn JR, Wilson CB. Regulation of interferon-gamma during innate and adaptive immune responses. *Adv Immunol.* (2007) 96:41–101. doi: 10.1016/S0065-2776(07)96002-2
48. Lamberti Y, Gorgojo J, Massillo C, Rodriguez ME. *Bordetella pertussis* entry into respiratory epithelial cells and intracellular survival. *Pathog Dis.* (2013) 69:194–204. doi: 10.1111/2049-632X.12072
49. Steed LL, Setareh M, Friedman RL. Intracellular survival of virulent *Bordetella pertussis* in human polymorphonuclear leukocytes. *J Leukoc Biol.* (1991) 50:321–30.
50. Friedman RL, Nordensson K, Wilson L, Akporiaye ET, Yocum DE. Uptake and intracellular survival of *Bordetella pertussis* in human macrophages. *Infect Immun.* (1992) 60:4578–85.
51. Connelly CE, Sun Y, Carbonetti NH. Pertussis toxin exacerbates and prolongs airway inflammatory responses during *Bordetella pertussis* infection. *Infect Immun.* (2012) 80:4317–32. doi: 10.1128/IAI.00808-12
52. Mitchell G, Isberg RR. Innate immunity to intracellular pathogens: balancing microbial elimination and inflammation. *Cell Host Microbe.* (2017) 22:166–75. doi: 10.1016/j.chom.2017.07.005
53. MacMicking JD. Immune control of phagosomal bacteria by p47 GTPases. *Curr Opin Microbiol.* (2005) 8:74–82. doi: 10.1016/j.mib.2004.12.012
54. Feng CG, Weksberg DC, Taylor GA, Sher A, Goodell MA. The p47 GTPase Lrg-47 (Irgm1) links host defense and hematopoietic stem cell proliferation. *Cell Stem Cell* (2008) 2:83–9. doi: 10.1016/j.stem.2007. 10.007
55. Santiago HC, Feng CG, Bafica A, Roffe E, Arantes RM, Cheever A, et al. Mice deficient in LRG-47 display enhanced susceptibility to *Trypanosoma cruzi* infection associated with defective hemopoiesis and intracellular control of parasite growth. *J Immunol.* (2005) 175:8165–72. doi: 10.4049/jimmunol.175.12.8165
56. Feng CG, Zheng L, Lenardo MJ, Sher A. Interferon-inducible immunity-related GTPase Irgm1 regulates IFN gamma-dependent host defense, lymphocyte survival and autophagy. *Autophagy* (2009) 5:232–4. doi: 10.4161/auto.5.2.7445
57. Ryan M, Murphy G, Ryan E, Nilsson L, Shackley F, Gothefors L, et al. Distinct T-cell subtypes induced with whole cell and acellular pertussis vaccines in children. *Immunology* (1998) 93:1–10.
58. Ausiello CM, Urbani F, la Sala A, Lande R, Cassone A. Vaccine- and antigen-dependent type 1 and type 2 cytokine induction after primary vaccination of infants with whole-cell or acellular pertussis vaccines. *Infect Immun.* (1997) 65:2168–74.
59. Redhead K, Watkins J, Barnard A, Mills KH. Effective immunization against *Bordetella pertussis* respiratory infection in mice is dependent on induction of cell-mediated immunity. *Infect Immun.* (1993) 61:3190–8.
60. Mills KH, Barnard A, Watkins J, Redhead K. Cell-mediated immunity to *Bordetella pertussis*: role of Th1 cells in bacterial clearance in a murine respiratory infection model. *Infect Immun.* (1993) 61:399–410.
61. Patrone L, Damore MA, Lee MB, Malone CS, Wall R. Genes expressed during the IFN gamma-induced maturation of pre-B cells. *Mol Immunol.* (2002) 38:597–606. doi: 10.1016/S0161-5890(01)00097-9
62. Plotkin SA, Orenstein WA, Offit PA. *Plotkin's Vaccines.* 7th ed. Philadelphia, PA: Elsevier (2018).
63. Gregg KA, Harberts E, Gardner FM, Pelletier MR, Cayatte C, Yu L, et al. Rationally designed TLR4 ligands for vaccine adjuvant discovery. *MBio* (2017) 8:e00492-17. doi: 10.1128/mBio.00492-17

10

Role of the Multidrug Resistance Efflux Pump MexCD-OprJ in the *Pseudomonas aeruginosa* Quorum Sensing Response

***Manuel Alcalde-Rico*[1]*, Jorge Olivares-Pacheco*[1*†]*, Carolina Alvarez-Ortega*[1†]*, Miguel Cámara*[2]* and José Luis Martínez*[1*]**

[1] Centro Nacional de Biotecnología, Consejo Superior de Investigaciones Científicas, Madrid, Spain, [2] Centre for Biomolecular Sciences, School of Life Sciences, University of Nottingham, Nottingham, United Kingdom

***Correspondence:**
Jorge Olivares-Pacheco
jorge.olivares@pucv.cl
José Luis Martínez
jlmtnez@cnb.csic.es

Multidrug efflux pumps constitute a category of antibiotic resistance determinants that are a part of the core bacterial genomes. Given their conservation, it is conceivable that they present functions beyond the extrusion of antibiotics currently used for therapy. *Pseudomonas aeruginosa* stands as a relevant respiratory pathogen, with a high prevalence at hospitals and in cystic fibrosis patients. Part of its success relies on its low susceptibility to antibiotics and on the production of virulence factors, whose expression is regulated in several cases by quorum sensing (QS). We found that overexpression of the MexCD-OprJ multidrug efflux pump shuts down the *P. aeruginosa* QS response. Our results support that MexCD-OprJ extrudes kynurenine, a precursor of the alkyl-quinolone signal (AQS) molecules. Anthranilate and octanoate, also AQS precursors, do not seem to be extruded by MexCD-OprJ. Kynurenine extrusion is not sufficient to reduce the QS response in a mutant overexpressing this efflux pump. Impaired QS response is mainly due to the extrusion of 4-hydroxy-2-heptylquinoline (HHQ), the precursor of the *Pseudomonas* Quinolone Signal (PQS), leading to low PQS intracellular levels and reduced production of QS signal molecules. As the consequence, the expression of QS-regulated genes is impaired and the production of QS-regulated virulence factors strongly decreases in a MexCD-OprN *P. aeruginosa* overexpressing mutant. Previous work showed that MexEF-OprJ, another *P. aeruginosa* efflux pump, is also able of extruding kynurenine and HHQ. However, opposite to our findings, the QS defect in a MexEF-OprN overproducer is due to kynurenine extrusion. These results indicate that, although efflux pumps can share some substrates, the affinity for each of them can be different. Although the QS response is triggered by population density, information on additional elements able of modulating such response is still scarce. This is particularly important in the case of *P. aeruginosa* lung chronic infections, a situation in which QS-defective mutants are accumulated. If MexCD-OprJ overexpression alleviates the cost associated to triggering the QS response when un-needed, it could be possible that MexCD-OprJ antibiotic resistant overproducer strains might be selected even in the absence of antibiotic selective pressure, acting as antibiotic resistant cheaters in heterogeneous *P. aeruginosa* populations.

Keywords: *Pseudomonas aeruginosa*, quorum sensing, antibiotic resistance, multidrug efflux pump, MexCD-OprJ

INTRODUCTION

Pseudomonas aeruginosa is a free-living microorganism able to survive in different environments that not only plays an ecological role in natural ecosystems (Green et al., 1974; Romling et al., 1994; Morales et al., 2004; Walker et al., 2004), but it is also an important causative agent of infections in patients with underlying diseases (Obritsch et al., 2005; Driscoll et al., 2007; Martinez-Solano et al., 2008; Talwalkar and Murray, 2016). The characteristic low susceptibility to antibiotics of this organism relies on several factors (Fajardo et al., 2008). Particularly relevant is the activity of chromosomally-encoded multidrug resistance (MDR) efflux pumps (Vila and Martínez, 2008; Hernando-Amado et al., 2016). Further, the acquisition of mutation-driven resistance is common in this opportunistic pathogen, particularly along chronic infections (Oliver et al., 2015; Palmer and Whiteley, 2015; Lopez-Causape et al., 2018), where the constitutive overexpression of MDR efflux pumps is one of the biggest problems to eradicate these infections (Vila and Martínez, 2008; Vila et al., 2011; Hernando-Amado et al., 2016). Efflux pumps exhibit different functions, with physiological and ecological significances that go beyond their activity as antibiotic resistance elements (Piddock, 2006; Martinez et al., 2009; Alcalde-Rico et al., 2016; Hernando-Amado et al., 2016). In the case of *P. aeruginosa*, an opportunistic pathogen not fully adapted to human hosts (Alonso et al., 1999; Morales et al., 2004), these functions should be of relevance for the success of *P. aeruginosa* as a respiratory infectious pathogen.

Pseudomonas aeruginosa harbors several efflux systems that belong to different families (Stover et al., 2000). The most studied because of their clinical relevance are MexAB-OprM (Li et al., 1995), MexCD-OprJ (Poole et al., 1996; Kohler et al., 1997), MexEF-OprN (Kohler et al., 1997), and MexXY (Aires et al., 1999; Mine et al., 1999). They all belong to the *Resistance-Nodulation-Division* (RND) family of MDR systems (Hernando-Amado et al., 2016). Mutants that exhibit constitutive overexpression of each of these efflux pumps are selected upon treatment with antibiotics; the mutations are frequently located in the regulatory elements adjacent to the respective operon encoding for these MDR systems (Llanes et al., 2004; Sobel et al., 2005; Jeannot et al., 2008; Zaborskyte et al., 2017).

The unregulated overexpression of an efflux system not only contributes to antibiotic resistance but may also have pleiotropic effects in the bacterial physiology. We have recently reported that overexpression of RND systems in *P. aeruginosa* leads to an excessive internalization of protons that acidify the cytoplasm, which causes a biological cost in absence of oxygen or nitrate, since both are necessary to compensate for the intracellular H^+ accumulation (Olivares et al., 2014; Olivares Pacheco et al., 2017). In addition to these non-specific effects, other effects might be due to the unregulated extrusion of intracellular compounds, some of which may be relevant for the ecological behavior of *P. aeruginosa* (Blanco et al., 2016). Indeed, different studies have shown that overexpression of MDR efflux pumps may challenge the *P. aeruginosa* quorum sensing (QS) response (Evans et al., 1998; Kohler et al., 2001; Linares et al., 2005; Olivares et al., 2012), which is in turn determinant for modulating several physiological processes, including bacterial pathogenicity, in response to population density (Williams et al., 2007).

In *P. aeruginosa*, the QS-signaling network consists of three main interconnected regulatory systems: Las, Rhl, and Pqs, which synthetize and respond to the autoinducers *N*-(3-oxododecanoyl)-L-homoserine lactone (3-oxo-C12-HSL), *N*-butanoyl-L-homoserine lactone (C4-HSL), and the 2-alkyl-4(1*H*)-quinolones (AQs) *Pseudomonas* Quinolone Signal (PQS, or its immediate precursor 2-heptyl-4-hydroxyquinoline, HHQ), respectively (Williams and Camara, 2009). These autoinducers are able to bind to their respective transcriptional regulators, namely LasR, RhlR and PqsR, thus controlling the expression of a large number of genes including those responsible for their own synthesis: *lasI, rhlI,* and *pqsABCDE,* respectively.

Some *P. aeruginosa* RND systems have been associated with QS. MexAB-OprM is induced by C4-HSL (Maseda et al., 2004) and has been proposed to extrude 3-oxo-C12-HSL and other 3-oxo-HSL related compounds (Evans et al., 1998; Pearson et al., 1999; Minagawa et al., 2012). MexEF-OprN is able to efflux HHQ (Lamarche and Déziel, 2011) and kynurenine (Olivares et al., 2012), both precursors of the PQS autoinducer signal (Farrow and Pesci, 2007; Palmer et al., 2013). In agreement with these findings, the antibiotic resistant mutants that overproduce MexAB-OprM or MexEF-OprN have been associated with a low production of QS-controlled virulence factors (Evans et al., 1998; Pearson et al., 1999; Sanchez et al., 2002; Olivares et al., 2012). Some studies have demonstrated that acquisition of antibiotic resistance due to constitutive overexpression of *mexCD-oprJ* correlates with a decrease in the production of several virulence factors, some of them controlled by QS (Sanchez et al., 2002; Linares et al., 2005; Jeannot et al., 2008; Stickland et al., 2010). However, the underlying reasons for this correlation remain to be elucidated. In this work, we analyzed in depth the production of each QS signal molecule (QSSM) and the expression levels of the genes controlled by these regulation systems in order to understand how overexpression of MexCD-OprJ could be affecting the *P. aeruginosa* QS response, and consequently the behavior of this bacterial pathogen in the infected patient.

MATERIALS AND METHODS

Bacterial Strains, Plasmids, Primers, and Culture Conditions

The *Escherichia coli* and *P. aeruginosa* strains and the plasmids used in this work, are listed in the **Table 1**. The primers used are listed in the **Table 2**.

Unless other conditions are specified, experiments were carried out at 37°C in 100 ml flasks containing 25 ml of LB broth (Lennox). The *E. coli* strains carrying plasmids with ampicillin (Amp^R) or tetracycline (Tc^R) resistance genes were grown in LB medium with 100 μg/ml of ampicillin or 10 μg/ml of tetracycline, respectively. For determining the effect of different carbon sources on *P. aeruginosa* growth, overnight cultures were washed with M63 medium containing $MgSO_4$ 1 mM and diluted to an OD_{600} = 0.01 in clear bottom 96-well plates containing 150 μl/well of M63 with the corresponding carbon source at a final concentration of 10 mM. The growth of each strain was measured at 37°C using a multi-plate reader.

Whole Genome Sequence of the *nfxB** Strain and Generation of a *nfxB** Δ*mexD* Mutant

The *nfxB** mutant was fully sequenced at Parque Científico de Madrid using Illumina technology as described (Garcia-Leon et al., 2014). Two ≈1000 bp DNA regions adjacent to the fragment of *mexD* to be deleted were amplified by PCR using the primers listed in **Table 2**. The amplicons were purified and used together for a nested PCR reaction in which a recombinant 2058 bp DNA was generated and cloned into pGEM-t Easy (pGEM-T-Δ*mexD*). *E. coli* OmniMax^{TM} cells were transformed with this plasmid and the sequence of the construction was verified by Sanger sequencing. The fragment was excised using HindIII and subcloned into pEX18Ap. The resulting pEX18Ap-Δ*mexD* construction was incorporated into *E. coli* S17-1λ *pir* by transformation. Introduction of the deleted allele into *P. aeruginosa nfxB** was performed by conjugation using S17-1λ *pir* (pEX18Ap-Δ*mexD*) as donor strain as described (Hoang et al., 1998). *mexD* deletion was confirmed by PCR using the primers described in **Table 2**.

Analysis of the Production of QS-Regulated Virulence Factors

The secretion of elastase and protease IV was measured after 20 h of incubation of the bacterial cultures in LB at 37°C following the methods described in Kessler and Safrin (2014). Rhamnolipids detection was carried out as described (Wittgens et al., 2011). Pyocyanin was determined as detailed (Essar et al., 1990). For the swarming motility assay, O/N cultures were washed with sterile 0.85% NaCl and diluted to an OD_{600} = 1.0. Five-microliters drops were poured on the center of Petri dishes containing 25 ml of a defined medium (0.5% casamino acids, 0.5% bacto agar, 0.5% glucose, 3.3 mM K_2HPO_4, and 3 mM $MgSO_4$), which were incubated 16 h at 37°C.

RNA Extraction and Real-Time RT-PCR

RNA was obtained using the RNeasy mini kit (QIAGEN) as described (Olivares et al., 2012). After treatment with DNase (Olivares et al., 2012), the presence of DNA contamination was checked by PCR using *rplU* primers. Real-time RT-PCR was performed as described in Olivares et al. (2012) using the primers listed in **Table 2**. The experiments were carried out in triplicate. The $2^{-\Delta\Delta Ct}$ method (Livak and Schmittgen, 2001) was used for quantifying the results, normalizing the results to the housekeeping gene, *rpsL*.

Thin Layer Chromatography (TLC) and Time Course Monitoring of QSSMs Accumulation

Bacterial O/N cultures were washed with fresh LB medium and diluted to an OD_{600} = 0.01 for subsequent growth. For TLC assays, the QSSMs extractions were carried out as described (Fletcher et al., 2007a). For time course assays, this protocol was optimized to simultaneous monitoring QSSMs accumulation and cell density. For each extraction time, 1.8 ml aliquots from cultures were centrifuged (7,000 × *g*, 10 min at 4°C). The supernatants were filtered through 0.22 μm pore size membrane and the cellular pellets were resuspended in 1.8 ml of methanol HPLC grade to extract the QSSMs. 900 μl of cell-free supernatants were used to extract the QSSMs by adding 600 μl of acidified ethyl acetate twice. The resulting acidified ethyl acetate extracts were dried and subsequently dissolved in 900 μl of methanol HPLC grade.

Alkyl-quinolone signal (AQs) were detected by TLC as described (Fletcher et al., 2007a) using the PAO1 CTX::P_{pqsA}-*lux* biosensor strain. C4-HSL and 3-oxo-C12-HSL were analyzed using the JM109-pSB536 (RhlR- based biosensor) and JM109-pSB1142 (LasR-based biosensor) biosensor strains, respectively (Yates et al., 2002). The image processing software "ImageJ" was used for densitometry analysis of the light spots.

For time course accumulation assays, flat white 96-well plates with optical bottom were filled with a mix containing 5 μl of sample and 195 μl of a 1/100 dilution of the corresponding O/N biosensor cultures. The experiments were carried out on a multi-plate luminometer/spectrophotometer reader. The highest relative light units (RLU = luminescence/OD_{600} ratio) obtained for each biosensor strain and the OD_{600} in which the samples were taken from *P. aeruginosa* cultures were represented.

Analysis by HPLC-MS of Kynurenine and Anthranilate Accumulation in Cell-Free Supernatants

Bacterial strains were grown in M63 containing succinate (10 mM) and tryptophan (10 mM). After 24 h at 37°C, the supernatants were filtered through a 0.22 μm pore size membrane and lyophilized. 100 mg of each sample were resuspended in 2 ml of 3 mM ammonium acetate and dissolved in H_2O/methanol (50/50). The amounts of anthranilate and kynurenine were determined by HPLC-MS at Laboratorio de Cromatografía-SIdI from the Universidad Autónoma de Madrid.

Insertion of the Reporter Construction, miniCTX::P*pqsA-lux*, in the Chromosome of *P. aeruginosa* and Analysis of *pqsABCDE* Expression

The insertion of the miniCTX::P*pqsA-lux* reporter into the chromosomes of the different *P. aeruginosa* strains was carried out by conjugation as described (Hoang et al., 1998) using *E. coli* S17-1λ *pir* containing miniCTX::P*pqsA-lux* (Fletcher et al., 2007b) as donor strain. The resulting *P. aeruginosa* reporter strains were inoculated in flat white 96-well plates with optical bottom containing 200 μL of LB with or without 4 mM anthranilate at an initial OD_{600} = 0.01. The growth (OD_{600}) and the bioluminescence emitted by the P*pqsA-luxCDABE* construction was monitored using a multi-plate reader.

Statistical Analysis

At least three biological replicates were analyzed in each experiment. Statistical significance was evaluated by using a

TABLE 1 | Bacterial strains and plasmids used in the present work.

Bacterial strain/plasmids	Description	Reference/origin
Escherichia coli		
One Shot OmniMax™ 2 T1	Host strain used for the maintenance of cloning plasmids: F′ *pro*AB *lacI*^{q} *lacZ*ΔM15 *Tn*10(Tet^R) Δ(*ccd*AB) *mcr*A, Δ(*mrr,hsd*RMS-*mcr*BC) ϕ80(*lacZ*)ΔM15 Δ(*lacZYA-argF*)U169 *end*A1 recA1 *sup*E44 *thi*-1 *gyr*A96 *rel*A1 *ton*A *pan*D	Invitrogen
S17-1λ *pir*	Conjugative donor strain used for transferring plasmids to *P. aeruginosa* acceptor strains by conjugation assays: F$^-$ *thi pro hsdR hsdM*$^+$ *recA* RP42-Tc::Mu-Km::Tn7	Simon et al., 1986
S17 miniCTX::*PpqsA-lux*	S17-1λ *pir* strain containing the miniCTX::*PpqsA-lux* plasmid	Fletcher et al., 2007a,b
JM109-pSB1142 (LasR-based Biosensor)	Biosensor strain used for detecting the QS signal, 3-oxo-C12-HSL, produced by *P. aeruginosa* strains	Winson et al., 1998
JM109-pSB536 (RhlR-based Biosensor)	Biosensor strain used for detecting the QS signal, C4-HSL, produced by *P. aeruginosa* strains	Swift et al., 1997
Pseudomonas aeruginosa		
PAO1	Wild-type PAO1-V clinic strain given from the lab of V. de Lorenzo	Linares et al., 2005
PAO1 miniCTX::*PpqsA-lux* (*PAO1_PpqsA*)	PAO1-V strain with the reporter construction *PpqsA-luxCDABE* inserted in the specific *attB* site of the chromosome	Present work
JFL28 (*nfxB**)	Spontaneous resistant mutant obtained from PAO1-V strain, which overproduces the MexCD-OprJ efflux system by punctual inactivating mutation in *nfxB* gene	Linares et al., 2005
JFL28 miniCTX::*PpqsA-lux* (*nfxB*_PpqsA*)	JFL28 strain with the reporter construction *PpqsA-luxCDABE* inserted in the specific *attB* site of the chromosome	Present work
*nfxB** Δ*mexD*	JFL28 strain with an inactive MexCD-OprJ efflux system by partial deletion of the *mexD* gene	Present work
PAO1 CTX::P$_{pqsA}$-*lux::pqsA* (PqsR-based Biosensor)	PAO1-Δ*pqsA* strain with the reporter construction *PpqsA-luxCDABE* inserted in the specific *attB* site of the chromosome. Used for detecting the AQs produced by other *P. aeruginosa* strains	Fletcher et al., 2007a,b
Plasmid		
pGEM-T Easy	Commercial plasmid used for cloning optimization of PCR products (Amp^R)	Promega
pGEM-T-Δ*mexD*	pGEM-T Easy vector with the flanking DNA sequences of a 2058 bp inner region of *mexD* gene (Amp^R)	Present work
pEX18Ap	Plasmid with conjugative properties used for deleting genes in *P. aeruginosa* by homolog recombination. Amp^R	Hoang et al., 1998
pEX18Ap-Δ*mexD*	pEX18Ap vector with the flanking DNA sequences of a 2058 bp inner region of *mexD* gene used for deleting *mexD* gene in *P. aeruginosa* strains. Amp^R	Present work
Mini-CTX-*lux-PpqsA*	Plasmid derived from mini-CTX-*lux* Becher and Schweizer (2000) in which the expression of the *luxCDABE* operon is under the transcriptional control of the *pqsABCDE* promoter region of *P. aeruginosa*. Tc^R	Fletcher et al., 2007a,b
pSB1142	Plasmid carried by the LasR-Bioreporter strain necessary for detecting 3-oxo-C12-HSL. Tc^R	Winson et al., 1998
pSB536	Plasmid carried by the RhlR-Bioreporter strain necessary for detecting C4-HSL. Amp^R	Swift et al., 1997

Student's two-tailed test with a confidence interval of 95%. The differences were considered significant for P-values < 0.05 ($^*P < 0.05$; $^{**}P < 0.01$; $^{***}P < 0.001$). The quantification of the areas under the curves was carried out using the GraphPad Prim software and the mean of each biological replicates were used to calculate statistical significance.

RESULTS

Increased expression of efflux pumps due to mutations in their regulators can produce different changes in bacterial physiology. In most cases, the phenotypes observed in this kind of mutants are attributed to the activity of the overexpressed efflux pump. However, in other instances, the mutations in the local regulator itself might have effects on the bacterial physiology, which affect bacterial virulence and are independent of the activity of the efflux pump (Tian et al., 2009a,b). To address this possibility, we used a previously described mutant that overexpresses MexCD-OprJ (Linares et al., 2005). To discard the possibility that other mutations besides those in the *mexCD-oprJ* repressors might have been selected in this strain during its stay in the laboratory, the genome of the mutant was fully sequenced. Only the already described *nfxB* mutation (Linares et al., 2005) was found. From this mutant, an *nfxB**Δ*mexD* strain, which keeps the *nfxB* mutation in addition to a partial deletion of the *mexD* gene, was generated. By comparing *nfxB** and *nfxB**Δ*mexD* strains, we were able to define more precisely which phenotypes depend on the activity of the efflux pump and which are solely due to the inactivation of the NfxB repressor, independently of the activity of the efflux pump.

Overexpression of MexCD-OprJ Results in a Decrease in the Production of QS-Controlled Virulence Factors in *P. aeruginosa*

Swarming motility and the production of elastase, proteinase IV, pyocyanin, and, rhamnolipids were analyzed to establish

TABLE 2 | Collection of primers used in the present work.

Name	Sequence	Description
HindIII_*mexD*_Fw *mexD*_int_Rev	5′-CCCAAGCTTCGAGGTGCGCGCGCGGGTGGCCGGC-3′ 5′-GCGAGCCTGCAGCAGCGCTTATTCGGACATCGGAAAATCC-3′	Amplification of the DNA flanking region "Up" for deleting *mexD* gene
*mexD*_int_Fw HindIII_*mexD*_Rev	5′-GGATTTTCCGATGTCCGAATAAGCGCTGCTGCAGGCTCGC-3′ 5″-CCCAAGCTTCAGACGAAACAGATAGGTACGAACA-3′	Amplification of the DNA flanking region "Down" for deleting *mexD* gene
Δ*mexD*_check_Fw Δ*mexD*_check_Rev	5′-GGTGAAGATCGTGCCGAAG-3′ 5′-ATTGGTGAAGTCGTTGATCA-3′	To check the deletion of the *mexD* gene
M13_Fw M13_Rev	5′-CACGACGTTGTAAAACGAC-3′ 5′-GGATAACAATTTCACACAGG-3′	To check the insertion of cloning DNA fragment into pGEM-t Easy vector
*rplU*_Fwd *rplU*_Rev	5′-CGCAGTGATTGTTACCGGTG-3′ 5′-AGGCCTGAATGCCGGTGATC-3′	To check DNA contamination of RNA samples
*rpsL*_Fwd *rpsL*_Rev	5′-GCAAGCGCATGGTCGACAAGA-3′ 5′-CGCTGTGCTCTTGCAGGTTGTGA-3′	Real-time RT-PCR (Housekeeping)
*lasA*_Fwd *lasA*_Rev	5′-ATGGACCAGATCCAGGTGAG-3′ 5′-CGTTGTCGTAGTTGCTGGTG-3′	Real-time RT-PCR
*lasB*_Fwd *lasB*_Rev	5′-ATCGGCAAGTACACCTACGG-3′ 5′-ACCAGTCCCGGTACAGTTTG-3′	Real-time RT-PCR
*rhlA*_Fwd *rhlA*_Rev	5′-CGAGGTCAATCACCTGGTCT-3′ 5′-GACGGTCTCGTTGAGCAGAT-3′	Real-time RT-PCR
*rhlB*_Fwd *rhlB*_Rev	5′-GAGCGACGAACTGACCTACC-3′ 5′-GGGAATCCCGTACTTCTCGT-3′	Real-time RT-PCR
*lecA*_Fwd *lecA*_Rev	5′-ATAACGAAGCAGGGCAGGTA-3′ 5′-TTGCCAATCTTCATGACCAG-3′	Real-time RT-PCR
*phzB1*_Fwd *phzB1*_Rev	5′-AACGAACTTCGCGAAAAGAA-3′ 5′-TTTGTCTTTGCCACGAATGA-3′	Real-time RT-PCR
*phzB2*_Fwd *phzB2*_Rev	5′-GCGAGACGGTGGTCAAGTAT-3′ 5′-AATCCGGGAAGCATTTCAG-3′	Real-time RT-PCR
*phzS*_Fwd *phzS*_Rev	5′-CAAGTCGCTGGTGAACTGG-3′ 5′-CGGGTACTGCAGGATCAACT-3′	Real-time RT-PCR
*mexG*_Fwd *mexG*_Rev	5′-GGCGAAGCTGTTCGACTATC-3′ 5′-AGAAGGTGTGGACGATGAGG-3′	Real-time RT-PCR
*lasI*_Fwd *lasI*_Rev	5′-CTACAGCCTGCAGAACGACA-3′ 5′-ATCTGGGTCTTGGCATTGAG-3′	Real-time RT-PCR
*rhlI*_Fwd *rhlI*_Rev	5′-CTCTCTGAATCGCTGGAAGG-3′ 5′-GACGTCCTTGAGCAGGTAGG-3′	Real-time RT-PCR
*pqsA*_Fwd *pqsA*_Rev	5′-CAATACACCTCGGGTTCCAC-3′ 5′-TGAACCAGGGAAAGAACAGG-3′	Real-time RT-PCR
*pqsD*_Fwd *pqsD*_Rev	5′-CATGTGATCTGCCATCAACC-3′ 5′-AGCCGTAGGTCAGGACCAG-3′	Real-time RT-PCR
*pqsE*_Fwd *pqsE*_Rev	5′-GACATGGAGGCTTACCTGGA-3′ 5′-CTCAGTTCGTCGAGGGATTC-3′	Real-time RT-PCR
*phnB*_Fwd *phnB*_Rev	5′-CACTCGCTGGTGGTCAGTC-3′ 5′-AGAGTAGAGCGTTCTCCAGCA-3′	Real-time RT-PCR
*pqsH*_Fwd *pqsH*_Rev	5′-ATGTCTACGCGACCCTGAAG-3′ 5′-AACTCCTCGAGGTCGTTGTG-3′	Real-time RT-PCR

whether or not MexCD-OprJ affects the production of *P. aeruginosa* QS-regulated virulence elements. As **Figure 1** shows and in agreement with previous studies (Sanchez et al., 2002; Stickland et al., 2010), the *nfxB** strain exhibits a decrease in swarming motility and in the production of all analyzed virulence factors in comparison with the wild-type PAO1 strain. The fact that the deletion of *mexD* fully restores the production of QS-regulated virulence factors in an *nfxB** background, indicates that the observed impairment is solely due to the activity of MexCD-OprJ,

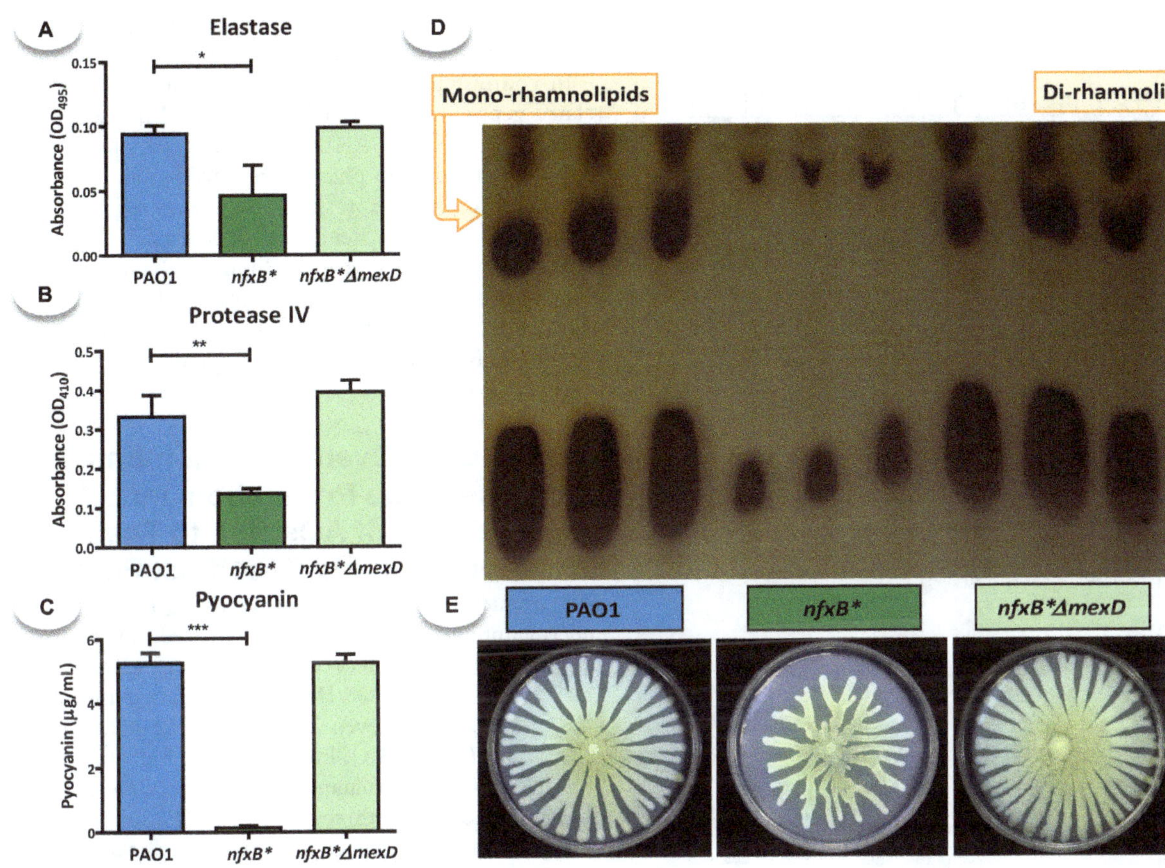

FIGURE 1 | Overexpression of the MexCD-OprJ efflux pump results in a decrease in the production of different virulence factors regulated by the QS system. The elastase **(A)**, protease IV **(B)**, pyocyanin **(C)**, rhamnolipids, **(D)** and swarming **(E)** assays were conducted as described in Methods using cultures of the PAO1, *nfxB** and *nfxB** Δ*mexD* strains. Statistical significances were evaluated by using a Student's two-tailed test and considered significant if $P < 0.05$, with a confidence interval of 95% (*$P < 0.05$; **$P < 0.01$; ***$P < 0.001$). *nfxB** presented a lower production of all tested virulence factors that the parental wild-type PAO1. The deletion of *mexD* in strain *nfxB*mexD* restores the phenotypes to the levels of the wild-type strain, indicating that the defects in the expression of virulence factors were solely due to the activity of the *mexCD-oprJ* efflux pump.

independently of the potential activity of the NfxB regulator protein.

Overproduction of the MexCD-OprJ Efflux System Results in a Lower Expression of QS- Regulated Genes

Expression of a set of QS-regulated genes (Pearson et al., 1997; Deziel et al., 2003, 2005; Dietrich et al., 2006; Rampioni et al., 2016) was analyzed to determine if a low production of virulence factors in the *nfxB** mutant correlates with a deregulated expression of QS-regulated genes. LasB controls elastase production (Pearson et al., 1997; Kessler and Safrin, 2014). RhlA and RhlB are implicated in rhamnolipids biosynthesis (Pearson et al., 1997; Deziel et al., 2003), which in turn is important for swarming motility (Deziel et al., 2003). PhzB1, PhzB2, and PhzS are implicated in pyocyanin biosynthesis and the MexGHI-OpmD efflux pump has been described to be regulated by this phenazine (Dietrich et al., 2006). As shown in **Figure 2A**, the expression levels of the tested genes are lower in the *nfxB** strain than in PAO1. In addition, the expression of these genes is restored to PAO1 levels, even overcoming them, upon *mexD* deletion in the *nfxB** strain, further confirming that *mexCD-oprJ* overexpression is what causes an impaired QS response in the *nfxB** mutant. These results are in agreement with the lower production of virulence factors observed in *nfxB** (**Figure 1**).

To gain more insights on the reasons for this impaired QS-response, we analyzed the expression of genes responsible for the production of both families of autoinducers AHLs (*lasI* and *rhlI*) (Pesci et al., 1997) and AQs (*pqsABCDE-phnAB* and *pqsH*) (Gallagher et al., 2002). This was performed along the exponential growth phase when expression of these QS biosynthesis genes starts, and in early stationary phase, when the Pqs-system is fully active (Lepine et al., 2003). As shown in **Figures 2B,C**, expression of the genes responsible for the synthesis of PQS and HHQ exhibit a marked decrease in the *nfxB** strain at both time points. These changes were restored to wild-type levels upon MexCD-OprJ inactivation in an *nfxB** background. *pqsA*, from the *pqsABCDE* operon responsible for the biosynthesis of AQs (Gallagher et al., 2002), exhibits the sharpest decrease

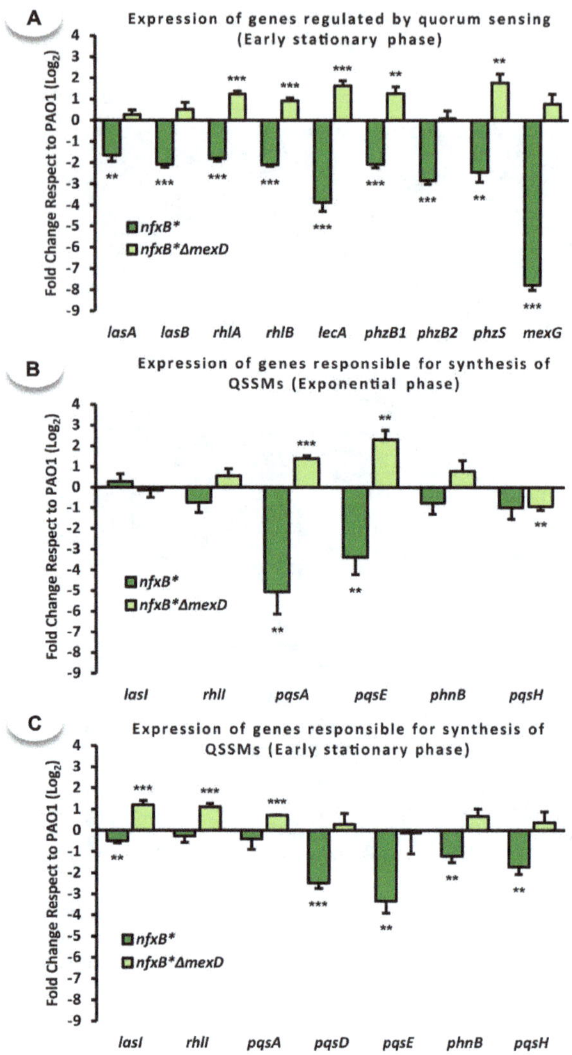

FIGURE 2 | Overexpression of the MexCD-OprJ efflux system affects the expression levels of QS-regulated genes. Transcriptional analysis by real-time RT-PCR of **(A)** genes regulated by quorum sensing (QS) response (*lasA*, *lasB*, *rhlA*, *rhlB*, *lecA*, *phzB1*, *phzB2*, *phzS*, and *mexG*) and **(B,C)** genes responsible for QSSMs production (*lasI*, *rhlI*, *pqsA*, *pqsD*, *pqsE*, *phnB*, and *pqsH*) from samples obtained in **(B)** exponential (OD_{600} = 0.6) and **(A,C)** early stationary phase of growth (OD_{600} = 2.5) in PAO1, *nfxB** and *nfxB** Δ*mexD* strains grown in LB medium. Statistical significances were evaluated by using a Student's two-tailed test and considered significant if $P < 0.05$, with a confidence interval of 95% (*$P < 0.05$; **$P < 0.01$; ***$P < 0.001$). The results showed that the genes implicated in the synthesis of PQS *pqsA* and *pqsE* were expressed at lower level in the *nfxB** strain than in the wild-type PAO1 strain at exponential phase of growth **(B)**. In early stationary growth phase **(A,C)**, the expression levels of the PQS-biosynthesis genes (*pqsD*, *pqsE*, *phnB,* and *pqsH*), as well as all of the analyzed QS-regulated genes, were significantly lower in the *nfxB** strain than in the PAO1 wild-type. The deletion of *mexD* in strain *nfxB*mexD* restores or even increase the levels of expression to those of the wild-type strain, indicating that these defects were solely due to the activity of the MexCD-OprJ efflux pump.

in expression during exponential growth phase (**Figure 2B**). Expression of *phnB*, implicated in the synthesis of anthranilate through the chorismic acid pathway (Farrow and Pesci, 2007; Palmer et al., 2013), as well as *pqsH*, which codify the enzyme responsible for the conversion of HHQ into PQS (Gallagher et al., 2002), decreases more in early stationary phase (**Figures 2B,C**).

In contrast to the strong variations in expression of PQS-related genes, the activity of MexCD-OprJ had a minor impact on the expression of AHLs-related genes in both exponential and stationary growth phases. The *nfxB** strain did not present alterations in *rhlI* expression, the gene responsible for the synthesis of C4-HSL, neither in exponential (**Figure 2B**) nor in stationary phase of growth (**Figure 2C**). A similar behavior was observed for *lasI*, the gene responsible for the synthesis of 3-oxo-C12-HSL, detecting just a slight decreased expression in the *nfxB** strain during early stationary growth phase (**Figures 2B,C**).

MexCD-OprJ Overexpression Entails a Decrease in the Production and Accumulation of AQs Due to Their Extrusion Through This Efflux Pump

The production and accumulation of PQS and HHQ in both supernatant and cellular extracts decreased in the *nfxB** mutant (**Figure 3A**). This effect is directly dependent on MexCD-OprJ activity, since PQS/HHQ accumulation increased in the *nfxB** Δ*mexD* strain, even overcoming the wild-type levels in cell extracts (**Figure 3A**). Interestingly, the proportion of HHQ present in the supernatants with respect to cell-extracts is different among the three strains. As **Figure 3B** shows, the *nfxB** mutant has a higher supernatant/cell extract HHQ ratio than PAO1. Further, the deletion of *mexD* in the *nfxB** strain produced the opposite effect, decreasing the HHQ ratio to lower values than those of the wild-type strain, suggesting that MexCD-OprJ may be extruding HHQ, affecting the progressive intracellular accumulation of this signal. Since the expression of the *pqsABCDE-phnAB* operon, responsible of AQs biosynthesis (Gallagher et al., 2002), is activated in presence of PQS/HHQ (Wade et al., 2005; Hazan et al., 2010; Rampioni et al., 2016), we postulate that HHQ extrusion by MexCD-OprJ could be the main cause for the lower production of AQs observed in the *nfxB** strain, ultimately resulting in a defective QS-system.

Overexpression of MexCD-OprJ Produces Minor Effects in the Synthesis of 3-oxo-C12-HSL and C4-HSL Autoinducers

Since the Las, Rhl, and Pqs regulation systems are highly interconnected (McKnight et al., 2000; Diggle et al., 2003; Kasper et al., 2016), we wanted to know whether or not the excessive HHQ extrusion through MexCD-OprJ in the *nfxB** mutant could be also affecting the production of the QS signals, 3-oxo-C12-HSL (autoinducer signal for Las system) and C4-HSL (autoinducer signal for Rhl system). As shown in **Figures 4A–C,F**, both intracellular and extracellular amounts of 3-oxo-C12-HSL are slightly higher in *nfxB** cultures than in either the wild-type PAO1 strain or the *nfxB** Δ*mexD*

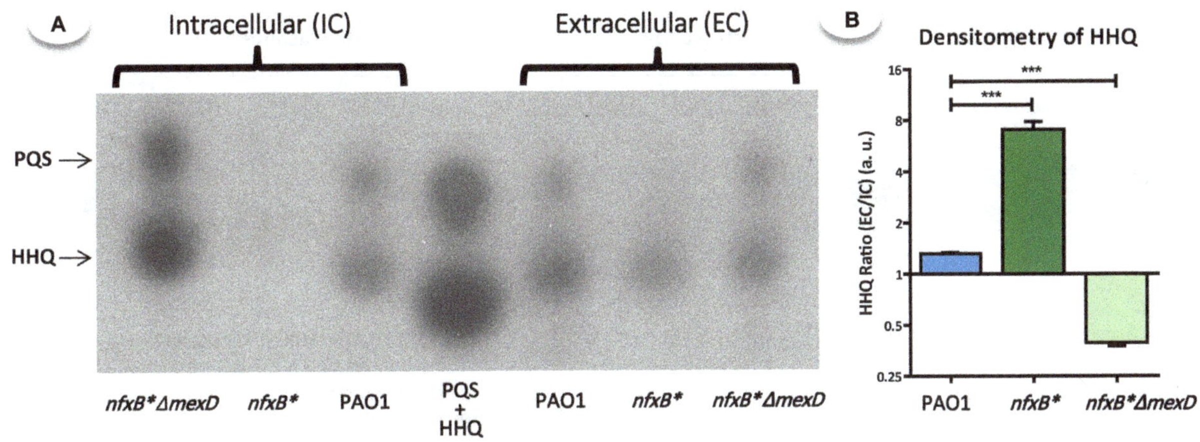

FIGURE 3 | PQS and HHQ production is impaired in the strain that overproduces the MexCD-OprJ efflux pump. **(A)** To determine the accumulation levels of the autoinducers synthesized by *Pseudomonas aeruginosa,* a technique based on TLC coupled with a PqsR-based biosensor was used. The samples were extracted from cultures in early stationary phase (OD_{600} = 2.5). **(B)** The TLC-spots corresponding to HHQ were quantified by densitometry and the ratio between the HHQ present in the supernatant respect to cell extract was calculated and represented. Statistical significances were evaluated by using a Student's two-tailed test and considered significant if $P < 0.05$, with a confidence interval of 95% (*$P < 0.05$; **$P < 0.01$; ***$P < 0.001$). As shown, overexpression of the MexCD-OprJ efflux system in *nfxB** strongly reduces the production of PQS and HHQ as compared with PAO1 and *nfxB** Δ*mexD* strains. Furthermore, the analysis by densitometry of the HHQ ratio shows that this defect in AQs production is likely caused by an excessive extrusion of HHQ through MexCD-OprJ.

mutant. The opposite effect was observed for C4-HSL; the *nfxB** mutant accumulates slightly lower extracellular levels of this QS signal during late exponential phase (**Figure 4D**), reaching the levels of extracellular accumulation observed in both PAO1 and *nfxB**Δ*mexD* in early stationary phase (**Figures 4E,F**). This variation may also exist inside the cell due to the ability of C4-HSL to freely diffuse through cytoplasmic membrane (Pearson et al., 1999). Altogether, these results indicate that overexpression of MexCD-OprJ leads to minor alterations of AHLs production. These changes might be due to the strongly impaired production of PQS and HHQ.

MexCD-OprJ Is Able to Extrude Kynurenine but Not Anthranilate, Both Precursors of AQs Signals

Our results indicate that the impaired QS response associated to the overexpression of the MexCD-OprJ efflux pump is mainly caused by a decreased production of PQS and HHQ, likely due to an excessive HHQ extrusion through this efflux system. The MexEF-OprN efflux pump is able to extrude both HHQ and its precursor kynurenine (Lamarche and Déziel, 2011; Olivares et al., 2012); extrusion of the latter is the main cause for the impaired QS response observed in MexEF-OprN overproducer strains (Olivares et al., 2012). A similar situation might also apply to MexCD-OprJ.

One of the immediate precursors of AQs in *P. aeruginosa* is anthranilate, which can < be synthetized either by PhnAB from chorismic acid or by kynurenine pathway when tryptophan is present in the medium (Deziel et al., 2004; Farrow and Pesci, 2007). Since the kynurenine pathway is the main source of anthranilate for AQs production when bacteria grow in rich LB medium (Farrow and Pesci, 2007), it could be possible that extrusion of some of the biosynthetic intermediates through MexCD-OprJ might affect the AQs production in *nfxB**. To test this hypothesis, we first analyzed the growth kinetic of the strains PAO1, *nfxB**, and *nfxB**Δ*mexD* in minimal medium containing tryptophan, kynurenine, or succinate as the sole carbon source. As shown in **Figure 5A**, the *nfxB** mutant presents a growth defect in both tryptophan or kynurenine as the sole carbon source when compared to PAO1. These results strongly suggest extrusion of one or more intermediates of the kynurenine pathway through the MexCD-OprJ efflux system. As shown (**Figure 5A**) deletion of *mexD* in this mutant was enough to restore the wild-type growth rate, indicating that the observed growth defects, and the potential extrusion of these intermediates was solely due to the activity of MexCD-OprJ.

To analyze this possibility, we looked for the presence of kynurenine and anthranilate in the supernatants of PAO1 and *nfxB** cultures. We observed a lower amount of anthranilate and a higher accumulation of kynurenine in the supernatants of *nfxB** cultures (**Figure 5B**). Altogether, these results show that MexCD-OprJ is able to extrude kynurenine, but not anthranilate.

The Low Levels of PQS and HHQ Observed in the *nfxB** Strain Is Not Just Due to Kynurenine Extrusion

Having established that the constitutive overexpression of MexCD-OprJ efflux pump leads to a decrease in the extracellular accumulation of anthranilate, we wondered whether a low intracellular availability of anthranilate could be the cause of the impaired PQS and HHQ production observed in the *nfxB** strain. To address this possibility, we grew PAO1 and *nfxB** in

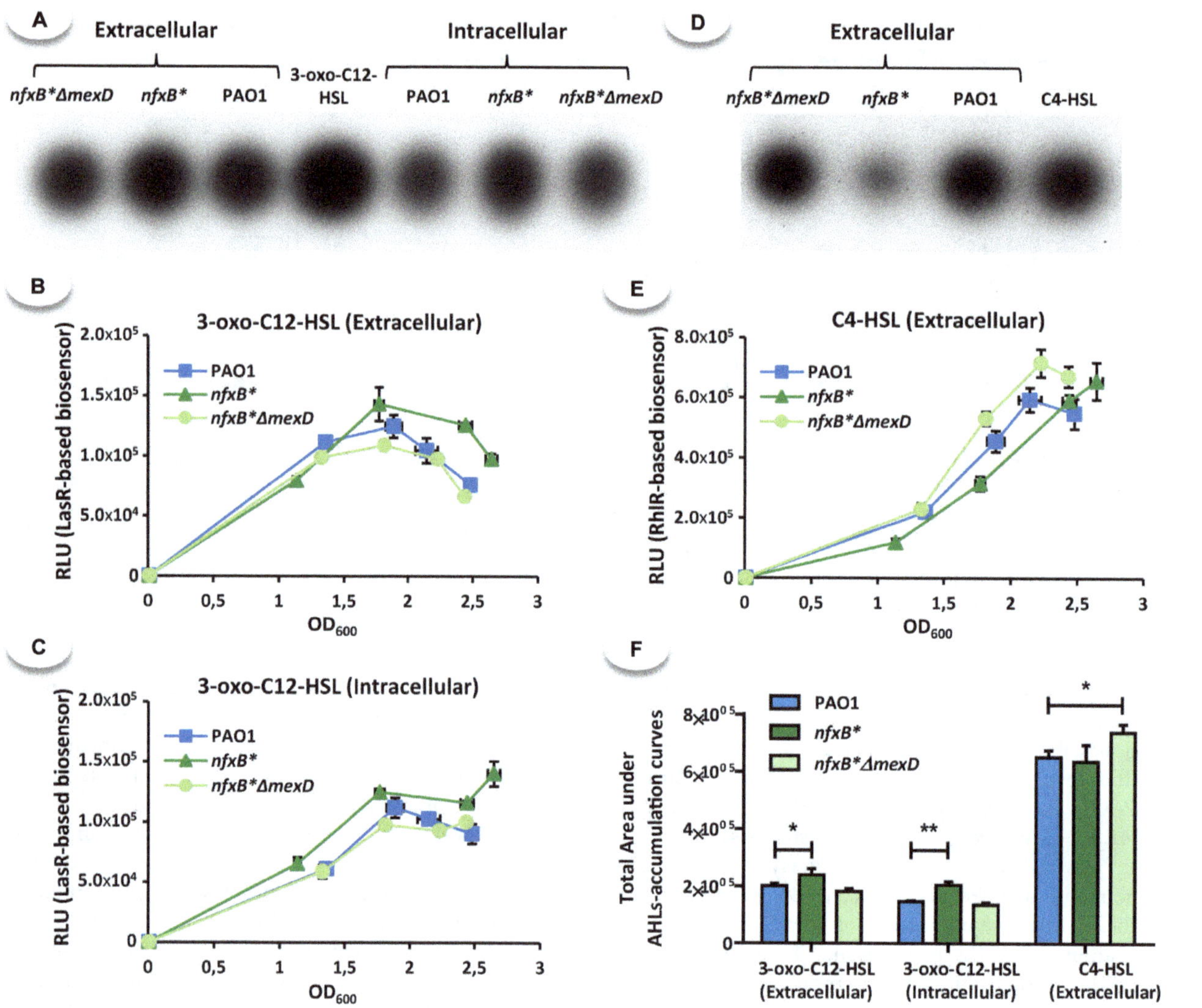

FIGURE 4 | The *nfxB** mutant displays minor alterations in the kinetic of accumulation of 3-oxo-C12-HSL autoinducer. TLCs **(A,D)** and time course accumulation assays **(B,C,E)** were used to determine the accumulation of either 3-oxo-C12-HSL or C4-HSL autoinducer compounds. The samples for the TLC assays were extracted from cultures in late exponential phase (OD_{600} = 1.7) and the samples for the time course assay were taken at different time along the cell cycle (4, 5, 6, and 7 h post-inoculation). The area under the curve of each time course assay was calculated **(F)** and statistical significances were evaluated by using a Student's two-tailed test with a confidence interval of 95% ($^*P < 0.05$; $^{**}P < 0.01$; $^{***}P < 0.001$). As shown, the overexpression of MexCD-OprJ has a slightly but significant effect on 3-oxo-C12-HSL accumulation. The *nfxB** strain presented higher levels of 3-oxo-C12-HSL than PAO1 and *nfxB** Δ*mexD* both outside **(A,B,F)** and inside the cells **(A,C,F)**. In contrast, the supernatant accumulation of C4-HSL in late exponential phase was lower in the MexCD-OprJ overexpressing mutant as compared with PAO1 and *nfxB** Δ*mexD* strains **(D,E)**. However, the quantification of total area under the curves **(F)** only showed a significant increase in *nfxB** Δ*mexD* strain respect to both PAO1 and *nfxB**.

LB medium supplemented with 1 mM anthranilate and analyzed the production and accumulation of these two signals. As shown in **Figure 5C**, anthranilate supplementation does not restore PQS/HHQ production to wild-type levels in the *nfxB** strain. In addition, our results indicate that the *nfxB** strain continues to extrude HHQ at higher levels than those observed in the wild-type strain under these conditions (**Figure 5D**).

We entertained the possibility that a higher anthranilate concentration was needed to restore AQs production to wild-type levels in *nfxB**. To this end, we supplemented LB medium with up to 4 mM anthranilate and analyzed the activation of the *pqsABCDE* promoter in real-time in both PAO1 and *nfxB**. As shown in **Figure 5E**, a higher concentration of anthranilate did not restore the activation of the *pqsABCDE* promoter in the *nfxB** strain. These results indicate that a low anthranilate concentration caused by kynurenine extrusion is not the main underlying cause for the impaired PQS and HHQ production observed in this strain. These results further support the notion that an excessive, non-physiological, extrusion of HHQ caused by the overexpression of MexCD-OprJ is likely the main cause for the lower accumulation and production of HHQ and PQS in the multidrug resistant *nfxB** mutants.

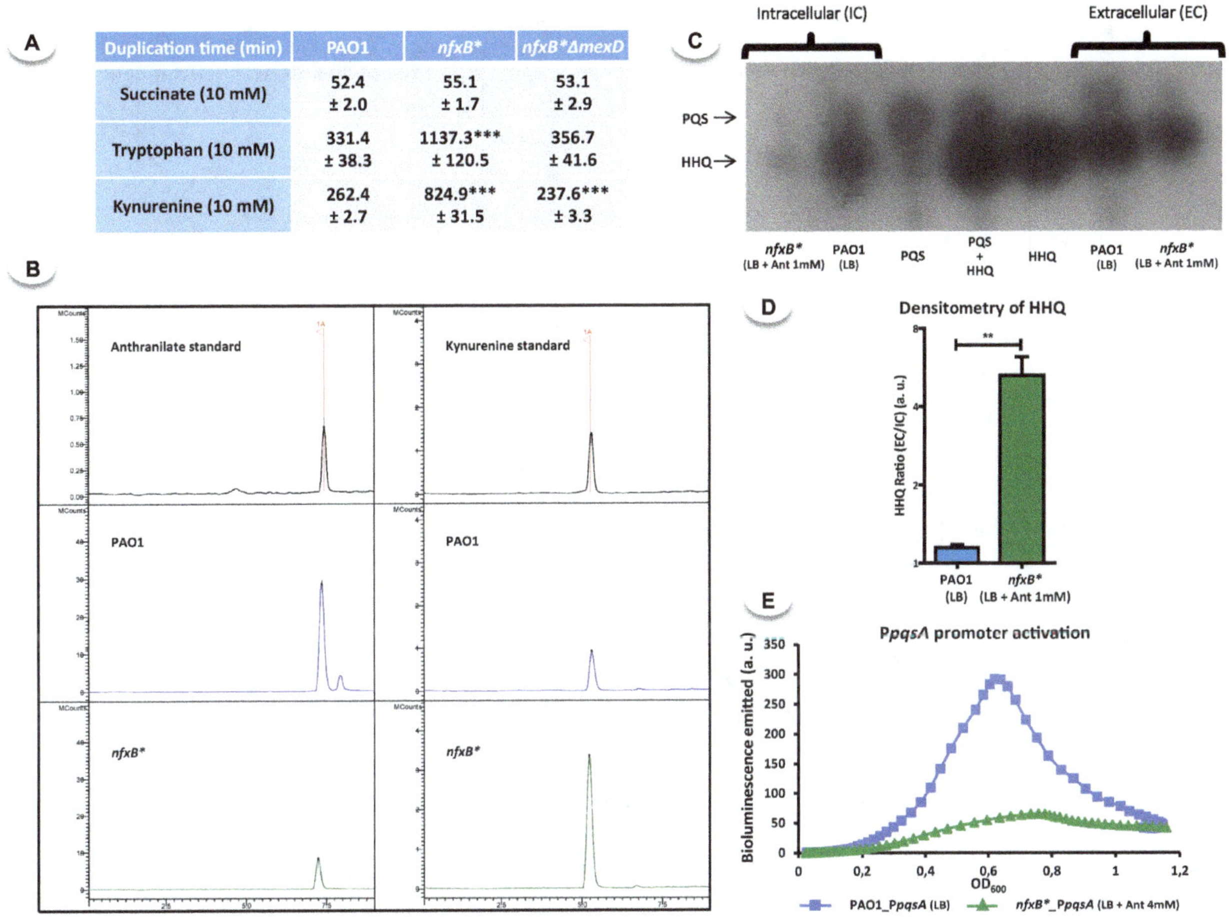

FIGURE 5 | Impaired intracellular accumulation of anthranilate produced by an excessive kynurenine extrusion through MexCD-OprJ is not the cause for lower AQs production of the *nfxB** mutant. Statistical significances were evaluated by using a Student's two-tailed test and considered significant if $P < 0.05$, with a confidence interval of 95% (*$P < 0.05$; **$P < 0.01$; ***$P < 0.001$). **(A)** The duplication time of PAO1, *nfxB**, and *nfxB** Δ*mexD* strains growing in minimal medium with succinate (control), tryptophan or kynurenine (both anthranilate precursors) as sole carbon sources was determined. As shown, the *nfxB** mutant presents an impaired growth in both tryptophan and kynurenine, and deletion of *mexD* gene restored the growth rate in *nfxB** mutant, suggesting these compounds might be substrates of MexCD-OprJ. **(B)** Anthranilate and kynurenine accumulation in cell-free supernatants was quantified by HPLC-MS from PAO1 and *nfxB** cultures grown along 24 h in M63 minimal medium with succinate (10 mM) and tryptophan (10 mM) as sole carbon sources. Left panels anthranilate, right panels kynurenine. As shown, the supernatants from *nfxB** cultures contained more kynurenine and less anthranilate than those from the wild-type PAO1 strain, indicating that kynurenine is a substrate of MexCD-OprJ and anthranilate is not extruded by this efflux pump. **(C)** The production of AQs in PAO1 and *nfxB** strains growing in LB medium supplemented with anthranilate 1 mM was analyzed in early stationary phase ($OD_{600} = 2.5$) by TLC. **(D)** The extracellular vs. intracellular HHQ ratios were calculated measuring each one of the HHQ spots obtained in the TLC-assays by densitometry. **(E)** Real-time *pqsABCDE* expression was analyzed in both PAO1 and *nfxB** strains growing in LB medium and LB supplemented with anthranilate 4 mM respectively, using a chromosomal insertion of the reporter construction *PpqsA::luxCDABE*. The results show that anthranilate supplementation of LB medium does not restore the AQs production in the *nfxB** strain **(C,E)**, reinforcing our hypothesis that HHQ extrusion **(D)** rather than kynurenine extrusion through MexCD-OprJ is the main cause for the QS-defective response of the *nfxB** strain.

The Low Production of AQs Associated to MexCD-OprJ Overexpression Is Not Caused by an Impaired Intracellular Accumulation of Octanoate

Octanoate is the other direct precursor of PQS and HHQ (Dulcey et al., 2013). Once we established that anthranilate synthesis is not the limiting step in the production of AQs by the *nfxB** strain, we wondered whether a hypothetical low production or intracellular accumulation of octanoate might be affecting the AQs production in this strain. For that purpose, we measured the progressive accumulation of AQs in both cell-free supernatants and cellular extracts from PAO1, *nfxB**, and *nfxB** Δ*mexD* cultures grown in LB supplemented with 5 mM octanoate.

In agreement with previous findings (Dulcey et al., 2013), we found that the intracellular accumulation of AQs (**Figure 6A**) and pyocyanin production (**Figure 7**) increase when octanoate is added. However, these increases were similar in all strains, and both the pyocyanin production and the absolute AQs levels reached inside cells were still lower in *nfxB** than in PAO1 or in *nfxB** Δ*mexD*. These results indicate that a lower availability of octanoate is not the cause of the impaired QS response displayed by the *nfxB** strain.

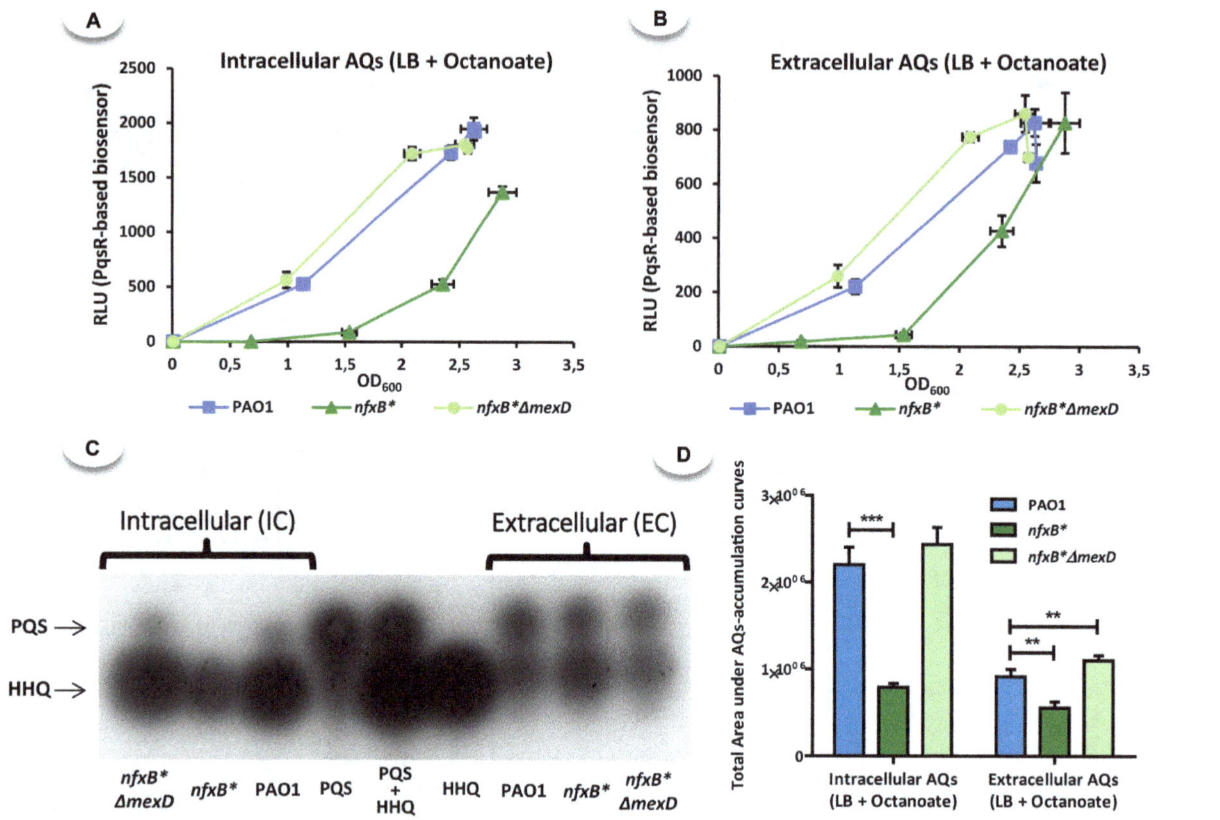

FIGURE 6 | LB supplementation with octanoate increased the AQs production in PAO1, *nfxB**, and *nfxB** Δ*mexD* strains but, in the case of *nfxB**, but the accumulation levels remain being lower in *nfxB** than observed in the other strains. To determine the time course production of AQs in PAO1, *nfxB**, and *nfxB** Δ*mexD* strains, we extracted these compounds from both the cells **(A)** and the cell-free supernatants **(B)** at different times along the cell cycle (4, 5, 6, and 7 h post-inoculation). Additionally, the last points of time course extractions were analyzed by TLC **(C)** in order to know the proportion of PQS and HHQ present on each AQs-extracts. The total area under each time course accumulation curve was quantified **(D)** and statistical significances were evaluated by using a Student's two-tailed test and considered significant if $P < 0.05$, with a confidence interval of 95% (*$P < 0.05$; **$P < 0.01$; ***$P < 0.001$). The results show that supplementation of LB with 5 mM octanoate, even allowing *nfxB** strain to accumulate levels of AQs out of the cells near to those in PAO1 and *nfxB** Δ*mexD* **(B–D)**, was insufficient to restore the intracellular accumulation of PQS and HHQ **(A,C,D)**. Furthermore, the fact that in TLC assay **(C)**, the spot corresponding with HHQ present in *nfxB** supernatant is slightly higher than that in PAO1 and *nfxB** Δ*mexD*, together with the evident low intracellular accumulation of HHQ in the *nfxB** strain, confirm our hypothesis that MexCD-OprJ is able to extrude HHQ.

It is worth mentioning that, although the *nfxB** supernatants exhibit a delay in AQs accumulation in the presence of 5 mM octanoate, the supernatants from all three strains exhibit similar levels when the cultures reach high cell densities ($OD_{600} > 2.5$) (**Figure 6B**). In contrast, the intracellular AQs accumulation remains lower in the *nfxB** strain (**Figure 6A**). In the same way, the quantification of the areas under the curve for AQs-accumulation shows that the differences observed in these strains are lower in the supernatants when compared to cell extracts (**Figure 6D**). Further, the analysis by TLC of AQs extracted from the last point of the time course assay showed that, while the intracellular accumulation of PQS and HHQ remained being lower in the case of *nfxB**, the extracellular accumulation of these two AQs were similar among PAO1, *nfxB** and *nfxB**Δ*mexD* cultures (**Figure 6C**). These results further reinforce the hypothesis that MexCD-OprJ is able to extrude HHQ (and likely PQS as well), and confirm that overexpression of this system adversely affects the intracellular accumulation of AQs. This extrusion can be considered the bottleneck that precludes a proficient PQS production as well as the onset of a proper QS response in *nfxB**-type mutants.

DISCUSSION

In the current work, we demonstrate that a *P. aeruginosa nfxB** mutant, which overexpresses the MexCD-OprJ efflux pump, exhibits an impaired QS response due the extrusion of HHQ. Specifically, this non-physiological extrusion leads to a decrease in the expression of the *pqsABCDE* operon responsible for AQs synthesis, which affects AQs-dependent and the PqsE-dependent regulons that comprise the genes involved in swarming motility, and in the production of pyocyanin, rhamnolipids, and proteases among others (Hazan et al., 2010; Rampioni et al., 2010, 2016).

The QS response in *P. aeruginosa* consists mainly on the Las, Rhl, and Pqs systems which are dependent on

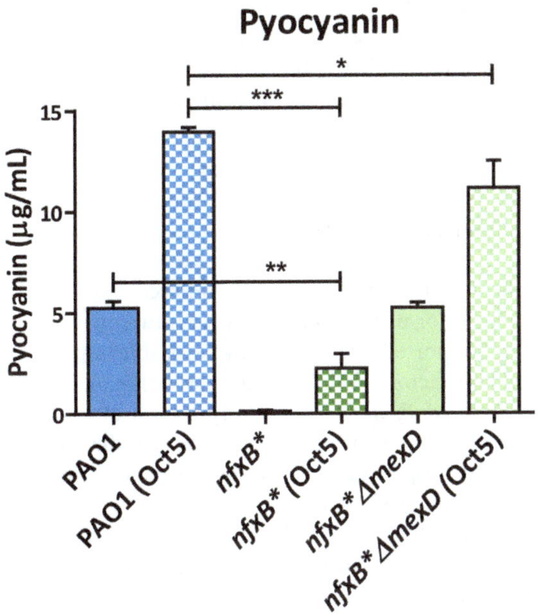

FIGURE 7 | LB supplementation with octanoate increased the pyocyanin production in all analyzed strains, but *nfxB** remained producing lower levels than those observed in PAO1 when grew in LB medium. For pyocyanin assay, the strains were grown in LB medium with or without octanoate (5 mM) along a time lapse of 20 h and the pyocyanin was extracted with chloroform-based protocol as is described in Methods. Statistical significances were evaluated by using a Student's two-tailed test and considered significant if $P < 0.05$, with a confidence interval of 95% (*$P < 0.05$; **$P < 0.01$; ***$P < 0.001$). The results show that supplementation of LB with 5 mM octanoate, even allowing *nfxB** strain increase the pyocyanin production, was insufficient to reach the levels produced by PAO1 in LB without octanoate. This indicate that a hypothetical low intracellular accumulation of octanoate is not the main cause for defective pyocyanin production observed in *nfxB** strain.

the 3-oxo-C12-HSL, C4-HSL, and PQS/HHQ autoinducers, respectively (Williams and Camara, 2009). The cross-regulation between these QS-systems is hierarchically understood, with the Las system located at the top, activating the other two QS systems, and followed by the Pqs-dependent activation of the Rhl-system, and by the Rhl-dependent repression of the Pqs-system (Dubern and Diggle, 2008; Williams and Camara, 2009). However, evidence exists that the hierarchy and the relationship between these QS-systems may be modulated depending on environmental conditions and the activity of global regulators as MvaT or RsmA among others (Choi et al., 2011; Mellbye and Schuster, 2014; Hammond et al., 2016; Maura et al., 2016; Welsh and Blackwell, 2016). In addition, recent studies have highlighted the relevant role of the feedback-regulation between Las, Rhl, and Pqs systems as well as the relevance of the PqsE and RhlR regulators (Deziel et al., 2005; Farrow et al., 2008; Dekimpe and Deziel, 2009; Hazan et al., 2010; Rampioni et al., 2010, 2016). Indeed, it has been demonstrated that the expression of approximately 90% of the genes in the AQs-regulon may be regulated through *pqsE* induction (Hazan et al., 2010). Likewise, the non-virulent phenotype prompted by the absence of AQs synthesis may be by-passed through *pqsE* induction, restoring the full *P. aeruginosa* virulence (Deziel et al., 2005; Hazan et al., 2010; Rampioni et al., 2010). Further, the regulation of several QS-dependent factors could be redundant. In such a way, the production of elastase, rhamnolipids, or pyocyanin, which are mainly under the control of Las, Rhl, and Pqs systems, respectively, are also regulated by PqsE independently of AQs production (Deziel et al., 2005; Hazan et al., 2010; Rampioni et al., 2010, 2016). In addition, expression of *rhlR* increases upon *pqsE* induction at the same time that some functions of PqsE as a QS-regulator are dependent on RhlR and C4-HSL production, thus establishing a complex feedback regulation loop (Hazan et al., 2010). Even more, exogenous addition of C4-HSL to the cultures may partially complement some of the phenotypes impaired in a *pqsE* mutant, such as pyocyanin production (Farrow et al., 2008; Hazan et al., 2010; Rampioni et al., 2010). Recent work indicates that PqsE is an alternative ligand synthase and PqsE and RhlR function as a QS-autoinducer synthase–receptor pair able of regulate the *P. aeruginosa* QS response independently of RhlI (Mukherjee et al., 2018).

Given this role of PqsE as one of the main elements in the QS regulatory network, we postulate that a reduced production of PQS and HHQ, together with a decreased *pqsE* expression, are the main causes for the lack of QS-response associated to the constitutive overexpression of the MexCD-OprJ efflux system. In this work, we show that expression of QS-regulated genes decreases in an *nfxB** antibiotic resistant mutant and that inactivation of the MexCD-OprJ efflux pump in this background restores expression of these genes to wild-type levels, being even higher in some cases (**Figure 2**). Similar results were obtained with some QS-regulated phenotypes such as the production of elastase, protease IV, pyocyanin, rhamnolipids, and swarming motility (**Figure 1**), indicating that the alterations in the QS-response displayed by the *nfxB** mutant are directly caused by the increased expression and activity of the MexCD-OprJ efflux system. We also demonstrated that loss of function of NfxB leads to an excessive extrusion of HHQ through the overexpressed MexCD-OprJ efflux pump, resulting in a low intracellular accumulation. Expression of *pqsABCDE* during exponential and early stationary growth phases is subjected to a positive feed-back transcriptional regulation under the control of the PqsR-(PQS/HHQ) complex (Rampioni et al., 2016). Therefore, the non-physiological HHQ extrusion through MexCD-OprJ may abrogate this positive feed-back regulation and directly cause the decrease in *pqsABCDE-phnAB* expression (**Figure 2**) and the AQs synthesis impairment (**Figure 3**) observed in the *nfxB** mutant. We also showed that this defective AQs accumulation could not be restored by adding either anthranilate or octanoate, the two PQS/HHQ main precursors (**Figures 5, 6**), reinforcing the concept that the main cause for the defective QS-response associated to *nfxB* mutations is an excessive extrusion of HHQ through MexCD-OprJ, and not of metabolic precursors as kynurenine, also extruded by MexCD-OprJ. Additionally, the presence of similar levels of PQS in the supernatants of PAO1, *nfxB** and *nfxB**Δ*mexD* growing in presence of octanoate, together with the absence of this autoinducer signal in the cell-extracts of *nfxB** (**Figure 6C**) suggests that PQS could also be a MexCD-OprJ substrate.

To sum up, here we show that the AQs production is affected by the increased efflux of HHQ by the MexCD-OprJ RND system overexpressed in the *nfxB** ciprofloxacin-resistant mutants. To note here that this type of antibiotic resistant mutants that are isolated *in vivo* from ciprofloxacin-treated patients (Jeannot et al., 2008). As a consequence, expression of the Pqs-regulon, which also comprises those PqsE-regulated genes in a PQS-independent way (Rampioni et al., 2010, 2016), is strongly altered in an *nfxB** mutant. This alteration may have minor collateral effects on the AHLs-dependent QS systems and is likely the main cause for the low virulence profile observed in antibiotic resistant mutants overproducing MexCD-OprJ.

Previous work has shown that the *P. aeruginosa* MDR efflux pump MexEF-OprN is able of extruding kynurenine and HHQ as well (Lamarche and Déziel, 2011; Olivares et al., 2012). However, different to the situation with MexCD-OprJ, the reason for the impairment in the QS response of a MexEF-OprN overexpressing mutant was mainly the extrusion of kynurenine (Olivares et al., 2012), the HHQ precursor. Similarly, both efflux pumps can accommodate the same antibiotics, although the affinity for each of them can be different. Indeed, overexpression of whatever these two efflux systems increases ciprofloxacin and chloramphenicol resistance but at different levels, being MexCD-OprJ more efficient extruding ciprofloxacin and MexEF-OprN extruding chloramphenicol (Linares et al., 2005). It has been shown that, in addition to contributing to a coordinated response of the bacterial population, several QS signal molecules (Williams, 2007; Pacheco and Sperandio, 2009; Martinez, 2014) are also involved in inter-specific communication. For example, it has been shown that AQs may function as antimicrobial compounds against *Staphylococcus aureus*, a bacterial species commonly detected together *P. aeruginosa* in polymicrobial infections (Mashburn et al., 2005; Nguyen et al., 2015; Nguyen and Oglesby-Sherrouse, 2016). Further, HHQ also is able to induce apoptosis in human mesenchymal stem cells (Holban et al., 2014), and to impair the production of several factors implicated in the innate immune response affecting the binding of the nuclear factor-κβ to its targets (Kim et al., 2010). The fact that in this work we demonstrate that MexCD-OprJ is able to extrude HHQ, altering the accumulation level of the autoinducer signals produced by *P. aeruginosa*, opens a new perspective over the potential functions of this RND efflux system in the interactions between this opportunistic pathogen and other co-existing species (including the human host); a hypothesis that remain to be explored.

The activation of the QS-response implies an increase in expression of 100s of genes, and it has been estimated that this consumes approximately 10% of *P. aeruginosa* metabolic resources (Haas, 2006). Under this panorama, QS-defective mutants, which are unable to produce different exoproducts such as siderophores or proteases relevant for nutrients uptake, could be cheaters supported by neighbor bacteria able to produce these QS-dependent factors (Wilder et al., 2011; Pollak et al., 2016). The evolution of *P. aeruginosa* along the chronic infection of the lungs of cystic fibrosis patients involves a radiative evolution, with different morphotypes, including QS-deficient mutants, co-existing in the lung of each patient (LaFayette et al., 2015). It is conceivable that the mutants lacking a proficient QS response remain in the population because they can obtain the benefits brought about by an appropriate QS response carried out by co-existing bacteria without the cost associated with it. In agreement with this hypothesis, it might be possible that antibiotic resistance mediated by MexCD-OprJ overproduction allows *nfxB** mutants to function as cheaters in the mixed populations colonizing the lung of the infected patient. This feature may have important implications concerning the persistence of antibiotic resistant mutants even in the absence of selection (Knoppel et al., 2017).

AUTHOR CONTRIBUTIONS

MA-R performed the experimental work. JO-P and JM designed the study. MA-R, JO-P, MC, CA-O, and JM contributed to the interpretation of the results and in writing the article.

ACKNOWLEDGMENTS

Thanks are given to Diana Palenzuela for her help in the assays of quorum-sensing regulated phenotypes.

REFERENCES

1. Aires, J. R., Kohler, T., Nikaido, H., and Plesiat, P. (1999). Involvement of an active efflux system in the natural resistance of *Pseudomonas aeruginosa* to aminoglycosides. *Antimicrob. Agents Chemother.* 43, 2624–2628. doi: 10.1128/ AAC.43.11.2624
2. Alcalde-Rico, M., Hernando-Amado, S., Blanco, P., and Martinez, J. L. (2016). Multidrug efflux pumps at the crossroad between antibiotic resistance and bacterial virulence. *Front. Microbiol.* 7:1483. doi: 10.3389/ fmicb.2016 .01483
3. Alonso, A., Rojo, F., and Martinez, J. L. (1999). Environmental and clinical isolates of *Pseudomonas aeruginosa* show pathogenic and biodegradative properties irrespective of their origin. *Environ. Microbiol.* 1, 421–430. doi: 10.1046/j.1462- 2920.1999.00052.x
4. Becher, A., and Schweizer, H. P. (2000). Integration-proficient *Pseudomonas aeruginosa* vectors for isolation of single-copy chromosomal lacZ and lux gene fusions. *Biotechniques* 29, 948–950. doi: 10.2144/00295bm04
5. Blanco, P., Hernando-Amado, S., Reales-Calderon, J. A., Corona, F., Lira, F., Alcalde-Rico, M., et al. (2016). Bacterial multidrug efflux pumps: much more than antibiotic resistance determinants. *Microorganisms* 4:E14. doi: 10.3390/ microorganisms4010014
6. Choi, Y., Park, H. Y., Park, S. J., Park, S. J., Kim, S. K., Ha, C., et al. (2011). Growth phase-differential quorum sensing regulation of anthranilate metabolism in *Pseudomonas aeruginosa*. *Mol. Cells* 32, 57–65. doi: 10.1007/ s10059-011-2322-6

7. Dekimpe, V., and Deziel, E. (2009). Revisiting the quorum-sensing hierarchy in *Pseudomonas aeruginosa*: the transcriptional regulator RhlR regulates LasR- specific factors. *Microbiology* 155, 712–723. doi: 10.1099/mic.0.022764-0
8. Deziel, E., Gopalan, S., Tampakaki, A. P., Lepine, F., Padfield, K. E., Saucier, M., et al. (2005). The contribution of MvfR to *Pseudomonas aeruginosa* pathogenesis and quorum sensing circuitry regulation: multiple quorum sensing-regulated genes are modulated without affecting lasRI, rhlRI or the production of N-acyl-L-homoserine lactones. *Mol. Microbiol.* 55, 998–1014. doi: 10.1111/j.1365-2958.2004.04448.x
9. Deziel, E., Lepine, F., Milot, S., He, J., Mindrinos, M. N., Tompkins, R. G., et al. (2004). Analysis of *Pseudomonas aeruginosa* 4-hydroxy-2- alkylquinolines (HAQs) reveals a role for 4-hydroxy-2-heptylquinoline in cell- to-cell communication. *Proc. Natl. Acad. Sci. U.S.A.* 101, 1339–1344. doi: 10. 1073/pnas.0307694100
10. Deziel, E., Lepine, F., Milot, S., and Villemur, R. (2003). rhlA is required for the production of a novel biosurfactant promoting swarming motility in *Pseudomonas aeruginosa*: 3-(3-hydroxyalkanoyloxy)alkanoic acids (HAAs), the precursors of rhamnolipids. *Microbiology* 149, 2005–2013. doi: 10.1099/mic.0. 26154-0
11. Dietrich, L. E., Price-Whelan, A., Petersen, A., Whiteley, M., and Newman, D. K. (2006). The phenazine pyocyanin is a terminal signalling factor in the quorum sensing network of *Pseudomonas aeruginosa*. *Mol. Microbiol.* 61, 1308–1321. doi: 10.1111/j.1365-2958.2006.05306.x
12. Diggle, S. P., Winzer, K., Chhabra, S. R., Worrall, K. E., Camara, M., and Williams, P. (2003). The *Pseudomonas aeruginosa* quinolone signal molecule overcomes the cell density-dependency of the quorum sensing hierarchy, regulates rhl-dependent genes at the onset of stationary phase and can be produced in the absence of LasR. *Mol. Microbiol.* 50, 29–43. doi: 10.1046/j.1365- 2958.2003.03672.x
13. Driscoll, J. A., Brody, S. L., and Kollef, M. H. (2007). The epidemiology, pathogenesis and treatment of *Pseudomonas aeruginosa* infections. *Drugs* 67, 351–368. doi: 10.2165/00003495-200767030-00003
14. Dubern, J. F., and Diggle, S. P. (2008). Quorum sensing by 2-alkyl-4-quinolones in *Pseudomonas aeruginosa* and other bacterial species. *Mol. Biosyst.* 4, 882–888. doi: 10.1039/b803796p
15. Dulcey, C. E., Dekimpe, V., Fauvelle, D. A., Milot, S., Groleau, M. C., Doucet, N., et al. (2013). The end of an old hypothesis: the pseudomonas signaling molecules 4-hydroxy-2-alkylquinolines derive from fatty acids, not 3-ketofatty acids. *Chem. Biol.* 20, 1481–1491. doi: 10.1016/j.chembiol.2013. 09.021
16. Essar, D. W., Eberly, L., Hadero, A., and Crawford, I. P. (1990). Identification and characterization of genes for a second anthranilate synthase in *Pseudomonas aeruginosa*: interchangeability of the two anthranilate synthases and evolutionary implications. *J. Bacteriol.* 172, 884–900. doi: 10.1128/jb.172.2.884-900.1990
17. Evans, K., Passador, L., Srikumar, R., Tsang, E., Nezezon, J., and Poole, K. (1998). Influence of the MexAB-OprM multidrug efflux system on quorum sensing in *Pseudomonas aeruginosa*. *J. Bacteriol.* 180, 5443–5447.
18. Fajardo, A., Martinez-Martin, N., Mercadillo, M., Galan, J. C., Ghysels, B., Matthijs, S., et al. (2008). The neglected intrinsic resistome of bacterial pathogens. *PLoS One* 3:e1619. doi: 10.1371/journal.pone.0001619
19. Farrow, J. M. III, and Pesci, E. C. (2007). Two distinct pathways supply anthranilate as a precursor of the *Pseudomonas* quinolone signal. *J. Bacteriol.* 189, 3425– 3433. doi: 10.1128/JB.00209-07
20. Farrow, J. M. III, Sund, Z. M., Ellison, M. L., Wade, D. S., Coleman, J. P., and Pesci, E. C. (2008). PqsE functions independently of PqsR-*Pseudomonas* quinolone signal and enhances the rhl quorum-sensing system. *J. Bacteriol.* 190, 7043–7051. doi: 10.1128/JB.00753-08
21. Fletcher, M. P., Diggle, S. P., Camara, M., and Williams, P. (2007a). Biosensor-based assays for PQS, HHQ and related 2-alkyl-4-quinolone quorum sensing signal molecules. *Nat. Protoc.* 2, 1254–1262.
22. Fletcher, M. P., Diggle, S. P., Crusz, S. A., Chhabra, S. R., Camara, M., and Williams, P. (2007b). A dual biosensor for 2-alkyl-4-quinolone quorum-sensing signal molecules. *Environ. Microbiol.* 9, 2683–2693.
23. Gallagher, L. A., Mcknight, S. L., Kuznetsova, M. S., Pesci, E. C., and Manoil, C. (2002). Functions required for extracellular quinolone signaling by *Pseudomonas aeruginosa*. *J. Bacteriol.* 184, 6472–6480. doi: 10.1128/JB.184.23. 6472-6480.2002
24. Garcia-Leon, G., Salgado, F., Oliveros, J. C., Sanchez, M. B., and Martinez, J. L. (2014). Interplay between intrinsic and acquired resistance to quinolones in *Stenotrophomonas maltophilia*. *Environ. Microbiol.* 16, 1282–1296. doi: 10. 1111/1462-2920.12408
25. Green, S. K., Schroth, M. N., Cho, J. J., Kominos, S. K., and Vitanza-Jack, V. B. (1974). Agricultural plants and soil as a reservoir for *Pseudomonas aeruginosa*. *Appl. Microbiol.* 28, 987–991.
26. Haas, D. (2006). Cost of cell-cell signalling in *Pseudomonas aeruginosa*: why it can pay to be signal-blind. *Nat. Rev. Microbiol.* 4:562; author rely 562.
27. Hammond, J. H., Hebert, W. P., Naimie, A., Ray, K., Van Gelder, R. D., Digiandomenico, A., et al. (2016). Environmentally endemic *Pseudomonas aeruginosa* strains with mutations in lasR are associated with increased disease severity in corneal ulcers. *mSphere* 1:e00140-16. doi: 10.1128/mSphere.001 40-16
28. Hazan, R., He, J., Xiao, G., Dekimpe, V., Apidianakis, Y., Lesic, B., et al. (2010). Homeostatic interplay between bacterial cell-cell signaling and iron in virulence. *PLoS Pathog.* 6:e1000810. doi: 10.1371/journal.ppat.1000810
29. Hernando-Amado, S., Blanco, P., Alcalde-Rico, M., Corona, F., Reales-Calderon, J. A., Sanchez, M. B., et al. (2016). Multidrug efflux pumps as main players in intrinsic and acquired resistance to antimicrobials. *Drug Resist. Updat.* 28, 13–27. doi: 10.1016/j.drup.2016.06.007
30. Hoang, T. T., Karkhoff-Schweizer, R. R., Kutchma, A. J., and Schweizer, H. P. (1998). A broad-host-range Flp-FRT recombination system for site-specific excision of chromosomally-located DNA sequences: application for isolation of unmarked *Pseudomonas aeruginosa* mutants. *Gene* 212, 77–86. doi: 10.1016/ S0378-1119(98)00130-9
31. Holban, A. M., Bleotu, C., Chifiriuc, M. C., Bezirtzoglou, E., and Lazar, V. (2014). Role of *Pseudomonas aeruginosa* quorum sensing (QS) molecules on the viability and cytokine profile of human mesenchymal stem cells. *Virulence* 5, 303–310. doi: 10.4161/viru.27571
32. Jeannot, K., Elsen, S., Kohler, T., Attree, I., Van Delden, C., and Plesiat, P. (2008). Resistance and virulence of *Pseudomonas aeruginosa* clinical strains overproducing the MexCD-OprJ efflux pump. *Antimicrob. Agents Chemother.* 52, 2455–2462. doi: 10.1128/AAC.01107-07
33. Kasper, S. H., Bonocora, R. P., Wade, J. T., Musah, R. A., and Cady, N. C. (2016). Chemical inhibition of kynureninase reduces *Pseudomonas aeruginosa* quorum sensing and virulence factor expression. *ACS Chem. Biol.* 11, 1106–1117. doi: 10.1021/acschembio.5b01082
34. Kessler, E., and Safrin, M. (2014). Elastinolytic and proteolytic enzymes. *Methods Mol. Biol.* 1149, 135–169. doi: 10.1007/978-1-4939-0473-0_13
35. Kim, K., Kim, Y. U., Koh, B. H., Hwang, S. S., Kim, S. H., Lepine, F., et al. (2010). HHQ and PQS, two *Pseudomonas aeruginosa* quorum-sensing molecules, down-regulate the innate immune responses through the nuclear factor- kappaB pathway. *Immunology* 129, 578–588. doi: 10.1111/j.1365-2567.2009.0 3160.x
36. Knoppel, A., Nasvall, J., and Andersson, D. I. (2017). Evolution of antibiotic resistance without antibiotic exposure. *Antimicrob. Agents Chemother.* 61:e01495-17. doi: 10.1128/AAC.01495-17
37. Kohler, T., Michea-Hamzehpour, M., Henze, U., Gotoh, N., Curty, L. K., and Pechere, J. C. (1997). Characterization of MexE-MexF-OprN, a positively regulated multidrug efflux system of *Pseudomonas aeruginosa*. *Mol. Microbiol.* 23, 345–354. doi: 10.1046/j.1365-2958.1997.2281594.x
38. Kohler, T., Van Delden, C., Curty, L. K., Hamzehpour, M. M., and Pechere, J. C. (2001). Overexpression of the MexEF-OprN multidrug efflux system affects cell-to-cell signaling in *Pseudomonas aeruginosa*. *J. Bacteriol.* 183, 5213–5222. doi: 10.1128/JB.183.18.5213-5222.2001
39. LaFayette, S. L., Houle, D., Beaudoin, T., Wojewodka, G., Radzioch, D., Hoffman, L. R., et al. (2015). Cystic fibrosis-adapted *Pseudomonas aeruginosa* quorum sensing lasR mutants cause hyperinflammatory responses. *Sci. Adv.* 1:e1500199. doi: 10.1126/sciadv.1500199
40. Lamarche, M. G., and Déziel, E. (2011). MexEF-OprN efflux pump exports the *Pseudomonas* quinolone signal (PQS) precursor HHQ (4-hydroxy-2- heptylquinoline). *PLoS One* 6:e24310. doi: 10.1371/journal.pone.0024310
41. Lepine, F., Deziel, E., Milot, S., and Rahme, L. G. (2003). A stable isotope dilution assay for the quantification of the *Pseudomonas* quinolone signal in *Pseudomonas aeruginosa* cultures. *Biochim. Biophys. Acta* 1622, 36–41. doi: 10.1016/S0304-4165(03) 00103-X

42. Li, X. Z., Nikaido, H., and Poole, K. (1995). Role of mexA-mexB-oprM in antibiotic efflux in *Pseudomonas aeruginosa*. *Antimicrob. Agents Chemother.* 39, 1948– 1953. doi: 10.1128/AAC.39.9.1948
43. Linares, J. F., Lopez, J. A., Camafeita, E., Albar, J. P., Rojo, F., and Martinez, J. L. (2005). Overexpression of the multidrug efflux pumps MexCD-OprJ and MexEF-OprN is associated with a reduction of type III secretion in *Pseudomonas aeruginosa*. *J. Bacteriol.* 187, 1384–1391. doi: 10.1128/JB.187.4. 1384-1391.2005
44. Livak, K. J., and Schmittgen, T. D. (2001). Analysis of relative gene expression data using real-time quantitative PCR and the 2- ⊠ ⊠ CT Method. *Methods* 25, 402–408. doi: 10.1006/meth.2001.1262
45. Llanes, C., Hocquet, D., Vogne, C., Benali-Baitich, D., Neuwirth, C., and Plesiat, P. (2004). Clinical strains of *Pseudomonas aeruginosa* overproducing MexAB-OprM and MexXY efflux pumps simultaneously. *Antimicrob. Agents Chemother.* 48, 1797–1802. doi: 10.1128/AAC.48.5.1797-1802.2004
46. Lopez-Causape, C., Rubio, R., Cabot, G., and Oliver, A. (2018). Evolution of the *Pseudomonas aeruginosa* aminoglycoside mutational resistome in vitro and in the cystic fibrosis setting. *Antimicrob. Agents Chemother.* 62, e2583–e2517. doi: 10.1128/AAC.02583-17
47. Martinez, J. L. (2014). Interkingdom signaling and its consequences for human health. *Virulence* 5, 243–244. doi: 10.4161/viru.28073
48. Martinez, J. L., Sanchez, M. B., Martinez-Solano, L., Hernandez, A., Garmendia, L., Fajardo, A., et al. (2009). Functional role of bacterial multidrug efflux pumps in microbial natural ecosystems. *FEMS Microbiol. Rev.* 33, 430–449. doi: 10.1111/ j.1574-6976.2008.00157.x
49. Martinez-Solano, L., Macia, M. D., Fajardo, A., Oliver, A., and Martinez, J. L. (2008). Chronic *Pseudomonas aeruginosa* infection in chronic obstructive pulmonary disease. *Clin. Infect. Dis.* 47, 1526–1533. doi: 10.1086/593186
50. Maseda, H., Sawada, I., Saito, K., Uchiyama, H., Nakae, T., and Nomura, N. (2004). Enhancement of the mexAB-oprM efflux pump expression by a quorum- sensing autoinducer and its cancellation by a regulator, MexT, of the mexEF- oprN efflux pump operon in *Pseudomonas aeruginosa*. *Antimicrob. Agents Chemother.* 48, 1320–1328. doi: 10.1128/AAC.48.4.1320-1328.2004
51. Mashburn, L. M., Jett, A. M., Akins, D. R., and Whiteley, M. (2005). *Staphylococcus aureus* serves as an iron source for *Pseudomonas aeruginosa* during in vivo coculture. *J. Bacteriol.* 187, 554–566. doi: 10.1128/JB.187.2.554-566.2005
52. Maura, D., Hazan, R., Kitao, T., Ballok, A. E., and Rahme, L. G. (2016). Evidence for direct control of virulence and defense gene circuits by the Pseudomonas aeruginosa quorum sensing regulator. MvfR. *Sci. Rep.* 6:34083. doi: 10.1038/ srep34083
53. McKnight, S. L., Iglewski, B. H., and Pesci, E. C. (2000). The *Pseudomonas* quinolone signal regulates rhl quorum sensing in *Pseudomonas aeruginosa*. *J. Bacteriol.* 182, 2702–2708. doi: 10.1128/JB.182.10.2702-2708.2000
54. Mellbye, B., and Schuster, M. (2014). Physiological framework for the regulation of quorum sensing-dependent public goods in *Pseudomonas aeruginosa*. *J. Bacteriol.* 196, 1155–1164. doi: 10.1128/JB.01223-13
55. Minagawa, S., Inami, H., Kato, T., Sawada, S., Yasuki, T., Miyairi, S., et al. (2012). RND type efflux pump system MexAB-OprM of *Pseudomonas aeruginosa* selects bacterial languages, 3-oxo-acyl-homoserine lactones, for cell-to-cell communication. *BMC Microbiol.* 12:70. doi: 10.1186/1471-2180-12-70
56. Mine, T., Morita, Y., Kataoka, A., Mizushima, T., and Tsuchiya, T. (1999). Expression in *Escherichia coli* of a new multidrug efflux pump, MexXY, from *Pseudomonas aeruginosa*. *Antimicrob. Agents Chemother.* 43, 415–417. doi: 10. 1128/AAC.43.2.415
57. Morales, G., Wiehlmann, L., Gudowius, P., Van Delden, C., Tummler, B., Martinez,
58. J. L., et al. (2004). Structure of *Pseudomonas aeruginosa* populations analyzed by single nucleotide polymorphism and pulsed-field gel electrophoresis genotyping. *J. Bacteriol.* 186, 4228–4237. doi: 10.1128/JB.186.13.4228-4237. 2004
59. Mukherjee, S., Moustafa, D. A., Stergioula, V., Smith, C. D., Goldberg, J. B., and Bassler, B. L. (2018). The PqsE and RhlR proteins are an autoinducer synthase- receptor pair that control virulence and biofilm development in *Pseudomonas aeruginosa*. *Proc. Natl. Acad. Sci. U.S.A.* 115, E9411–E9418. doi: 10.1073/pnas. 1814023115
60. Nguyen, A. T., Jones, J. W., Ruge, M. A., Kane, M. A., and Oglesby-Sherrouse, A. G. (2015). Iron depletion enhances production of antimicrobials by *Pseudomonas aeruginosa*. *J. Bacteriol.* 197, 2265–2275. doi: 10.1128/JB.00072-15
61. Nguyen, A. T., and Oglesby-Sherrouse, A. G. (2016). Interactions between *Pseudomonas aeruginosa* and *Staphylococcus aureus* during co-cultivations and polymicrobial infections. *Appl. Microbiol. Biotechnol.* 100, 6141–6148. doi: 10. 1007/s00253-016-7596-3
62. Obritsch, M. D., Fish, D. N., Maclaren, R., and Jung, R. (2005). Nosocomial infections due to multidrug-resistant *Pseudomonas aeruginosa*: epidemiology and treatment options. *Pharmacotherapy* 25, 1353–1364. doi: 10.1592/phco. 2005.25.10.1353
63. Olivares, J., Alvarez-Ortega, C., Linares, J. F., Rojo, F., Kohler, T., and Martinez, L. (2012). Overproduction of the multidrug efflux pump MexEF-OprN does not impair *Pseudomonas aeruginosa* fitness in competition tests, but produces specific changes in bacterial regulatory networks. *Environ. Microbiol.* 14, 1968– 1981. doi: 10.1111/j.1462-2920.2012.02727.x
64. Olivares, J., Alvarez-Ortega, C., and Martinez, J. L. (2014). Metabolic compensation of fitness costs associated with overexpression of the multidrug efflux pump MexEF-OprN in *Pseudomonas aeruginosa*. *Antimicrob. Agents Chemother.* 58, 3904–3913. doi: 10.1128/AAC.00121-14
65. Olivares Pacheco, J., Alvarez-Ortega, C., Alcalde Rico, M., and Martinez, J. L. (2017). Metabolic compensation of fitness costs is a general outcome for antibiotic-resistant *Pseudomonas aeruginosa* mutants overexpressing efflux pumps. *mBio* 8:e00500-17. doi: 10.1128/mBio.00500-17
66. Oliver, A., Mulet, X., Lopez-Causape, C., and Juan, C. (2015). The increasing threat of *Pseudomonas aeruginosa* high-risk clones. *Drug Resist. Updat.* 2, 41–59. doi: 10.1016/j.drup.2015.08.002
67. Pacheco, A. R., and Sperandio, V. (2009). Inter-kingdom signaling: chemical language between bacteria and host. *Curr. Opin. Microbiol.* 12, 192–198. doi: 10.1016/j.mib.2009.01.006
68. Palmer, G. C., Jorth, P. A., and Whiteley, M. (2013). The role of two *Pseudomonas aeruginosa* anthranilate synthases in tryptophan and quorum signal production. *Microbiology* 159, 959–969. doi: 10.1099/mic.0.063065-0
69. Palmer, G. C., and Whiteley, M. (2015). Metabolism and Pathogenicity of *Pseudomonas aeruginosa* Infections in the lungs of Individuals with cystic fibrosis. *Microbiol Spectr.* 3, 1–20. doi: 10.1128/microbiolspec.MBP-0003-2014 Pearson, J. P., Pesci, E. C., and Iglewski, B. H. (1997). Roles of *Pseudomonas aeruginosa* las and rhl quorum-sensing systems in control of elastase and rhamnolipid biosynthesis genes. *J. Bacteriol.* 179, 5756–5767. doi: 10.1128/jb. 179.18.5756-5767.1997
70. Pearson, J. P., Van Delden, C., and Iglewski, B. H. (1999). Active efflux and diffusion are involved in transport of *Pseudomonas aeruginosa* cell-to-cell signals. *J. Bacteriol.* 181, 1203–1210.
71. Pesci, E. C., Pearson, J. P., Seed, P. C., and Iglewski, B. H. (1997). Regulation of las and rhl quorum sensing in *Pseudomonas aeruginosa*. *J. Bacteriol.* 179, 3127–3132. doi: 10.1128/jb.179.10.3127-3132.1997
72. Piddock, L. J. (2006). Multidrug-resistance efflux pumps - not just for resistance. *Nat. Rev. Microbiol.* 4, 629–636. doi: 10.1038/nrmicro1464
73. Pollak, S., Omer-Bendori, S., Even-Tov, E., Lipsman, V., Bareia, T., Ben-Zion, I., et al. (2016). Facultative cheating supports the coexistence of diverse quorum- sensing alleles. *Proc. Natl. Acad. Sci. U.S.A.* 113, 2152–2157. doi: 10.1073/pnas. 1520615113
74. Poole, K., Gotoh, N., Tsujimoto, H., Zhao, Q., Wada, A., Yamasaki, T., et al. (1996). Overexpression of the mexC-mexD-oprJ efflux operon in nfxB-type multidrug- resistant strains of *Pseudomonas aeruginosa*. *Mol. Microbiol.* 21, 713–724. doi: 10.1046/j.1365-2958.1996.281397.x
75. Rampioni, G., Falcone, M., Heeb, S., Frangipani, E., Fletcher, M. P., Dubern, J. F., et al. (2016). Unravelling the genome-wide contributions of specific 2-Alkyl- 4-quinolones and PqsE to quorum sensing in *Pseudomonas aeruginosa*. *PLoS Pathog.* 12:e1006029. doi: 10.1371/journal.ppat.1006029
76. Rampioni, G., Pustelny, C., Fletcher, M. P., Wright, V. J., Bruce, M., Rumbaugh, P., et al. (2010). Transcriptomic analysis reveals a global alkyl-quinolone- independent regulatory role for PqsE in facilitating the environmental adaptation of *Pseudomonas aeruginosa* to plant and animal hosts. *Environ. Microbiol.* 12, 1659–1673. doi: 10.1111/j.1462-2920.2010.02214.x
77. Romling, U., Wingender, J., Muller, H., and Tummler, B. (1994). A major *Pseudomonas aeruginosa* clone common to patients and aquatic habitats. *Appl. Environ. Microbiol.* 60, 1734–1738.

78. Sanchez, P., Linares, J. F., Ruiz-Diez, B., Campanario, E., Navas, A., Baquero, F., et al. (2002). Fitness of in vitro selected *Pseudomonas aeruginosa* nalB and nfxB multidrug resistant mutants. *J. Antimicrob. Chemother.* 50, 657–664. doi: 10.1093/jac/dkf185
79. Simon, R., O'connell, M., Labes, M., and Puhler, A. (1986). Plasmid vectors for the genetic analysis and manipulation of rhizobia and other gram-negative bacteria. *Methods Enzymol.* 118, 640–659. doi: 10.1016/0076-6879(86)18106-7
80. Sobel, M. L., Neshat, S., and Poole, K. (2005). Mutations in PA2491 (mexS) promote MexT-dependent mexEF-oprN expression and multidrug resistance in a clinical strain of *Pseudomonas aeruginosa. J. Bacteriol.* 187, 1246–1253. doi: 10.1128/JB.187.4.1246-1253.2005
81. Stickland, H. G., Davenport, P. W., Lilley, K. S., Griffin, J. L., and Welch, M. (2010). Mutation of nfxB causes global changes in the physiology and metabolism of *Pseudomonas aeruginosa. J. Proteome Res.* 9, 2957–2967. doi: 10.1021/ pr9011415
82. Stover, C. K., Pham, X. Q., Erwin, A. L., Mizoguchi, S. D., Warrener, P., Hickey, M. J., et al. (2000). Complete genome sequence of *Pseudomonas aeruginosa* PAO1, an opportunistic pathogen. *Nature* 406, 959–964. doi: 10.1038/35023079 Swift, S., Karlyshev, A. V., Fish, L., Durant, E. L., Winson, M. K., Chhabra,
83. S. R., et al. (1997). Quorum sensing in Aeromonas hydrophila and Aeromonas salmonicida: identification of the LuxRI homologs AhyRI and AsaRI and their cognate N-acylhomoserine lactone signal molecules. *J. Bacteriol.* 179, 5271–5281. doi: 10.1128/jb.179.17.5271-5281.1997
84. Talwalkar, J. S., and Murray, T. S. (2016). The approach to *Pseudomonas aeruginosa* in cystic fibrosis. *Clin. Chest. Med.* 37, 69–81. doi: 10.1016/j.ccm.2015.10.004 Tian, Z. X., Fargier, E., Mac Aogain, M., Adams, C., Wang, Y. P., and O'gara, F.
85. (2009a). Transcriptome profiling defines a novel regulon modulated by the LysR-type transcriptional regulator MexT in *Pseudomonas aeruginosa. Nucleic Acids Res.* 37, 7546–7559. doi: 10.1093/nar/gkp828
86. Tian, Z. X., Mac Aogain, M., O'connor, H. F., Fargier, E., Mooij, M. J., Adams, C., et al. (2009b). MexT modulates virulence determinants in *Pseudomonas aeruginosa* independent of the MexEF-OprN efflux pump. *Microb. Pathog.* 47, 237–241. doi: 10.1016/j.micpath.2009.08.003
87. Vila, J., Fabrega, A., Roca, I., Hernandez, A., and Martinez, J. L. (2011). Efflux pumps as an important mechanism for quinolone resistance. *Adv. Enzymol. Relat. Areas Mol. Biol.* 77, 167–235. doi: 10.1002/9780470920541.ch5
88. Vila, J., and Martínez, J. L. (2008). Clinical impact of the over-expression of efflux pump in nonfermentative gram-negative bacilli, development of efflux pump inhibitors. *Curr. Drug Targets* 9, 797–807. doi: 10.2174/138945008785747806
89. Wade, D. S., Calfee, M. W., Rocha, E. R., Ling, E. A., Engstrom, E., Coleman, J. P., et al. (2005). Regulation of *Pseudomonas* quinolone signal synthesis in *Pseudomonas aeruginosa. J. Bacteriol.* 187, 4372–4380. doi: 10.1128/JB.187.13. 4372-4380.2005
90. Walker, T. S., Bais, H. P., Deziel, E., Schweizer, H. P., Rahme, L. G., Fall, R., et al. (2004). *Pseudomonas aeruginosa*-plant root interactions. pathogenicity, biofilm formation, and root exudation. *Plant Physiol.* 134, 320–331. doi: 10.1104/pp. 103.027888
91. Welsh, M. A., and Blackwell, H. E. (2016). Chemical genetics reveals environment-specific roles for quorum sensing circuits in *Pseudomonas aeruginosa. Cell Chem. Biol.* 23, 361–369. doi: 10.1016/j.chembiol.2016.01.006
92. Wilder, C. N., Diggle, S. P., and Schuster, M. (2011). Cooperation and cheating in *Pseudomonas aeruginosa*: the roles of the las, rhl and pqs quorum-sensing systems. *ISME J.* 5, 1332–1343. doi: 10.1038/ismej.2011.13
93. Williams, P. (2007). Quorum sensing, communication and cross-kingdom signalling in the bacterial world. *Microbiology* 153, 3923–3938. doi: 10.1099/ mic.0.2007/012856-0
94. Williams, P., and Camara, M. (2009). Quorum sensing and environmental adaptation in *Pseudomonas aeruginosa*: a tale of regulatory networks and multifunctional signal molecules. *Curr. Opin. Microbiol.* 12, 182–191. doi: 10.1016/j.mib.2009.01.005
95. Williams, P., Winzer, K., Chan, W. C., and Camara, M. (2007). Look who's talking: communication and quorum sensing in the bacterial world. *Philos. Trans. R. Soc. Lond. B Biol. Sci.* 362, 1119–1134. doi: 10.1098/rstb.2007.2039
96. Winson, M. K., Swift, S., Fish, L., Throup, J. P., Jorgensen, F., Chhabra, S. R., et al. (1998). Construction and analysis of luxCDABE-based plasmid sensors for investigating N-acyl homoserine lactone-mediated quorum sensing. *FEMS Microbiol. Lett.* 163, 185–192. doi: 10.1111/j.1574-6968.1998.tb13044.x
97. Wittgens, A., Tiso, T., Arndt, T. T., Wenk, P., Hemmerich, J., Muller, C., et al. (2011). Growth independent rhamnolipid production from glucose using the non-pathogenic Pseudomonas putida KT2440. *Microb Cell Fact* 10:80. doi: 10.1186/1475-2859-10-80
98. Yates, E. A., Philipp, B., Buckley, C., Atkinson, S., Chhabra, S. R., Sockett, R. E., et al. (2002). N-acylhomoserine lactones undergo lactonolysis in a pH-, temperature-, and acyl chain length-dependent manner during growth of *Yersinia pseudotuberculosis* and *Pseudomonas aeruginosa. Infect. Immun.* 70, 5635–5646. doi: 10.1128/IAI.70.10.5635-5646.2002
99. Zaborskyte, G., Andersen, J. B., Kragh, K. N., and Ciofu, O. (2017). Real- time monitoring of nfxB mutant occurrence and dynamics in *Pseudomonas aeruginosa* biofilm exposed to subinhibitory concentrations of ciprofloxacin. *Antimicrob. Agents Chemother.* 61:e02292-16. doi: 10.1128/AAC.02292-16

11

EF-Tu from Non-Typeable *Haemophilus influenzae* is an Immunogenic Surface-Exposed Protein Targeted by Bactericidal Antibodies

*Oskar Thofte, Yu-Ching Su, Marta Brant, Nils Littorin, Benjamin Luke Duell, Vera Alvarado, Farshid Jalalvand and Kristian Riesbeck**

Clinical Microbiology, Department of Translational Medicine, Faculty of Medicine, Lund University, Malmö, Sweden

Correspondence:
Kristian Riesbeck
kristian.riesbeck@med.lu.se

Non-typeable *Haemophilus influenzae* (NTHi), a commensal organism in pre-school children, is an opportunistic pathogen causing respiratory tract infections including acute otitis media. Adults suffering from chronic obstructive pulmonary disease (COPD) are persistently colonized by NTHi. Previous research has suggested that, in some bacterial species, the intracellular elongation factor thermo-unstable (EF-Tu) can moonlight as a surface protein upon host encounter. The aim of this study was to determine whether EF-Tu localizes to the surface of *H. influenzae*, and if such surface-associated EF-Tu is a target for bactericidal antibodies. Using flow cytometry, transmission immunoelectron microscopy, and epitope mapping, we demonstrated that EF-Tu is exposed at the surface of NTHi, and identified immunodominant epitopes of this protein. Rabbits immunized with whole-cell NTHi produced significantly more immunoglobulin G (IgG) directed against EF-Tu than against the NTHi outer membrane proteins D and F as revealed by enzyme-linked immunosorbent assays. Chemical cleavage of NTHi EF-Tu by cyanogen bromide (CNBr) followed by immunoblotting showed that the immunodominant epitopes were located within the central and C-terminal regions of the protein. Peptide epitope mapping by dot blot analysis further revealed four different immunodominant peptide sequences; EF-Tu$^{41-65}$, EF-Tu$^{161-185}$, EF-Tu$^{221-245}$, and EF-Tu$^{281-305}$. These epitopes were confirmed to be surface-exposed and accessible by peptide-specific antibodies in flow cytometry. We also analyzed whether antibodies raised against NTHi EF-Tu cross-react with other respiratory tract pathogens. Anti-EF-Tu IgG significantly detected EF-Tu on unencapsulated bacteria, including the Gram-negative *H. parainfluenzae, H. haemolyticus, Moraxella catarrhalis* and various Gram-positive *Streptococci* of the oral microbiome. In contrast, considerably less EF-Tu was observed at the surface of encapsulated bacteria including *H. influenzae* serotype b (Hib) and *Streptococcus pneumoniae* (e.g., serotype 3 and 4). Removal of the capsule, as exemplified by Hib RM804, resulted in increased EF-Tu surface density. Finally, anti-NTHi EF-Tu IgG promoted complement-dependent bacterial killing of NTHi and other unencapsulated Gram-negative bacteria as well as opsonophagocytosis of Gram-positive bacteria. In conclusion, our data demonstrate that NTHi EF-Tu is surface-exposed and recognized by antibodies mediating host innate immunity against NTHi in addition to other unencapsulated respiratory tract bacteria.

Keywords: antibody response, elongation factor Tu (EF-Tu), epitope mapping, *Haemophilus influenzae* (Hi), immunization, rabbit, opsonophagocytosis, serum resistance

INTRODUCTION

The Gram-negative bacterium *Haemophilus influenzae* is subdivided into two categories based on the presence of a polysaccharide capsule; the encapsulated *H. influenzae* is classified as serotypes a-f and unencapsulated non-typeable *H. influenzae* (NTHi). Introduction of a vaccine against *H. influenzae* type b (Hib) in the 1990s substantially reduced Hib infections. NTHi is currently the most common cause of *Haemophilus* infections in humans, and any vaccine against NTHi does not exist. The bacterium is rarely invasive, causing sepsis predominantly in the elderly or in patients with co-morbidities (1). However, NTHi is commonly associated with respiratory tract infections. Pre-school children, harboring NTHi, *Moraxella catarrhalis*, and *Streptococcus pneumoniae* as commensals, are at the highest risk. In this age group, NTHi often causes acute otitis media (AOM) and sinusitis, occasionally upon co-infection with the common cold viruses (2). In the adult population, NTHi mainly infects and persistently colonizes patients with chronic obstructive pulmonary disease (COPD) (3). However, more virulent or antimicrobial-resistant sequence types of NTHi, such as sequence type (ST) 14, can cause severe sinusitis, bronchitis, and pneumonia in healthy adults (4).

Recent research, exploring prevention of NTHi infections, has identified several protein-based NTHi outer membrane proteins that potentially also can be used as vaccine candidates (5–7). One example is the adhesin *H. influenzae* protein F that interacts with the extracellular matrix proteins laminin and vitronectin, the latter of which inhibits the terminal pathway of complement activation (8, 9). Another example is Protein D, an enzyme with glycerophosphodiesterase activity that is currently included as a carrier protein in a 10-valent conjugated pneumococcal vaccine (Synflorix®) (10, 11).

Elongation factor thermo unstable (EF-Tu) is an essential bacterial protein that constitutes up to 5% of the total cell content (12). In *E. coli*, the genes *tufA* and *tufB* encode 40- to 45-kDa EF-Tu proteins, each containing three structural domains and varying only in their C-termini (13). EF-Tu, which binds various guanosine-containing polyphosphates, functions in polypeptide elongation with aminoacyl transfer RNAs and guanosine triphosphate. Early studies have shown that EF-Tu is located at the surface in *E. coli* (14). Subsequent studies have demonstrated that EF-Tu is surface-exposed in other bacterial species, including Gram-negative *Acinetobacter baumanii*, *Borrelia burgdorferi* and *Pseudomonas aeruginosa* (15–17), and Gram-positive *Staphylococcus aureus* and *Streptococcus pneumoniae* (18, 19). Extracellular localization of the translation elongation factor 1 (Tef1) of *Candida albicans*, an ortholog of EF-Tu, has also been reported (20).

Extracellular EF-Tu was initially considered a contaminant from the cytoplasm due to its high abundance in the cell. However, EF-Tu was eventually recognized as a moonlighting protein playing several roles depending on the bacterial species in question. In addition to EF-Tu, other proteins initially identified as intracellular have been described to have extracellular functions (21). EF-Tu-dependent interactions with several host molecules have been verified both biochemically and functionally. For example, *P. aeruginosa*, commonly infecting chronic wounds and patients suffering from cystic fibrosis, uses EF-Tu to attract human plasma proteins such as Factor H, Factor H-like protein, and plasminogen, thereby manipulating the activation of the alternative complement pathway (17). Moreover, *S. pneumoniae* EF-Tu has been found to increase bacterial survival in the presence of host components (19). Extracellular matrix proteins represent other putative targets for bacterial EF-Tu; *Lactobacillus casei* and *Mycoplasma pneumoniae* use EF-Tu as a receptor for fibronectin (22–24).

The moonlighting function of EF-Tu in exploiting the endogenous inhibitors of the complement system represents one of the strategies used by pathogens to evade host innate immunity (17, 19). Evasion of the complement system is also important for the pathogenicity of NTHi (25). However, the host, unable to modify the innate defense system *per se*, also relies on the adaptive immune system and the generation of high-affinity antibodies. Production of a wide repertoire of antibodies against bacterial proteins, such as EF-Tu, begins in the first year after birth and continues throughout life as a strategy to defend against intruding bacteria. Interestingly, an immunoproteome analysis revealed that infection with Shiga toxin-producing *E. coli* (STEC) significantly increased levels of serum immunoglobulin G (IgG) directed against EF-Tu (26). Sera from patients suffering from meningococcal disease also contain higher concentrations of IgG against EF-Tu (27).

Considering these findings, the present study sought to determine whether EF-Tu is also present on the surface of the respiratory pathogen NTHi. Moreover, we wanted to assess whether an immune response against EF-Tu is elicited after exposure to NTHi cells. We also determined whether anti-NTHi EF-Tu IgG recognizes other bacterial species in the respiratory tract microbiome.

RESULTS

Unencapsulated *Haemophilus influenzae* Displays EF-Tu at the Cell Surface

To analyze whether *H. influenzae* carries EF-Tu at its cell surface, we raised anti-EF-Tu polyclonal antibodies (pAbs) by immunizing rabbits with manufactured recombinant EF-Tu derived from *H. influenzae*. Rabbit pAbs, produced as a result of an immune response elicited by recombinant EF-Tu, readily detected EF-Tu on the cell surface of clinical NTHi strains, albeit at different levels, as revealed by flow cytometry (**Figures 1A,B**) and transmission immunoelectron microscopy (TEM) (**Figure 1C**). In contrast to NTHi, encapsulated *H. influenzae* type b (Hib) strain Eagan and harbored less surface-exposed EF-Tu (**Figure 1D**). Hib MinnA carried, however, EF-Tu to the same level as NTHi. Importantly, removal of the capsule from Hib Eagan promoted exposure of EF-Tu, as evidenced by the unencapsulated mutant Hib Eagan designated RM804 (**Figures 1E,F**). These results suggested that mainly unencapsulated *H. influenzae*, that is, NTHi contains antibody-accessible EF-Tu on its outer membrane.

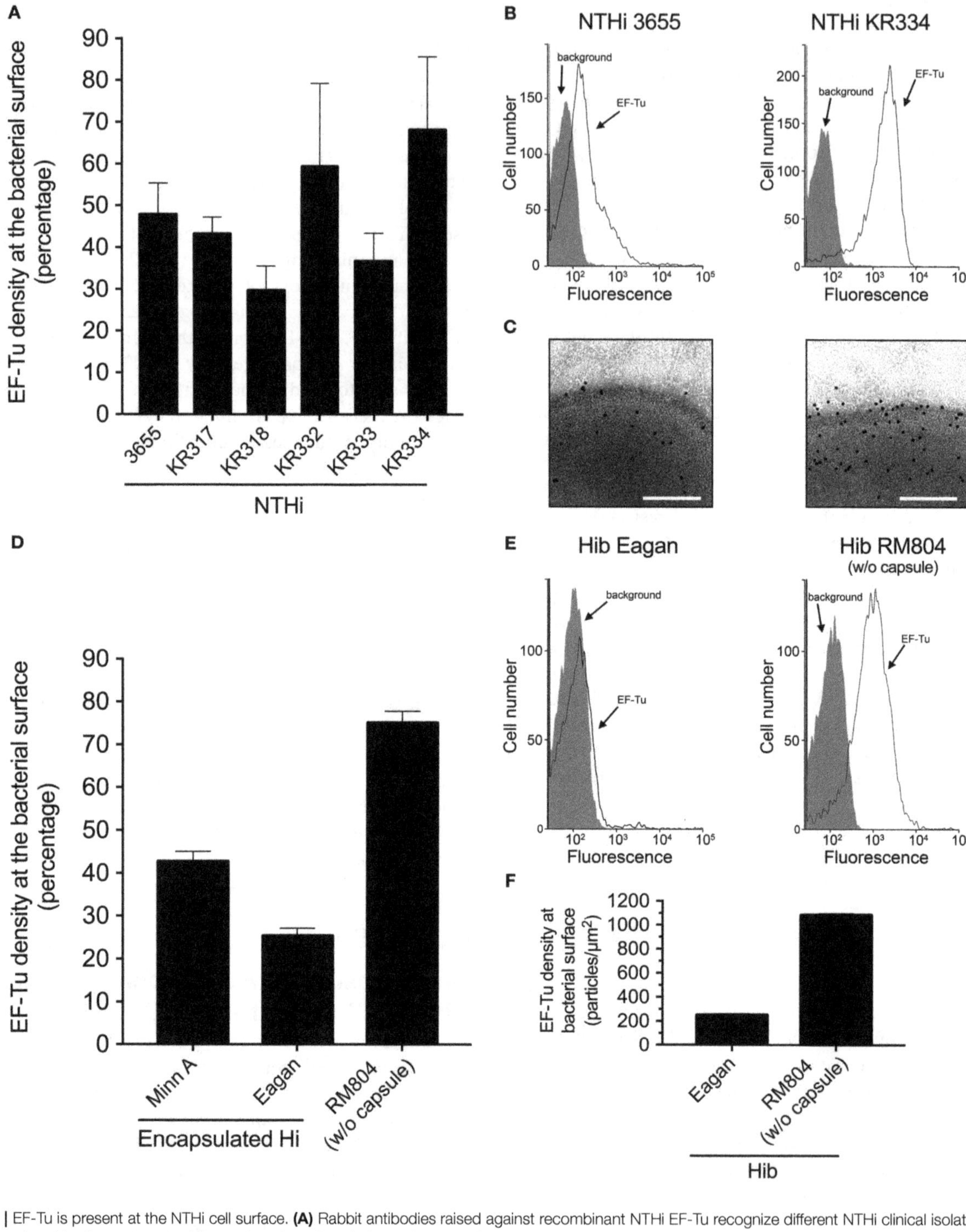

FIGURE 1 | EF-Tu is present at the NTHi cell surface. **(A)** Rabbit antibodies raised against recombinant NTHi EF-Tu recognize different NTHi clinical isolates. NTHi ($n = 6$) were analyzed by flow cytometry. Mean values from three independent experiments are shown and error bars represent standard error of the mean (SEM). **(B)** Representative flow cytometry profiles of NTHi 3655 and KR334. **(C)** Localization of EF-Tu in NTHi 3655 and KR334 was analyzed by transmission electron microscopy (TEM). **(D)** Encapsulated *H. influenzae* represented by *H. influenzae* type b (MinnA and Eagan) as compared to the non-encapsulated mutant *H. influenzae* RM804 based upon Hib Eagan. **(E)** Representative flow cytometry profiles of Hib Eagan and the capsule mutant Hib RM804. **(F)** Surface concentration of EF-Tu on Hib Eagan and RM804 as measured by TEM. Anti-EF-Tu IgG was used in all experiments. Antibodies were affinity purified from rabbits that had been immunized with recombinant NTHi EF-Tu produced in *E. coli*. Flow cytometry analyses were performed using *H. influenzae* incubated with rabbit anti-EF-Tu IgG followed by secondary FITC-conjugated goat anti-IgG pAbs. Background represents bacteria incubated with only the secondary antibody, and was defined as $< 2\%$ of positive bacterial cells. Error bars indicate SEM. For TEM visualization, a gold-labeled secondary antibody was used.

EF-Tu Is Highly Immunogenic in Rabbits Immunized With Whole NTHi Cells

We next assessed the NTHi-induced immune response against EF-Tu. Rabbits were immunized with heat-killed whole NTHi bacterial cells 3655 and KR317, followed by enzyme-linked immunosorbent assays (ELISAs) of pre-immune and convalescent anti-NTHi sera against three different NTHi antigens (**Figure 2**). Recombinant NTHi proteins F and D, both of which are surface-exposed in NTHi and accessible by antibodies, were used as positive controls, whereas an *E. coli* lysate was included as a negative control representing the expression host of recombinant NTHi proteins and possible contaminants from *E. coli* (8, 10). Interestingly, in this particular experimental model, recombinant EF-Tu seemed to be immunodominant resulting in 2-fold more IgG directed against EF-Tu than against proteins F and D.

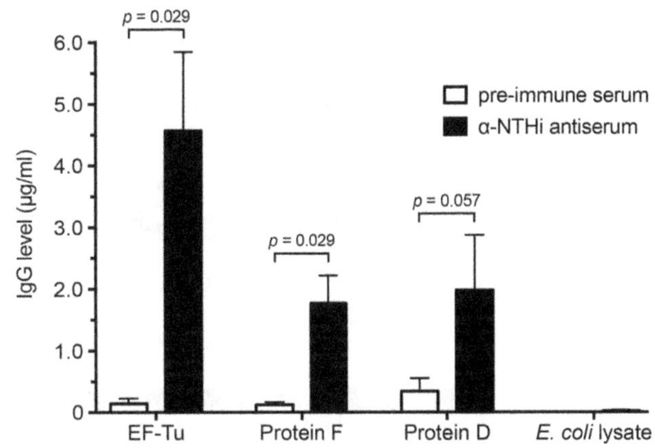

FIGURE 2 | High concentrations of anti-EF-Tu IgG is produced in rabbits immunized with whole NTHi. Mean values of anti-EF-Tu IgG levels are shown for 4 rabbits that were immunized with 3 doses of whole-cell NTHi 3655 or KR334. Sera were harvested 4 weeks after the last immunization, and reactivity against recombinant affinity-purified EF-Tu, protein F, and protein D was analyzed by ELISA using HRP-conjugated goat-anti rabbit antibodies. An *E. coli* lysate was included as a negative control. Significance was assessed using the Mann-Whitney *U*-test, and error bars indicate SEM.

The Immunodominant Epitopes of EF-Tu Are Located Within Its Central and C-Terminal Regions

Prokaryotic EF-Tu consists of three domains (12) (**Figure 3A**). Several segments of EF-Tu are predicted *in silico* to be exposed to the environment and to be antigenic, with the potential to be targeted by host antibodies (**Supplementary Figure 1**). To identify the immunodominant epitopes of *H. influenzae* EF-Tu, we subjected recombinant NTHi EF-Tu purified from *E. coli* to chemical cleavage by CNBr. This procedure resulted in production of 4 major fragments with molecular weights of 12, 13, 20, and 25 kDa (designated a to d in **Figure 3B**). Cleaved EF-Tu was subjected to immunoblotting with rabbit anti-EF-Tu pAbs (**Figure 3C**). Anti-EF-Tu IgG recognized full-length recombinant EF-Tu ($\approx$45.8 KDa) and the two larger fragments. The 25- and 20-kDa EF-Tu fragments (a and b) were subsequently isolated from the gel (**Figure 3B**) for peptide fingerprinting and identification. These two fragments were identified as spanning NTHi EF-Tu residues glutamate-128 to arginine-334 (E^{128}-R^{334}) and E^{156}-R^{334}, respectively (**Figure 3A**, lower panel). We hence concluded that rabbit serum recognized the middle portion of EF-Tu, comprising the C-terminal part of domain 1, the complete domain 2, and the N-terminal portion of domain 3.

To further pin-point the target sequences of anti-EF-Tu IgG, a series of synthetic peptides spanning the entire EF-Tu molecule were synthesized (**Figure 4A**). Peptide epitope mapping (**Supplementary Figure 2**) was performed using purified pAbs from rabbits immunized with recombinant EF-Tu or sera from rabbits immunized with whole NTHi. Semi-quantitative dot blot analysis of anti-EF-Tu pAbs revealed that some of the highest levels of reactivity were against peptides ID 3, 9, 12, and 15 (**Figure 4B**; red bars and boxes), corresponding to sequences EF-Tu^{41-65}, EF-$Tu^{161-185}$, EF-$Tu^{221-245}$, and EF-$Tu^{281-305}$, respectively (**Figure 4A** and **Supplementary Figure 3**). In contrast, serum from a rabbit immunized with whole NTHi (**Figure 2**) mainly detected full-length (native) EF-Tu (**Figure 4B**; blue bars).

Based on the results above, we delineated the potential surface-exposed, antigenic parts of EF-Tu as indicated in **Figure 4C**. To examine whether the regions corresponding to sequences in peptide ID 3, 9, 12, and 15 were accessible within the EF-Tu molecule on the bacterial surface, we analyzed NTHi by flow cytometry using affinity-purified anti-peptide Abs. All four immunogenic regions were readily detected by the peptide-specific Abs (**Figure 4D**). Antibodies directed against peptide ID 12 resulted in the strongest signal that was comparable to the one obtained with IgG against full-length recombinant EF-Tu. Taken together, these data revelaed that the immunodominant epitopes of surface-associated EF-Tu are accessible by the host humoral immune system.

Anti-NTHi EF-Tu Antibodies Are Bactericidal

The immune response elicited by immunization with recombinant NTHi EF-Tu prompted us to test whether antibodies directed against EF-Tu can induce complement-dependent killing of NTHi cells. Following the pre-incubation of bacteria with serum from rabbits immunized with recombinant EF-Tu and the addition of an external complement source, C3 deposition was analyzed by flow cytometry (**Figure 5A**). Clear shifts were observed with EF-Tu antiserum compared to control pre-immune serum samples, suggesting initiation of the classical complement activation pathway.

To validate the findings on C3 deposition, we also performed serum bactericidal activity (SBA) assays. Affinity-purified Abs directed against full-length EF-Tu and peptides ID 3, 9, 12, and 15 were incubated with NTHi followed by the addition of complement. Approximately 40% of NTHi were killed following incubation with antibodies directed against

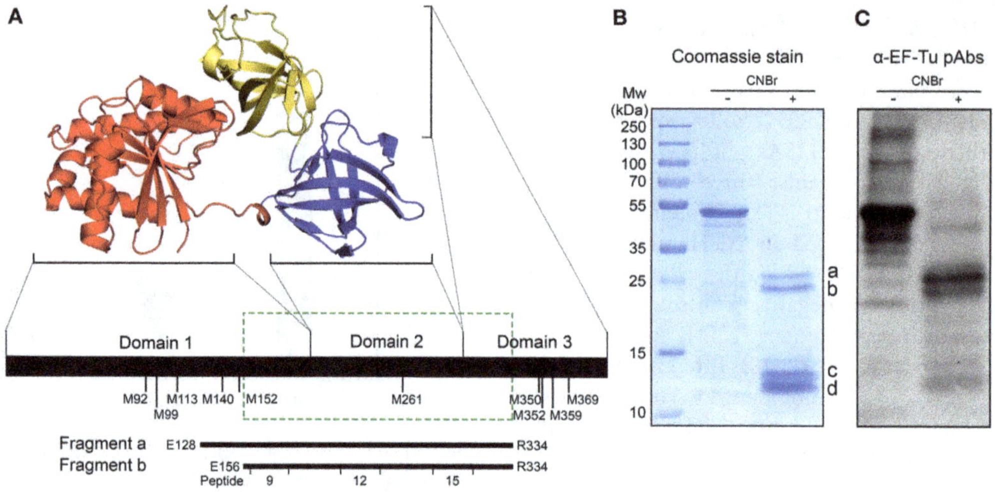

FIGURE 3 | Anti-EF-Tu antibodies mainly target a region comprising the EF-Tu C-terminal part of domain 1, the complete domain 2, and the N-terminal part of domain 3. **(A)** Schematic organization of EF-Tu domains 1–3. The 3-dimensional structure of EF-Tu is based upon PDB 1dg1 (28, 29). Methionine (M) residues where CNBr cleavage can occur are indicated below the horizontal line. Fragments a and b represent two products of EF-Tu cleavage by CNBr, spanning glutamate-128 to arginine-334 (E^{128}-R^{334}) and E^{156}-R^{334} residues of EF-Tu. The green box indicates the experimentally determined immunodominant region of EF-Tu. **(B)** Recombinant NTHi EF-Tu was digested with CNBr and subjected to analysis by SDS-PAGE and Coomassie staining to determine the fragmentation pattern. The indicated cleaved bands a and b were in-gel trypsin digested, excised, and sequenced to identify the corresponding fragments depicted in **(A)**. The CNBr-digested EF-Tu was also subjected to Western blotting with affinity-purified rabbit anti-EF-Tu pAbs **(C)**. Secondary HRP-conjugated anti-IgG pAbs were used for detection in Western blot.

specific surface-exposed parts of EF-Tu (**Figure 5B**). The serum bactericidal activity of the anti-peptide Abs, except for peptide ID 15, was similar to that of IgG pAbs directed against the full-length EF-Tu molecule. The combination of the four anti-peptide antibodies did not, however, exhibit enhanced efficacy relative to the individual antibodies. Taken together, these data demonstrated that Abs directed against EF-Tu trigger the innate immune defense resulting in complement activation, as evidenced by C3b generation and bacterial killing.

Anti-NTHi EF-Tu pAbs Recognize Unencapsulated Respiratory Tract Bacteria and Promote Antibody-Dependent Killing

Since anti-EF-Tu pAbs clearly recognized NTHi and elicited a bactericidal effect (**Figure 1**, **5B**), we subsequently investigated whether the anti-EF-Tu pAbs could also recognize other bacterial species with homologous EF-Tu proteins (**Supplementary Figure 3**). Multiple Gram-negative and Gram-positive bacterial species, including pathogens and commensals, were subjected to flow cytometry analyses followed by assessment of SBA or opsonophagocytosis. Anti-EF-Tu pAbs detected EF-Tu molecules on *H. parainfluenzae*, *H. haemolyticus*, and *Moraxella catarrhalis*, but did not bind encapsulated *N. meningitidis*. Moreover, the anti-EF-Tu pAbs recognized various unencapsulated *Streptococci* from the oral microbiome, but not the encapsulated *S. pneumoniae* (**Figure 6A**). Finally, a set of clinical *Escherichia coli* isolates (KR714-716) were not detected by anti-EF-Tu IgG that was in bright contrast to the unencapsulated laboratory strains *E. coli* BL21 and DH5α that significantly carried EF-Tu at the surface.

Subsequent SBA assays revealed that antibodies against NTHi EF-Tu promoted the killing of NTHi and unencapsulated Hib RM804 (**Figure 6B**), but not of the encapsulated Hib Eagan that did not have any surface-exposed EF-Tu. In addition, *H. haemolyticus, H. parainfluenzae*, and *M. catarrhalis* were targeted for antibody-dependent complement attack, but at levels lower than NTHi and RM804 (**Figure 6B**). The effects of anti-NTHi EF-Tu IgG against Gram-positive, unencapsulated *S. sanguinis*, *S. salivarius*, and *S. parasanguinis* were also tested in an opsonophagocytosis assay (OPA) using the phagocytic cell line HL60 pre-activated with dimethylformamide. Phagocytes exhibited significant killing activity against the unencapsulated *Streptococcus* species, but not against encapsulated *S. pneumoniae* (**Figure 6C**). Taken together, IgG directed against NTHi EF-Tu recognized most unencapsulated bacteria derived from the upper respiratory tract microbiome and promoted EF-Tu IgG-dependent killing via SBA and opsonophagocytosis.

DISCUSSION

We found that antibody-accessible EF-Tu is associated with the surface of NTHi cells using flow cytometry and TEM (**Figures 1A–C**). This is in agreement with previous observations with other bacteria from the gastrointestinal and respiratory tracts displaying surface-associated EF-Tu (15–19). Our findings support the role of EF-Tu as a moonlighting protein that possibly mediates interactions with the host extracellular matrix and

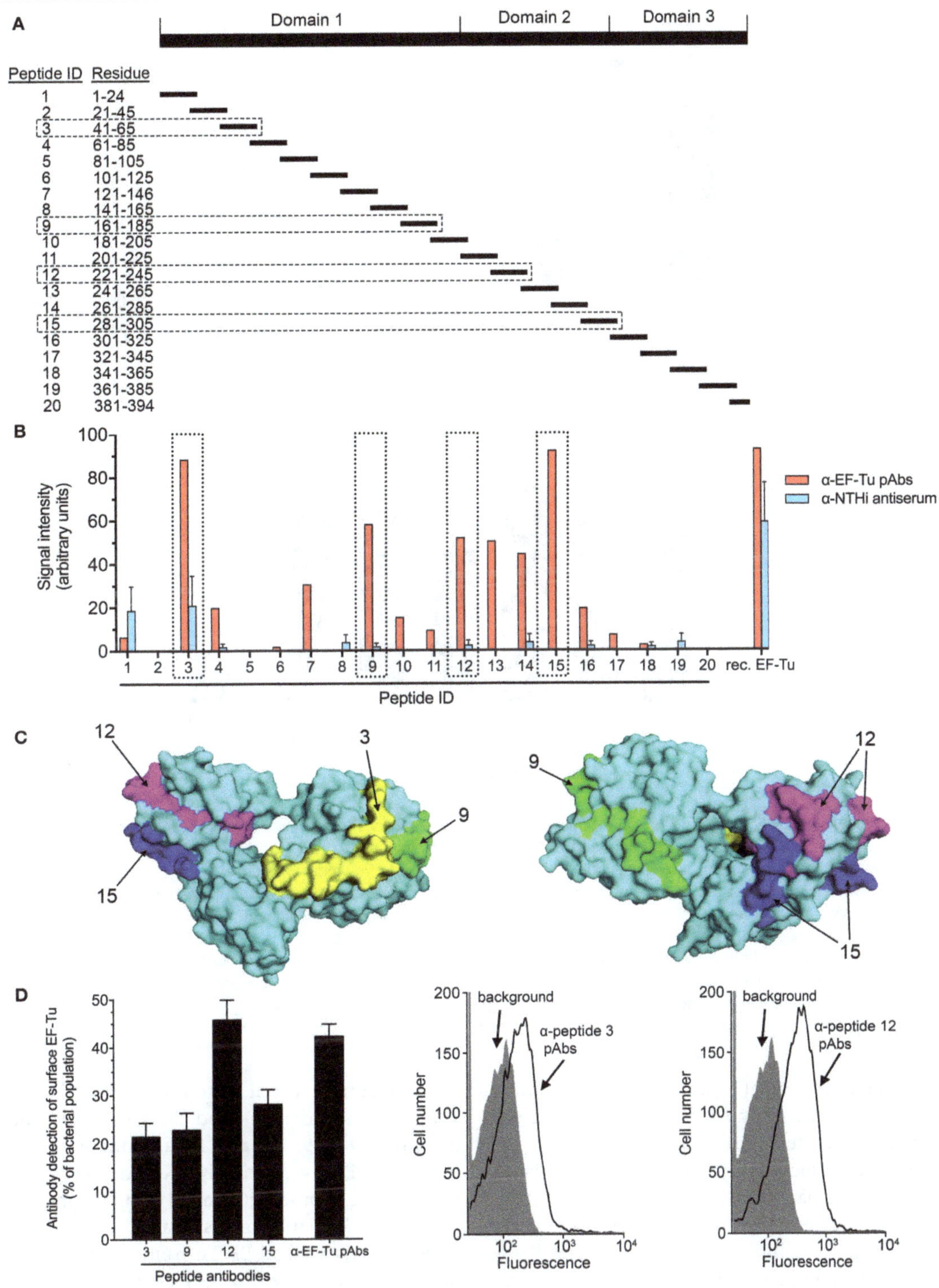

FIGURE 4 | Four main immunoreactive epitopes are detected at the surface of EF-Tu. **(A)** Map of the synthetic peptides covering the EF-Tu protein sequence that were used for epitope mapping. **(B)** The reactivity of anti-EF-Tu pAbs from rabbits ($n = 4$) immunized with recombinant EF-Tu, and of sera from rabbits immunized with whole NTHi (3655 or 334) ($n = 5$) were tested against synthetic EF-Tu peptides using a dot blot (**Supplementary Figure 2**). Mean values obtained by scanning densitometry are shown. **(C)** The surface-exposed peptides ID 3, 9, 12, and 15 are indicated on the model of the EF-Tu crystal structure (Protein Data Bank entry 1dg1). These peptides corresponded to EF-Tu$^{41-65}$, EF-Tu$^{161-185}$, EF-Tu$^{221-245}$, and EF-Tu$^{281-305}$. Peptides ID 9, 12, and 15 were located within the CNBr-generated fragments indicated in **Figure 4A**. **(D)** Specific antibodies against peptides ID 3, 9, 12, and 15 recognize EF-Tu on the surface of NTHi 3655, as revealed by flow cytometry. Mean values from 9 experiments are shown. The anti-peptide antibodies were affinity-purified from sera obtained from rabbits immunized with full-length recombinant EF-Tu. Error bars indicate SEM. Representative flow cytometry results are shown for anti-peptide Abs directed against peptide ID 3 and 12. Flow cytometry analysis was performed using NTHi 3655 cells incubated with the anti-EF-Tu IgG or peptide-specific antibodies followed by secondary FITC-conjugated pAbs. Background represents bacteria incubated with secondary antibody only.

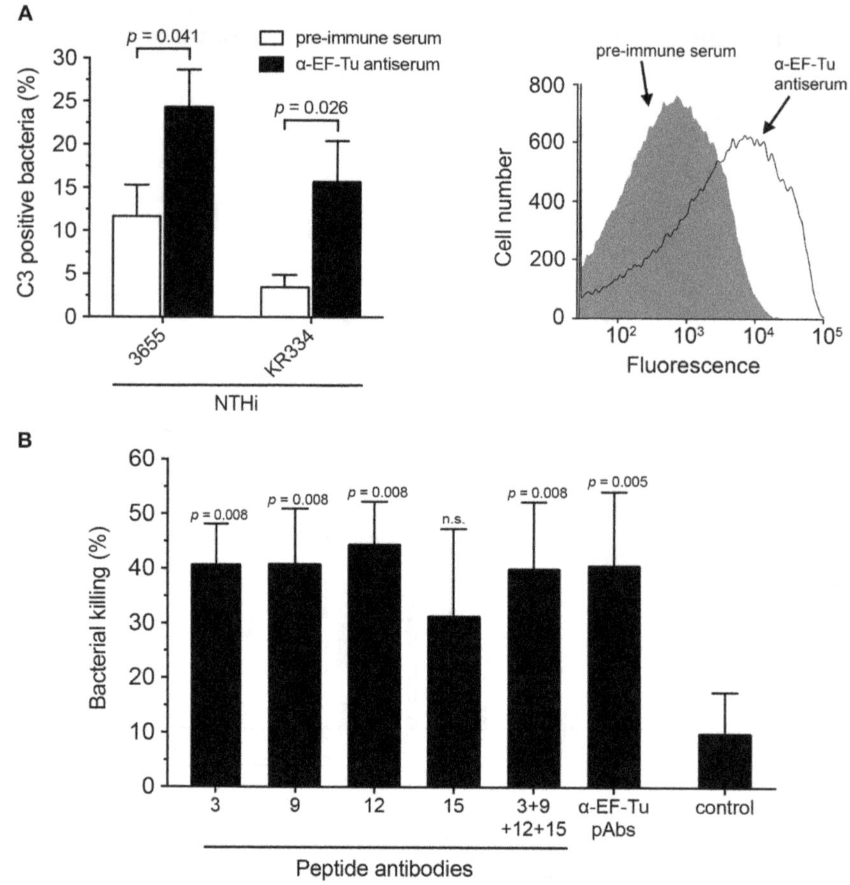

FIGURE 5 | Antibodies directed against EF-Tu are functional and induce bactericidal activity via complement activation. **(A)** C3 deposition was assessed in the presence of rabbit antiserum against full-length EF-Tu. NTHi strains KR334 and 3655 were incubated with EF-Tu antiserum, and baby rabbit complement was used as a complement source. Flow cytometry analysis was performed using a specific anti-C3 antibody. Pre-immune serum was used as a negative control. Mean values from 6 experiments are shown. A representative flow cytometry profile is also shown. Background represents bacteria incubated with the secondary antibody only. **(B)** Serum bactericidal activity (SBA) was performed to assess NTHi killing induced by anti-EF-Tu antibodies. Rabbit antibodies directed against full-length EF-Tu or peptide ID 3, 9, and 12 significantly induced the classical pathway of complement activation in the presence of baby rabbit complement. Bacterial killing represents differences between incubation with active or heat-inactivated baby rabbit complement. Control represents bacterial killing from baby rabbit complement with the non-related anti-OprG pAb detecting a *Pseudomonas aeruginosa* outer membrane protein. Mean values from 5 separate experiments are indicated. Statistical significances were calculated using the Mann-Whitney test. Error bars indicate SEM.

components of the innate immunity (21, 24). In conjunction with previous reports, our observations underscore the importance of EF-Tu surface exposure in bacterial fitness and virulence.

Considering the immunogenicity of surface-associated EF-Tu in various mammalian hosts, we sought to identify the immunodominant sequences and surface-exposed parts of NTHi EF-Tu. Epitope mapping of NTHi EF-Tu based on CNBr-fragmented EF-Tu and peptide libraries unveiled several immunogenic regions, corresponding to peptides ID 3, 9, 12, and 15 (**Figures 3**, **4** and **Supplementary Figure 2**). The antigenic properties of these peptide sequences were predicted *in silico* by B-cell epitope analysis (**Supplementary Figure 1A**), and was in concordance with our mapping data. Furthermore, using bioinformatic analyses, these peptides were also predicted to be accessible at the protein surface (**Figure 4C** and **Supplementary Figure 1**). Surface accessible antigen determinants or B-cell epitopes are crucial for an appropriate antibody response (30), and these collective findings establish peptides ID 3, 9, 12, and 15 as immunodominant sequences of NTHi EF-Tu. Similarly, Kolberg *et al.* showed that a monoclonal mouse IgG raised against pneumococcal EF-Tu recognized EF-Tu domains 2 and 3 (31). In contrast, Pyclik *et al.* recently studied EF-Tu from *Streptococcus agalactiae* and found two sequences to be recognized by human antibodies; ^{28}LTAAITTVLARRLP^{41} (slightly overlapping NTHi EF-Tu peptide ID 3 on domain 1) and ^{294} GQVLAKPGSINPHTKF^{309} (corresponding to NTHi EF-Tu peptide ID 15). This discrepancy could be due to hitherto unknown proteolytic processing events on the bacterial surface (24). Interestingly, we found peptide ID 3 to be the only peptide detected by both α-EF-Tu pAb and the α-NTHi serum (**Figure 4B**). IgG antibodies directed against peptide ID 3 provided, however, the weakest signal

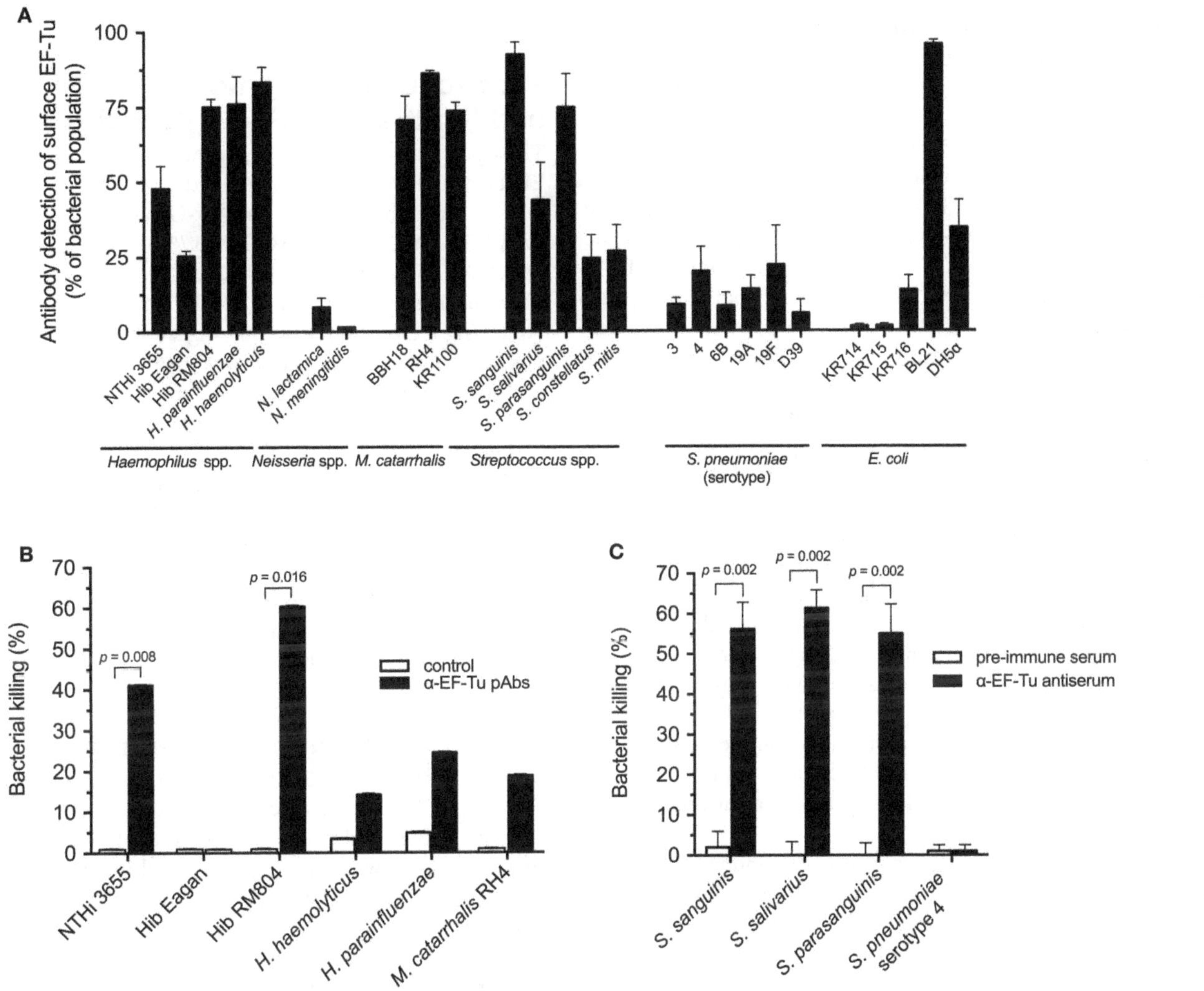

FIGURE 6 | Multiple bacterial species are recognized by NTHi anti-EF-Tu antibodies, but exhibit differential susceptibilities to antibody-mediated bactericidal activity. **(A)** The indicated bacterial species were tested for detection by anti-NTHi EF-Tu pAbs using flow cytometry. Mean values from at least three different experiments are shown. **(B)** Anti-EF-Tu IgG-dependent bactericidal activity against indicated Gram-negative species was tested using the SBA assay. For the SBA assay, the indicated bacterial cells were combined with purified anti-EF-Tu IgG and baby rabbit complement, followed by determination of CFU after overnight incubation. Mean values from 5 independent experiments are shown. **(C)** The Gram-positive *S. sanguinis*, *S. salivarius*, and *S. parasanguinis*, but not *S. pneumoniae* were killed by HL60 cells when pre-incubated with rabbit anti-NTHi EF-Tu antiserum. Gram-positive bacteria with highest levels of surface-associated EF-Tu, as revealed by flow cytometry, were selected for these experiments. Mean values from 6 independent experiments are shown. *S. pneumoniae* reference strain D39 in panel **A** belongs to serotype 2 (**Table 1**). Statistical significance was calculated using the Mann-Whitney test. Error bars indicate SEM.

in flow cytometry analysis of whole NTHi (**Figure 4D**), suggesting that the protein structure is slightly altered *in vivo* with other parts (epitopes) exposed of the EF-Tu molecule.

The immunoreactive properties of EF-Tu has been thoroughly evaluated (24, 32, 33). However, a high titer of specific antibodies does not always translate to increased protection of the host (34). An example of this is the study done by Carrasco *et al.* who showed that EF-Tu in *Borrelia burgdorferi* is highly immunogenic, but the antibodies produced are not bactericidal during Lyme borreliosis (16). This is alluded to the finding that the EF-Tu is not accessible at the *B. burgdorferi* bacterial surface. We found that serum from rabbits immunized with recombinant NTHi EF-Tu, when supplemented with active baby rabbit complement, was able to significantly increase the deposition of complement factor C3 on the bacterial surface (**Figure 5A**). In addition, purified antibodies against full-length NTHi EF-Tu and peptide ID 3, 9 and 12 significantly increased bacterial killing by complement activation in the SBA assay (**Figure 5B**). These results can be interpreted as further evidence of that EF-Tu and the indicated peptide sequences are indeed accessible at the bacterial surface. This also makes it interesting to further study whether immunization with NTHi EF-Tu can generate protection against colonization or infection with NTHi *in vivo*.

The high similarity (and function) of EF-Tu between different bacterial species (**Supplementary Figure 3**) warrants the speculation of cross-reactivity, especially between *Haemophilus* species that share EF-Tu sequence, and its potential implications on the microbiome. Flow cytometry analysis indicated that antibodies against NTHi EF-Tu also cross-react with various unencapsulated species, supporting surface display of EF-Tu in general. As expected, EF-Tu was not detectable on the surface of most encapsulated bacteria, including *H. influenzae* type b (Hib) *N. meningitides*, or pneumococci (**Figures 1D–F, 6A**). This underscores previous suggestions that the capsule of pneumocci and meningococci shields surface-associated EF-Tu from antibody dectection (31). There was a clear correlation between EF-Tu recognition and differences in antibody-dependent bacterial killing (**Figures 6A,B**) for *H. influenzae* strains. However, despite being recognized by anti-EF-Tu antibodies at the same level as NTHi, *H. haemolyticus*, *H. parainfluenzae*, and *M. catarrhalis* were less susceptible to the antibody-dependent bactericidal activity as compared to NTHi suggesting that C1q binding and further activation of the classical pathway of complement activation was not maximally initiated. Our results thus suggested that species-specific differences exist regarding EF-Tu surface exposure. However, the full extent of cross-reacivity with the upper respiratory tract microbiota, but also the gut microbiome must be further studied. In particular, commensal bacteria not expressing IgA1 protease might be subjected to a negative selective pressure by secreted IgA specific for surface-exposed EF-Tu.

In conclusion, we have shown that EF-Tu moonlights at the surface of NTHi, and that the protein is highly immunogenic with immunodominant epitopes residing primarily at the C-terminal half of the molecule. IgG raised against NTHi EF-Tu can cross-react with and promote antibody-dependent killing of other bacterial species, albeit at rates different from those observed for NTHi. We propose that the adaptive immune response against surface EF-Tu is highly important in the context of respiratory tract infections in order to protect the host from attack and consequently infection.

MATERIALS AND METHODS

Bacteria and Culture Conditions

Bacteria used in the present study are listed in **Table 1**. NTHi was grown at 37°C in a humid atmosphere containing 5% CO_2 on chocolate agar or in brain heart infusion (BHI) broth supplemented with 2 µg/mL nicotinamide adenine dinucleotide NAD (Sigma-Aldrich, St Louis, MO, United States) and 10 µg/mL hemin (Merck, Darmstadt, Germany). *E. coli* was cultured in Luria-Bertani (LB) broth or on LB agar. All other strains were cultured on chocolate agar or in BHI at 37°C with 5% CO_2. Clinical isolates were obtained from Clinical Microbiology (Laboratory Medicine, Lund, Sweden). Type strains were from the American Type Culture Collection (ATCC; Manassas, VA, United States) or Culture Collection of the University of Gothenburg (CCUG; Department of Clinical Bacteriology, Sahlgrenska Hospital, Gothenburg, Sweden).

Production of Recombinant NTHi EF-Tu and Synthesis of EF-Tu Peptides

The open reading frame of the gene encoding full-length NTHi EF-Tu (EDJ92442.1) was amplified from NTHi 3655 genomic DNA using the primer pair 5′-GGGGCGGATCCGATGTC TAAAGAAAAATTTGAACGTA-3′/5′-GGCGGAAGCTTTTT GATGATTTTCGCAACAACGCCA-3′ containing restriction enzyme sites *Bam*HI and *Hin*dIII (underlined), respectively. Following restriction enzyme digestion, the resulting DNA fragment (1214 base pairs) was cloned into the expression vector pET26(b)+ (Novagen, Merck Darmstadt, Germany) for recombinant protein production as described previously (8). Briefly, the resulting plasmid was transformed into *E. coli* DH5α, followed by DNA sequencing. Recombinant proteins were thereafter produced in *E. coli* BL21 (DE3) and purified by affinity chromatography using Ni-NTA agarose. For NTHi epitope mapping, 20- to 25-residue-long peptides, overlapping by 5 residues and together covering the entire EF-Tu sequence, were synthesized by Genscript (Piscataway, NJ). These peptides were also used for affinity-purification of Abs from the rabbit anti-EF-Tu antiserum as described below.

Antisera and Antibody Preparation

Rabbit anti-NTHi 3655, anti-NTHi 334, anti-EF-Tu sera and rabbit anti-EF-Tu pAbs were prepared as previously described (8) with some modifications. Briefly, rabbits were immunized subcutaneously with 200 µg of recombinant EF-Tu in 0.5 ml saline or with 10^9 CFU of indicated heat-killed NTHi strains with 0.5 ml incomplete Freund's adjuvant. The animals were boosted 3 times every 4 weeks with alum used as an adjuvant. Blood was drawn 2 weeks after the last immunization. Rabbit pAbs against EF-Tu and antibodies against specific EF-Tu peptides (**Supplementary Figure 3A**) were further affinity purified using EF-Tu or synthetic peptides (peptide ID: 3, 9, 12, and 15) coupled to CNBr-activated Sepharose™ (GE Healthcare Biosciences, Chicago, IL).

Flow Cytometry

Bacteria grown for 3 h or overnight at 35.5°C with 5% CO_2, were adjusted to 10^9 CFU/ml in PBS containing 1% bovine serum albumin (BSA). Samples containing 2×10^7 bacteria were incubated for 1 h on ice with 2 µg of rabbit anti-EF-Tu pAb or EF-Tu peptide specific antibodies, washed, and incubated for 20 min on ice with fluorescein isothiocyanate (FITC)-conjugated swine anti-rabbit antibodies (Dako, Glostrup, Denmark). Samples were washed with phosphate-buffered saline (PBS) and resuspended in 300 µl PBS for analysis on a FACSverse™ flow cytometer (Becton-Dickson, Franklin Lakes, NJ).

Transmission Electron Microscopy (TEM)

TEM was used to visualize the localization of EF-Tu on the bacterial surface. The *H. influenzae* NTHi 3655, NTHi KR334, Hib Eagan, and Hib RM804 strains were incubated with gold-labeled rabbit anti-EF-Tu pAbs, subjected to negative staining with uranyl formate, and visualized using a Jeol JEM 1230 electron microscope (JEOL, Tokyo, Japan) operated at 60 kV accelerating voltage. Images were recorded with a Gatan Multiscan 791 CCD camera (Gatan, Pleasanton, CA).

ELISA

Following the addition of 0.5 μg of purified recombinant EF-Tu, protein F (8), or protein D (41) in 0.1 M Tris (pH 9) per well, Nunc PolySorp 96-well microtiter plates (Thermo Fisher Scientific, Waltham, MA) were incubated overnight at 4°C. After 4 washes, the plates were blocked for 1 h at RT with 250 μl PBS with tween 20 (PBST) with 1% BSA per well. After washing, the samples were incubated for 1 h at RT with sera diluted 1:100 in PBST with 2.5% BSA and subsequently washed 3 times. HRP-conjugated goat anti-rabbit pAbs (Dako, Glostrup, Denmark) were added for 1 h at RT, with 4 washes following the incubation. At all steps, each wash was performed for 5 min using PBST. Antibody-antigen complexes were detected

TABLE 1 | Bacterial species used in the present study.

Reference strain or clinical isolate	Serotype/group	Number	Site of origin	Clinical diagnosis/remarks	Age (year)	Reference
GRAM-NEGATIVE SPECIES						
H. influenzae	Type b (Hib)	Eagan (18095)	Cerebrospinal fluid	Meningitis/ encapuslated		CCUG[a]
	Type b (Hib)	RM804		Capsule-deficient mutant of Eagan		(35)
	Type b (Hib)	MinnA	Cerebrospinal fluid	Laboratory reference strain		(36)
Non-typeable *H. influenzae* (NTHi)		KR317	Nasopharynx	Bronchitis	55	This study
		KR318	Nasopharynx	Bronchitis	49	This study
		KR332	Nasopharynx	Upper respiratory tract infection	3	This study
		KR333	Nasopharynx	Sinusitis	68	This study
		KR334	Nasopharynx	Conjunctivitis	2	This study
		3655	Middle ear	Acute otitis media		(37)
H. parainfluenzae		13788	Oral cavity	Reference strain		CCUG
H. haemolyticus		KR161	Throat	Normal flora		This study
Moraxella catarrhalis		BBH18	Blood	Sepsis		(38)
		RH4	Blood	Sepsis		(39)
		KR1100	Nasopharynx	Bronchitis	85	This study
Neisseria lactamica		23972		Reference strain		ATCC[b]
N. meningitides	Serogroup A	3269	Spinal fluid	Meningitis		CCUG
	Serogroup B	MC58				National Reference lab., Örebro, Sweden
	Serogroup C	KR822	Spinal fluid	Meningitis		This study
	Serogroup C	FAM20				(40)
Escherichia coli		KR714	Urine	Urinary tract infection	6	This study
		KR715	Urine	Urinary tract infection	63	This study
		KR716	Urine	Urinary tract infection	59	This study
		BL21		Laboratory strain		
		DH5α		Laboratory strain		
GRAM-POSITIVE SPECIES						
Streptococcus pneumoniae	ST2[c]	D39		Reference strain		ATCC
	ST3	6303		Reference strain		ATCC
	ST4	KR440	Blood	Pneumonia, sepsis	73	This study
	ST6B	1350	Cerebrospinal fluid	Meningits, otitis/ Reference strain		CCUG
	ST19A	KR1148	Nasopharynx	AOM	2	This study
	ST19F	49619		Reference strain		ATCC
S. sanguinis		KR1143		Normal flora	60	This study
S. parasanguinis		KR1144		Normal flora	45	This study
S. salivarius		KR1145		Normal flora	68	This study
S. constellatus		KR1146		Normal flora	64	This study
S. mitis		KR1147		Normal flora	64	This study

[a] *CCUG; Culture collection University of Gothenburg (Sweden) (www.ccug.se).*
[b] *ATCC; American type culture collection (www.atcc.org).*
[c] *ST; serotype.*

using a hydrogen peroxide/3,3′,5,5′-tetramethylbenzidine (TMB) substrate solution, with reactions stopped with 1 M sulfuric acid, followed by determination of the absorbance at optical density 450 nm.

Cyanogen Bromide Digestion

Full-length EF-Tu was treated with 1 μg cyanogen bromide (CNBr) in 70% formic acid per 5 μg of protein. Samples were incubated for 2 h at 25°C in a vacuum centrifuge. Lyophilized samples were resuspended in phosphate-buffered saline (PBS).

SDS-PAGE and Western Blotting

Samples with full-length EF-Tu or CNBr-digested EF-Tu were separated on a 12% polyacrylamide gel and either stained with Coomassie Brilliant Blue R-250 (Bio-Rad, Munich, Germany) or transferred onto a 0.45-μm Immobilon-P PVDF Membrane (Millipore, Bedford, MA, United States) at 16 V for 15 h. Following blocking in 5% skim milk in PBST, membranes were incubated at room temperature (RT) for 1 h with rabbit α-EF-Tu pAbs diluted 1:1,000 in 5 ml PBST with 5% skim milk. Following three washes in PBS, the membranes were incubated for 1 h with horseradish peroxidase (HRP)-conjugated swine anti-rabbit pAbs (Dako, Glostrup, Denmark). The membranes were thereafter washed in PBS with 0.05% Tween 20 (PBST), developed using Pierce™ Enhanced Chemiluminescence (ECL) Western Blotting Substrate (Thermo Scientific, Waltham, MA), and visualized on a BioRad ChemiDoc™.

Peptide-Based Epitope Mapping

To identify epitopes recognized by the anti-EF-Tu IgG, EF-Tu peptides (20 μg; peptide ID 1-20; **Figure 4A**) or full-length EF-Tu (0.05, 0.5 and 5 μg) were coated onto nitrocellulose (NC) membranes. The membranes were dried for 30 min at 37°C, stained with Ponceuau S, and thereafter blocked for 1 h at RT in PBST with 1% BSA and 1% casein. The membranes were then incubated overnight at 4°C with sera diluted 1:100 in PBST with 1% BSA and 1% casein. The membranes were incubated with HRP-conjugated swine anti-rabbit pAbs (Dako) for 20 min at RT, with 4 washes (10 min each) in PBST performed prior to and following the incubation. Membranes were developed using Pierce™ ECL Western Blot substrate and visualized on a BioRad ChemiDoc™. Pixel densities of the dot blot images were assessed using ImageJ® version 1.51.

Structural Modeling

The 3D structure of NTHi EF-Tu was modeled by SWISS-MODEL (42–45) automated server against homologous templates available in the Protein Data Bank (PDB; available at: http:/www.rcsb.org). Three-dimensional model were elucidated using the program PyMOL (available at: http://www.pymol.org/).

Serum Bactericidal Activity (SBA) and Determination of C3 Deposition

Susceptibility of antibody-exposed bacterial cells to complement-mediated killing was measured using a modified SBA assay as previously described (8). Briefly, 4×10^4 CFU of indicated bacterial strains were resuspended in Hank's balanced salt solution with 2% heat-inactivated baby rabbit complement (Nordic BioSite AB, Täby, Sweden) followed by incubation with 2.5 μg rabbit anti-EF-Tu pAbs or peptide-specific antibodies for 30 min at RT. In some experiments, anti-OprG pAb detecting a *Pseudomonas aeruginosa* outer membrane protein (Riesbeck *et al.*, unpublished) was included as a control pAb not recognizing NTHi. After the addition of active or heat-inactivated baby rabbit complement to a final concentration of 2.5%, samples were incubated for 1 h at 37°C with gentle shaking. Aliquots (10 μl) from the reaction mixtures were plated on chocolate agar, and CFUs were determined after overnight incubation. To determine C3 deposition at the bacterial surface, NTHi 3655 cells were incubated with pre-immune or anti-EF-Tu sera from the same rabbit, followed by the addition of 4% baby rabbit complement as described above. The cells were thereafter stained with FITC-conjugated goat anti-rabbit C3 pAbs (MP Biomedicals, Santa Ana, CA, United States), followed by analysis using a FACSverse™ flow cytometer.

Opsonophagocytosis Assay (OPA)

Antibody functionality and bacterial survival in opsonophagocytosis was determined by an OPA as previously described (46). HL60 cells (kindly provided by Prof. Urban Gullberg, Lund University) were cultured in RPMI 1640 medium supplemented with 10% fetal bovine serum and GlutaMAX (Gibco, Life Technologies, Carlsbad, CA). Cells were differentiated by adding 0.91% dimethylformamide for 5–6 days. Granulocytes expressing CD35 were detected by flow cytometry and viability was determined using trypan blue staining. Bacteria were added in duplicates to 3-fold serial serum dilutions, starting at 1:4 serum concentration, and incubated in microtiter plates for 30 min at 700 rpm to promote antibody binding. Following the addition of differentiated HL60 cells and baby rabbit complement serum, the plates were incubated for 45 min at 37°C with 5% CO_2 and at 700 rpm to allow for phagocytosis. The contents were thereafter transferred to blood agar plates and grown overnight. The assays were done using EF-Tu antiserum and pre-immune serum as the negative control. Killing by effector cells was verified in each experiment using pneumococci and in-house quality control serum from volunteers immunized with a pneumococcal conjugate vaccine (Prevenar13).

Statistics

Mann-Whitney U-test was used for nonparametric data sets and differences were considered statistically significant at $p \leq 0.05$. All analyses were performed using GraphPad PrismR version 7.0 (GraphPad Software, La Jolla, CA).

AUTHOR CONTRIBUTIONS

Y-CS and KR planned the study. OT, Y-CS, MB, NL, BD, VA, and FJ contributed to the experimental work. OT, Y-CS, and KR wrote the manuscript.

ACKNOWLEDGMENTS

We are grateful to Mrs. Kerstin Norrman and Ms. Emma Mattsson for excellent technical assistance, and the Clinical Microbiology laboratory at Labmedicin Skåne (Lund, Sweden) for providing clinical isolates.

REFERENCES

1. Resman F, Ristovski M, Forsgren A, Kaijser B, Kronvall G, Medstrand P, et al. Increase of β-lactam-resistant invasive *Haemophilus influenzae* in Sweden, 1997 to 2010. *Antimicrob Agents Chemother* (2012) 56:4408–15. doi: 10.1128/AAC.00415-12
2. Pichichero ME. Ten-year study of acute otitis media in Rochester, NY. *Pediatr Infect Dis J.* (2016) 35:1027–32. doi: 10.1097/INF.0000000000001216
3. Ahearn CP, Gallo MC, Murphy TF. Insights on persistent airway infection by non-typeable *Haemophilus influenzae* in chronic obstructive pulmonary disease. *Pathog Dis.* (2017) 75:1–18. doi: 10.1093/femspd/ftx042
4. Månsson V, Skaare D, Riesbeck K, Resman F. The spread and clinical impact of ST14CC-PBP3 type IIb/A, a clonal group of non-typeable *Haemophilus influenzae* with chromosomally mediated β-lactam resistance-a prospective observational study. *Clin Microbiol Infect.* (2017) 23:209.e1–209.e7. doi: 10.1016/j.cmi.2016.11.006
5. Khan MN, Ren D, Kaur R, Basha S, Zagursky R, Pichichero ME. Developing a vaccine to prevent otitis media caused by nontypeable *Haemophilus influenzae. Expert Rev Vaccines* (2016) 15:863–78. doi: 10.1586/14760584.2016.1156539
6. Jalalvand F, Riesbeck K. *Haemophilus influenzae*: recent advances in the understanding of molecular pathogenesis and polymicrobial infections. *Curr Opin Infect Dis.* (2014) 27:268–74. doi: 10.1097/QCO.0000000000000056
7. Duell BL, Su YC, Riesbeck K. Host-pathogen interactions of nontypeable *Haemophilus influenzae*: from commensal to pathogen. *FEBS Lett.* (2016) 590:3840–53. doi: 10.1002/1873-3468.12351
8. Su YC, Jalalvand F, Mörgelin M, Blom AM, Singh B, Riesbeck K. *Haemophilus influenzae* acquires vitronectin via the ubiquitous Protein F to subvert host innate immunity. *Mol Microbiol.* (2013) 87:1245–66. doi: 10.1111/mmi.12164
9. Jalalvand F, Littorin N, Su YC, Riesbeck K. Impact of immunization with Protein F on pulmonary clearance of nontypeable *Haemophilus influenzae* . *Vaccine* (2014) 32:2261–4. doi: 10.1016/j.vaccine.2014.02.082
10. Forsgren A, Riesbeck K, Janson H. Protein D of *Haemophilus influenzae* : a protective nontypeable *H. influenzae* antigen and a carrier for pneumococcal conjugate vaccines. *Clin Infect Dis.* (2008) 46:726–31. doi: 10.1086/527396
11. Clarke C, Bakaletz LO, Ruiz-Guiñazú J, Borys D, Mrkvan T. Impact of protein D-containing pneumococcal conjugate vaccines on non-typeable *Haemophilus influenzae* acute otitis media and carriage. *Expert Rev Vaccines* (2017) 16:1–14. doi: 10.1080/14760584.2017.1333905
12. Jacobson GR, Rosenbusch JP. Abundance and membrane association of elongation factor Tu in *E. coli*. *Nature* (1976) 261:23–6.
13. Kavaliauskas D, Nissen P, Knudsen CR. The busiest of all ribosomal assistants: elongation factor Tu. *Biochemistry* (2012) 51:2642–51. doi: 10.1021/bi300077s
14. Dombou M, Bhide SV, Mizushima S. Appearance of elongation factor Tu in the outer membrane of sucrose-dependent spectinomycin-resistant mutants of *Escherichia coli*. *Eur J Biochem.* (1981) 113:397–403. doi: 10.1111/j.1432-1033.1981.tb05079.x
15. Koenigs A, Zipfel PF, Kraiczy P. Translation elongation factor Tuf of *Acinetobacter baumannii* is a plasminogen-binding protein. *PLoS ONE* (2015) 10:e0134418. doi: 10.1371/journal.pone.0134418
16. Carrasco SE, Yang Y, Troxell B, Yang X, Pal U, Yang XF. *Borrelia burgdorferi* elongation factor EF-Tu is an immunogenic protein during Lyme borreliosis. *Emerg Microbes Infect.* (2015) 4:e54. doi: 10.1038/emi.2015.54
17. Kunert A, Losse J, Gruszin C, Hühn M, Kaendler K, Mikkat S, et al. Immune evasion of the human pathogen *Pseudomonas aeruginosa*: elongation factor Tuf is a factor H and plasminogen binding protein. *J. Immunol.* (2007) 179:2979–88. doi: 10.4049/jimmunol.179.5.2979
18. Brady RA, Leid JG, Camper AK, Costerton JW, Shirtliff ME. Identification of *Staphylococcus aureus* proteins recognized by the antibody-mediated immune response to a biofilm infection. *Infect Immun.* (2006) 74:3415–26. doi: 10.1128/IAI.00392-06
19. Mohan S, Hertweck C, Dudda A, Hammerschmidt S, Skerka C, Hallström T, et al. Tuf of *Streptococcus pneumoniae* is a surface displayed human complement regulator binding protein. *Mol Immunol.* (2014) 62:249–64. doi: 10.1016/j.molimm.2014.06.029
20. Crowe JD, Sievwright IK, Auld GC, Moore NR, Gow NAR, Booth NA. *Candida albicans* binds human plasminogen: identification of eight plasminogen-binding proteins. *Mol Microbiol.* (2003) 47:1637–51. doi: 10.1046/j.1365-2958.2003.03390.x
21. Wang W, Jeffery CJ. An analysis of surface proteomics results reveals novel candidates for intracellular/surface moonlighting proteins in bacteria. *Mol Biosyst.* (2016) 12:1420–31. doi: 10.1039/C5MB00550G
22. Dallo SF, Kannan TR, Blaylock MW, Baseman JB. Elongation factor Tu and E1 beta subunit of pyruvate dehydrogenase complex act as fibronectin binding proteins in *Mycoplasma pneumoniae. Mol Microbiol.* (2002) 46:1041–51. doi: 10.1046/j.1365-2958.2002.03207.x
23. Muñoz-Provencio D, Pérez-Martínez G, Monedero V. Identification of surface proteins from *Lactobacillus casei* BL23 able to bind fibronectin and collagen. *Probiotics Antimicrob Proteins* (2011) 3:15–20. doi: 10.1007/s12602-011-9065-8
24. Widjaja M, Harvey KL, Hagemann L, Berry IJ, Jarocki VM, Raymond BBA, et al. Elongation factor Tu is a multifunctional and processed moonlighting protein. *Sci Rep.* (2017) 7:11227. doi: 10.1038/s41598-017-10644-z
25. Hallström T, Riesbeck K. *Haemophilus influenzae* and the complement system. *Trends Microbiol.* (2010) 18:258–65. doi: 10.1016/j.tim.2010.03.007
26. Montero D, Orellana P, Gutiérrez D, Araya D, Salazar JC, Prado V, et al. Immunoproteomic analysis to identify Shiga toxin-producing *Escherichia coli* outer membrane proteins expressed during human infection. *Infect Immun.* (2014) 82:4767–77. doi: 10.1128/IAI.02030-14
27. Mendum TA, Newcombe J, McNeilly CL, McFadden J. Towards the immunoproteome of *Neisseria meningitidis*. *PLoS ONE* (2009) 4:e5940. doi: 10.1371/journal.pone.0005940
28. Heffron SE, Moeller R, Jurnak F. Solving the structure of *Escherichia coli* elongation factor Tu using a twinned data set. *Acta Crystallogr D Biol Crystallogr* (2006) 62:433–8. doi: 10.1107/S0907444906004021
29. Abel K, Yoder MD, Hilgenfeld R, Jurnak F. An alpha to beta conformational switch in EF-Tu. *Structure* (1996) 4:1153–9. doi: 10.1016/S0969-2126(96)00123-2
30. Van Regenmortel MHV. Antigenicity and immunogenicity of synthetic peptides. *Biologicals* (2001) 29:209–13. doi: 10.1006/biol.2001.0308
31. Kolberg J, Hammerschmidt S, Frank R, Jonák J, Sanderová H, Aase A. The surface-associated elongation factor Tu is concealed for antibody binding on viable pneumococci and meningococci. *FEMS Immunol Med Microbiol.* (2008) 53:222–30. doi: 10.1111/j.1574-695X.2008.00419.x
32. Pyclik M, Górska S, Brzozowska E, Dobrut A, Ciekot J, Gamian A, et al. Epitope Mapping of *Streptococcus agalactiae* elongation factor Tu protein recognized by human sera. *Front Microbiol.* (2018) 9:125. doi: 10.3389/fmicb.2018.00125
33. Jiang F, He J, Navarro-Alvarez N, Xu J, Li X, Li P, et al. Elongation factor Tu and heat shock protein 70 are membrane-associated proteins from *Mycoplasma ovipneumoniae* capable of inducing strong immune response in mice. *PLoS ONE* (2016) 11:e0161170. doi: 10.1371/journal.pone.0161170

34. McIntosh EDG, Bröker M, Wassil J, Welsch JA, Borrow R. Serum bactericidal antibody assays–The role of complement in infection and immunity. *Vaccine* (2015) 33:4414–21. doi: 10.1016/j.vaccine.2015.07.019
35. Kroll JS, Moxon ER. Capsulation and gene copy number at the cap locus of *Haemophilus influenzae* type b. *J Bacteriol.* (1988) 170:859–64. doi: 10.1128/jb.170.2.859-864.1988
36. Ahrén IL, Williams DL, Rice PJ, Forsgren A, Riesbeck K. The importance of a beta-glucan receptor in the nonopsonic entry of nontypeable *Haemophilus influenzae*into human monocytic and epithelial cells. *J Infect Dis.* (2001) 184:150–8. doi: 10.1086/322016
37. Su YC, Mukherjee O, Singh B, Hallgren O, Westergren-Thorsson G, Hood D, et al. *Haemophilus influenzae* P4 Interacts with extracellular matrix proteins promoting adhesion and serum resistance. *J Infect Dis.* (2016) 213:314–23. doi: 10.1093/infdis/jiv374
38. de Vries SPW, van Hijum SAFT, Schueler W, Riesbeck K, Hays JP, Hermans PWM, et al. Genome analysis of *Moraxella catarrhalis* strain BBH18, [corrected] a human respiratory tract pathogen. *J Bacteriol.* (2010) 192:3574–83. doi: 10.1128/JB.00121-10
39. Möllenkvist A, Nordström T, Halldén C, Christensen JJ, Forsgren A, Riesbeck K. The *Moraxella catarrhalis* immunoglobulin D-binding protein MID has conserved sequences and is regulated by a mechanism corresponding to phase variation. *J Bacteriol.* (2003) 185:2285–95. doi: 10.1128/JB.185.7.2285-2295.2003
40. Albiger B, Johansson L, Jonsson AB. Lipooligosaccharide-deficient *Neisseria meningitidis* shows altered pilus-associated characteristics. *Infect Immun.* (2003) 71:155–62. doi: 10.1128/IAI.71.1.155-162.2003
41. Janson H, Hedén LO, Grubb A, Ruan MR, Forsgren A. Protein D, an immunoglobulin D-binding protein of *Haemophilus influenzae*: cloning, nucleotide sequence, and expression in *Escherichia coli*. *Infect Immun.* (1991) 59:119–25.
42. Waterhouse A, Bertoni M, Bienert S, Studer G, Tauriello G, Gumienny R, et al. SWISS-MODEL: homology modelling of protein structures and complexes. *Nucleic Acids Res.* (2018) 46:W296–303. doi: 10.1093/nar/gky427
43. Bienert S, Waterhouse A, de Beer TAP, Tauriello G, Studer G, Bordoli L, et al. The SWISS-MODEL repository-new features and functionality. *Nucleic Acids Res.* (2017) 45:D313–9. doi: 10.1093/nar/gkw1132
44. Guex N, Peitsch MC, Schwede T. Automated comparative protein structure modeling with SWISS-MODEL and Swiss-PdbViewer: a historical perspective. *Electrophoresis* (2009) 30 (Suppl. 1):S162–73. doi: 10.1002/elps.200900140
45. Benkert P, Biasini M, Schwede T. Toward the estimation of the absolute quality of individual protein structure models. *Bioinformatics* (2011) 27:343–50. doi: 10.1093/bioinformatics/btq662
46. Nahm MH, Briles DE, Yu X. Development of a multi-specificity opsonophagocytic killing assay. *Vaccine* (2000) 18:2768–71. doi: 10.1016/S0264-410X(00)00044-X

12

Protective Regulatory T Cell Immune Response Induced by Intranasal Immunization with the Live-Attenuated Pneumococcal Vaccine SPY1 *via* the Transforming Growth Factor-β1-Smad2/3 Pathway

Hongyi Liao[1,2†], *Xiaoqiong Peng*[3†], *Lingling Gan*[4], *Jiafu Feng*[4], *Yue Gao*[1,2], *Shenghui Yang*[1,2], *Xuexue Hu*[1,2], *Liping Zhang*[5], *Yibing Yin*[1,2], *Hong Wang*[1,2] *and Xiuyu Xu*[5*]

[1] *Key Laboratory of Diagnostic Medicine Designated by the Ministry of Education, Chongqing Medical University, Chongqing, China,* [2] *School of Laboratory Medicine, Chongqing Medical University, Chongqing, China,* [3] *Department of Ultrasound, The First Affiliated Hospital of Chongqing Medical University, Chongqing, China,* [4] *Department of Clinical Laboratory, Mianyang Central Hospital, Mianyang, Sichuan, China,* [5] *Department of Laboratory Medicine, The First Affiliated Hospital of Chongqing Medical University, Chongqing, China*

Correspondence:
Xiuyu Xu
xuxiuyu85@126.com

† *These authors have contributed equally to this work.*

Vaccine effectiveness is mainly determined by the mechanism mediating protection, emphasizing the importance of unraveling the protective mechanism for novel pneumococcal vaccine development. We previously demonstrated that the regulatory T cell (Treg) immune response has a protective effect against pneumococcal infection elicited by the live-attenuated pneumococcal vaccine SPY1. However, the mechanism underlying this protective effect remains unclear. In this study, a short synthetic peptide (P17) was used to downregulate Tregs during immunization and subsequent challenges in a mouse model. In immunized mice, increase in immune cytokines (IL-12p70, IL-4, IL-5, and IL-17A) induced by SPY1 were further upregulated by P17 treatment, whereas the decrease in the infection-associated inflammatory cytokine TNF-α by SPY1 was reversed. P17 also inhibited the increase in the immunosuppressive cytokine IL-10 and inflammatory mediator IL-6 in immunized mice. More severe pulmonary injuries and more dramatic inflammatory responses with worse survival in P17-treated immunized mice indicated the indispensable role of the Treg immune response in protection against pneumococcal infection by maintaining a balance among acquired immune responses stimulated by SPY1. Further studies revealed that the significant elevation of active transforming growth factor β (TGF-β)1 by SPY1 vaccination activated FOXP3, leading to increased frequencies of $CD4^+CD25^+Foxp3^+$ T cells. Moreover, SPY1 vaccination elevated the levels of Smad2/3 and phosphor-Smad2/3 and downregulated the negative regulatory factor Smad7 in a time-dependent manner during pneumococcal infection, and these changes were reversed by P17 treatment. These results illustrate that SPY1-stimulated TGF-β1 induced the generation of SPY1-specific Tregs *via* the Smad2/3 signaling pathway. In addition, SPY1-specific Tregs may participate in protection *via* the enhanced expression of PD-1 and CTLA-4. The data presented here extend our understanding of how the SPY1-induced acquired Treg immune response contributes to protection elicited by live-attenuated vaccines and may be helpful for the evaluation of live vaccines and other mucosal vaccine candidates.

Keywords: ***Streptococcus pneumoniae*, vaccine, protective mechanism, transforming growth factor β1, regulatory T cells**

INTRODUCTION

Streptococcus pneumoniae, an important opportunistic pathogen that colonizes the human oral and nasopharyngeal cavities, is the leading cause of pneumonia in the elderly, immunocompromised, and children younger than 5 years (1, 2). Vaccination is an effective means of preventing pneumococcal disease (3). Currently, both injection and the intranasal administration of pneumococcal vaccines are recommended by the WHO (4). However, intranasal administration can stimulate mucosal immune responses, unlike the conventional systemic delivery of vaccines using a needle and syringe. Furthermore, the mucosal delivery of vaccines can induce systemic immunity, similar to that induced by injection-based vaccination. Mucosal vaccination is pain-free, reduces the risk of needle reuse, and reduces the burden on healthcare professionals, among other benefits (5). However, commercial pneumococcal polysaccharide vaccines and conjugate vaccines are constrained by limited serotype coverage, high-cost, and vaccine serotype replacement (6, 7); accordingly, it is necessary to develop novel vaccine candidates who can overcome these disadvantages. Due to the strong antigenicity and comprehensive serotype coverage promised by a wide range of antigenic molecules, whole-cell pneumococcal vaccines are regarded as ideal vaccine candidates (8, 9). Importantly, vaccine effectiveness is mainly dependent on the underlying protective mechanism; therefore, unraveling this mechanism is critical for novel pneumococcal vaccine development.

Streptococcus pneumoniae strain SPY1 is a live-attenuated pneumococcal vaccine. We have systematically described the extremely reduced virulence, reliable genetic stability, high safety, and excellent protection against pneumococcal infection in a mouse model (10). Humoral and Th2–Th17 T cell immune responses are indispensable for the protection induced by SPY1 (11). We have also surprisingly detected a protective role of the regulatory T cell (Treg) immune response elicited by SPY1, which has not previously been described for *S. pneumoniae* vaccines (11). These findings highlight the importance of the development of novel pneumococcal vaccines that can induce a protective Treg response, which is vital for the maintenance of immune homeostasis as well as for limiting infection-associated inflammation and facilitating the resolution of tissue damage post-infection. However, the mechanism underlying the activation of the SPY1-induced Treg response is still unknown.

As a pleiotropic cytokine, transforming growth factor β (TGF-β) is essential for the differentiation of Tregs in innate immunity (12). TGF-β could induce the expression of Foxp3 and the conversion of $CD4^+CD25^-$ T cells to $CD4^+CD25^+$ T cells, promoting Treg proliferation and subsequent immunosuppression (13–15). In our previous study, a short peptide P17 (KRIWFIPRSSWYERA) was introduced to inhibit the production of TGF-β1 and to downregulate Tregs (11, 16, 17). As expected, treatment with P17 significantly impairs the effectiveness of SPY1 in colonization and invasive infection models, suggesting the importance of SPY1-induced TGF-β1 for the protective Treg immune response in acquired immunity. Several signaling pathways, including Smad-dependent and Smad-independent pathways, have potential roles in the activation of Tregs mediated by activated TGF-β1, and the specific functional pathway varies among experimental models (18–21). Previous research has shown that the percentage of Tregs is elevated in SPY1-vaccinated mice; however, signaling mechanism by which TGF-β1 mediates the differentiation of Tregs is unknown.

In this study, the mechanism underlying the protective Treg response activated by vaccination with SPY1 was explored. The inhibition of TGF-β1 dramatically attenuated the SPY1-induced protection against pulmonary injuries caused by pneumococcal colonization. In addition, SPY1-induced TGF-β1 is essential for the balance among systemic protective immune responses triggered by SPY1 vaccination. The activation of the TGF-β1-Smad2/3 signaling pathway is responsible for the generation of Tregs, which are involved in SPY1 protection *via* the elevated expression of CTLA-4 and PD-1. These findings and those of our previous studies provide insight into the proximal mechanism mediating the protection elicited by the SPY1-induced acquired Treg immune response and may contribute to a more comprehensive evaluation of live vaccines and other mucosal vaccines.

MATERIALS AND METHODS

Mice

Female C57BL/6 mice (6–8 weeks) were purchased from the animal center of Chongqing Medical University, Chongqing, China. Mice were kept under specific pathogen-free conditions at the animal facilities of Chongqing Medical University during the time of the experiments. All animal experiments were performed in accordance with the guidelines of the Institutional Animal Care and Use Committee of Chongqing Medical University.

Bacterial Strains and Immunogen Preparation

Streptococcus pneumoniae strain NCTC 7466 (D39, serotype 2) was obtained from the National Collection of Type Cultures (NCTC; London, UK). The *S. pneumoniae* clinical isolate CMCC 31693 (serotype 19F) was obtained from the National Center for Medical Culture Collections (CMCC; Beijing,

China). SPY1 is a novel live-attenuated *S. pneumoniae* vaccine candidate strain with definite serotype-independent protection against pneumococcal infection (10), and its basic protective mechanism has been described in our previous research (11). All pneumococcal strains were grown in casein-based medium with yeast extract (C + Y medium) or on Columbia sheep blood agar plates at 37°C in 5% CO_2. To prepare the immunogens, SPY1 was grown at 37°C in 5% CO_2 in C + Y medium to approximately 2×10^8 CFU/ml. After centrifugation and washing (twice), sediments were resuspended in sterile phosphate-buffered saline (PBS). The final vaccine mixture for routine immunization contained 1×10^8 CFU of SPY1 and 1 µg of adjuvant cholera toxin (CT; Sigma-Aldrich, St. Louis, MO, USA) per 20-µl dose.

Immunization of Mice and Challenge

C57BL/6 mice were anesthetized with ethyl ether and then intranasally administered the vaccine (group CT + SPY1) or adjuvant alone (group CT) four times at 1-week intervals. One week after the last vaccination, mice were intranasally challenged with either strain 19F (1×10^8 CFU) or strain D39 (1×10^8 CFU). To investigate the roles and related mechanisms of the SPY1-induced Treg immune response, as shown in **Figure 1A**, during the whole vaccination period of 28 days, half of the mice in the CT + SPY1 group were randomly chosen and treated with an intraperitoneal injection of 100 µg of peptide P17 daily to downregulate Tregs (group CT + SPY1 + P17), as described previously (11). The other half of mice in the CT + SPY1 group received sterile PBS as a control. Similarly, mice from CT group were also injected with P17 or PBS daily. In addition to 28 days of P17 treatment, on the day of challenge, the P17-treated mice received 500 µg of P17 twice at 2 and 4 h before challenge (**Figure 1A**). The peptide P17 (KRIWFIPRSSWYERA; purity >95%, as determined by high performance liquid chromatography) was synthesized by GL Biochem (Shanghai, China).

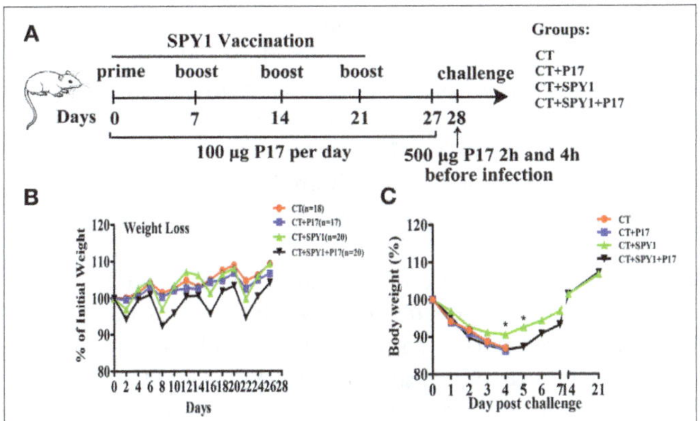

FIGURE 1 | Regulatory T cell (Treg) downregulator P17 eliminates SPY1-elicited protection against invasive *S. pneumonia* infection. **(A)** Mice were intranasally immunized with SPY1 plus CT or with CT alone for four times at 1-week intervals. During the whole vaccination progress of 28 days in all, half of mice from group CT + SPY1 were randomly chosen to be intraperitoneally injected with 100 µg of peptide P17 daily and the other half of mice in group CT + SPY1 received sterile phosphate-buffered saline (PBS) as control. Similarly, mice from CT group were also injected with P17 or PBS daily. On day 28, mice were intranasally challenged with pneumococcal strains. **(B)** Mice body weight were monitored every other day during the vaccination procedure, and the weight data were expressed as the percentages of initial mice weights measured at day 0 of vaccination. On day 28, mice were intranasal challenged with 1×10^8 CFU of pneumococcal strain D39, and the body weights of live mice were monitored for consecutive 21 days after infection **(C)**. $^*p < 0.05$.

Flow Cytometry

Mouse lungs were removed and cell suspensions were prepared. For Treg ($CD4^+CD25^+Foxp3^+$) detection, lung cells were first incubated with CD16/CD32 and stained with anti-mouse CD4-FITC (clone RM4-5; eBioscience, San Diego, CA, USA) and anti-mouse CD25-APC (clone PC61.5; eBioscience). Then, these cells were fixed and permeabilized in Fix/Perm buffer and subsequently incubated with anti-mouse Foxp3-PE (clone FJK-16S; eBioscience), according to the instructions provided with the Mouse Regulatory T Cell Staining Kit (eBioscience) for the intracellular Foxp3 analysis. To analyze the expression of PD-1 and CTLA-4, cells were stained with anti-mouse CD279 (PD-1)-APC/Cy7 (clone 29F.1A12; BioLegend, San Diego, CA, USA) and anti-mouse CD152 (CTLA-4)-PerCP/Cy5.5 (clone UC10-4B9; BioLegend). All the samples were analyzed using a Becton Dickinson FACSCalibur flow cytometer (Franklin Lakes, NJ, USA).

RNA Extraction and Quantitative Real-Time PCR

Mouse lungs were removed at different time points after pneumococcal 19F challenge, and total RNA was extracted using RNAiso Plus reagent (Takara Bio, Dalian, China) following the manufacturer's instructions. For reverse transcription, 1 µg of total RNA was reverse-transcribed into cDNA, and the PrimeScript™ RT Reagent Kit (Takara Bio) was used for reverse transcription. PCR amplification was performed on the Bio-Rad CFX96 Real-Time system using SYBR Premix Ex Taq™ (Takara Bio). The $2^{-\Delta\Delta Ct}$ method was used to determine the specific Ct value of each target gene. Quantitative real-time PCR for each target gene were repeated three times. The PCR primers were synthesized by Sangon (Shanghai, China) and the sequences are listed in Table S1 in Supplementary Material. All genes were murine in origin.

Protein Extraction and Western Blot Analysis

Lungs were collected at different time points after pneumococcal 19F challenge, and proteins were extracted by adding the appropriate volume of whole-cell lysates [RIPA buffer (Beyotime, Shanghai, China): PMSF: phosphatase inhibitor (BioTools, Jupiter, FL, USA) = 100:10:1]. For the detection of Smad2/3, phosphor-Smad2/3, and Smad7 at the protein levels, the same concentrations of total cellular extracts were separated by 10% SDS-PAGE, subjected to electrophoresis, and transferred to PVDF membranes (Millipore, Bedford, MA, USA) by electroblotting. After they were blocked with 5% skim milk for 2 h at room temperature, membranes were incubated overnight at 4°C with primary antibodies, including anti-mouse β-actin, anti-mouse Smad2/3, anti-mouse phosphor-Smad2/3 (Cell Signaling Technology, Danvers, MA, USA), and anti-mouse Smad7 antibodies (Abcam, Cambridge, UK), followed by incubation with an HRP-conjugated secondary antibody for 1 h at room temperature. The Enhanced Chemiluminescence (ECL) Western Blotting System (GE Healthcare, Little Chalfont, UK) was used to detect the target bands. The band intensities were quantified using Quantity One (Bio-Rad Laboratories, Hercules, CA, USA).

Cytokine Assays

Mouse lungs and spleens were fully homogenized and centrifuged, and the supernatants were collected for cytokine measurement. In addition, mouse splenocytes were plated in 24-well tissue culture plates in 1 ml of DMEM with 10% fetal calf serum (HyClone, Logan, UT, USA) (2×10^7 cells/well) after red blood cells were removed by hemolysis. Cultured splenocytes were stimulated with 70% ethanol-inactivated SPY1 (equivalent to 10^7 CFU/ml), and the supernatants were harvested at different time points for cytokine measurement. Levels of IL-6, TNF-α, IL-12p70, IFN-γ, IL-4, IL-5, IL-17A, and IL-10 in homogenate supernatants and splenocyte supernatants were measured using an enzyme-linked immunosorbent assay (ELISA) kit (BioLegend) in accordance with the manufacturer's protocols. Samples were diluted when required.

Immunofluorescence Assay

At 24 h post-pneumococcal 19F challenge, mouse lungs were removed and fixed in 4% paraformaldehyde for 24 h and permeated in 20% sucrose for 24 h. Then, the tissues were frozen in OCT at −20°C and cryo-cut for slides. For Smad2/3 staining, after thawing and blocking with goat serum and subsequent washing with PBS, slides were covered with an anti-Smad2/3 antibody (Cell Signaling Technology) at 4°C overnight, followed by incubation with Fluorescein-Conjugated Goat Anti-Rat IgG (ZSGB-bio, Beijing, China). DAPI was used to stain cell nuclei for 2 h at room temperature in the dark. The cell morphology and fluorescence intensities were observed using an ECLIPSE 80i microscope equipped with a Nikon INTENSILIGHT C-HGFI. The percentages of lung cells with positive Smad2/3 expression were calculated by counting 100 cells per slide (three mice per group).

Lung Histology and Immunohistochemistry

On day 7 after the last immunization, mice were intranasally challenged with 1×10^8 CFU of pneumococcal strain 19F. Mice were sacrificed and lung tissues were removed at 6, 12, and 24 h post-infection. After fixation in buffered 10% formalin, lungs were sectioned and embedded in paraffin, and 5-μm sections were cut. The sections were stained with hematoxylin and eosin (Sigma-Aldrich) and then examined using a light microscope. The degrees of peribronchial inflammation were graded semi-quantitatively following previously described methods (22).

For immunohistochemistry, sections were retrieved in citrate buffer for 5 min. After natural cooling, sections were incubated with 3% H_2O_2 and washed three times with PBS, followed by incubation with an anti-FOXP3 antibody (BioLegend) and Rabbit anti-TGF-β1 polyclonal antibody (OmnimAbs, Alhambra, CA, USA) and treatment with streptavidin horseradish peroxidase chemistry according to standard protocols. The mean IODs (integral optical density) of TGF-β1 expression were measured using Image-Pro Plus (Media Cybernetics, Silver Spring, MD, USA).

Data Analysis and Statistics

Statistical analyses were performed using GraphPad Prism 5 (GraphPad Software, La Jolla, CA, USA). Unpaired Student's *t*-tests were used to compare two independent groups. One-way ANOVA was utilized for multiple comparisons. Differences at $p < 0.05$ were considered statistically significant.

RESULTS

Treg Downregulator P17 Eliminates SPY1-Elicited Protection Against Invasive *S. pneumoniae* Infection

In this study, female C57BL/6 mice were intranasally immunized according to the vaccination schedule described in **Figure 1A**. During the vaccination process, half of the immunized mice were intraperitoneally injected with 100 μg of the short synthetic peptide P17 to downregulate Treg activity, and the body weights of all mice were observed every other day. Compared with the CT group, mice in the SPY1 group lost more body weight in the first several days after the first vaccination, and body weight in the of SPY1 group recovered quickly to the level of the CT group (**Figure 1B**). However, we observed greater body weight loss in mice in the CT + SPY1 + P17 group than in the CT + SPY1 group during the vaccination period (**Figure 1B**), which may be due to the disruption of the immune regulatory response caused by P17 administration.

On day 28, mice were intranasally challenged with *S. pneumoniae* strain D39. Greater body weight loss was observed in non-immunized mice than in immunized mice on day 4 post-challenge (**Figure 1C**). Beginning at day 5 post-D39 infection, body weights of mice belonging to the SPY1-immunized group began to increase, finally recovering to the weights recorded before infection, illustrating the protection elicited by SPY1, to some extent (**Figure 1C**). The body weights of mice in the P17-treated SPY1-immunized group also recovered on day 5 post-infection; however, the degree of body weight increase was significantly lower than that in the SPY1-immunized group (**Figure 1C**). More importantly, compared with other mouse groups, SPY1-immunized mice survived for longer after lethal *S. pneumoniae* strain D39 infection (Figure S1 in Supplementary Material), consistent with our previous results (11). Collectively, these data demonstrated that the Treg downregulator P17 can markedly eliminate SPY1-elicited protection against invasive *S. pneumoniae* infection, highlighting the importance of the protective Treg immune response.

P17 Treatment Disturbs the Immune Responses Triggered by SPY1 Vaccination

To further investigate the influence of P17 administration on the specific immune responses induced by SPY1, concentrations of immune and inflammatory cytokines in mouse splenocyte supernatants after stimulation by inactivated SPY1 were determined on day 7 after the last immunization. Coincident with our previous results (11), stimulation with inactivated SPY1 induced higher levels of IL-6, IL-12p70, IL-4, IL-5, and IL-17A in immunized mice than in non-immunized mouse (**Figure 2**). Elevated levels of IL-10 in immunized mice indicated the activation of an immunoregulatory response elicited by SPY1 (**Figure 2**). We detected a disturbance in the SPY1-activated immune responses in P17-treated immunized mice, which was attributed to the inhibition of immunosuppressive Tregs by P17. The increase in immune cytokines (IL-12p70, IL-4, IL-5, and IL-17A) induced by SPY1 were further upregulated by P17 treatment, whereas the decrease in the infection-associated inflammatory cytokine TNF-α by SPY1 was reversed. Furthermore, P17 also inhibited the increase in the immunosuppressive cytokine IL-10 and inflammatory mediator IL-6 (23) in immunized mice (**Figure 2**).

P17 Treatment Significantly Impairs SPY1-Induced Protection Against Pulmonary Injury Caused by Pneumococcal Colonization

Previously, we established the negative effect of P17 on SPY1-specific protection against *S. pneumoniae* infection, including improved survival rates and reduced bacterial loads in the nasopharynx and lungs (11). In this study, to explore the protective roles of the SPY1-stimulated Treg immune response in more detail, differences in mouse pulmonary damage after pneumococcal colonization among groups were evaluated based on lung morphological observations and histopathological analyses. Moderate inflammatory cell recruitment to the pulmonary interstitium around airways and blood vessels and slight damage to alveolar structural integrity were observed in SPY1-immunized mice post-intranasal challenge with pneumococcal strain 19 F (**Figures 3A,B**; Figure S2 in Supplementary Material). By contrast, more severe pulmonary injuries were found in the CT control group, with extensive inflammatory cell infiltration in peribronchial as well as perivascular spaces and in the alveoli, disappearance of alveolar structural integrity, and obvious hemorrhage. Similar serious pulmonary injuries were also detected in P17-treated immunized mice, since the immune modulatory response was markedly suppressed. Consistent with these results, compared with other groups, a remarkably lower peribronchial inflammation score was observed in SPY1-immunized mice (**Figure 3C**). Simultaneously, pulmonary levels of cytokines representing different immune responses triggered by SPY1 vaccination were evaluated. As shown in **Figure 3D**, compared with non-immunized mice, a decrease in the inflammatory cytokine TNF-α and increase in immune cytokines, including IL-6, IL-12p70, IL-4, IL-5, IL-17A, and IL-10, were found in immunized mouse lung homogenates, indicating elevated, but controlled SPY1-induced immune responses, which are beneficial for fighting

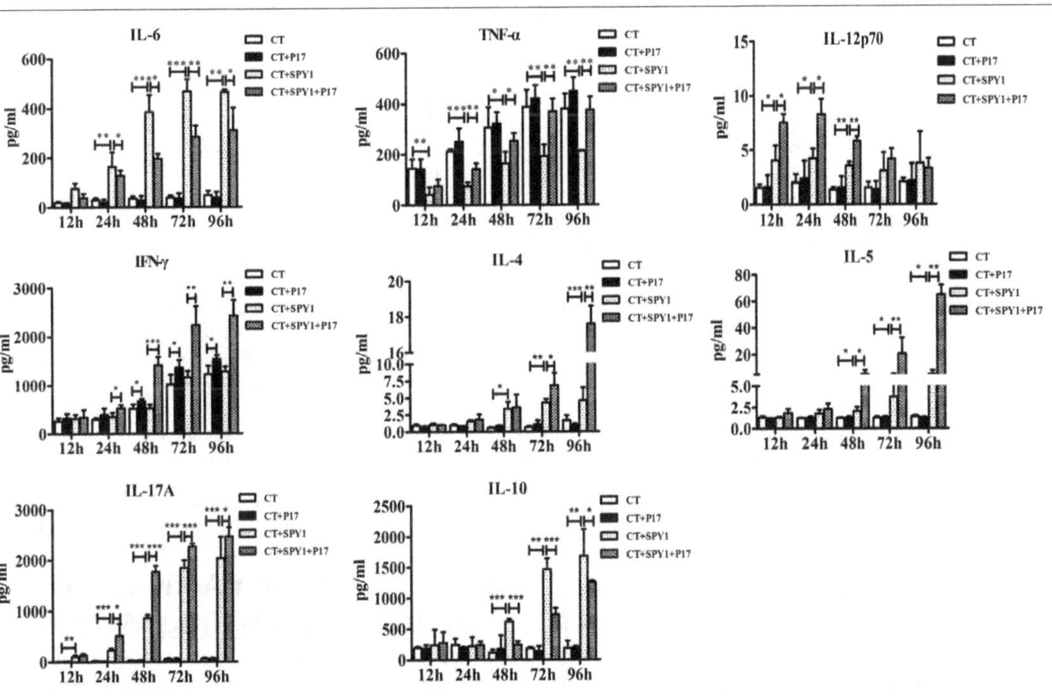

FIGURE 2 | P17 treatment strikes the balance among systemic protective immune responses triggered by SPY1 vaccination. On day 7 after the last immunization, mice splenocytes were isolated and stimulated with 70% ethanol-inactivated SPY1. Splenocytes treated with Concanavalin A served as positive control. Concentrations of cytokines including IL-6, TNF-α, IL-12p70, IFN-γ, IL-4, IL-5, IL-17A, and IL-10 in supernatants of stimulated splenocytes were analyzed by enzyme-linked immunosorbent assay. All data were presented as the mean ± SD of three independent experiments. *$p < 0.05$; **$p < 0.01$; ***$p < 0.001$.

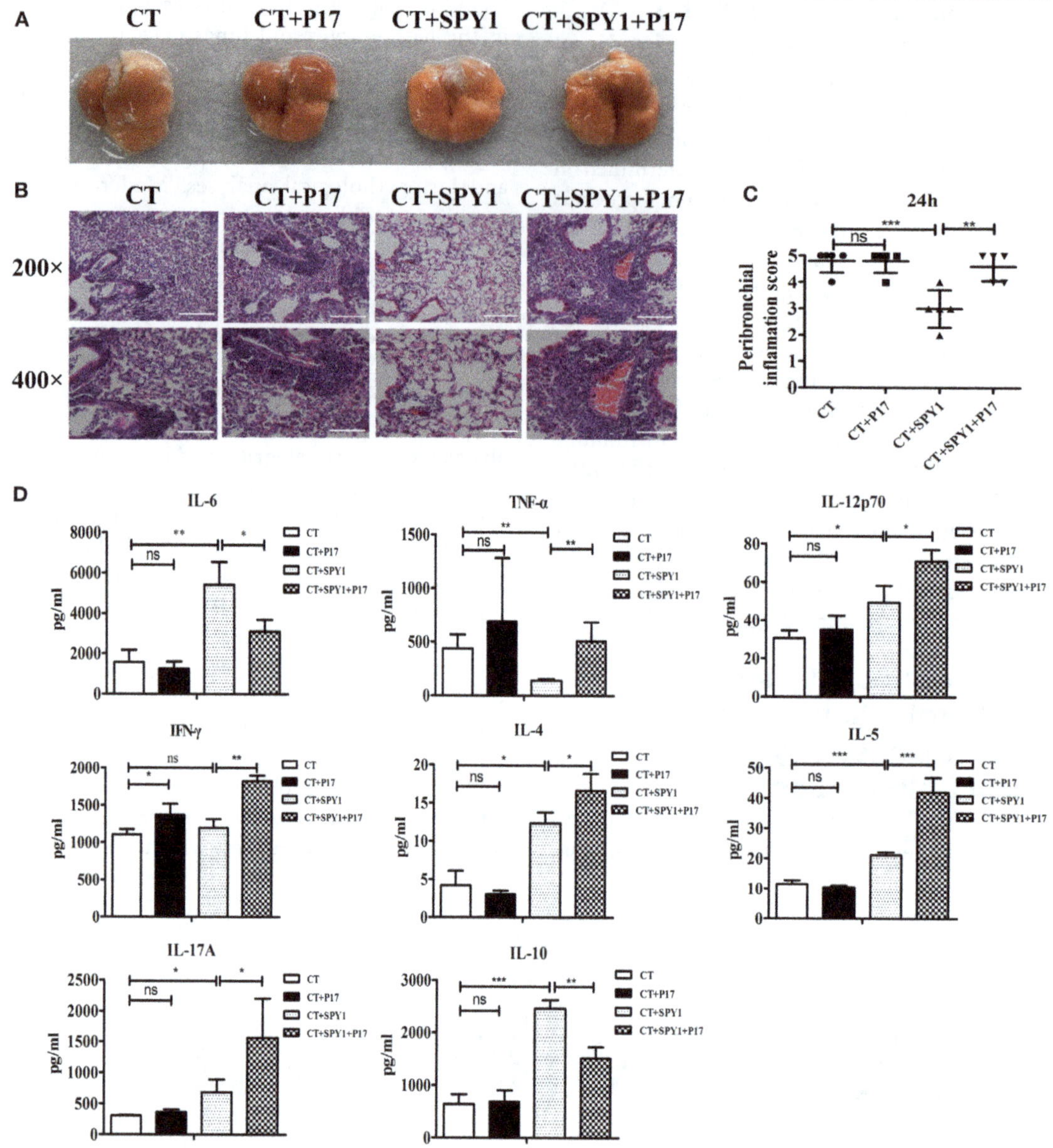

FIGURE 3 | P17 treatment significantly impairs the SPY1-induced acquired protection against pulmonary injury caused by pneumococcal colonization. On day 7 after the last immunization, mice were intranasal challenged with 1 × 10^8 CFU of pneumococcal strain 19F. Mice were sacrificed and lung tissues were removed at 24 h post-intranasal infection with pneumococcal strain 19F. **(A)** Lungs appearance post-infection. **(B)** Pathological analyses were done by hematoxylin and eosin staining, with lung sections examined under light microscopy at 200× (scale bar = 100 μm) and 400× (scale bar = 50 μm) magnification. **(C)** Scores of peribronchial inflammations were semi-quantitatively graded, and data were shown as mean ± SD of scores of five mice per group. **(D)** Concentrations of cytokines including IL-6, TNF-α, IL-12p70, IFN-γ, IL-4, IL-5, IL-17A, and IL-10 in lung homogenates collected at 48 h post-infection were detected by enzyme-linked immunosorbent assay, and the data were shown as mean ± SD (each experiment was individually performed three times). *$p < 0.05$; **$p < 0.01$; ***$p < 0.001$.

against pneumococcal colonization. By contrast, due to the downregulation of the immune-suppressive cytokine IL-10 and consequent immune imbalance caused by P17 treatment, mice showed drastic and uncontrolled pulmonary immune responses as well as infection-associated inflammation, characterized by even higher concentrations of TNF-α, IL-12p70, IFN-γ, IL-4, IL-5, and IL-17A (**Figure 3D**), consistent with the degrees of pulmonary injury described above.

SPY1 Vaccination Activates the Expression of the Treg Molecule FOXP3

In our previous study, we were surprised to detect a protective role of the SPY1-specific Treg immune response during pneumococcal infection (11). In this study, to comprehensively analyze the mechanism underlying the activation of Tregs by vaccination, the expression of the transcription factor Foxp3, a characteristic molecule in the Treg immune pathway, was first examined. Flow cytometry results showed a significant increase ($p < 0.01$) in CD4$^+$CD25$^+$Foxp3$^+$ T cells in immunized mouse lungs; however, P17 treatment could reverse the increase in Foxp3-positive cells to a level similar to that in the CT control group (**Figure 4A**). More importantly, the *foxp3* mRNA level was significantly higher in SPY1-immunized mice than in the CT control group, and the upregulation was reversed by P17 treatment (**Figure 4B**). The inhibition of FOXP3 in SPY1-vaccinated mice by P17 treatment was also verified by immunohistochemical staining of lung tissues (**Figure 4C**). Thus, these results demonstrated that SPY1 triggers a FOXP3 response.

SPY1 Vaccination Stimulates TGF-β1 Production

Transforming growth factor β is a vital cytokine for the differentiation of Tregs (14). To identify the mechanism underlying the generation of SPY1-specific Tregs, the production of TGF-β1, one of the three isoforms expressed mainly in the immune system in immunized mice, was evaluated. As shown in **Figures 5A,B**, substantial increases in the concentrations of active TGF-β1 in lung homogenates as well as spleen homogenates in immunized mice were observed by ELISA. Splenocytes from mice immunized with SPY1 expressed significantly more active TGF-β1 in response to inactivated SPY1 *in vitro* than that of splenocytes from CT-treated control mice (**Figure 5C**), illustrating the stimulation of TGF-β1. Further verifying the production of SPY1-stimulated TGF-β1, *tgf-β1* mRNA, levels were higher in immunized mouse lungs after intranasal infection with pneumococcal strain 19F than in the CT-treated control group, reaching peak levels at 12 h post-infection (**Figure 5D**). Immunohistochemical staining of mouse lung tissues with TGF-β1 antibodies also proved the activation of TGF-β1 by vaccination with SPY1 (**Figures 5E,F**; Figure S3 in Supplementary Material), with a remarkable increase in the percentage of TGF-β1-positive lung cells from SPY1-immunized mice in a time-dependent manner (**Figure 5G**). More importantly, all of the trends indicating an increase in active TGF-β1 in immunized mice were obviously inhibited by the administration of P17, providing further evidence that SPY1 vaccination could stimulate the production of TGF-β1.

TGF-β1-Smad2/3 Signaling Participates in the Generation of SPY1-Specific Tregs

Classic TGF-β-inducing intracellular signaling is mediated by SMAD family proteins, and the differentiation of Tregs from naïve T cells is mainly regulated by the TGF-β/Smad pathway (24). To explore the specific signaling pathway involving in the differentiation of SPY1-induced Tregs, dynamic changes in *Smad* mRNA in mouse lungs post-pneumococcal infection were detected. As shown in **Figures 6A–C**, compared with CT-treated mice, the expression levels of *smad2*, *smad3*, and *smad4* mRNA were substantially higher in immunized mice at 6 and 12 h post-pneumococcal strain 19F infection and were also significantly higher than those in P17-treated SPY1-vaccinated mice. A relatively low level of *smad7*, which is a negative regulator in the TGF-β signaling pathway, was detected in immunized mice (**Figure 6D**). Moreover, P17 treatment significantly upregulated the expression of *smad7* in the immunized group, since P17 injection could block TGF-β

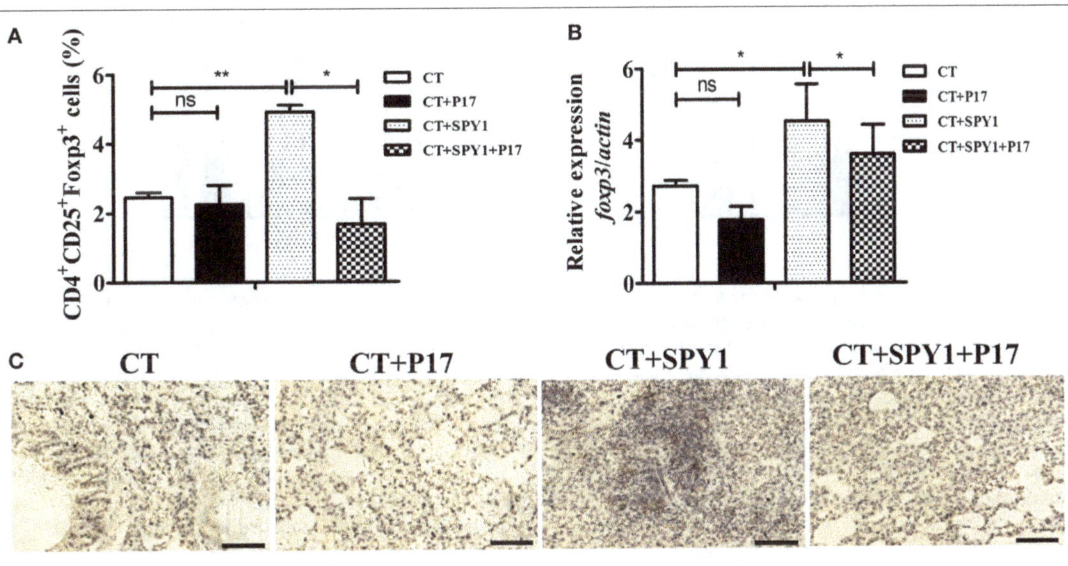

FIGURE 4 | SPY1 vaccination activates the expression of regulatory T cells (Tregs) molecule Foxp3. **(A)** On day 7 after the last immunization, mice lungs were aseptically removed and homogenized, and single lung cell was stained with anti-mouse CD4-FITC and anti-mouse CD25-APC, followed by anti-mouse Foxp3-APC according to the manufacturer's instructions. Cells were analyzed using a Becton Dickinson FACSCalibur flow cytometer then. The percentages of CD4$^+$ T cells which were CD25$^+$Foxp3$^+$ Treg were calculated. **(B)** On day 7 after the last immunization, mice lungs were aseptically removed, and total RNA were extracted. Expression of *foxp3* mRNA was analyzed by quantitative real-time PCR. Data were shown as mean ± SD from three independent experiments. **(C)** On day 7 after the last immunization, mice lungs were aseptically removed, and lung sections were stained with anti-FOXP3 antibody followed by streptavidin horseradish peroxidase chemistry. Then, the sections were examined under light microscopy at 100x magnification. Scale bar = 100 μm. Images were representative of staining observed in the lungs of mice within the group (n = 4–6 mice). $^*p < 0.05$; $^{**}p < 0.01$.

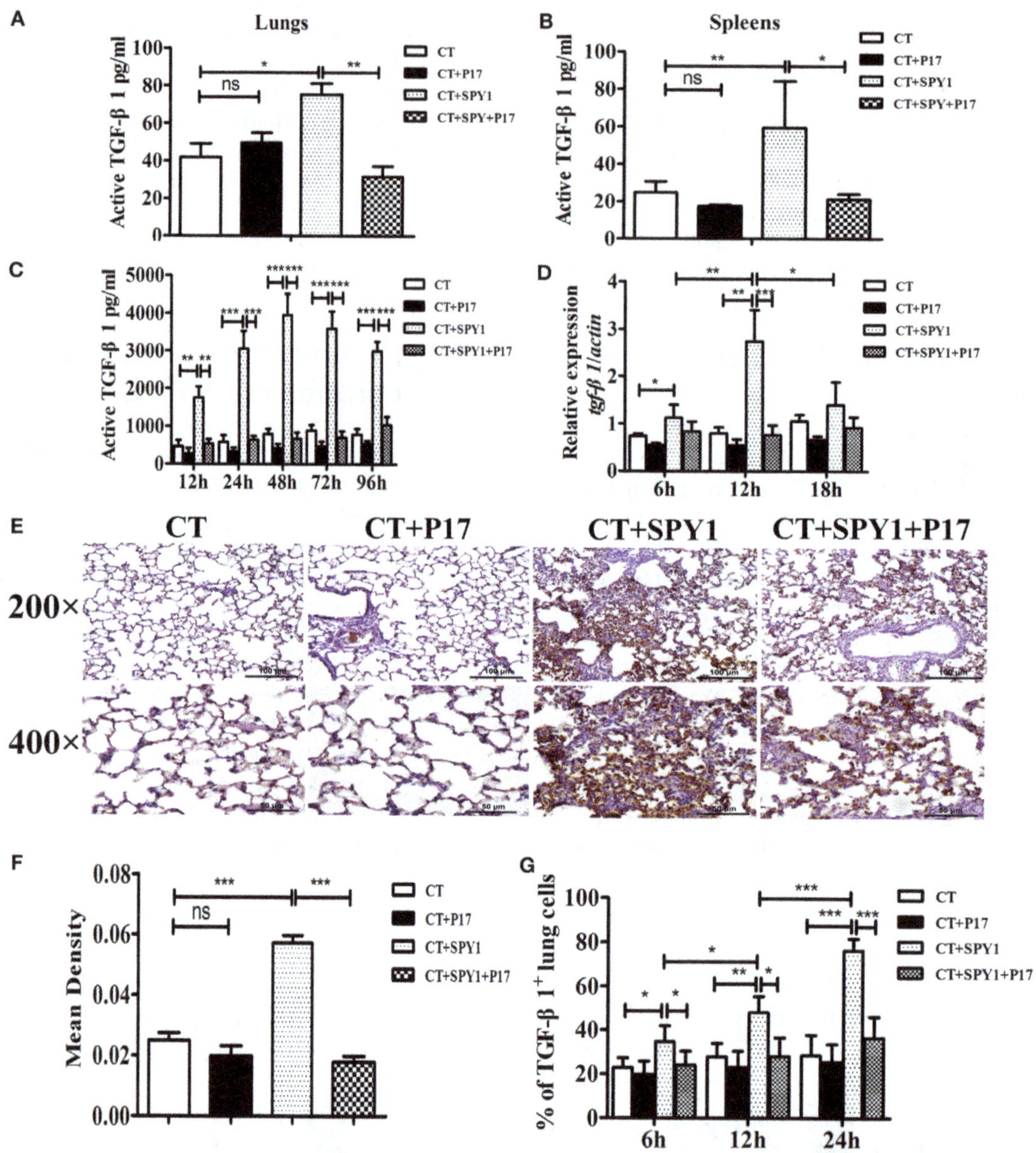

FIGURE 5 | SPY1 vaccination stimulates the production of transforming growth factor β (TGF-β)1. On day 7 after the last immunization, mice were sacrificed and concentrations of active TGF-β1 in lungs **(A)** and spleens **(B)** were determined by enzyme-linked immunosorbent assay (ELISA). **(C)** Splenocytes were isolated and stimulated with 70% ethanol-killed SPY1, and the level of active TGF-β1 in splenocytes supernatants was also detected by ELISA. **(D)** Mice were intranasal challenged with 1×10^8 CFU of pneumococcal strain 19F on day 7 after the last immunization, and expression of *tgf-β1* mRNA in lungs were analyzed by quantitative real-time PCR at 6, 12, and 18 h post-infection, respectively. **(E)** At 24 h post-pneumococcal 19F infection, immunohistochemical staining with anti-TGF-β1 polyclonal antibody was utilized to detect expression of TGF-β1 in lung tissues. Lung sections were examined under light microscopy at magnification 200x (scale bar = 100 μm) and 400x (scale bar = 50 μm). **(F)** The mean IODs of TGF-β1 expression were measured and calculated by Image-Pro Plus. Data were shown as mean ± SD of IODs of five mice per group. **(G)** Expressions of TGF-β1 in mice lungs at 6, 12, and 24 h post 19F infection were determined by immunohistochemical staining, and percentages of lung cells with positive TGF-β1 expressions were calculated by counting 100 cells of each lung section with three slides per time point (three mice per group). Data were shown as the mean ± SD from three independent experiments. $^{*}p < 0.05$; $^{**}p < 0.01$; $^{***}p < 0.001$.

signaling. Furthermore, total Smad2/3, phosphorylated Smad2/3, and Smad7 protein expression levels were analyzed by western blotting (**Figures 6E–H**). Consistent with the observed mRNA expression changes, the expression of Smad2/3 was upregulated in immune mice and downregulated in P17-injected mice at 12 and 18 h post-infection. The stimulation of the TGF-β1/Smad pathway in mouse lungs by SPY1 vaccination was also established by an immunofluorescence assay, indicating significant differences in the percentages of cells expressing Smad2/3 between immunized mice and P17-treated immunized mice (**Figures 6I,J**). We further evaluated whether other SMAD-independent pathways were involved in the stimulation of SPY1-specific Tregs, but the mRNA expression levels of various signaling molecules including *p38 mapk*, *akt*, *mtor*, and *pi3k*, did not differ significantly among

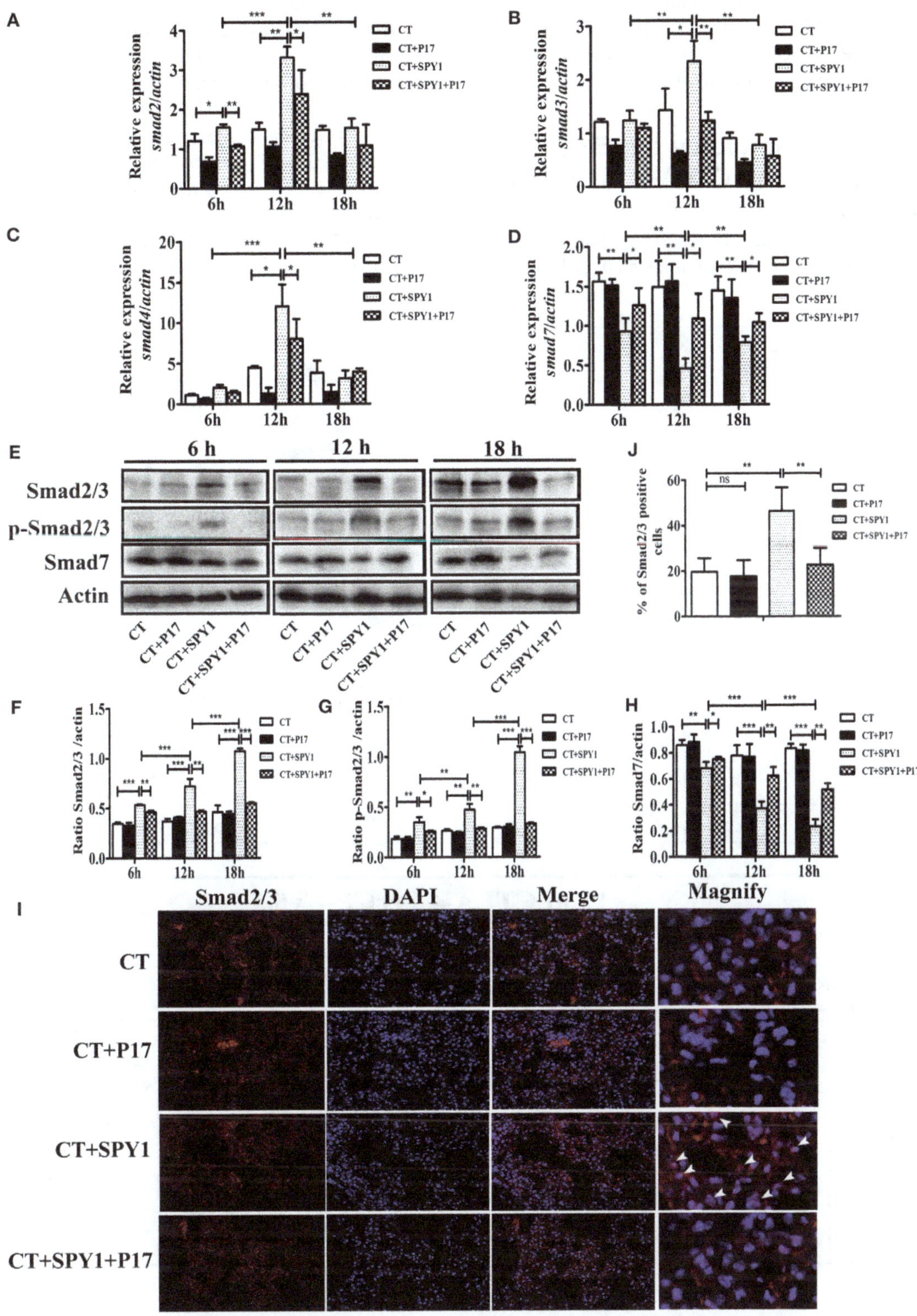

FIGURE 6 | Transforming growth factor β (TGF-β)1-Smad2/3 signaling participates in generation of SPY1-specific regulatory T cells (Tregs). Mice were intranasal challenged with pneumococcal strain 19F on day 7 after the last immunization, and the lungs were aseptically removed at 6, 12, and 18 h post-infection. **(A–D)** Expression of *smad2*, *smad3*, *smad4*, and *smad7* in lungs were analyzed by quantitative real-time PCR. The productions of Smad2/3, phosphor-Smad2/3, and Smad7 in lungs were, respectively, determined by western blot **(E)** and the related band intensities were shown in histograms **(F–H)**. **(I)** The expression of Smad2/3 in lungs at 24 h post-infection was examined by immunofluorescence assay with anti-Smad2/3 antibody. Lung sections were examined under light microscopy at magnification 400×. **(J)** Statistical analysis of the percentages of lung cells with positive Smad2/3 expression was performed by counting 100 cells per slide (three mice per group). Data were shown as the mean ± SD from three independent experiments. *$p < 0.05$; **$p < 0.01$; ***$p < 0.001$.

groups (data not shown). Taken together, these results confirmed that SPY1 vaccination could activate the TGF-β1-Smad2/3 signal pathway to induce a SPY1-specific Treg response and, as a consequence, protection during pneumococcal infection.

SPY1 Vaccination Stimulates the Elevated Expression of PD-1 and CTLA-4 on Tregs in Immunized Mice

As an immune response balance factor, Tregs play roles in immunosuppression *via* multiple Treg-associated cell surface molecules and secreted molecules (25). Therefore, to investigate the specific effectors of SPY1-induced Tregs, the expression of PD-1 and CTLA-4 on $CD4^+CD25^+Foxp3^+$ cells was examined by flow cytometry (**Figure 7A**). As shown in **Figures 7B,C**, the percentages of $PD\text{-}1^+CD4^+CD25^+Foxp3^+$ and $CTLA\text{-}4^+CD4^+CD25^+Foxp3^+$ cells were both significantly higher in SPY1-immunized mice than in the CT control group, while treatment with P17 (CT + SPY1 + P17 group) reversed the upregulation of immunosuppressive factors. Taken together, these results indicated that PD-1 and CTLA-4 are involved in the SPY1-specific immune modulatory response.

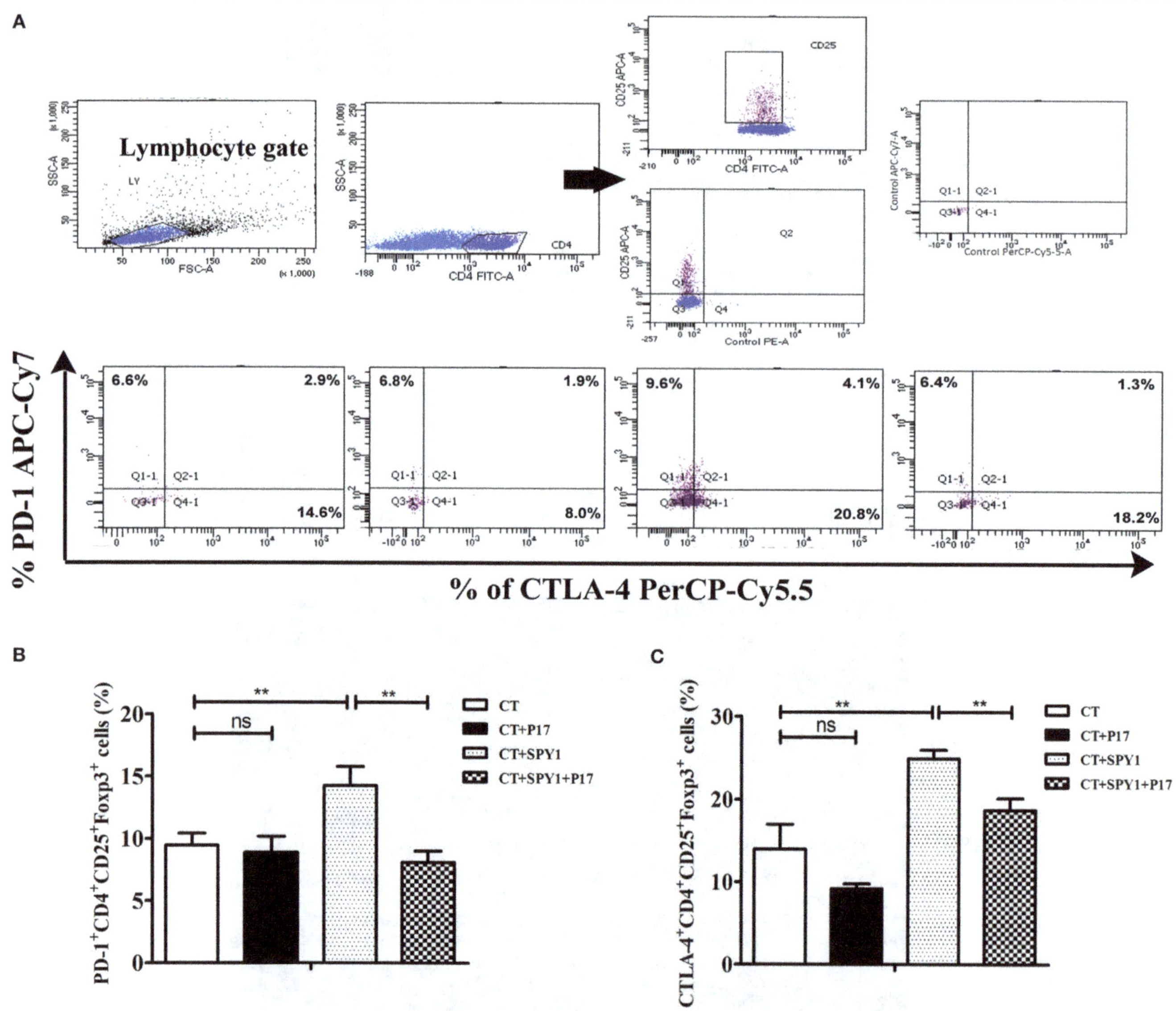

FIGURE 7 | SPY1 vaccination stimulates elevating expression of PD-1 and CTLA-4 on regulatory T cells (Tregs) in immune mice. **(A)** Mice were intranasal challenged with pneumococcal strain 19F on day 7 after the last immunization, and mice lungs were removed on day 3 post-infection. The relative expression of PD-1 and CTLA-4 on $CD4^+CD25^+Foxp3^+$ cells were analyzed by flow cytometry with antibodies including anti-mouse CD279(PD-1)-APC/Cy7, anti-mouse CD152(CTLA-4)-PerCP/Cy5.5, anti-mouse CD4-FITC, anti-mouse CD25-APC, and anti-mouse Foxp3-PE, respectively. The procedure was as describe in Section "Materials and Methods." Percentages of $PD\text{-}1^+CD4^+CD25^+Foxp3^+$ cells **(B)** and $CTLA\text{-}4^+CD4^+CD25^+Foxp3^+$ cells **(C)** in mice lung of triplicate samples were calculated. Data were shown as the mean ± SD. $^{**}p < 0.01$.

DISCUSSION

Investigations of the mechanism underlying immune protection are crucial for novel vaccine development. We have previously detected protective roles of the acquired Treg response induced by the novel live-attenuated pneumococcal vaccine SPY1 during pneumococcal infection. In this study, we clarified the mechanism mediating the protective Treg response.

Pneumococcal conjugate vaccines reduce the risk of nasopharyngeal colonization by the serotypes included in the vaccine (3). However, their wide application is restricted by the limited serotypes, high cost, serotype replacement, etc. Compared with pneumococcal conjugate vaccines, pneumococcal whole-cell vaccines may be a better choice for developing countries, since they retained whole molecules which act as pathogen-associated molecular patterns recognized by host antigen-presenting cells and are presented in their natural configuration (9). Various procedures are used for vaccination, even for live-attenuated vaccines. In an investigation of the live-attenuated cholera vaccine VCUSM21P, administration twice at an interval of 14 days yielded acceptable protection (26). Other studies have found that live-attenuated hepatitis A vaccines H2 and LA-1 virus strains exert satisfactory protection with a single dose administered by subcutaneous injection (27). Based on our previous exploration of SPY1 vaccination, we observed a robust humoral and cellular immune response after intranasal vaccination with SPY1 four times, inducing robust immune responses (11, 28). In our previous work, the differences in immune responses and protective efficacies of SPY1 by intraperitoneal immunization and intranasal immunization were evaluated. Intraperitoneal immunization and intranasal immunization both induced elevations in IL-10, IL-4, and IL-17A; however, the levels of IL-17A in splenocyte supernatants and nasal washes as well as secretory IgA in saliva in intranasally immunized mice were significantly higher than those in intraperitoneally immunized mice, suggesting better protection against pneumococcal colonization in an intranasal immunization model (10). In addition, intranasal immunization provided increased protection against lethal pneumococcal challenge at 3 months post-vaccination, and the survival rates for the intranasal immunization model and intraperitoneal immunization model were 100 and 75%, respectively, and this difference can probably be explained by the more rapid clearance of the subcutaneously injected vaccine (29).

Vaccine adjuvants can be used to enhance immunogenicity, accelerate the immune response, increase the duration of protection, and so on (30). For live-attenuated vaccines, some studies have shown that the antigenicity and immunogenicity of vaccine strains, such as live-attenuated *Yersinia pestis* against pneumonic plague are strong enough so that the adjuvant is not necessary (31). However, other studies have shown the indispensable role of adjuvants for vaccination with live-attenuated vaccines, such as the cholera vaccine candidate VCUSM21P (26) and H5N1 live-attenuated influenza vaccines (32). In our previous research, we have evaluated the vaccination of SPY1 without adjuvant CT; however, the protective effect was not as efficient as that obtained by CT (data not published). We used adjuvant CT, as in our other studies of SPY1 (10, 11). However, the toxicity of CT limits its application in humans, making the development of safe and nontoxic adjuvants that induce protective immunity essential for the nasal immunization of SPY1 in humans. We have developed safe and effective mucosal adjuvants as CT alternatives, such as the mast cell activator compound 48/80 (C48/80) (33) and CaPi mineralized shell (34). Coupled with these nontoxic adjuvants, protection induced by SPY1 or its derived vaccine SPY1ΔlytA is as efficient as that obtained with CT, ensuring the future application of SPY1 in humans.

The balance between immune response activation essential for host defense and immune suppression restricting excessive host damage caused by the immune response should be strictly regulated during pathogen invasion. In this study, P17, which downregulates Tregs, influenced the systemic protective immune response elicited by SPY1 immunization. P17 treatment significantly upregulated levels of the infection-associated inflammatory cytokine TNF-α and immune cytokines (IL-12p70, IFN-γ, IL-4, IL-5, and IL-17A) and downregulated concentrations of the immunosuppressive cytokine IL-10 and inflammatory mediator IL-6 (23) secreted by splenocytes of SPY1-immunized mice. Correspondently, compared with SPY1-immunized mice not treated with P17, we observed more severe pulmonary injuries in P17-treated immunized mice during pneumococcal infection. Moreover, the changes in cytokines in immunized mouse lung homogenates were in line with those in splenocytes mentioned above. These data indicated that the SPY1-specific Treg immune response could inhibit uncontrolled pulmonary immune responses and infection-associated inflammation and thereby limit excessive immunopathology in immunized mice, resulting in acquired immune homeostasis, which is necessary for vaccination-induced protection against pneumococcal infection. P17 suppressed the increase in IFN-γ; however, the elevation of IFN-γ in immunized mice was not SPY1-specific (no significant differences in the IFN-γ increase were detected between the CT group and CT + SPY1 group) and were probably caused by CT, consistent with the results of our previous study (11) and other reports (35). As a crucial pro-inflammatory cytokine (36), IL-12p70 is elevated by SPY1-infected dendritic cells co-cultured with $CD4^+$ cells (37), consistent with the results of this study. Several studies have suggested that IL-6 is a pro-inflammatory cytokine in infection (38); however, other studies have shown that IL-6-deficient mice exhibit impaired resistance against *S. pneumoniae* (23), *Listeria monocytogenes* (23, 39), and *Escherichia coli* (40), implying that IL-6 inhibits inflammation. Taken together, these findings suggest that IL-6 is a dual cytokine. As one of the immunosuppressive cytokines secreted by Tregs, the roles of IL-10 in infection are unclear. IL-10 impairs the immunosuppressive activity of Tregs in murine models of schistosomiasis japonica or asthma (41). However, during remission stage in mice with lymphocytic choriomeningitis virus infection, IL-10 produced by Tregs promotes the maturation of memory $CD8^+$ T cells, which is beneficial for host defense against secondary infections by intracellular pathogens (42). Similarly, in this study, dramatically elevated expression of IL-10 and palliative pulmonary injuries was observed in SPY1-immunized mice, indicating the beneficial effect of IL-10 on immunoprotection of SPY1-specific Tregs.

There are three main types of $CD4^+$ regulatory cells, i.e., Tr1, $CD4^+$ Th3, and $CD4^+CD25^+Foxp3^+$ T cells (43). Most studies have focused on $CD4^+CD25^+Foxp3^+$ T cells, which are indispensable for the maintenance of the immunologic balance (44). SPY1 could induce the Treg immune response involved in protection against pneumococcal infection (11). In this study, we showed that the expression of Foxp3, a key transcription factor belonging to the Treg immune pathway, mediates the activation of SPY1-specific Tregs. Obviously upregulated Foxp3 attributed to SPY1 vaccination was detected, suggesting that $CD4^+CD25^+$ $Foxp3^+$ T cells are the major type of SPY1-specific Tregs.

Regulatory T cell differentiation is mainly regulated by TGF-β/Smad signaling (24). Smad2 and Smad3 contribute to Foxp3 induction *via* different mechanisms, Smad3 directly interacts with an enhancer region of *Foxp3*, i.e., CNS1 (45), and the interaction is believed to be necessary for sustaining normal $Foxp3^+$ Treg numbers in the mouse gut but not in other organs (46). Smad2 has a relatively lower affinity to DNA than Smad3, and it cannot directly interact with CNS1 (47). However, the absence of Smad2 significantly decreases the upregulation of Foxp3 on T cells (48) and the deletion of both Smad2 and Smad3 could completely abolish the induction of Foxp3 by TGF-β (49), illustrating the synergetic effects of Smad2 and Smad3 in Treg induction. We observed increased levels of Smad2 and Smad3 as well as decreased levels of the negative regulatory factor Smad7 in the SPY1 vaccination group. These changes in Smads were significantly reversed by P17 treatment due to the inhibition of TGF-β1, illustrating that SPY1-stimulated TGF-β1 induced the generation of SPY1-specific Tregs *via* the Smad2/3 signaling pathway. Given that several Smad-independent pathways are also responsible for the induction of Tregs *via* TGF-β in different experiment models (18–21), the levels of *p38 mapk, akt, mtor,* and *pi3k* in pulmonary tissues were determined by real-time PCR, and no significant differences were detected among the control group, P17-treated SPY1-immunized group, and non-P17-treated immunized group (data not shown). Nevertheless, we cannot rule out the potential roles of other unknown signaling pathways in the generation of SPY1-specific Tregs for the immunoprotection in mice.

As foremost costimulatory inhibitors, PD-1 and CTLA-4 play key roles in the suppressive activity of Tregs (25, 50). We observed enhanced expression of PD-1 and CLTA-4 on SPY1-specific Tregs and their subsequent roles in immunoprotection elicited by SPY1-specific Tregs together with increased IL-10. TGF-β is believed to be another important inhibitory cytokine secreted by Tregs; however, its suppressive function remains contentious (47). Some research has revealed that TGF-β1 is redundant for Treg suppressor functions (51), but Ming et al. (52) showed that Treg-derived TGF-β1 is essential for controlling inflammatory-bowel disease. Therefore, the role of TGF-β1 in the immunoprotective function of SPY1-specific Tregs may be complicated.

Despite their crucial role in immune homeostasis and in the prevention of autoimmunity, the function of Tregs in infection is still controversial. Tregs are detrimental to hosts by restricting the effector T cell immune response during early tuberculosis (53). In some cases, virus or bacteria-specific Tregs not only prevent pathogen elimination but also promote a generalized state of immune suppression *in vivo*, making the host more susceptible to secondary infections with other pathogens (54). However, growing evidence has suggested that interactions between pathogens and Tregs are mutually beneficial to the pathogen and host, which allows persistent infection, conferring the maintenance of long-term memory and resistance to reinfection in a model of *Leishmania major* infection (55). Furthermore, emerging evidence suggests that Tregs can be beneficial to the host by restricting an overly robust inflammatory response, which causes excessive collateral damage to self-tissues (56), and by promoting the reparation of damaged tissues (57). Accordingly, Tregs should be established to regulate immune responses by maintaining homeostasis for efficient vaccination (58), highlighting the importance of considering vaccine-induced protective Tregs in the design of vaccine candidates.

In addition to Tregs and the regulatory cytokines IL-10 and IL-6, other cells including myeloid-derived suppressor cells, regulatory B cells (Bregs), regulatory γδ T cells, and immunosuppressive plasmocytes, as well as the cytokine IL-35 have immunosuppressive functions. Bregs have strong immunosuppressive effects and can negatively regulate immune responses in malignant tumors (59), infections (60), and autoimmune diseases (61) by multiple mechanisms. IL-35 is a vital anti-inflammatory cytokine that not only induces Bregs but also serves as an important effector of Bregs, participating in the regulation of the immune response *via* a positive feedback network. The immunosuppressive effects of Bregs and IL-35 have been found in innate immunity model against infection but not in an acquired immunity model with vaccination, and we cannot exclude the potential roles of other immunosuppressive cells and cytokines in the immune protective effect of SPY1.

As identified using a phage-displayed peptide library, peptide P17 is an effective inhibitor of Tregs by inhibiting TGF-β1, and its effect and specificity on Tregs have been well documented in various models, including in an invasive pneumococcal infection model (17, 62). P17 inhibits TGF-β1, TGF-β2, and TGF-β3 activity according to a previous study (17). Being predominantly expressed in the immune system, TGF-β1 is believed to be a crucial pleiotropic cytokine with potent immunoregulatory properties (24). The binding of P17 to TGF-β1 is stronger than binding to other isoforms of TGF-β (17). Therefore, in this study, we focused on TGF-β1. In follow-up work, the protective effect of SPY1-specific Tregs may be further established by evaluating a co-culture of TGF-β1 with mice splenocytes *in vitro* or by supplying mice with recombinant TGF-β1 *in vivo*. In addition, depletion of regulatory T cell mice (63) can be used to further evaluate the protection and related mechanisms of SPY1-induced acquired Treg immune responses in future studies.

To conclude, we characterized the mechanism underlying the protective role of vaccine-specific Treg immune response in response to the novel live-attenuated pneumococcal vaccine SPY1 in a mouse model. Immunization with SPY1 stimulated the activation of TGF-β1 *via* the Smad2/3 signaling pathway, which led to the production of $Foxp3^+$ Tregs and the subsequent upregulation of the costimulatory inhibitors PD-1 and CTLA-4. The activated SPY1-specific Treg immune response maintained the beneficial immune balance among the infection-associated inflammatory cytokine TNF-α, immune cytokines IL-6, IL-12p70, IL-4, IL-5, and IL-17A, as well as the immunoregulatory cytokine IL-10, and further alleviated excessive pulmonary injury, resulting in decreased bacterial colonization, elevated survival rates, and prolonged survival. Our results indicated that a protective immune response is elicited by vaccine-specific Tregs *via* the TGF-β1-Smad2/3 pathway. These findings may contribute to the comprehensive assessment of live vaccines and other mucosal vaccine candidates.

AUTHOR CONTRIBUTIONS

HL, XP, and LG were in charge of the whole project and participated in manuscript drafting. YG, SY, XH, and LG contributed to lab work and data analyses. JF, LZ, HW, YY, and XX revised the paper critically. All the authors have reviewed the manuscript.

ACKNOWLEDGMENTS

This work was supported by National Natural Science Foundation of China (31500749) and Chongqing Natural Science Foundation (cstc2015jcyjA10102).

REFERENCES

1. Liu L, Oza S, Hogan D, Perin J, Rudan I, Lawn JE, et al. Global, regional, and national causes of child mortality in 2000-13, with projections to inform post-2015 priorities: an updated systematic analysis. *Lancet* (2015) 385(9966):430–40. doi:10.1016/S0140-6736(14)61698-6
2. Mitchell AM, Mitchell TJ. *Streptococcus pneumoniae*: virulence factors and variation. *Clin Microbiol Infect* (2010) 16(5):411–8. doi:10.1111/j.1469-0691.2010.03183.x
3. Cilloniz C, Amaro R, Torres A. Pneumococcal vaccination. *Curr Opin Infect Dis* (2016) 29(2):187–96. doi:10.1097/QCO.0000000000000246
4. Giudice EL, Campbell JD. Needle-free vaccine delivery. *Adv Drug Deliv Rev* (2006) 58(1):68–89. doi:10.1016/j.addr.2005.12.003
5. Shakya AK, Chowdhury MYE, Tao W, Gill HS. Mucosal vaccine delivery: current state and a pediatric perspective. *J Control Release* (2016) 240: 394–413. doi:10.1016/j.jconrel.2016.02.014
6. Flasche S, Van Hoek AJ, Sheasby E, Waight P, Andrews N, Sheppard C, et al. Effect of pneumococcal conjugate vaccination on serotype-specific carriage and invasive disease in England: a cross-sectional study. *PLoS Med* (2011) 8(4):e1001017. doi:10.1371/journal.pmed.1001017
7. Balsells E, Guillot L, Nair H, Kyaw MH. Serotype distribution of *Streptococcus pneumoniae* causing invasive disease in children in the post-PCV era: a systematic review and meta-analysis. *PLoS One* (2017) 12(5):e0177113. doi:10.1371/journal.pone.0177113
8. Rosch JW, Iverson AR, Humann J, Mann B, Gao G, Vogel P, et al. A live-attenuated pneumococcal vaccine elicits CD4+ T-cell dependent class switching and provides serotype independent protection against acute otitis media. *EMBO Mol Med* (2014) 6(1):141–54. doi:10.1002/emmm.201202150
9. Pichichero ME. Pneumococcal whole-cell and protein-based vaccines: changing the paradigm. *Expert Rev Vaccines* (2017) 16(12):1181–90. doi:10.1080/14760584.2017.1393335
10. Wu K, Yao R, Wang H, Pang D, Liu Y, Xu H, et al. Mucosal and systemic immunization with a novel attenuated pneumococcal vaccine candidate confer serotype independent protection against *Streptococcus pneumoniae* in mice. *Vaccine* (2014) 32(33):4179–88. doi:10.1016/j.vaccine.2014.05.019
11. Xu X, Wang H, Liu Y, Wang Y, Zeng L, Wu K, et al. Mucosal immunization with the live attenuated vaccine SPY1 induces humoral and Th2-Th17-regulatory T cell cellular immunity and protects against pneumococcal infection. *Infect Immun* (2015) 83(1):90–100. doi:10.1128/IAI.02334-14
12. Sanjabi S, Oh SA, Li MO. Regulation of the immune response by TGF-beta: from conception to autoimmunity and infection. *Cold Spring Harb Perspect Biol* (2017) 9(6):a022236. doi:10.1101/cshperspect.a022236
13. Chen W, Jin W, Hardegen N, Lei KJ, Li L, Marinos N, et al. Conversion of peripheral CD4+CD25- naive T cells to CD4+CD25+ regulatory T cells by TGF-beta induction of transcription factor Foxp3. *J Exp Med* (2003) 198(12):1875–86. doi:10.1084/jem.20030152
14. Huber S, Schramm C, Lehr HA, Mann A, Schmitt S, Becker C, et al. Cutting edge: TGF-beta signaling is required for the in vivo expansion and immunosuppressive capacity of regulatory CD4+CD25+ T cells. *J Immunol* (2004) 173(11):6526–31. doi:10.4049/jimmunol.173.11.6526
15. Marie JC, Letterio JJ, Gavin M, Rudensky AY. TGF-beta1 maintains suppressor function and Foxp3 expression in CD4+CD25+ regulatory T cells. *J Exp Med* (2005) 201(7):1061–7. doi:10.1084/jem.20042276
16. Dotor J, Lopez-Vazquez AB, Lasarte JJ, Sarobe P, Garcia-Granero M, Riezu-Boj JI, et al. Identification of peptide inhibitors of transforming growth factor beta 1 using a phage-displayed peptide library. *Cytokine* (2007) 39(2):106–15. doi:10.1016/j.cyto.2007.06.004
17. Gil-Guerrero L, Dotor J, Huibregtse IL, Casares N, Lopez-Vazquez AB, Rudilla F, et al. In vitro and in vivo down-regulation of regulatory T cell activity with a peptide inhibitor of TGF-beta1. *J Immunol* (2008) 181(1):126–35. doi:10.4049/jimmunol.181.1.126
18. Zhao M, Zhang H, Liu X, Jiang Y, Ren L, Hu X. The effect of TGF-beta on Treg cells in adverse pregnancy outcome upon *Toxoplasma gondii* infection. *Front Microbiol* (2017) 8:901. doi:10.3389/fmicb.2017.00901
19. Huber S, Schrader J, Fritz G, Presser K, Schmitt S, Waisman A, et al. P38 MAP kinase signaling is required for the conversion of CD4+CD25- T cells into iTreg. *PLoS One* (2008) 3(10):e3302. doi:10.1371/journal.pone.0003302
20. Derynck R, Zhang YE. Smad-dependent and Smad-independent pathways in TGF-beta family signalling. *Nature* (2003) 425(6958):577–84. doi:10.1038/nature02006
21. Haxhinasto S, Mathis D, Benoist C. The AKT-mTOR axis regulates de novo differentiation of CD4+Foxp3+ cells. *J Exp Med* (2008) 205(3):565–74. doi:10.1084/jem.20071477
22. Blanquiceth Y, Rodriguez-Perea AL, Tabares Guevara JH, Correa LA, Sanchez MD, Ramirez-Pineda JR, et al. Increase of frequency and modulation of phenotype of regulatory T cells by atorvastatin is associated with decreased lung inflammatory cell infiltration in a murine model of acute allergic asthma. *Front Immunol* (2016) 7:620. doi:10.3389/fimmu.2016.00620
23. van der Poll T, Keogh CV, Guirao X, Buurman WA, Kopf M, Lowry SF. Interleukin-6 gene-deficient mice show impaired defense against pneumococcal pneumonia. *J Infect Dis* (1997) 176(2):439–44. doi:10.1086/514062
24. Yoshimura A, Wakabayashi Y, Mori T. Cellular and molecular basis for the regulation of inflammation by TGF-beta. *J Biochem* (2010) 147(6):781–92. doi:10.1093/jb/mvq043
25. Kawai K, Uchiyama M, Hester J, Wood K, Issa F. Regulatory T cells for tolerance. *Hum Immunol* (2017) 79(5):294–303. doi:10.1016/j.humimm.2017.12.013
26. Murugaiah C, Nik Mohd Noor NZ, Mustafa S, Manickam R, Pattabhiraman L. Construction and evaluation of *V. cholerae* O139 mutant, VCUSM21P, as a safe live attenuated cholera vaccine. *PLoS One* (2014) 9(2):e81817. doi:10.1371/journal.pone.0081817
27. Xu Z-Y, Wang X-Y. Live attenuated hepatitis A vaccines developed in China. *Hum Vaccin Immunother* (2013) 10(3):659–66. doi:10.4161/hv.27124
28. Qiu Y, Zhang X, Wang H, Zhang X, Mo Y, Sun X, et al. Heterologous prime-boost immunization with live SPY1 and DnaJ protein of *Streptococcus pneumoniae* induces strong Th1 and Th17 cellular immune responses in mice. *J Microbiol* (2017) 55(10):823–9. doi:10.1007/s12275-017-7262-1
29. Tarahomjoo S. Recent approaches in vaccine development against *Streptococcus pneumoniae*. *J Mol Microbiol Biotechnol* (2014) 24(4):215–27. doi:10.1159/000365052
30. Mohan T, Verma P, Rao DN. Novel adjuvants & delivery vehicles for vaccines development: a road ahead. *Indian J Med Res* (2013) 138(5):779–95.

31. Zhang X, Qi Z, Du Z, Bi Y, Zhang Q, Tan Y, et al. A live attenuated strain of *Yersinia pestis* DeltayscB provides protection against bubonic and pneumonic plagues in mouse model. *Vaccine* (2013) 31(22):2539–42. doi:10.1016/j.vaccine.2013.03.054
32. Zheng D, Yi Y, Chen Z. Development of live-attenuated influenza vaccines against outbreaks of H5N1 influenza. *Viruses* (2012) 4(12):3589–605. doi:10.3390/v4123589
33. Zeng L, Liu Y, Wang H, Liao P, Song Z, Gao S, et al. Compound 48/80 acts as a potent mucosal adjuvant for vaccination against *Streptococcus pneumoniae* infection in young mice. *Vaccine* (2015) 33(8):1008–16. doi:10.1016/j.vaccine.2015.01.013
34. Zhang X, Cui J, Wu Y, Wang H, Wang J, Qiu Y, et al. *Streptococcus pneumoniae* attenuated strain SPY1 with an artificial mineral shell induces humoral and Th17 cellular immunity and protects mice against pneumococcal infection. *Front Immunol* (2017) 8:1983. doi:10.3389/fimmu.2017.01983
35. Meza-Sanchez D, Perez-Montesinos G, Sanchez-Garcia J, Moreno J, Bonifaz LC. Intradermal immunization in the ear with cholera toxin and its non-toxic beta subunit promotes efficient Th1 and Th17 differentiation dependent on migrating DCs. *Eur J Immunol* (2011) 41(10):2894–904. doi:10.1002/eji.201040997
36. Thompson A, Orr SJ. Emerging IL-12 family cytokines in the fight against fungal infections. *Cytokine* (2018). doi:10.1016/j.cyto.2018.05.019
37. Gao S, Zeng L, Zhang X, Wu Y, Cui J, Song Z, et al. Attenuated *Streptococcus pneumoniae* vaccine candidate SPY1 promotes dendritic cell activation and drives a Th1/Th17 response. *Immunol Lett* (2016) 179:47–55. doi:10.1016/j.imlet.2016.08.008
38. Ataie-Kachoie P, Pourgholami MH, Richardson DR, Morris DL. Gene of the month: interleukin 6 (IL-6). *J Clin Pathol* (2014) 67(11):932–7. doi:10.1136/jclinpath-2014-202493
39. Kopf M, Baumann H, Freer G, Freudenberg M, Lamers M, Kishimoto T, et al. Impaired immune and acute-phase responses in interleukin-6-deficient mice. *Nature* (1994) 368(6469):339–42. doi:10.1038/368339a0
40. Dalrymple SA, Slattery R, Aud DM, Krishna M, Lucian LA, Murray R. Interleukin-6 is required for a protective immune response to systemic *Escherichia coli* infection. *Infect Immun* (1996) 64(8):3231–5.
41. He L, Zhou S, Qi Q, Chi Y, Zhu J, Xu Z, et al. The regulation of regulation: interleukin-10 increases CD4(+) CD25(+) regulatory T cells but impairs their immunosuppressive activity in murine models with schistosomiasis japonica or asthma. *Immunology* (2018) 153(1):84–96. doi:10.1111/imm.12813
42. Laidlaw BJ, Cui W, Amezquita RA, Gray SM, Guan T, Lu Y, et al. Production of IL-10 by CD4(+) regulatory T cells during the resolution of infection promotes the maturation of memory CD8(+) T cells. *Nat Immunol* (2015) 16(8):871–9. doi:10.1038/ni.3224
43. Zhao H, Liao X, Kang Y. Tregs: where we are and what comes next? *Front Immunol* (2017) 8:1578. doi:10.3389/fimmu.2017.01578
44. Sakaguchi S, Powrie F. Emerging challenges in regulatory T cell function and biology. *Science* (2007) 317(5838):627–9. doi:10.1126/science.1142331
45. Zheng Y, Josefowicz S, Chaudhry A, Peng XP, Forbush K, Rudensky AY. Role of conserved non-coding DNA elements in the Foxp3 gene in regulatory T-cell fate. *Nature* (2010) 463(7282):808–12. doi:10.1038/nature08750
46. Schlenner SM, Weigmann B, Ruan Q, Chen Y, von Boehmer H. Smad3 binding to the foxp3 enhancer is dispensable for the development of regulatory T cells with the exception of the gut. *J Exp Med* (2012) 209(9):1529–35. doi:10.1084/jem.20112646
47. Kelly A, Houston SA, Sherwood E, Casulli J, Travis MA. Regulation of innate and adaptive immunity by TGFbeta. *Adv Immunol* (2017) 134:137–233. doi:10.1016/bs.ai.2017.01.001
48. Martinez GJ, Zhang Z, Reynolds JM, Tanaka S, Chung Y, Liu T, et al. Smad2 positively regulates the generation of Th17 cells. *J Biol Chem* (2010) 285(38):29039–43. doi:10.1074/jbc.C110.155820
49. Takimoto T, Wakabayashi Y, Sekiya T, Inoue N, Morita R, Ichiyama K, et al. Smad2 and Smad3 are redundantly essential for the TGF-beta-mediated regulation of regulatory T plasticity and Th1 development. *J Immunol* (2010) 185(2):842–55. doi:10.4049/jimmunol.0904100
50. Jain N, Nguyen H, Chambers C, Kang J. Dual function of CTLA-4 in regulatory T cells and conventional T cells to prevent multiorgan autoimmunity. *Proc Natl Acad Sci U S A* (2010) 107(4):1524–8. doi:10.1073/pnas.0910341107
51. Fahlen L, Read S, Gorelik L, Hurst SD, Coffman RL, Flavell RA, et al. T cells that cannot respond to TGF-beta escape control by CD4(+)CD25(+) regulatory T cells. *J Exp Med* (2005) 201(5):737–46. doi:10.1084/jem.20040685
52. Li MO, Wan YY, Flavell RA. T cell-produced transforming growth factor-beta1 controls T cell tolerance and regulates Th1- and Th17-cell differentiation. *Immunity* (2007) 26(5):579–91. doi:10.1016/j.immuni.2007.03.014
53. Shafiani S, Tucker-Heard G, Kariyone A, Takatsu K, Urdahl KB. Pathogen-specific regulatory T cells delay the arrival of effector T cells in the lung during early tuberculosis. *J Exp Med* (2010) 207(7):1409–20. doi:10.1084/jem.20091885
54. Roquilly A, McWilliam HEG, Jacqueline C, Tian Z, Cinotti R, Rimbert M, et al. Local modulation of antigen-presenting cell development after resolution of pneumonia induces long-term susceptibility to secondary infections. *Immunity* (2017) 47(1):135–47.e5. doi:10.1016/j.immuni.2017.06.021
55. Belkaid Y, Piccirillo CA, Mendez S, Shevach EM, Sacks DL. CD4+CD25+ regulatory T cells control *Leishmania major* persistence and immunity. *Nature* (2002) 420(6915):502–7. doi:10.1038/nature01152
56. Fulton RB, Meyerholz DK, Varga SM. Foxp3+ CD4 regulatory T cells limit pulmonary immunopathology by modulating the CD8 T cell response during respiratory syncytial virus infection. *J Immunol* (2010) 185(4):2382–92. doi:10.4049/jimmunol.1000423
57. Arpaia N, Green JA, Moltedo B, Arvey A, Hemmers S, Yuan S, et al. A distinct function of regulatory T cells in tissue protection. *Cell* (2015) 162(5):1078–89. doi:10.1016/j.cell.2015.08.021
58. Brezar V, Godot V, Cheng L, Su L, Levy Y, Seddiki N. T-regulatory cells and vaccination "pay attention and do not neglect them": lessons from HIV and cancer vaccine trials. *Vaccines (Basel)* (2016) 4(3):30. doi:10.3390/vaccines4030030
59. Shen M, Sun Q, Wang J, Pan W, Ren X. Positive and negative functions of B lymphocytes in tumors. *Oncotarget* (2016) 7(34):55828–39. doi:10.18632/oncotarget.10094
60. Fillatreau S. Regulatory roles of B cells in infectious diseases. *Clin Exp Rheumatol* (2016) 34(4 Suppl 98):1–5.
61. Ray A, Dittel BN. Mechanisms of regulatory B cell function in autoimmune and inflammatory diseases beyond IL-10. *J Clin Med* (2017) 6(1):E12. doi:10.3390/jcm6010012
62. Neill DR, Fernandes VE, Wisby L, Haynes AR, Ferreira DM, Laher A, et al. T regulatory cells control susceptibility to invasive pneumococcal pneumonia in mice. *PLoS Pathog* (2012) 8(4):e1002660. doi:10.1371/journal.ppat.1002660
63. Lahl K, Loddenkemper C, Drouin C, Freyer J, Arnason J, Eberl G, et al. Selective depletion of Foxp3+ regulatory T cells induces a scurfy-like disease. *J Exp Med* (2007) 204(1):57–63. doi:10.1084/jem.20061852

13

Impact of Host Genetics and Biological Response Modifiers on Respiratory Tract Infections

Alicia Lacoma [1], Lourdes Mateo [2], Ignacio Blanco [3], Maria J. Méndez [4], Carlos Rodrigo [5], Irene Latorre [1], Raquel Villar-Hernandez [1], Jose Domínguez [1†] and Cristina Prat [1†]*

[1] Servei de Microbiologia, Hospital Universitari Germans Trias i Pujol, Institut d'Investigació Germans Trias i Pujol, Universitat Autònoma de Barcelona, CIBER Enfermedades Respiratorias, Barcelona, Spain, [2] Servei de Reumatologia, Hospital Universitari Germans Trias i Pujol, Institut d'Investigació Germans Trias i Pujol, Universitat Autònoma de Barcelona, Barcelona, Spain, [3] Clinical Genetics and Genetic Counseling Program, Hospital Universitari Germans Trias i Pujol, Institut d'Investigació Germans Trias i Pujol, Barcelona, Spain, [4] Servei de Pediatria, Hospital Universitari Germans Trias i Pujol, Institut d'Investigació GermansTrias i Pujol, Universitat Autònoma de Barcelona, Barcelona, Spain, [5] Servei de Pediatria, Hospital Universitari Vall d'Hebron, Vall d'Hebron Institut de Recerca, Facultat de Medicina, Unitat Docent Germans Trias i Pujol, Universitat Autònoma de Barcelona, Barcelona, Spain

***Correspondence:**
Cristina Prat
cprat.germanstrias@gencat.cat

† These authors are co-senior authors of this study

Host susceptibility to respiratory tract infections (RTI) is dependent on both genetic and acquired risk factors. Repeated bacterial and viral RTI, such as pneumonia from encapsulated microorganisms, respiratory tract infections related to respiratory syncytial virus or influenza, and even the development of bronchiectasis and asthma, are often reported as the first symptom of primary immunodeficiencies. In the same way, neutropenia is a well-known risk factor for invasive aspergillosis, as well as lymphopenia for *Pneumocystis,* and mycobacterial infections. However, in the last decades a better knowledge of immune signaling networks and the introduction of next generation sequencing have increased the number and diversity of known inborn errors of immunity. On the other hand, the use of monoclonal antibodies targeting cytokines, such as tumor necrosis factor alpha has revealed new risk groups for infections, such as tuberculosis. The use of biological response modifiers has spread to almost all medical specialties, including inflammatory diseases and neoplasia, and are being used to target different signaling networks that may mirror some of the known immune deficiencies. From a clinical perspective, the individual contribution of genetics, and/or targeted treatments, to immune dysregulation is difficult to assess. The aim of this article is to review the known and newly described mechanisms of impaired immune signaling that predispose to RTI, including new insights into host genetics and the impact of biological response modifiers, and to summarize clinical recommendations regarding vaccines and prophylactic treatments in order to prevent infections.

Keywords: immunogenetics, biological response modifiers, respiratory tract infections, primary immunodeficiencies, inborn errors

EPIDEMIOLOGY AND PATHOGENESIS OF RESPIRATORY TRACT INFECTIONS

Acute and chronic respiratory tract infections (RTI) are one of the most frequent causes of infections and antimicrobial prescription, and the leading cause of death in developing countries (1, 2). Pneumonia accounts for 1.3 million deaths annually in children <5 years of age (3). In 2017, 1.6 million people died of tuberculosis (TB). Children (aged <15 years) accounted for 15% of total deaths, higher than their share of estimated cases, suggesting poorer access to diagnosis and treatment. About 1.7 billion people, 23% of the world's population, are estimated to have a latent TB infection (4). The control of latent TB, a stage in which a person is infected with *Mycobacterium tuberculosis* plays an important role in disease control, since dormant bacilli are a reservoir of potential TB cases (5). Viral acute RTI are estimated to cause 75% of acute diseases in children, and is the main reason for hospitalization worldwide (6). The annual prevalence in an otherwise healthy child is from 3 to 10 infections (7). Early and recurrent lower RTI are linked to a higher risk to develop asthma or bronchiectasis (8–10). However, bronchiectasis secondary to recurrent and severe infections alone have declined, with an increasing proportion of patients being recognized as having underlying conditions predisposing to its development (11).

Improvements in immunization programs and the wide availability of antimicrobials, have led to optimism for most of the devastating infectious diseases. Always without forgetting that alleviation of poverty is crucial, the combination of genetic versatility and ecological opportunism of the microbial world appears to have been under-estimated (12). Some emerging pathogens, such as *Legionella*, avian influenza, and coronavirus species were described in the past decades (13). Ethnic variations in the incidence of RTI have also been reported, suggesting genetic susceptibility to disease (14). Most children, on reaching 2 years of age, have been in contact with the most common respiratory viruses, such as respiratory syncytial virus (RSV), but while some develop a mild disease, others develop severe bronchiolitis (15). Influenza viruses cause mild to moderate respiratory illness in most people, but some develop fatal infections. The virulence factors encoded by viral genes can explain seasonal or geographical differences at a population level, but are unlikely to account for inter-individual clinical variability (16). TB outcome depends on the pathogen and extrinsic elements, as well as on host factors that are still unclear (17).

As regards bacteria, focusing on those species whose normal ecological niche is the airways, therapeutic decisions are a daily clinical challenge (18). The shift from commensalism to infection is shaped by host intrinsic (genetics) and extrinsic factors (for example, diet and exposure to cigarette smoke and environmental pollution) and by bacterial features that also contribute to inter-individual variability (19). Bacteria develop adaptive mechanisms (at genetic/phenotypic level) in order to survive in a hostile environment, such as the respiratory tract (20, 21). Whether pathogen virulence generates clinical symptoms depends on how well the immune system limits its impact. Recently, changes in gut and lung microbiome composition (dysbiosis) have also been related to dysfunctional immune modulation (22).

IMMUNE RESPONSE TO RESPIRATORY TRACT INFECTIONS

Respiratory immune responses are complex, and inborn errors can be present at any level. Essential pathways can be summarized as follows: Firstly, the pathogen has to be detected by host cells. This identification relies on a set of pathogen associated molecular profiles that bind to pattern recognition receptors (PRR). PRR can be found as transmembrane, cytosolic or extracellular components. Among PRRs, it is important to mention toll-like receptors (TLR), nucleotide-binding oligomerization domain-containing (NOD) receptor, NOD-like receptors (NLR), RIG-I-Like Receptors (RLR), and receptor CD14 because of their importance during respiratory infections (23). Depending on the PRR, different intracellular signaling pathways are activated (24). Most of the signaling pathways converge on signaling hubs, such as transcription nuclear factor κβ (NF-κβ), interferon regulatory factor families (IRF3, IRF7), and mitogen-activated protein kinase, leading to the induction of gene expression encoding adhesion molecules, pro-inflammatory cytokines, chemokines, and type I interferon, among others. NLRs directly trigger inflammasome assembly and caspase-1 activation, leading to interleukin (IL)-1β and IL-18 processing (25). Type III interferons, also termed IFN-λ, have been recently identified as regulators of immunity and homeostasis in the respiratory tract (26) during infections, as well as during chronic lung diseases, such as asthma and chronic obstructive pulmonary disease (COPD) (27). Alveolar macrophages and dendritic cells (DC) have an important role sensing microbes and thus activating lung epithelial cells and neutrophils. These are essential for the defense against bacteria, viruses, and *Aspergillus* (28, 29), as well as in the pathogenesis of acute lung injury. In a recent study, patterns of differentially expressed cellular genes shared by several respiratory pathogens were searched using transcriptomics (30). Most of the commonly up-regulated host genes were related to the innate immune response and/or apoptosis, with Toll-like, RIG-I-like, and NLR among the top 10 signalers. Some of the genes showed a high degree of interconnection and possible redundancy to respiratory viral and bacterial infections. The adaptive immune response requires the activation of antigen-specific T and B lymphocytes to trigger protective cellular and humoral responses. Most of the T lymphocyte subsets, along with B lymphocytes and DC, are essential for immune defense and/or regulation (31). In particular, the protective immunity against *M. tuberculosis* depends on $CD4^+$ T-helper1 lymphocytes that mainly secrete interferon-gamma (IFN-γ), IL-2, and tumor necrosis factor alpha (TNF-α), which leads to macrophage activation, cytokine production, and bacterial control (32). HIV-revealed T-cell lymphopenia as a well-defined risk group for *Pneumocystis jirovecii* pneumonia (PJP), but also in other situations where CD4 lymphocyte count is lower, such as renal transplant recipients (33).

GENETIC SUSCEPTIBILITY TO RESPIRATORY TRACT INFECTIONS

The study of susceptibility to lower respiratory tract infections is complex, and requires different approaches. There are three main elements playing a role: host genetic background (in relation to lung tissue functionality and immune response), pathogen virulence determinants, and environmental factors.

Early life (children under 5 years of age) is a challenging period because pulmonary tissue and the immune system are still in a maturation process while being continuously exposed to airborne antigens (34). However, the occurrence of life-threatening bacterial/viral/fungal infection in an otherwise healthy individual deserves further immunological and genetic studies (35, 36). Complications during upper RTI include sinusitis and otitis media, and in the lower airways, pneumonia, bronchitis, as well as the development of bronchiectasis, interstitial lung diseases, organizing pneumonia, and hyperreactive airway diseases (37). Indeed, genetic susceptibility for the concomitant illnesses that predispose to RTI can also play a role, including congenital defects of the airways, familial congenital bronchiectasis or tracheobronchomegaly (11). As regards impaired mucociliary clearance, cystic fibrosis is the most common autosomal recessive disorder and primary cause of bronchiectasis in the developed world. Mutations are well-defined, but its severity is influenced by genes involving inflammatory and anti-inflammatory mediators (38, 39). Other disorders include ciliopathies and disorders of humoral immunity. Alpha 1-antitrypsin is a circulating serine protease inhibitor (serpin) made in the liver that plays an important role in modulating immunity, inflammation, apoptosis, and possibly cellular senescence programs and its deficiency is considered the genetic cause of COPD, but there are other genetic factors that may affect disease activity and outcomes, even in patients without this deficiency (27).

High-throughput whole genome sequencing technologies and novel bioinformatics tools are revealing the sequence and annotation of the complete human genome, as well as genome-wide maps of polymorphic microsatellite markers and single nucleotide polymorphisms (SNP). In order to characterize genetic susceptibility, two complementary approaches can be envisaged: whole genome association studies (WGAS) for the identification of variants with high population frequency but low impact at individual level in terms of risk of infection (although SNP identification can potentially be later included in healthcare planning protocols); and mechanistic studies for identifying disease-causing mutations with deleterious effects, related to a high risk of infection at individual level, although its frequency in general population is low. Many genetic variants have been associated with complex human diseases and traits, but often confer relatively small increases in risk (40). According to a recent review, there are more than 300 primary immunodeficiency disorders (PIDs), most of them monogenic conditions with Mendelian inheritance, that are mainly associated with crucial defects in adaptive immunity (31). Innate immune responses are largely redundant, with pleiotropic nature of some gene products (31), thus most of the defects can be potentially counterbalanced. According to the literature, there is another view suggesting that while patients with broad immunodeficiencies may present with one of their many infections, the phenotype of particular inborn errors of immunity is very narrow, with susceptibility to only one specific infection (36, 41, 42). A set of inborn errors affecting "primarily" innate immunity, exercise their effect on the adaptive immune response (41). The range and nature of infections depend on several factors. The improving recognition of immune dysregulation diseases, autoinflammatory disorders, and interferonopathies leads to changes in terminology. The annual report of the authoritative International Union of Immunological Societies (43) has categorized and listed (as of February 2017) 354 inborn errors of immunity, and those with a predominant RTI phenotype have been included in **Table 1**.

Despite the limitations of molecular genetic studies in pulmonary infections, several associations have been described between SNPs and bacterial pneumonia and mycobacterial infections (14, 45). Polymorphisms affecting community-acquired pneumonia including, among others, those related to mannose-binding lectin and the IgG2 Fc gamma receptor II, and are discussed extensively elsewhere (14). The genetic contribution for the propensity to develop severe RSV infection was estimated to account for ~20% of the variance in RSV disease severity. Several studies have attempted to link candidate host SNPs to disease severity, mostly in chemokine receptors and PRRs (46, 47).

As regards TB, SNPs are frequently found in loci involving TLR-2, TNF-α, IL-12, and IFN-γ, and their corresponding receptors (45). Genetic variations in dendritic cell-specific ICAM-3 grabbing non-integrin have been linked with reduced risk of developing TB (48). Mendelian susceptibility to mycobacterial disease is a syndrome characterized by susceptibility to weakly virulent mycobacteria, including the attenuated vaccine Bacillus Calmette-Guerin (BCG) strain and non-tuberculous mycobacteria (NTM). Different gene mutations have been identified, most of which are related to IFN-γ-mediated immunity (49–51). Using exome and transcriptome sequencing, three rare loss-of-function variants have been recently characterized in theIFIH1 gene. These encode a RIG-I-like receptor involved in the sensing of viral RNA (52). The deficiency causes a primary immunodeficiency manifested in extreme susceptibility to common respiratory RNA viruses. Interestingly, human primary immunodeficiency disorders (PID) affecting T and B cells were not found to predispose to severe influenza. However, human IRF7 was shown to be essential for IFN-α/β- and IFN-λ-dependent protective immunity against primary influenza *in vivo* (53).

IMPACT OF BIOLOGICAL RESPONSE MODIFIERS IN RESPIRATORY TRACT INFECTIONS AND TUBERCULOSIS

Biological response modifiers (BRM) are substances that interact with and modify the host immune system by acting on a therapeutic target considered important in the pathogenic

TABLE 1 | Reported risk of infection and recommended prophylaxis according to functional classification of biologicals-based on ESCMID consensus document (44) and to categorization of inborn errors of immunity-based on International Union of Immunological Societies annual report (43).

	Reported risk of infection	**Recommendations**			
		TB screening and prophylaxis	**Pneumocystis prophylaxis**	**Pneumococcal/ capsulated bacteria vaccination**	**Influenza vaccination**
TARGETED AGENT					
Anti-tumor necrosis factor-α agents	Two to four increase in the risk of active TB compared to healthy patients and other granulomatous conditions Rate of *Legionella* 37-fold higher. Histoplasmosis and coccidioidomycosis	Yes	No	Yes	Yes
Interleukins, immunoglobulins and complement factors	IL-1 family, moderate risk of infection, IL-6 and IL-6 receptor (JAK), similar to TNF. Neutropenia in some cases C5 targeted, *Aspergillus* encapsulated bacteria, specially *Neisseria*, IL-17 upper respiratory tract infections and *Candida* IgE helminth infection, *Strongyloides*	Yes	No	Yes	Yes
Cell surface receptors/associated signaling pathways	Drug induced neutropenia Skin and soft tissue infections and sometimes pneumonia Overall risk of infection low for epidermal growth factor	Optional	No	Age appropriate	Yes
Intracellular signaling pathways	Increased overall risk of infection, cytomegalovirus and hepatitis B reactivation Difficult to distinguish from the risk of the underlying disease Cases of *Pneumocystis*, invasive fungal infection nocardiosis, mainly JAK	Yes	Yes	Age appropriate	Yes
Lymphoid cells surface antigens (CD19, CD20, CD52)	Can cause IgG hypogammaglobulinaemia and neutropenia Evidence of catheter related bacteremia, severe respiratory tract infection, hepatitis B reactivation and varicella zoster	Yes	Yes	Age appropriate	Yes
Lymphoid/Myeloid cells surface antigens (CD22, CD30, CD33, CD38, CD40, SLAMF-7, CCR4)	Similar to anti CD20	Optional	Yes	Age appropriate	Yes
Immune checkpoint inhibitors, cell adhesion inhibitors, sphingosine-1-phosphate receptor modulators and proteasome inhibitors	Associated T cell lymphopenia but no opportunistic infections reported Risk of varicella zoster virus	Yes	Yes	Yes	Yes
INBORN ERRORS OF IMMUNITY					
Severe combined immune deficiency:	Severe opportunistic disseminated infections in early childhood	Non-applicable	Yes	No	No (cohabitants)
Less severe combined immune deficiency	Some related to recurrent respiratory tract infections	Optional	Yes	Yes	Yes
Combined immune deficiencies with syndromic features e.g., Wiscot Aldrich and those altering DNA reparation	Recurrent infections	Optional	No	Yes	Yes
Humoral immune deficiencies Antibody deficiencies	Repeated respiratory tract infections (pneumonia, sinusitis, otitis, ...)	Optional	No	Yes	Yes
Defects of phagocyte number or function	Fungal and bacterial infections, pulmonary abscesses, aspergillosis	No	No	Yes	Yes
Defects in intrinsic and innate immunity	Pyogenic bacterial infections	In selected cases	No (*)	Yes	Yes
Autoinflammatory diseases	No clear predisposition to infection	No	No	Yes	Yes
Complement deficiencies	Disseminated infections (meningitis/sepsis) by capsulated microorganisms and *Neisseria*	No	No (*)	Yes	Yes

**Antibiotic prophylaxis to prevent bacterial infections.*

process of the disease. Monoclonal antibodies (mAbs) are now established as therapies for malignancies, transplant rejection, several immune disorders from most organ systems, and even infectious diseases (54). Safety problems related to immunomodulation and infection have been identified in some cases (55). The use of mAb indirectly provides insights into the function of the molecule to combat particular pathogens, increasing our knowledge of the immune system (56). A recent consensus document has reviewed the groups of drugs according to the targeted site of action, the expected impact on susceptibility to infection, the evidence of risk, and the recommendation of prevention strategies. It is also important to mention the influence of previous or concomitant therapies, underlying conditions, and the accumulative exposure to the agent (44). As regards lower RTI, treatment with BRM results in an increased risk is reported for pneumonia, influenza-related complications, TB and NTM, *Pneumocystis,* and fungal infections, such as histoplasmosis, taking into account the impact of geographical variations on incidence rates (57). The knowledge obtained from experience with the prescription of BRM may be particularly valuable for the understanding of some genetic inborn errors, as the type of infections acquired as a side effect may help to identify which genetic defects favors a similar infectious phenotype. With the current knowledge and because of pleiotropic effects, it is not feasible to show how biological agents actually mimic some inborn errors of immunity, but several parallelisms can be inferred. We provide a Table containing the list of BRM according to their functional classification, and inborn errors categorized according to common infectious phenotypes (**Table 1**). Data presented are extracted from the respective consensus documents, and lists the main RTI and preventive recommendations.

Current recommendations should be focused on rheumatic diseases because of the greater experience in follow-up time (more than 15 years) and number of patients treated. Biological therapies targeting TNF-α, T cells, B cells, and various cytokines (including IL-6 and IL-1) have become essential for the treatment of rheumatic diseases [mainly rheumatoid arthritis (RA), ankylosing spondylitis, and psoriatic arthritis], as well as other immune-mediated diseases. Moreover, additional drugs with novel targets, including those that inhibit IL-12–IL-23, IL-17α, or the Janus activating kinase system have been introduced more recently. Immunomodulation offered by biological and non-biological disease-modifying therapies and prednisone contributes greatly to the increased risks of opportunistic infections (OI) (58, 59). In **Figure 1** we present the sites of action and associated risks of the most frequently prescribed BRM.

Two recent meta-analysis have calculated the relative risk of infection for rheumatic patients under biological treatment, with an odds ratio (OR) of 1.31–1.41 (60, 61). The absolute increase in the number of serious infections per 1,000 patients treated/year is six times higher than that observed with synthetic disease-modifying anti-rheumatic drugs (DMARDs). Different meta-analyses and national registries have confirmed the increase on the impact of any infections (20%), serious infections (40%), and TB (250%), associated with anti-TNF-α use (60). In addition, the risk of serious infections is highest during the first 6 months of therapy (62) (up to 4.5-fold risk), although, after 1 year this risk is no different from conventional DMARDs. Recurrent infections in RA are common. In a prospective observational cohort study, the baseline annual rate of a first serious infection was 4.6%. Additionally, 14% of this cohort experienced a recurrent episode/year during their follow-up, with the highest risk being within the first year (29%), and with respiratory infections being the most common (44% of all episodes) (63). Factors that have shown to be predictive of infection include, age, functional status, specific comorbidities (chronic renal/lung disease), corticosteroid treatment, number of previous DMARD, treatment failures, previous serious infections, and current treatment with anti-TNF-α inhibitors or non-biological DMARDs (64). Nevertheless, recent data suggest that patients having a serious infection and exposed to biological treatment have a significantly lower risk of sepsis and fatal outcome than patients treated with conventional DMARDs (62, 65). British and French national biological registries have reported OI rates of 200–270/100,000 in patients using anti-TNF-α therapies (66, 67). In particular, there is evidence of an increased risk of *M. tuberculosis*, herpes zoster, and *Listeria* infections. The overall incidence of OI is not significantly different considering drug classes; however, the rate of PJP is significantly higher in those patients using rituximab in comparison to anti-TNF-α therapy. The absolute risk of PJP is low, although corticosteroid exposure is a strong predictor. Current data do not support PJP prophylaxis for all rituximab users. However, it may be appropriate in certain high-risk individuals. Furthermore, rituximab-associated neutropenia and impaired antibody response is also well-described.

Pre-clinical and clinical evidence indicate that anti-TNF-α therapy (infliximab, adalimumab, golimumab, certolizumab pegol, and etanercept) is associated with a 2- to 4-fold increase in the risk of active tuberculosis and other granulomatous conditions. Risk seems to be lower for etanercept (68). Risk also depends on local TB prevalence: in the year 2000, Spanish investigators reported an estimated TB incidence of 1,893/100,000 person-years in patients with RA treated with infliximab (69). This rate is ~10- to 20-fold higher than the observed rate in naïve patients. These rates have decreased dramatically since the establishment of latent tuberculosis infection (LTBI) screening prior to biological therapy (67, 70). It is essential to rule out LTBI in such individuals in order to reduce the risk of active TB reactivation. Interferon-gamma release assays (IGRAs) are useful tools for LTBI diagnosis. They are more specific than the tuberculin skin test (TST) because they do not show cross-reactivity with BCG-vaccination or NTM sensitization (71–73). Moreover, these *in-vitro* assays incorporate a mitogen control that can detect the presence of anergy, common in patients on immunosuppressive therapy (74). However, the clinical performance of IGRAs is still controversial due to the variety of concomitant immunosuppressive drug-regimens used at the time of LTBI screening, population heterogeneity, and the severity of the disease itself (75). Therefore, the clinical accuracy of IGRAs seems to be differentially affected depending on the specific type

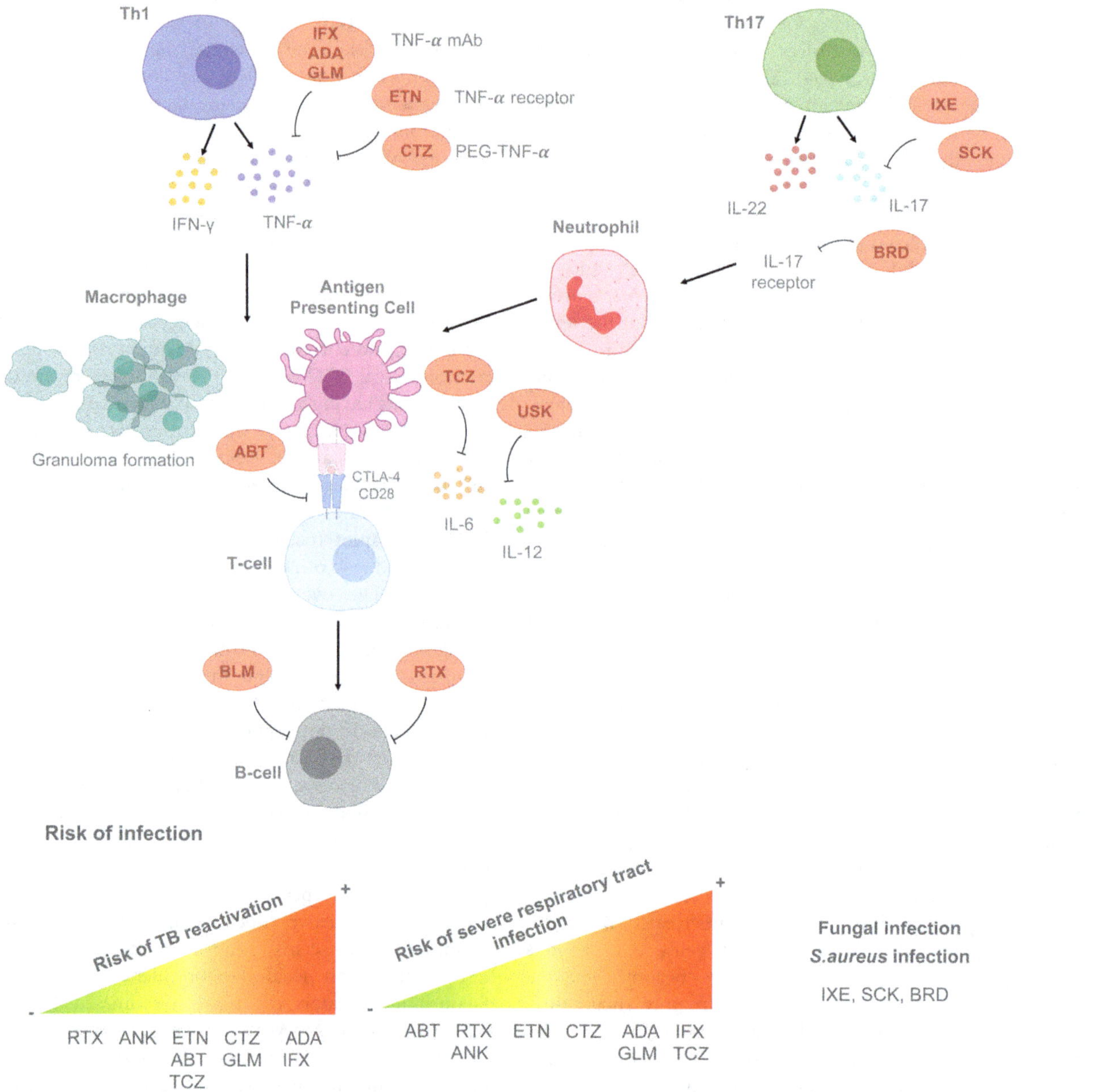

FIGURE 1 | Mode of action of biological response modifiers (BRM) according to cell type, cytokine and/or receptor targeted. Risk of developing infections according to the BRM considered is also shown. List of BRM. Anti-tumor necrosis factor-α (TNF-α) agents. ADA, adalimumab; CTZ, certolizumab; GLM, golimumab; IFX, infliximab; ETN, etanercept. Anti-interleukins, immunoglobulins, and complement factors. Anti IL-1, anakinra ANK; Anti IL-6: TCZ, tocilizumab; Anti IL-17: SCK, secukinumab; IXE, ixekizumab; BRD, brodalumab. Anti-IL12/23: USK, ustekinumab. Cell surface receptors/associated signaling pathways agents. Anti-CD28: ABT, abatacept; B-cell activating factor (BAFF): BLM, belimumab. Lymphoid cells surface antigens. Anti-CD20: RTX, rituximab. mAb, monoclonal antibody; PEG, polyethylene glycol; TB, tuberculosis; LTBI, latent tuberculosis infection.

of immune disorder. Crohn's disease and/or its concomitant drug-profile (such as azathioprine or high-dose corticosteroids) could negatively affect the clinical performance of IGRAs when compared with other immune-mediated diseases, such as psoriasis or inflammatory rheumatic diseases (76). Thus, it seems prudent and convenient to perform dual LTBI testing with TST and IGRAs (77). Patients with RA and underlying structural lung diseases are at increased risk of developing NTM infection (78), mostly *Mycobacterium avium*. In some countries, NTM infections are more common than TB after anti-TNF-α treatment. However, there are still no established recommendations as regards screening and prophylaxis (79). A baseline chest x-ray should be recommended prior to starting therapy, and in patients with chronic unexplained cough, further work-up should include chest computed tomography scans and culture of respiratory specimens.

Immunization strategies are recommended for all cases, regardless of whether the patient has PID or is receiving immunosuppressive treatment, and it is of importance to be vaccinated according to the national immunization routine schedules. For patients with anti-TNF-α treatment, pneumococcal and age-appropriate anti-viral vaccinations (i.e., influenza) should be administered (68). Immunization before and after BRM is well-established as regards inactivated vaccines, and precautions should be taken for live vaccines (57). However, even if response to vaccines is impaired in patients with PID (80), it may have an effect in patients receiving some BRM. This may be partially explained by the concept of trained immunity-based vaccines (81).

In conclusion, RTIs belong to the most common causes of infections in humans worldwide. The genetic contribution to severe RTIs may have been masked by other interventions (82). The inborn errors of innate immunity show us that the absence of a measurable immunological defect does not exclude an immunodeficiency (41). Further functional genetic studies are necessary in order to fully validate the impact of host genetics during lung infections. The knowledge obtained from experience with the prescription of BRM may be particularly valuable, as the infections acquired as a side effect may help to identify genetic defects with a similar infectious phenotype. In the meantime, recommendations based on biological rationale and clinical experience are mandatory in order to prevent re-emerging severe infections.

AUTHOR CONTRIBUTIONS

CP organized the structure and supervised the manuscript elaboration, revised literature and wrote a part of every chapter. AL revised literature, wrote the sections related to the immune response to infection and part of genetics, and edited the manuscript. IL, RV-H, and JD revised and wrote the aspects related to tuberculosis, and JD also supervised the manuscript elaboration. LM revised and wrote the section regarding the impact of biological response modifiers specially related to rheumatologic diseases. LM, AL, and RV-H prepared the figure. MM and CR revised aspects related to immunodeficiencies, and impact of BRM in children. IB revised host genetic factors. All authors revised and approved the final version of the manuscript.

REFERENCES

1. Ferkol T, Schraufnagel D. The global burden of respiratory disease. *Ann Am Thorac Soc.* (2014) 11:404–6. doi: 10.1513/AnnalsATS.201311-405PS
2. Mizgerd JP. Lung infection–a public health priority. *PLoS Med.* (2006) 3:e76. doi: 10.1371/journal.pmed.0030076
3. Walker CL, Rudan I, Liu L, Nair H, Theodoratou E, Bhutta ZA, et al. Global burden of childhood pneumonia and diarrhoea. *Lancet.* (2013) 381:1405–16. doi: 10.1016/S0140-6736(13)60222-6
4. World Health Organization. *Global Tuberculosis Report 2018 (WHO/CDS/TB/2018.20).* Geneva: World Health Organization.
5. Rustad TR, Sherrid AM, Minch KJ, Sherman DR. Hypoxia: a window into Mycobacterium tuberculosis latency. *Cell Microbiol.* (2009) 11:1151–9. doi: 10.1111/j.1462-5822.2009.01325.x
6. Nair H, Simoes EA, Rudan I, Gessner BD, Azziz-Baumgartner E, Zhang JS, et al. Global and regional burden of hospital admissions for severe acute lower respiratory infections in young children in 2010: a systematic analysis. *Lancet.* (2013) 381:1380–90. doi: 10.1016/S0140-6736(12)61901-1
7. Regamey N, Kaiser L, Roiha HL, Deffernez C, Kuehni CE, Latzin P, et al. Viral etiology of acute respiratory infections with cough in infancy: a community-based birth cohort study. *Pediatr Infect Dis J.* (2008) 27:100–5. doi: 10.1097/INF.0b013e31815922c8
8. Blanken MO, Rovers MM, Molenaar JM, Winkler-Seinstra PL, Meijer A, Kimpen JL, et al. Respiratory syncytial virus and recurrent wheeze in healthy preterm infants. *N Engl J Med.* (2013) 368:1791–9. doi: 10.1056/NEJMoa1211917
9. Henderson J, Hilliard TN, Sherriff A, Stalker D, Al Shammari N, Thomas HM. Hospitalization for RSV bronchiolitis before 12 months of age and subsequent asthma, atopy and wheeze: a longitudinal birth cohort study. *Pediatr Allergy Immunol.* (2005) 16:386–92. doi: 10.1111/j.1399-3038.2005.00298.x
10. Gern JE. Viral respiratory infection and the link to asthma. *Pediatr Infect Dis J.* (2008) 27(10 Suppl.):S97–103. doi: 10.1097/INF.0b013e318168b718
11. Gould CM, Freeman AF, Olivier KN. Genetic causes of bronchiectasis. *Clin Chest Med.* (2012) 33:249–63. doi: 10.1016/j.ccm.2012.03.002
12. McMichael A. Environmental and social influences on infectious diseases. In: Baquero F, Nombela C, Cassell G, Gutiérrez-Fuentes J, editors. *Evolutionary Biology of Bacterial and Fungal Pathogens.* Washington: American Society for Microbiology Press (2008). p. 31–8.
13. Morens DM, Folkers GK, Fauci AS. The challenge of emerging and re-emerging infectious diseases. *Nature.* (2004) 430:242–9. doi: 10.1038/nature02759
14. Affandi JS, Price P, Waterer G. Can immunogenetics illuminate the diverse manifestations of respiratory infections? *Ther Adv Respir Dis.* (2010) 4:161–76. doi: 10.1177/1753465810371484
15. Lambert L, Sagfors AM, Openshaw PJ, Culley FJ. Immunity to RSV in early-Life. *Front Immunol.* (2014) 5:466. doi: 10.3389/fimmu.2014.00466
16. Ciancanelli MJ, Abel L, Zhang SY, Casanova JL. Host genetics of severe influenza: from mouse Mx1 to human IRF7. *Curr Opin Immunol.* (2016) 38:109–20. doi: 10.1016/j.coi.2015.12.002
17. Bastos HN, Osorio NS, Gagneux S, Comas I, Saraiva M. The Troika host-pathogen-extrinsic factors in tuberculosis: modulating inflammation and clinical outcomes. *Front Immunol.* (2017) 8:1948. doi: 10.3389/fimmu.2017.01948
18. Cookson W, Cox MJ, Moffatt MF. New opportunities for managing acute and chronic lung infections. *Nat Rev Microbiol.* (2018) 16:111–20. doi: 10.1038/nrmicro.2017.122
19. Sen R, Nayak L, De RK. A review on host-pathogen interactions: classification and prediction. *Eur J Clin Microbiol Infect Dis.* (2016) 35:1581–99. doi: 10.1007/s10096-016-2716-7
20. Cullen L, McClean S. Bacterial adaptation during chronic respiratory infections. *Pathogens.* (2015) 4:66–89. doi: 10.3390/pathogens4010066
21. Prat C, Lacoma A. Bacteria in the respiratory tract-how to treat? Or do not treat? *Int J Infect Dis.* (2016) 51:113–22. doi: 10.1016/j.ijid.2016.09.005

22. Budden KF, Gellatly SL, Wood DL, Cooper MA, Morrison M, Hugenholtz P, et al. Emerging pathogenic links between microbiota and the gut-lung axis. *Nat Rev Microbiol.* (2017) 15:55–63. doi: 10.1038/nrmicro.2016.142
23. Mizgerd JP. Acute lower respiratory tract infection. *N Engl J Med.* (2008) 358:716–27. doi: 10.1056/NEJMra074111
24. Hancock RE, Nijnik A, Philpott DJ. Modulating immunity as a therapy for bacterial infections. *Nat Rev Microbiol.* (2012) 10:243–54. doi: 10.1038/nrmicro2745
25. Franchi L, Munoz-Planillo R, Nunez G. Sensing and reacting to microbes through the inflammasomes. *Nat Immunol.* (2012) 13:325–32. doi: 10.1038/ni.2231
26. Andreakos E, Salagianni M, Galani IE, Koltsida O. Interferon-lambdas: front-line guardians of immunity and homeostasis in the respiratory tract. *Front Immunol.* (2017) 8:1232. doi: 10.3389/fimmu.2017.01232
27. Egli A, Mandal J, Schumann DM, Roth M, Thomas B, Lorne Tyrrell D, et al. IFNLambda3/4 locus polymorphisms and IFNLambda3 circulating levels are associated with COPD severity and outcomes. *BMC Pulm Med.* (2018) 18:51. doi: 10.1186/s12890-018-0616-6
28. Dagenais TR, Keller NP. Pathogenesis of *Aspergillus fumigatus* in invasive aspergillosis. *Clin Microbiol Rev.* (2009) 22:447–65. doi: 10.1128/CMR.00055-08
29. Camp JV, Jonsson CB. A role for neutrophils in viral respiratory disease. *Front Immunol.* (2017) 8:550. doi: 10.3389/fimmu.2017.00550
30. Martinez I, Oliveros JC, Cuesta I, de la Barrera J, Ausina V, Casals C, et al. Apoptosis, toll-like, RIG-I-like and NOD-like receptors are pathways jointly induced by diverse respiratory bacterial and viral pathogens. *Front Microbiol.* (2017) 8:276. doi: 10.3389/fmicb.2017.00276
31. Fischer A, Rausell A. What do primary immunodeficiencies tell us about the essentiality/redundancy of immune responses? *Semin Immunol.* (2018) 36:13–6. doi: 10.1016/j.smim.2017.12.001
32. O'Garra A, Redford PS, McNab FW, Bloom CI, Wilkinson RJ, Berry MP. The immune response in tuberculosis. *Annu Rev Immunol.* (2013) 31:475–527. doi: 10.1146/annurev-immunol-032712-095939
33. Brunot V, Pernin V, Chartier C, Garrigue V, Vetromile F, Szwarc I, et al. An epidemic of *Pneumocystis jiroveci* pneumonia in a renal transplantation center: role of T-cell lymphopenia. *Transplant Proc.* (2012) 44:2818–20. doi: 10.1016/j.transproceed.2012.09.089
34. Lambert L, Culley FJ. Innate immunity to respiratory infection in early life. *Front Immunol.* (2017) 8:1570. doi: 10.3389/fimmu.2017.01570
35. Casanova JL, Abel L. The human model: a genetic dissection of immunity to infection in natural conditions. *Nat Rev Immunol.* (2004) 4:55–66. doi: 10.1038/nri1264
36. Casanova JL, Abel L. Human genetics of infectious diseases: Unique insights into immunological redundancy. *Semin Immunol.* (2018) 36:1–12. doi: 10.1016/j.smim.2017.12.008
37. Yazdani R, Abolhassani H, Asgardoon M, Shaghaghi M, Modaresi M, Azizi G, et al. Infectious and noninfectious pulmonary complications in patients with primary immunodeficiency disorders. *J Investig Allergol Clin Immunol.* (2017) 27:213–24. doi: 10.18176/jiaci.0166
38. Cutting GR. Modifier genes in Mendelian disorders: the example of cystic fibrosis. *Ann N Y Acad Sci.* (2010) 1214:57–69. doi: 10.1111/j.1749-6632.2010.05879.x
39. Corvol H, Blackman SM, Boelle PY, Gallins PJ, Pace RG, Stonebraker JR, et al. Genome-wide association meta-analysis identifies five modifier loci of lung disease severity in cystic fibrosis. *Nat Commun.* (2015) 6:8382. doi: 10.1038/ncomms9382
40. Manolio TA, Collins FS, Cox NJ, Goldstein DB, Hindorff LA, Hunter DJ, et al. Finding the missing heritability of complex diseases. *Nature.* (2009) 461:747–53. doi: 10.1038/nature08494
41. Bucciol G, Moens L, Bosch B, Bossuyt X, Casanova JL, Puel A, et al. Lessons learned from the study of human inborn errors of innate immunity. *J Allergy Clin Immunol.* (2019) 143:507–27. doi: 10.1016/j.jaci.2018.07.013
42. Casanova JL. Severe infectious diseases of childhood as monogenic inborn errors of immunity. *Proc Natl Acad Sci USA.* (2015) 112:E7128–37. doi: 10.1073/pnas.1521651112
43. Picard C, Bobby Gaspar H, Al-Herz W, Bousfiha A, Casanova JL, Chatila T, et al. International Union of Immunological Societies: 2017 Primary Immunodeficiency Diseases Committee report on inborn errors of immunity. *J Clin Immunol.* (2018) 38:96–128. doi: 10.1007/s10875-017-0464-9
44. Fernandez-Ruiz M, Meije Y, Manuel O, Akan H, Carratala J, Aguado JM, et al. ESCMID Study Group for Infections in Compromised Hosts (ESGICH) Consensus document on the safety of targeted and biological therapies: an infectious diseases perspective (Introduction). *Clin Microbiol Infect.* (2018) 24 Suppl. 2:S2–9. doi: 10.1016/j.cmi.2018.01.029
45. van Tong H, Velavan TP, Thye T, Meyer CG. Human genetic factors in tuberculosis: an update. *Trop Med Int Health.* (2017) 22:1063–71. doi: 10.1111/tmi.12923
46. Amanatidou V, Apostolakis S, Spandidos DA. Genetic diversity of the host and severe respiratory syncytial virus-induced lower respiratory tract infection. *Pediatr Infect Dis J.* (2009) 28:135–40. doi: 10.1097/INF.0b013e31818c8d17
47. Janssen R, Bont L, Siezen CL, Hodemaekers HM, Ermers MJ, Doornbos G, et al. Genetic susceptibility to respiratory syncytial virus bronchiolitis is predominantly associated with innate immune genes. *J Infect Dis.* (2007) 196:826–34. doi: 10.1086/520886
48. Barreiro LB, Neyrolles O, Babb CL, Tailleux L, Quach H, McElreavey K, et al. Promoter variation in the DC-SIGN-encoding gene CD209 is associated with tuberculosis. *PLoS Med.* (2006) 3:e20. doi: 10.1371/journal.pmed.0030020
49. Bustamante J, Arias AA, Vogt G, Picard C, Galicia LB, Prando C, et al. Germline CYBB mutations that selectively affect macrophages in kindreds with X-linked predisposition to tuberculous mycobacterial disease. *Nat Immunol.* (2011) 12:213–21. doi: 10.1038/ni.1992
50. Schurr E. The contribution of host genetics to tuberculosis pathogenesis. *Kekkaku.* (2011) 86:17–28.
51. Boisson-Dupuis S, Ramirez-Alejo N, Li Z, Patin E, Rao G, Kerner G, et al. Tuberculosis and impaired IL-23-dependent IFN-gamma immunity in humans homozygous for a common TYK2 missense variant. *Sci Immunol.* (2018) 3:eaau8714. doi: 10.1126/sciimmunol.aau8714
52. Asgari S, Schlapbach LJ, Anchisi S, Hammer C, Bartha I, Junier T, et al. Severe viral respiratory infections in children with IFIH1 loss-of-function mutations. *Proc Natl Acad Sci USA.* (2017) 114:8342–7. doi: 10.1073/pnas.1704259114
53. Ciancanelli MJ, Huang SX, Luthra P, Garner H, Itan Y, Volpi S, et al. Life-threatening influenza and impaired interferon amplification in human IRF7 deficiency. *Science.* (2015) 348:448–53. doi: 10.1126/science.aaa1578
54. Kaplon H, Reichert JM. Antibodies to watch in 2018. *MAbs.* (2018) 10:183–203. doi: 10.1080/19420862.2018.1415671
55. Hansel TT, Kropshofer H, Singer T, Mitchell JA, George AJ. The safety and side effects of monoclonal antibodies. *Nat Rev Drug Discov.* (2010) 9:325–38. doi: 10.1038/nrd3003
56. Davis BP, Ballas ZK. Biologic response modifiers: Indications, implications, and insights. *J Allergy Clin Immunol.* (2017) 139:1445–56. doi: 10.1016/j.jaci.2017.02.013
57. Davies HD, Committee On Infectious D. Infectious complications with the use of biologic response modifiers in infants and children. *Pediatrics.* (2016) 138:e2016120. doi: 10.1542/peds.2016-1209
58. Fisher MC, Greenberg JD. Assessing infection risk with biologic agents in RA: methodological challenges. *Nat Rev Rheumatol.* (2009) 5:288–91. doi: 10.1038/nrrheum.2009.51
59. Woodrick RS, Ruderman EM. Safety of biologic therapy in rheumatoid arthritis. *Nat Rev Rheumatol.* (2011) 7:639–52. doi: 10.1038/nrrheum.2011.145
60. Minozzi S, Bonovas S, Lytras T, Pecoraro V, Gonzalez-Lorenzo M, Bastiampillai AJ, et al. Risk of infections using anti-TNF agents in rheumatoid arthritis, psoriatic arthritis, and ankylosing spondylitis: a systematic review and meta-analysis. *Expert Opin Drug Saf.* (2016) 15(sup1):11–34. doi: 10.1080/14740338.2016.1240783
61. Singh JA, Cameron C, Noorbaloochi S, Cullis T, Tucker M, Christensen R, et al. Risk of serious infection in biological treatment of patients with rheumatoid arthritis: a systematic review and meta-analysis. *Lancet.* (2015) 386:258–65. doi: 10.1016/S0140-6736(14)61704-9
62. Galloway JB, Hyrich KL, Mercer LK, Dixon WG, Fu B, Ustianowski AP, et al. Anti-TNF therapy is associated with an increased risk of serious infections in patients with rheumatoid arthritis especially in the first 6 months of treatment: updated results from the British Society for Rheumatology Biologics Register with special emphasis on risks in the elderly. *Rheumatology (Oxford).* (2011) 50:124–31. doi: 10.1093/rheumatology/keq242

63. Subesinghe S, Rutherford AI, Byng-Maddick R, Leanne Hyrich K, Benjamin Galloway J. Recurrent serious infections in patients with rheumatoid arthritis-results from the British Society for Rheumatology Biologics Register. *Rheumatology (Oxford).* (2018) 57:651–5. doi: 10.1093/rheumatology/kex469
64. Zink A, Manger B, Kaufmann J, Eisterhues C, Krause A, Listing J, et al. Evaluation of the RABBIT Risk Score for serious infections. *Ann Rheum Dis.* (2014) 73:1673–6. doi: 10.1136/annrheumdis-2013-203341
65. Richter A, Listing J, Schneider M, Klopsch T, Kapelle A, Kaufmann J, et al. Impact of treatment with biologic DMARDs on the risk of sepsis or mortality after serious infection in patients with rheumatoid arthritis. *Ann Rheum Dis.* (2016) 75:1667–73. doi: 10.1136/annrheumdis-2015-207838
66. Mariette X, Gottenberg JE, Ravaud P, Combe B. Registries in rheumatoid arthritis and autoimmune diseases: data from the French registries. *Rheumatology (Oxford).* (2011) 50:222–9. doi: 10.1093/rheumatology/keq368
67. Rutherford AI, Patarata E, Subesinghe S, Hyrich KL, Galloway JB. Opportunistic infections in rheumatoid arthritis patients exposed to biologic therapy: results from the British Society for Rheumatology Biologics Register for Rheumatoid Arthritis. *Rheumatology (Oxford).* (2018) 57:997–1001. doi: 10.1093/rheumatology/key023
68. Baddley JW, Cantini F, Goletti D, Gomez-Reino JJ, Mylonakis E, San-Juan R, et al. ESCMID Study Group for Infections in Compromised Hosts (ESGICH) Consensus Document on the safety of targeted and biological therapies: an infectious diseases perspective (Soluble immune effector molecules [I]: anti-tumor necrosis factor-alpha agents). *Clin Microbiol Infect.* (2018) 24 Suppl. 2:S10–20. doi: 10.1016/j.cmi.2017.12.025
69. Gomez-Reino JJ, Carmona L, Valverde VR, Mola EM, Montero MD, Group B. Treatment of rheumatoid arthritis with tumor necrosis factor inhibitors may predispose to significant increase in tuberculosis risk: a multicenter active-surveillance report. *Arthritis Rheum.* (2003) 48:2122–7. doi: 10.1002/art.11137
70. Carmona L, Gomez-Reino JJ, Rodriguez-Valverde V, Montero D, Pascual-Gomez E, Mola EM, et al. Effectiveness of recommendations to prevent reactivation of latent tuberculosis infection in patients treated with tumor necrosis factor antagonists. *Arthritis Rheum.* (2005) 52:1766–72. doi: 10.1002/art.21043
71. Dominguez J, Ruiz-Manzano J, De Souza-Galvao M, Latorre I, Mila C, Blanco S, et al. Comparison of two commercially available gamma interferon blood tests for immunodiagnosis of tuberculosis. *Clin Vaccine Immunol.* (2008) 15:168–71. doi: 10.1128/CVI.00364-07
72. Ferrara G, Losi M, D'Amico R, Roversi P, Piro R, Meacci M, et al. Use in routine clinical practice of two commercial blood tests for diagnosis of infection with Mycobacterium tuberculosis: a prospective study. *Lancet.* (2006) 367:1328–34. doi: 10.1016/S0140-6736(06)68579-6
73. Latorre I, De Souza-Galvao M, Ruiz-Manzano J, Lacoma A, Prat C, Altet N, et al. Evaluating the non-tuberculous mycobacteria effect in the tuberculosis infection diagnosis. *Eur Respir J.* (2010) 35:338–42. doi: 10.1183/09031936.00196608
74. Dominguez J, Latorre I. Role of the T-cell interferon-gamma release assays in preventing reactivation of latent tuberculosis infection in immunosuppressed patients in treatment with anti-TNF agents. *J Crohns Colitis.* (2008) 2:250–4. doi: 10.1016/j.crohns.2008.05.007
75. Sester M, van Leth F, Bruchfeld J, Bumbacea D, Cirillo DM, Dilektasli AG, et al. Risk assessment of tuberculosis in immunocompromised patients. A TBNET study. *Am J Respir Crit Care Med.* (2014) 190:1168–76. doi: 10.1164/rccm.201405-0967OC
76. Latorre I, Minguez S, Carrascosa JM, Naves J, Villar-Hernandez R, Muriel B, et al. Immune-mediated inflammatory diseases differently affect IGRAs' accuracy for latent tuberculosis infection diagnosis in clinical practice. *PLoS One.* (2017) 12:e0189202. doi: 10.1371/journal.pone.0189202
77. Santin M, Garcia-Garcia JM, Rigau D, Altet N, Anibarro L, Casas I, et al. Executive summary of the guidelines for the use of interferon-gamma release assays in the diagnosis of tuberculosis infection. *Enferm Infecc Microbiol Clin.* (2016) 34:304–8. doi: 10.1016/j.eimc.2015.11.021
78. Winthrop KL, Chang E, Yamashita S, Iademarco MF, LoBue PA. Nontuberculous mycobacteria infections and anti-tumor necrosis factor-alpha therapy. *Emerg Infect Dis.* (2009) 15:1556–61. doi: 10.3201/eid1510.090310
79. Winthrop KL, Iseman M. Bedfellows: mycobacteria and rheumatoid arthritis in the era of biologic therapy. *Nat Rev Rheumatol.* (2013) 9:524–31. doi: 10.1038/nrrheum.2013.82
80. Mieves JF, Wittke K, Freitag H, Volk HD, Scheibenbogen C, Hanitsch LG. Influenza vaccination in patients with common variable immunodeficiency (CVID). *Curr Allergy Asthma Rep.* (2017) 17:78. doi: 10.1007/s11882-017-0749-3
81. Sanchez-Ramon S, Conejero L, Netea MG, Sancho D, Palomares O, Subiza JL. Trained immunity-based vaccines: a new paradigm for the development of broad-spectrum anti-infectious formulations. *Front Immunol.* (2018) 9:2936. doi: 10.3389/fimmu.2018.02936
82. Casanova JL. Human genetic basis of interindividual variability in the course of infection. *Proc Natl Acad Sci USA.* (2015) 112:E7118–27. doi: 10.1073/pnas.1521644112

14

The Role of Collectins and Galectins in Lung Innate Immune Defense

Cristina Casals[1,2*]*, María A. Campanero-Rhodes*[1,3]*, Belén García-Fojeda*[1,2] *and Dolores Solís*[1,3*]

[1] *Centro de Investigación Biomédica en Red de Enfermedades Respiratorias (CIBERES), Instituto de Salud Carlos III, Madrid, Spain,* [2] *Departamento de Bioquímica y Biología Molecular, Universidad Complutense de Madrid, Madrid, Spain,* [3] *Instituto de Química Física Rocasolano, CSIC, Madrid, Spain*

***Correspondence:**
Cristina Casals
ccasalsc@ucm.es
Dolores Solís
d.solis@iqfr.csic.es

Different families of endogenous lectins use complementary defense strategies against pathogens. They may recognize non-self glycans typically found on pathogens and/or host glycans. The collectin and galectin families are prominent examples of these two lectin categories. Collectins are C-type lectins that contain a carbohydrate recognition domain and a collagen-like domain. Members of this group include surfactant protein A (SP-A) and D (SP-D), secreted by the alveolar epithelium to the alveolar fluid. Lung collectins bind to several microorganisms, which results in pathogen aggregation and/or killing, and enhances phagocytosis of pathogens by alveolar macrophages. Moreover, SP-A and SP-D influence macrophage responses, contributing to resolution of inflammation, and SP-A is essential for tissue-repair functions of macrophages. Galectins also function by interacting directly with pathogens or by modulating the immune system in response to the infection. Direct binding may result in enhanced or impaired infection of target cells, or can have microbicidal effects. Immunomodulatory effects of galectins include recruitment of immune cells to the site of infection, promotion of neutrophil function, and stimulation of the bactericidal activity of infected macrophages. Moreover, intracellular galectins can serve as danger receptors, promoting autophagy of the invading pathogen. This review will focus on the role of collectins and galectins in pathogen clearance and immune response activation in infectious diseases of the respiratory system.

Keywords: respiratory pathogens, infection, inflammation, surfactant proteins, alternatively activated macrophages, autophagy, tissue repair, lung homeostasis

INTRODUCTION

Host defense in the lung is exceptionally, if not uniquely, challenging. The alveolar boundary is clearly the most vulnerable body interface. There are at least three important differences among the alveolar boundary and the upper respiratory tract, gut, and skin interfaces. First, the surface area to be defended is greater in the alveolar boundary (90 m^2) than in the gut (10 m^2) or skin (2 m^2) (1). Second, compared with the skin, gut, and upper respiratory tract, the bacterial biomass in the alveoli of healthy lungs is low (2). Third, there are physical barriers or harsh chemical environments in the skin (cornified epithelial layers) and gut (regular secretion of bile, which acts as an antiseptic detergent) but not in the delicate alveolar space. In addition, there is higher risk of pathogen dissemination at the alveolar boundary than at any other environmental boundary, since only two cell layers (the alveolar epithelium and the capillary endothelium) separate the invader from the bloodstream in order to facilitate gas exchange.

The innate immune system in the alveolar space is made up of a cellular arm [mainly alveolar macrophages (aMΦ) (1), but also epithelial (AEC), dendritic, and T cells (1, 3, 4)] and a humoral arm composed of antimicrobial proteins and peptides present in the alveolar fluid such as surfactant protein A (SP-A) and D (SP-D), lactoferrin, lysozyme, fibronectin, immunoglobulins, complement components, defensins, and cathelicidins, among others (5, 6). In this review we focus on the role of lung soluble collagenous C-type lectins (SP-A and SP-D) and galectins. SP-A and SP-D are principally secreted to the alveolar fluid by type II AECs and to the airway lumen by Club cells and submucosal cells (7). They are also detected in the trachea (8) and nasal mucosa (9), where they provide immune protection. Galectins are expressed in the lung by innate immune cells and epithelial cells. Galectins are present in the cytoplasm and nucleus, as well as extracellular space, although galectins lack a typical secretion signal peptide. They are secreted by direct translocation across the plasma membrane or through release in extracellular vesicles (10). Thus, they can function both inside and outside cells. The review describes biochemical and structural aspects of lung collectins and their role in antimicrobial immunity and alveolar immune homeostasis, and the involvement of galectins in the response to respiratory infectious diseases, including expression, binding to pathogens, modulatory effects on immune cells, and intracellular functions.

COLLECTINS

Biochemical and Structural Aspects

Collectins or collagenous C-type lectins are a family of proteins that contain a Ca^{2+}-dependent carbohydrate recognition domain (CRD) contiguous to a collagen-like triple helical domain. In humans, members of this group include SP-A and SP-D, secreted by the alveolar epithelium, nonciliated bronchiolar cells and other mucosal surfaces exposed to the external environment (7, 8, 11), mannan-binding lectin (MBL) secreted by hepatocytes to serum, and the recently discovered CL-L1, CL-K1, and CL-P1, present in the serum and several tissues (12, 13) (**Figure 1A**). Collectins are well-conserved oligomeric proteins, assembled in trimers or multiples of three subunits due to their collagen domains. The primary structure of each subunit consists of an N-terminal segment containing cysteine residues involved in oligomerization followed by a collagen-like region, an alpha helical coiled neck region, and a globular CRD with a calcium ion at the lectin site (**Figure 1A**). Lung collectins are modified after translation (cleavage of the signal peptide, proline hydroxylation, and N-linked glycosylation) (7, 15) and intracellularly assembled into oligomeric structures that, in the case of SP-A, resemble a flower bouquet of six trimers, while the assembly of SP-D resembles a cruciform of four trimers (**Figure 1A**). Supratrimeric oligomerization of lung collectins appears to be needed for many of their functions (16, 17) since it facilitates multivalent binding and increases the functional affinity of the globular domain for their ligands.

The CRDs of lung collectins bind to mannose and mannose-rich microbial glycoconjugates, such as yeast mannans and mycobacterial lipoarabinomannan. Besides, lung collectins recognize a wide variety of carbohydrates present in the surface of several microorganisms, including glucose, fucose, N-acetylglucosamine, and N-acetylmannosamine. Their globular domains recognize not only carbohydrates but also a broader repertoire of ligands, including proteins, nucleic acids, and lipids (7, 18, 19). Despite their similar CRDs, SP-A and SP-D show significant differences in ligand preferences, with SP-A ligands generally being more amphipathic (19, 20), and SP-D ligands richer in carbohydrates (20). These different preferences likely serve to extend the range of innate immune surveillance in the lung.

The collagen-like domains of collectins not only function as scaffolding that amplifies the ligand binding activities of globular domains but also are responsible for collectin binding to receptors in immune cells. Such receptors are involved in phagocytosis and clearance of microorganisms (7, 8, 12, 13) and biological/abiotic particles from the pulmonary environment (21–23), and in efferocytosis of dead cells (apoptotic/necrotic) (24, 25). Collagen-dependent functions of collectins are shared with other secreted defense collagens (C1q, ficolins, and adiponectin) (26). This group of proteins has a dual capacity to promote pathogen elimination and control inflammation (27–30). Moreover, they seem to activate molecular and cellular mechanisms that force a return to homeostasis (14).

Antimicrobial Immunity

SP-A and/or SP-D recognize a wide range of respiratory pathogens, including influenza A virus, respiratory syncytial virus, *Mycobacterium tuberculosis*, *Aspergillus fumigatus*, *Pseudomonas aeruginosa*, *Haemophilus influenzae* [see (8, 31) for reviews], and the parasitic helminth *Nippostrongylus brasiliensis* (32). SP-A- or SP-D-deficient mice show decreased microbe clearance and increased tissue markers of inflammation (14, 30–33), suggesting lung collectins' protective role in lung immune defense.

Lung collectins enhance the clearance of pathogens by four different mechanisms: (i) By aggregating pathogens to which they bind, which hinders their entry into epithelial cells and facilitates their removal, either by mucociliary clearance or by phagocytosis by aMΦs and recruited neutrophils (7, 8, 30, 31, 34). (ii) By binding to neutrophil extracellular traps (NET)-DNA and to bacteria simultaneously, thereby promoting bacterial trapping by the NETs (35). (iii) By enhancing phagocytosis of IgG-opsonized particles (36) and complement-coated particles (36, 37). (iv) By up-regulating expression of cell-surface receptors involved in microbial recognition, such as mannose receptor (38) and scavenger receptor SR-AI/II (39).

Data supporting direct antimicrobial activity of SP-A and SP-D are sparse (8, 31). Most respiratory pathogenic bacteria and fungi are resistant to SP-A and SP-D (8, 34, 40, 41). However, it is possible that cooperative interactions of lung collectins with other lung antimicrobial peptides enhance the microbicidal defense of the lungs. In this regard, we recently discovered synergic action between SP-A and SP-B^N, a secreted anionic antimicrobial peptide derived from SP-B proprotein. Interaction between SP-A and SP-B^N confers new antimicrobial properties, including the ability to bind, kill, and enhance phagocytosis of

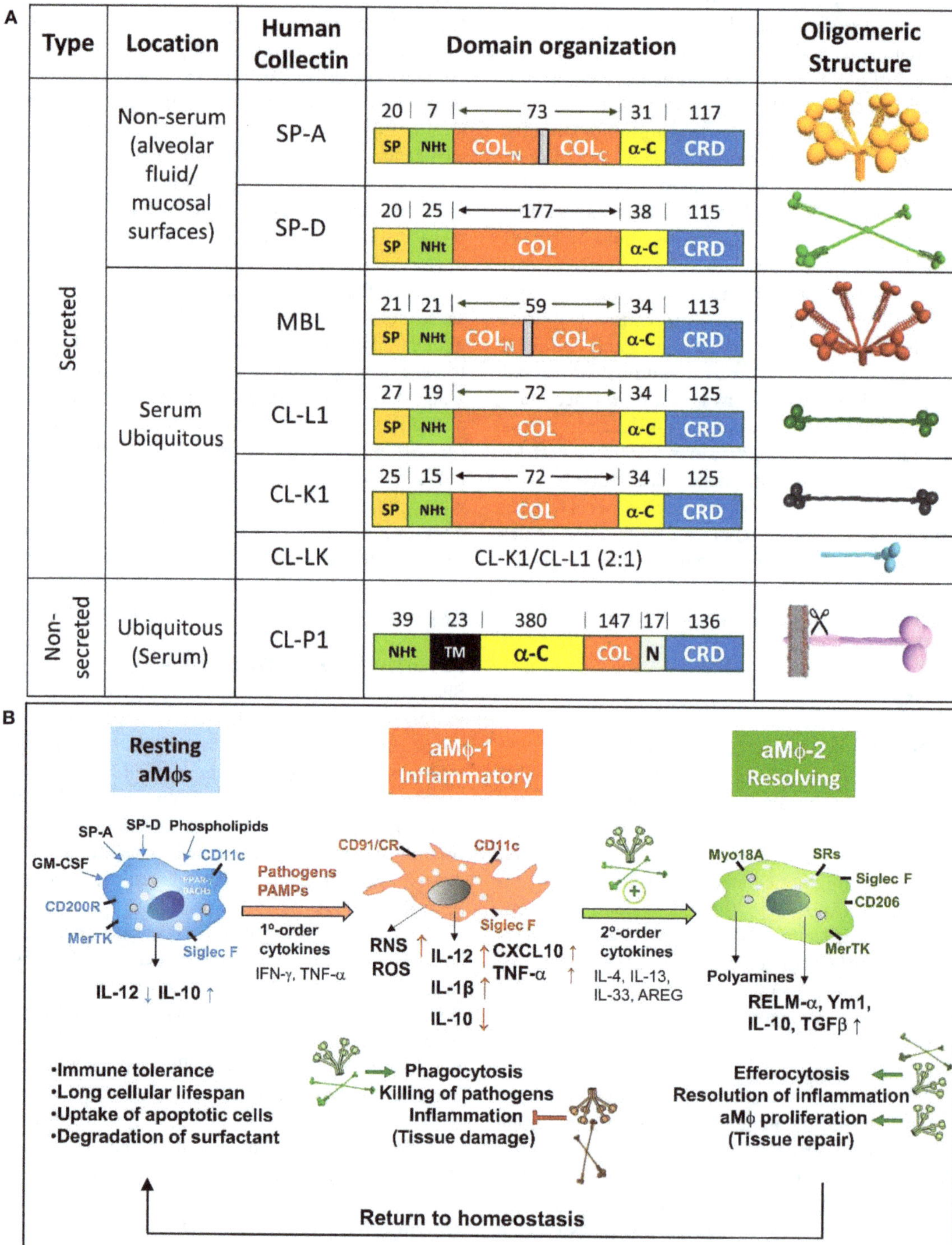

FIGURE 1 | (A) Structural analysis of human collectins. Domain organization of human collectin polypeptide chains and the number of amino acids covering each domain are shown. Interruptions in the collagen domain of SP-A and MBL are indicated. Three-dimensional models of collectin oligomers are also shown. Trimers of collectins are each built up by the association of three polypeptide chains, the collagen regions of which intertwine to form a collagen triple helix. Whereas all other collectins are soluble, CL-P1 is a transmembrane protein orientated with its N-terminal toward the cytosol. CL-P1 may be regarded as both a collectin and a scavenger receptor. The scissors symbol means the shedding of a soluble form of CL-P1 by a hitherto unknown mechanism, which results in the presence of soluble CL-P1 in the circulation. The molecules are not drawn to scale. SP, signal peptide; NHt, N-terminal domain; COL, collagen-like domain; α-C, α-helical coiled-coil domain; CRD, carbohydrate recognition domain; TM, transmembrane domain. **(B)** Role of lung collectins on sequential type 1 and type 2 immune responses following respiratory infection. Respiratory pathogens are detected by AECs and aMΦs, initiating an innate immune response to clear localized infections. The type 1 response is essential

(Continued)

FIGURE 1 | in controlling infection but also induces tissue damage. Stimulated tissue-resident lymphoid cells and AECs release appropriate second-order cytokines that initiate a two-tiered response. The type 2 response, amplified by lung collectins (14), modulates aMΦs toward an anti-inflammatory resolving phenotype involved in lung repair. The role of lung collectins in these homeostatic changes is shown by small green or red arrows, which mean SP-A/D-mediated activation or inhibition, respectively.

pathogenic *K. pneumoniae* K2 that is otherwise resistant to either protein alone (34). Moreover, therapeutic treatment with SP-A and SP-B^N protects against *K. pneumoniae* K2 infection *in vivo* due to SP-A/SP-B^N capability to both kill bacteria and modulate host inflammatory response (34). Yet a promising field to explore is the interaction of lung collectins with other lung antimicrobial peptides and antibiotics and the potential relevance of these interactions in innate host defense in the lung.

Alveolar Immune Homeostasis

The niche in which alveolar macrophages exist, rich in surfactant lipids, SP-A, and SP-D (42), has a considerable influence on many aspects of aMΦ phenotype (1, 43). Alveolar MΦs function as sentinels of a healthy state, promoting immune tolerance to innocuous antigens. During an infection, aMΦs recognize alarm signals such as IFN-γ and PAMPs, initiating proinflammatory responses and pathogen clearance (MΦ-1 phenotype) (**Figure 1B**), and collectins promote phagocytosis of pathogens by binding to the CD91/calreticulin receptor on aMΦs (44). However, host defense requires a balance between decreasing microbial burden and restricting tissue damage caused directly by pathogens or indirectly by the immune response (45). In this vein, lung collectins influence aMΦ responses to limit inflammation. First, they block the binding of TLR ligands to their receptors by direct interaction with TLR4, TLR2, the TLR co-receptor MD2, and CD14 (17, 30, 46) or by binding to TLR4/CD14 ligands (47, 48), acting as LPS scavengers *in vivo* (49). Second, they modify aMΦ response to TLR ligands by modulating signaling cascades. For example, SP-A and SP-D bind to SIRPα through their globular heads to initiate an SHP-1-dependent signaling pathway that blocks proinflammatory mediator production (44). In addition, SP-A increases the expression of negative regulators of TLR-signaling, such as IRAK-M (50) and β-arrestin 2 (51), and inhibits activation of NFκB, ERK, p38, and Akt in aMΦs (52, 53). Third, they reduce the production of reactive oxygen intermediates (54, 55) and for SP-D, this effect is mediated through its binding to the inhibitory receptor LAIR-1 (56). Fourth, SP-A limits inflammation by binding to IFN-γ, suppressing IFN-γ interaction with its receptor IFN-γR1 (57).

Besides limiting inflammation, lung collectins activate different mechanisms that contribute to disease resolution. After proinflammatory type 1 responses against invading pathogens, repair-associated type 2 responses must be initiated (58, 59). The tissue repair response is classically associated with the production of IL-4/IL-13 cytokines and the induction of alternatively activated macrophages (MΦ-2 phenotype) (**Figure 1B**). We recently found that defense collagens (SP-A and C1q) enhance IL-4/13-dependent alternative activation, proliferation, and tissue-repair functions of macrophages through binding to the myosin 18A receptor by their collagen domains (14). Loss of function studies using SP-A- and C1q-deficient mice demonstrated that SP-A and C1q are necessary to promote tissue repair during infection with the parasite *N. brasiliensis* and the Gram positive bacterium *Listeria monocytogenes,* respectively (14). SP-D also seems to be an important modulator of protective IL-4/13-induced aMΦ responses against *N. brasiliensis* (32). Interestingly, IL-4Rα signaling requires concomitant recognition of apoptotic cells to induce the tissue repair program in macrophages (60), suggesting that tissue repair is restricted to the damaged site. SP-A, SP-D, and C1q assist the recognition and clearance of apoptotic neutrophils by macrophages (24, 25, 61, 62), a mechanism that differs from classical phagocytosis and that leads to the production of anti-inflammatory cytokines (IL-10 and TGFβ) (63), contributing to host tolerance during lung infection.

In conclusion, pulmonary collectins provide immune protection against respiratory pathogens, promoting pathogen clearance, limiting inflammation, and activating molecular and cellular mechanisms that help to restore homeostasis. Much of what we know about the protective role of SP-A and SP-D has arisen from studies using SP-A– or SP-D–deficient mice in murine models of respiratory infections (14, 31–33) and other respiratory diseases (30, 31, 64).

GALECTINS

Galectins are a family of lectins sharing a CRD with β-sandwich fold and β-galactoside-binding ability (65, 66). Nevertheless, the glycan-binding preferences of different galectins may differ significantly, leading to functional divergences. To date, 16 mammalian galectins have been described, of which galectins 5, 6 (both found in rodents), 11, and 15 (found in ruminants) are not present in humans (**Figure S1**). Based on their structural organization (**Figure S1**), galectins are classified as proto type, composed of one or two identical CRDs forming non-covalent homodimers (e.g., Gal-1), chimera type, composed of one CRD linked to a non-lectin N-terminal region (Gal-3), and tandem-repeat type, containing two different CRDs covalently connected by a linker peptide (e.g., Gal-8 and -9). Galectins are widely expressed in epithelial and immune cells, and participate in different biological phenomena, including inflammation and immunity (67, 68).

The Expression of Galectins Is Altered in Respiratory Infections

An archetypal example is the accumulation of Gal-3 in the alveolar space of *Streptococcus pneumoniae*-infected mice (69). Gal-3 release also increases in the lungs of mice lethally infected with *Francisella novicida* (70). In patients infected with *M.*

tuberculosis, the plasma levels of Gal-9 are significantly increased (71). However, Gal-9 expression in macrophages generated in the presence of *M. tuberculosis* lipoarabinomannan is down-regulated, favoring bacterial intracellular growth (72).

The expression of galectins is also affected by respiratory viruses. As an example, Gal-1 is up-regulated in the lungs of influenza virus-infected mice, in correlation with the viral load (73). Interestingly, Gal-1 is differentially expressed in bronchoepithelial cells infected with 2009 A or seasonal H1N1 influenza virus, revealing strain-specific responses (74). Moreover, patients carrying genetic variants associated with higher Gal-1 expression are less susceptible to infection by avian influenza A (75).

Gal-3 levels in serum and lungs are augmented in infections by the fungus *Cryptococcus neoformans* (76), while plasma levels of Gal-9 are higher in severe infections by the parasite *Plasmodium falciparum* (77), and mRNA levels of Gal-9 in the lungs of *P. berghei*-infected mice are also increased (78).

Thus, the expression of galectins is altered in bacterial, viral, fungal, and parasitic respiratory infections, conceivably correlating with galectin-mediated defense mechanisms.

Galectins Bind to Different Respiratory Pathogens

Gal-3 binds mycolic acids (**Figure 2A**), the major constituents of mycobacterial cell wall, and could participate in their interaction with host cells (79). Gal-3 also binds lipopolysaccharides from different bacteria, including *K. pneumoniae* (80) and *P. aeruginosa* (81). Moreover, Gal-3 and Gal-8 bind to *K. pneumoniae* O1 cells and decrease bacterial viability, and the same occurs for Gal-8 and strain 2019 of non-typeable *H. influenzae* (NTHi) (82). Recently, binding of Gal-8 to other six different NTHi clinical isolates was detected (83), suggesting that this could be a general trait.

At the initial phase of infection by Nipah virus (NiV), Gal-1 bridges glycans of the envelope glycoprotein F (NiV-F) with those of host cells, thereby enhancing virus attachment. However, Gal-1 secreted in response to infection reduces NiV-F-mediated syncytia formation and production of progeny virus (84–86). This is a remarkable example of opposing effects of the same galectin on infection by a given pathogen. Moreover, Gal-1 binds to envelope glycoproteins of influenza virus, impairing infection. Cells treated with Gal-1 generate lower viral yields, and treatment of infected mice reduces viral load and lung inflammation (73). Conversely, Gal-1 could account for the increased susceptibility of influenza patients to subsequent infection with pneumococcus. Influenza infection results in desialylation of epithelial cell glycans and exposure of galactosyl moieties that serve as galectin ligands. As Gal-1 also binds to *S. pneumoniae*, it crosslinks the bacteria to the airway epithelial surface, enhancing pneumococcal adhesion (87).

As final example, Gal-3 binds to *C. neoformans* cells and delays fungal growth. Moreover, it exerts a lytic effect on fungal extracellular vesicles (76). Thus, Gal-3 has direct anti-*C. neoformans* effects.

Galectins Modulate the Immune Response to Infection

Accumulation of Gal-3 in the alveoli of pnemococcus-infected mice correlates with neutrophil extravasation (69). Consistently, less neutrophils are recruited in Gal-3$^{-/-}$ mice, which develop more severe pneumonia, and treatment with Gal-3 reduces the severity of infection (88, 89). Gal-3 bridges neutrophils to endothelial cells and activate neutrophils (**Figure 2B**), augmenting pneumococcus phagocytosis and delaying apoptosis. These effects are disabled by *Staphylococcus aureus* via degradation of Gal-3 with a bacterial protease (90). In contrast, Gal-3 deficiency confers resistance to *Rhodococcus equi* (91). Thus, Gal-3$^{-/-}$ mice exhibit higher bacteria lethal doses and production of IL-12 and IFN-γ. Moreover, Gal-3$^{-/-}$ macrophages show decreased bacterial replication and survival, and enhanced production of IL-1β and TLR2. Gal-3$^{-/-}$ mice lethally infected with *F. novicida*, however, show significantly reduced inflammatory response and leukocyte infiltration in the lungs, in parallel to improved lung architecture and survival (70), and the same is observed for Gal-9$^{-/-}$ mice (92). Thus, Gal-3 and Gal-9 function as proinflammatory alarmins in *F. novicida* infection.

Gal-9 also modulates the immune response through binding to TIM-3 receptor on neutrophils, macrophages and lymphocytes. For example, *P. aeruginosa* opsonization with Gal-9 enhances neutrophil-mediated killing via TIM-3 interactions inducing intracellular Ca^{2+} mobilization, neutrophil degranulation, and NADPH oxidase activity (93). Binding of Gal-9 expressed by *M. tuberculosis*-infected macrophages to TIM-3 also leads to restriction of intracellular bacterial growth through secretion of IL-1β, upregulation of TNF, and activation of caspase-3 (94–96). In contrast, Gal-9–TIM-3 binding decreases the levels of IL-17 in serum of mice infected with *K. pneumoniae*, resulting in reduced bacterial clearance (97).

Gal-9 binding to TIM-3 receptor on T lymphocytes decreases the immune response against viral infections. Influenza A virus-infected Gal-9$^{-/-}$ mice generate stronger humoral and CD8+ T-cell responses and cleared virus more rapidly than Gal-9$^{+/+}$ mice. Accordingly, selective blocking of the Gal-9–TIM-3 interaction in Gal-9$^{+/+}$ mice boosts the immune response (98). On the other hand, Gal-9 administered to mice infected with respiratory syncytial virus decreases the severity of lung pathology by increasing Tregs number and reducing the number of Th17 cells, IL-17 levels, and CD8+ T cell apoptosis (99). Similarly, Gal-9 injection into herpes simplex virus-infected mice increases Tregs number and decreases the levels of pro-inflammatory cytokines, improving the symptoms of inflammation (100), while intraperitoneal infusion of lactose, which prevents Gal-9 binding to TIM-3, reduces Treg function and augments CD8+ T cell responses (101).

In respiratory fungal infections, Gal-1 and Gal-3 play differential roles. Gal-1 modulates prostaglandin E2 and nitric oxide levels in *H. capsulatum* infection, contributing to phagocyte responses and thus exerting a protective effect (102). In contrast, Gal-3$^{-/-}$ mice clear *H. capsulatum* infection more efficiently than Gal-3$^{+/+}$ mice, likely due to a negative regulatory role

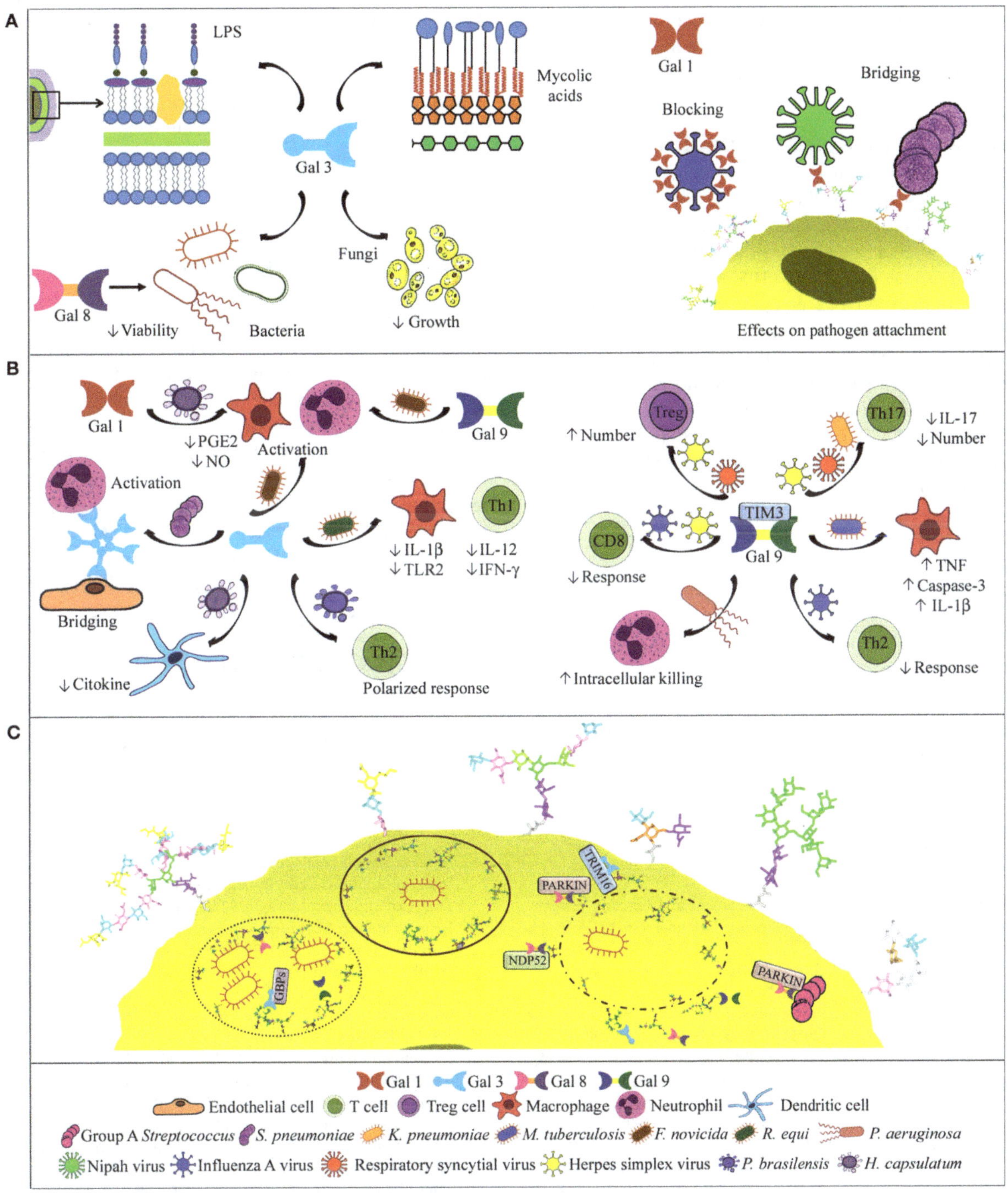

FIGURE 2 | Galectin activities in respiratory infections. **(A)** Binding to pathogens. Gal-3, the only chimera-type galectin described to date, binds bacterial mycolic acids, lipopolysaccharides, and cells, and also *C. neoformans* cells with antifungal effects. Gal-8 binds NTHi, decreasing bacterial viability (left side). Gal-1 binding to influenza virus blocks infection, while binding to NiV and *S. pneumoniae* bridges pathogen and host glycans (right side). **(B)** Effects on immune cells. Oligomerized Gal-3 can bridge neutrophils to endothelial cells. Depending on the pathogen, Gal-3 drives a Th2-polarized response, decreases macrophage and Th1 cell responses, or activates macrophages and/or neutrophils, similarly to Gal-9. In histoplasmosis, Gal-3 decreases cytokine production by dendritic cells, while Gal-1 modulates PGE2 and NO levels (left). Via TIM-3 binding, Gal-9 may promote bacterial killing by neutrophils or macrophages, decrease humoral and CD8+ cell responses or Th17 cells and IL-17 levels, and increase Treg cells (right). **(C)** Intracellular functions. Gal-3, -8, and -9 bind to host glycans in the luminal side of lysed phagosomes or permeable replicative vacuoles, and contribute to the autophagic response by recruiting NDP52, parkin, GBPs, or TRIM-16. Gal-8 also recruits parkin to group A *Streptococcus*.

of Gal-3 on cytokine production by dendritic cells (103). However, Gal-$3^{-/-}$ mice are more susceptible to *P. brasiliensis* infection and present a Th2-polarized immune response, clearly showing that Gal-3 effects depend on the particular pathogen (104).

Intracellular Activities of Galectins

After internalization into host cells, many bacteria lyse the phagosome and escape to the cytosol for establishing a replicative niche (**Figure 2C**). Galectins 3, 8, and 9 bind to damaged vacuoles that expose host glycans in the luminal side of the phagosome membrane (105, 106). Moreover, Gal-8 recruits the autophagy NDP52 receptor, activating phagosome degradation (106). Gal-8 also binds parkin, which targets damaged vesicles and bacteria for ubiquitination. Interestingly, Gal-3 diminishes the recruitment of Gal-8 and parkin to group A *Streptococcus*, which does not replicate in endothelial cells and organs of Gal-$3^{-/-}$ mice (107). Gal-8 also targets for degradation damaged endosomes in picornavirus and adenovirus infections (108, 109).

Other bacteria replicate within the phagosomes, as e.g., *Coxiella burnetii*. Yet, galectins 3, 8, and 9 accumulate in the luminal side of the vacuole membrane, revealing membrane permeability (110). Gal-3 and Gal-8 are also detected in replicative vacuoles of *Legionella pneumophila* (111) and mediate delivery of guanylate binding proteins, a family of antimicrobial GTPases induced by IFN-γ (112). Moreover, Gal-3 binds TRIM-16, further contributing to organizing the autophagic response. The Gal-3-TRIM-16 system operates in macrophages infected with *M. tuberculosis* strains causing phagosome damage, and is required for bacteria translocation to lysosomes. Accordingly, Gal-3 protects mice in acute and chronic *M. tuberculosis* infection (113, 114).

Summarizing, galectins play diverse roles in respiratory infections with sometimes disparate effects, which may benefit the host or the pathogen, depending on the specific galectin, pathogen, and host context.

CONCLUDING REMARKS

This review touched briefly on the important role of collectins and galectins in pathogen clearance and immune response activation. Lung collectins are critical in mediating a variety of immune and physiological responses during health and disease. Galectins also mediate effective antimicrobial and immunoregulatory activities but, if activated inappropriately, can act as potent inducers of immunopathology. It remains to be determined whether collectins and galectins can interact with each other and whether such collaborations harness a beneficial immune response to pathogens. A more complete understanding of the host factors that control microbial colonization will lead to improved therapies for respiratory infections.

AUTHOR CONTRIBUTIONS

CC, MC-R, BG-F, and DS contributed equally to the writing of this review article. CC and DS are co-corresponding authors.

REFERENCES

1. Kopf M, Schneider C, Nobs SP. The development and function of lung-resident macrophages and dendritic cells. *Nat Immunol.* (2015) 16:36–44. doi: 10.1038/ni.3052
2. Marsland BJ, Gollwitzer ES. Host-microorganism interactions in lung diseases. *Nat Rev Immunol.* (2014) 14:827–35. doi: 10.1038/nri3769
3. Whitsett JA, Alenghat T. Respiratory epithelial cells orchestrate pulmonary innate immunity. *Nat Immunol.* (2015) 16:27–35. doi: 10.1038/ni.3045
4. Chiu C. Openshaw PJ. Antiviral B cell and T cell immunity in the lungs. *Nat Immunol.* (2015) 16:18–26. doi: 10.1038/ni.3056
5. Zhang P, Summer WR, Bagby GJ, Nelson S. Innate immunity and pulmonary host defense. *Immunol Rev.* (2000) 173:39–51. doi: 10.1034/j.1600-065X.2000.917306.x
6. Iwasaki A, Foxman EF, Molony RD. Early local immune defences in the respiratory tract. *Nat Rev Immunol.* (2017) 17:7–20. doi: 10.1038/nri.2016.117
7. Wright JR. Immunoregulatory functions of surfactant proteins. *Nat Rev Immunol.* (2005) 5:58–68. doi: 10.1038/nri1528
8. Ordonez SR, Veldhuizen EJA, van Eijk M, Haagsman HP. Role of soluble innate effector molecules in pulmonary defense against fungal pathogens. *Front Microbiol.* (2017) 8:2098. doi: 10.3389/fmicb.2017.02098
9. Kim JK, Kim SS, Rha KW, Kim CH, Cho JH, Lee CH, et al. Expression and localization of surfactant proteins in human nasal epithelium. *Am J Physiol Lung Cell Mol Physiol.* (2007) 292:L879–84. doi: 10.1152/ajplung.00156.2006
10. Popa SJ, Stewart SE, Moreau K. Unconventional secretion of annexins and galectins. *Semin Cell Dev Biol.* (2018). doi: 10.1016/j.semcdb.2018.02.022. [Epub ahead of print].
11. Ujma S, Horsnell WG, Katz AA, Clark HW, Schäfer G. Non-pulmonary immune functions of surfactant proteins A and D. *J Innate Immun.* (2017) 9:3–11. doi: 10.1159/000451026
12. Hansen SW, Ohtani K, Roy N, Wakamiya N. The collectins CL-L1, CL-K1 and CL-P1, and their roles in complement and innate immunity. *Immunobiology* (2016) 221:1058–67. doi: 10.1016/j.imbio.2016.05.012
13. Howard M, Farrar CA, Sacks SH. Structural and functional diversity of collectins and ficolins and their relationship to disease. *Semin Immunopathol.* (2018) 40:75–85. doi: 10.1007/s00281-017-0642-0
14. Minutti CM, Jackson-Jones LH, García-Fojeda B, Knipper JA, Sutherland TE, Logan N, et al. Local amplifiers of IL-4Rα-mediated macrophage activation promote repair in lung and liver. *Science* (2017) 356:1076–80. doi: 10.1126/science.aaj2067
15. García-Verdugo I, Sánchez-Barbero F, Bosch FU, Steinhilber W, Casals C. Effect of hydroxylation, oligomerization, and N187-linked glycosylation on structural and biochemical properties of recombinant human SP-A1. *Biochemistry* (2003) 42:9532–42. doi: 10.1021/bi0347196

16. Sanchez-Barbero F, Rivas G, Steinhilber W, Casals C. Structural and functional differences among human surfactant proteins SP-A1, SP-A2, and coexpressed SP-A1/SP-A2. Role of supratrimeric oligomerization. *Biochem J.* (2007) 406:479–89. doi: 10.1042/BJ20070275
17. Yamada C, Sano H, Shimizu T, Mitsuzawa H, Nishitani C, Himi T, et al. Surfactant protein A directly interacts with TLR4 and MD-2 and regulates inflammatory cellular response. Importance of supratrimeric oligomerization. *J Biol Chem.* (2006) 281:21771–80. doi: 10.1074/jbc.M513041200
18. Palaniyar N, Nadesalingam J, Clark H, Shih MJ, Dodds AW, Reid KB. Nucleic acid is a novel ligand for innate, immune pattern recognition collectins surfactant proteins A and D and mannose-binding lectin. *J Biol Chem.* (2004) 279:32728–36. doi: 10.1074/jbc.M403763200
19. Casals C. Role of surfactant protein A (SP-A)/lipid interactions for SP-A functions in the lung. *Pediatr Pathol Mol Med.* (2001) 20:249–68. doi: 10.1080/15513810109168821
20. Rynkiewicz MJ, Wu H, Cafarella TR, Nikolaidis NM, Head JF, Seaton BA, et al. Differential ligand binding specificities of the pulmonary collectins are determined by the conformational freedom of a surface loop. *Biochemistry* (2017) 56:4095–105. doi: 10.1021/acs.biochem.6b01313
21. Erpenbeck VJ, Malherbe DC, Sommer S, Schmiedl A, Steinhilber W, Ghio AJ, et al. Surfactant protein D increases phagocytosis and aggregation of pollen-allergen starch granules. *Am J Physiol Lung Cell Mol Physiol.* (2005) 288:L692–8. doi: 10.1152/ajplung.00362.2004
22. Ruge CA, Kirch J, Ca-adas O, Schneider M, Perez-Gil J, Schaefer UF, et al. Uptake of nanoparticles by alveolar macrophages is triggered by surfactant protein A. *Nanomedicine* (2011) 7:690–3. doi: 10.1016/j.nano.2011.07.009
23. Lopez-Sanchez A, Sáenz A, Casals C. Surfactant protein A (SP-A)-tacrolimus complexes have a greater anti-inflammatory effect than either SP-A or tacrolimus alone on human macrophages-like U937 cells. *Eur J Pharm Biopharm.* (2011) 77:384–91. doi: 10.1016/j.ejpb.2010.12.013
24. Vandivier RW, Ogden CA, Fadok VA, Hoffmann PR, Brown KK, Botto M, et al. Role of surfactant proteins A, D, and C1q in the clearance of apoptotic cells *in vivo* and *in vitro*: calreticulin and CD91 as a common collectin receptor complex. *J Immunol.* (2002) 169:3978–86. doi: 10.4049/jimmunol.169.7.3978
25. Grabiec AM, Hussell T. The role of airway macrophages in apoptotic cell clearance following acute and chronic lung inflammation. *Semin Immunopathol.* (2016) 38:409–23. doi: 10.1007/s00281-016-0555-3
26. Tenner AJ. Membrane receptors for soluble defense collagens. *Curr Opin Immunol.* (1999) 11:34–41. doi: 10.1016/S0952-7915(99)80007-7
27. Orgeig S, Hiemstra PS, Veldhuizen EJ, Casals C, Clark HW, Haczku A, et al. Recent advances in alveolar biology: evolution and function of alveolar proteins. *Respir Physiol Neurobiol.* (2010) 173:S43–54. doi: 10.1016/j.resp.2010.04.023
28. Bohlson SS, O'Conner SD, Hulsebus HJ, Ho MM, Fraser DA. Complement, C1q, and C1q-related molecules regulate macrophage polarization. *Front Immunol.* (2014) 5:402–30. doi: 10.3389/fimmu.2014.00402
29. Nathan N, Taytard J, Duquesnoy P, Thouvenin G, Corvol H, Amselem S, et al. Surfactant protein A: a key player in lung homeostasis. *Int J Biochem Cell Biol.* (2016) 81:151–5. doi: 10.1016/j.biocel.2016.11.003
30. Sorensen GL. Surfactant protein D in respiratory and non-respiratory diseases. *Front Med.* (2018) 5:18. doi: 10.3389/fmed.2018.00018
31. Nayak A, Dodagatta-Marri E, Tsolaki AG, Kishore U. An insight into the diverse roles of surfactant proteins, SP-A and SP-D in innate and adaptive immunity. *Front Immunol.* (2012) 3:131. doi: 10.3389/fimmu.2012.00131
32. Thawer S, Auret J, Schnoeller C, Chetty A, Smith K, Darby M, et al. Surfactant protein-D is essential for immunity to helminth infection. *PLoS Pathog.* (2016) 12:e1005461. doi: 10.1371/journal.ppat.1005461
33. LeVine AM, Whitsett JA. Pulmonary collectins and innate host defense of the lung. *Microbes Infect.* (2001) 3:161–6. doi: 10.1016/S1286-4579(00)01363-0
34. Coya JM, Akinbi HT, Sáenz A, Yang L, Weaver TE, Casals C. Natural anti-infective pulmonary proteins: *in vivo* cooperative action of surfactant protein SP-A and the lung antimicrobial peptide SP-BN. *J Immunol.* (2015) 195:1628–36. doi: 10.4049/jimmunol.1500778
35. Douda DN, Jackson R, Grasemann H, Palaniyar N. Innate immune collectin surfactant protein D simultaneously binds both neutrophil extracellular traps and carbohydrate ligands and promotes bacterial trapping. *J Immunol.* (2011) 187:1856–65. doi: 10.4049/jimmunol.1004201
36. Tenner AJ, Robinson SL, Borchelt J, Wright JR. Human pulmonary surfactant protein (SP-A), a protein structurally homologous to C1q, can enhance FcR- and CR1-mediated phagocytosis. *J Biol Chem.* (1989) 64:13923–8.
37. Gil M, McCormack FX, Levine AM. Surfactant protein A modulates cell surface expression of CR3 on alveolar macrophages and enhances CR3-mediated phagocytosis. *J Biol Chem.* (2009) 284:7495–504. doi: 10.1074/jbc.M808643200
38. Beharka AA, Crowther JE, McCormack FX, Denning GM, Lees J, Tibesar E, et al. Pulmonary surfactant protein A activates a phosphatidylinositol 3-kinase/calcium signal transduction pathway in human macrophages: participation in the up-regulation of mannose receptor activity. *J Immunol.* (2005) 175:2227–36. doi: 10.4049/jimmunol.175.4.2227
39. Kuronuma K, Sano H, Kato K, Kudo K, Hyakushima N, Yokota S, et al. Pulmonary surfactant protein A augments the phagocytosis of *Streptococcus pneumoniae* by alveolar macrophages through a casein kinase 2-dependent increase of cell surface localization of scavenger receptor A. *J Biol Chem.* (2004) 279:21421–30. doi: 10.1074/jbc.M312490200
40. Zhang S, Chen Y, Potvin E, Sanschagrin F, Levesque RC, McCormack FX, et al. Comparative signature-tagged mutagenesis identifies Pseudomonas factors conferring resistance to the pulmonary collectin SP-A. *PLoS Pathog.* (2005) 1:259–68. doi: 10.1371/journal.ppat.0010031
41. Kuang Z, Hao Y, Hwang S, Zhang S, Kim E, Akinbi H, et al. The *Pseudomonas aeruginosa* flagellum confers resistance to pulmonary surfactant protein-A by impacting the production of exoproteases through quorum-sensing. *Mol Microbiol.* (2011) 79:1220–35. doi: 10.1111/j.1365-2958.2010.07516.x
42. Casals C, Cañadas O. Role of lipid ordered/disordered phase coexistence in pulmonary surfactant function. *Biochim Biophys Acta* (2012) 1818:2550–62. doi: 10.1016/j.bbamem.2012.05.024
43. Hussell T, Bell TJ. Alveolar macrophages: plasticity in a tissue-specific context. *Nat Rev Immunol.* (2014) 14:81–93. doi: 10.1038/nri3600
44. Gardai SJ, Xiao YQ, Dickinson M, Nick JA, Voelker DR, Greene KE, et al. By binding SIRPalpha or calreticulin/CD91, lung collectins act as dual function surveillance molecules to suppress or enhance inflammation. *Cell* (2003) 115:13–23. doi: 10.1016/S0092-8674(03)00758-X
45. Meunier I, Kaufmann E, Downey J, Divangahi M. Unravelling the networks dictating host resistance versus tolerance during pulmonary infections. *Cell Tissue Res.* (2017) 367:525–36. doi: 10.1007/s00441-017-2572-5
46. Sano H, Chiba H, Iwaki D, Sohma H, Voelker DR, Kuroki Y. Surfactant proteins A and D bind CD14 by different mechanisms. *J Biol Chem.* (2000) 275:22442–51. doi: 10.1074/jbc.M001107200
47. Kuan S, Rust K, Crouch E. Interactions of surfactant protein D with bacterial lipopolysaccharides. Surfactant protein D is an *Escherichia coli*-binding protein in bronchoalveolar lavage. *J Clin Invest.* (1992) 90:97–106. doi: 10.1172/JCI115861
48. García-Verdugo I, Sánchez-Barbero F, Soldau K, Tobias PS, Casals C. Interaction of surfactant protein A (SP-A) with bacterial rouge lipopolysaccharide (Re-LPS) and effects of SP-A on the binding of Re-LPS to CD14 and LPS binding protein. *Biochem J.* (2005) 391:115–24. doi: 10.1042/BJ20050529
49. van Rozendaal BA, van de Lest CH, van Eijk M, van Golde LM, Voorhout WF, van Helden HP, et al. Aerosolized endotoxin is immediately bound by pulmonary surfactant protein D *in vivo*. *Biochim Biophys Acta* (1999) 1454:261–9. doi: 10.1016/S0925-4439(99)00042-3
50. Nguyen HA, Rajaram MV, Meyer DA, Schlesinger LS. Pulmonary surfactant protein A and surfactant lipids upregulate IRAK-M, a negative regulator of TLR-mediated inflammation in human macrophages. *Am J Physiol Lung Cell Mol Physiol.* (2012) 303:L608–16. doi: 10.1152/ajplung.00067.2012
51. Sender V, Lang L, Stamme C. Surfactant protein-A modulates LPS-induced TLR4 localization and signaling via β-arrestin 2. *PLoS ONE* (2013) 8:e59896. doi: 10.1371/journal.pone.0059896
52. Moulakakis C, Steinhäuser C, Biedziak D, Freundt K, Reiling N, Stamme C. Surfactant protein A enhances constitutive immune functions of clathrin heavy chain and clathrin adaptor protein 2. *Am J Respir Cell Mol Biol.* (2016) 55:92–104. doi: 10.1165/rcmb.2015-0219OC

53. Henning LN, Azad AK, Parsa KV, Crowther JE, Tridandapani S, Schlesinger LS. Pulmonary surfactant protein A regulates TLR expression and activity in human macrophages. *J Immunol.* (2008) 180:7847–58. doi: 10.4049/jimmunol.180.12.7847
54. Crowther JE, Kutala VK, Kuppusamy P, Ferguson JS, Beharka AA, Zweier JL, et al. Pulmonary surfactant protein A inhibits macrophage reactive oxygen intermediate production in response to stimuli by reducing NADPH oxidase activity. *J Immunol.* (2004) 172:6866–74. doi: 10.4049/jimmunol.172.11.6866
55. Yoshida M, Korfhagen TR, Whitsett JA. Surfactant protein D regulates NF-kappaB and matrix metalloproteinase production in alveolar macrophages via oxidant-sensitive pathways. *J Immunol.* (2001) 166:7514–9. doi: 10.4049/jimmunol.166.12.7514
56. Olde Nordkamp MJ, van Eijk M, Urbanus RT, Bont L, Haagsman HP, Meyaard L. Leukocyte-associated Ig-like receptor-1 is a novel inhibitory receptor for surfactant protein D. *J Leukoc Biol.* (2014) 96:105–11. doi: 10.1189/jlb.3AB0213-092RR
57. Minutti CM, García-Fojeda B, Saenz A, De Las Casas-Engel M, Guillamat-Prats R, De Lorenzo A, et al. Surfactant protein A prevents IFN-gamma/IFN-gammaR interaction and attenuates classical activation of human alveolar macrophages. *J Immunol.* (2016) 197:590–8. doi: 10.4049/jimmunol.1501032
58. Allen JE, Sutherland TE. Host protective roles of type 2 immunity: parasite killing and tissue repair, flip sides of the same coin. *Semin Immunol.* (2014) 26:329–40. doi: 10.1016/j.smim.2014.06.003
59. Blériot C, Dupuis T, Jouvion G, Eberl G, Disson O, Lecuit M. Liver-resident macrophage necroptosis orchestrates type 1 microbicidal inflammation and type-2-mediated tissue repair during bacterial infection. *Immunity* (2015) 42:145–58. doi: 10.1016/j.immuni.2014.12.020
60. Bosurgi L, Cao YG, Cabeza-Cabrerizo M, Tucci A, Hughes LD, Kong Y, et al. Macrophage function in tissue repair and remodeling requires IL-4 or IL-13 with apoptotic cells. *Science* (2017) 356:1072–6. doi: 10.1126/science.aai8132
61. Jäkel A, Clark H, Reid KB, Sim RB. The human lung surfactant proteins A (SP-A) and D (SP-D) interact with apoptotic target cells by different binding mechanisms. *Immunobiology* (2010) 215:551–8. doi: 10.1016/j.imbio.2009.09.005
62. Jäkel A, Clark H, Reid KB, Sim RB. Surface-bound myeloperoxidase is a ligand for recognition of late apoptotic neutrophils by human lung surfactant proteins A and D. *Protein Cell* (2010) 1:563–72. doi: 10.1007/s13238-010-0076-0
63. Greenlee-Wacker MC. Clearance of apoptotic neutrophils and resolution of inflammation. *Immunol Rev.* (2016) 273:357–70. doi: 10.1111/imr.12453
64. Ledford JG, Addison KJ, Foster MW, Que LG. Eosinophil-associated lung diseases. A cry for surfactant proteins A and D help? *Am J Respir Cell Mol Biol.* (2014) 51:604–14. doi: 10.1165/rcmb.2014-0095TR
65. Johannes L, Jacob R, Leffler H. Galectins at a glance. *J Cell Sci.* (2018) 131:jcs208884. doi: 10.1242/jcs.208884
66. Dings RPM, Miller MC, Griffin RJ, Mayo KH. Galectins as molecular targets for therapeutic intervention. *Int J Mol Sci.* (2018) 19:E905. doi: 10.3390/ijms19030905
67. Liu FT, Rabinovich GA. Galectins: regulators of acute and chronic inflammation. *Ann N Y Acad Sci.* (2010) 1183:158–82. doi: 10.1111/j.1749-6632.2009.05131.x
68. Cerliani JP, Blidner AG, Toscano MA, Croci DO, Rabinovich GA. Translating the sugar code into immune and vascular signaling programs. *Trends Biochem Sci.* (2017) 42:255–73. doi: 10.1016/j.tibs.2016.11.003
69. Sato S, Ouellet N, Pelletier I, Simard M, Rancourt A, Bergeron MG. Role of galectin-3 as an adhesion molecule for neutrophil extravasation during streptococcal pneumonia. *J Immunol.* (2002) 168:1813–22. doi: 10.4049/jimmunol.168.4.1813
70. Mishra BB, Li Q, Steichen AL, Binstock BJ, Metzger DW, Teale JM, et al. Galectin-3 functions as an alarmin: pathogenic role for sepsis development in murine respiratory tularemia. *PLoS ONE* (2013) 8:e59616. doi: 10.1371/journal.pone.0059616
71. Shiratori B, Zhao J, Okumura M, Chagan-Yasutan H, Yanai H, Mizuno K, et al. Immunological roles of elevated plasma levels of matricellular proteins in Japanese patients with pulmonary tuberculosis. *Int J Mol Sci.* (2016) 18:E19. doi: 10.3390/ijms18010019
72. Chavez-Galan L, Ramon-Luing L, Carranza C, Garcia I, Sada-Ovalle I. Lipoarabinomannan decreases galectin-9 expression and tumor necrosis factor pathway in macrophages favoring *Mycobacterium tuberculosis* intracellular growth. *Front Immunol.* (2017) 8:1659. doi: 10.3389/fimmu.2017.01659
73. Yang ML, Chen YH, Wang SW, Huang YJ, Leu CH, Yeh NC, et al. Galectin-1 binds to influenza virus and ameliorates influenza virus pathogenesis. *J Virol.* (2011) 85:10010–20. doi: 10.1128/JVI.00301-11
74. Fang S, Zhang K, Wang T, Wang X, Lu X, Peng B, et al. Primary study on the lesions and specific proteins in BEAS-2B cells induced with the 2009 A (H1N1) influenza virus. *Appl Microbiol Biotechnol.* (2014) 98:9691–701. doi: 10.1007/s00253-014-5852-y
75. Chen Y, Zhou J, Cheng Z, Yang S, Chu H, Fan Y, et al. Functional variants regulating LGALS1 (Galectin 1) expression affect human susceptibility to influenza A(H7N9). *Sci Rep.* (2015) 5:8517. doi: 10.1038/srep08517
76. Almeida F, Wolf JM, da Silva TA, DeLeon-Rodriguez CM, Rezende CP, Pessoni AM, et al. Galectin-3 impacts *Cryptococcus neoformans* infection through direct antifungal effects. *Nat Commun.* (2017) 8:1968. doi: 10.1038/s41467-017-02126-7
77. Dembele BP, Chagan-Yasutan H, Niki T, Ashino Y, Tangpukdee N, Shinichi E, et al. Plasma levels of Galectin-9 reflect disease severity in malaria infection. *Malar J.* (2016) 15:403. doi: 10.1186/s12936-016-1471-7
78. Liu J, Huang S, Su XZ, Song J, Lu F. Blockage of Galectin-receptor interactions by alpha-lactose exacerbates plasmodium berghei-induced pulmonary immunopathology. *Sci Rep.* (2016) 6:32024. doi: 10.1038/srep32024
79. Barboni E, Coade S, Fiori A. The binding of mycolic acids to galectin-3: a novel interaction between a host soluble lectin and trafficking mycobacterial lipids? *FEBS Lett.* (2005) 579:6749–55. doi: 10.1016/j.febslet.2005.11.005
80. Mey A, Leffler H, Hmama Z, Normier G, Revillard JP. The animal lectin galectin-3 interacts with bacterial lipopolysaccharides via two independent sites. *J Immunol.* (1996) 156:1572–7.
81. Gupta SK, Masinick S, Garrett M, Hazlett LD. *Pseudomonas aeruginosa* lipopolysaccharide binds galectin-3 and other human corneal epithelial proteins. *Infect Immun.* (1997) 65:2747–53.
82. Stowell SR, Arthur CM, McBride R, Berger O, Razi N, Heimburg-Molinaro J, et al. Microbial glycan microarrays define key features of host-microbial interactions. *Nat Chem Biol.* (2014) 10:470–6. doi: 10.1038/nchembio.1525
83. Kalograiaki I, Euba B, Proverbio D, Campanero-Rhodes MA, Aastrup T, Garmendia J, et al. Combined bacteria microarray and quartz crystal microbalance approach for exploring glycosignatures of nontypeable *Haemophilus influenzae* and recognition by host lectins. *Anal Chem.* (2016) 88:5950–7. doi: 10.1021/acs.analchem.6b00905
84. Levroney EL, Aguilar HC, Fulcher JA, Kohatsu L, Pace KE, Pang M, et al. Novel innate immune functions for galectin-1: galectin-1 inhibits cell fusion by *Nipah virus* envelope glycoproteins and augments dendritic cell secretion of proinflammatory cytokines. *J Immunol.* (2005) 175:413–20. doi: 10.4049/jimmunol.175.1.413
85. Garner OB, Aguilar HC, Fulcher JA, Levroney EL, Harrison R, Wright L, et al. Endothelial galectin-1 binds to specific glycans on *Nipah virus* fusion protein and inhibits maturation, mobility, and function to block syncytia formation. *PLoS Pathog.* (2010) 6:e1000993. doi: 10.1371/journal.ppat.1000993
86. Garner OB, Yun T, Pernet O, Aguilar HC, Park A, Bowden TA, et al. Timing of galectin-1 exposure differentially modulates *Nipah virus* entry and syncytium formation in endothelial cells. *J Virol.* (2015) 89:2520–9. doi: 10.1128/JVI.02435-14
87. Nita-Lazar M, Banerjee A, Feng C, Amin MN, Frieman MB, Chen WH, et al. Desialylation of airway epithelial cells during influenza virus infection enhances pneumococcal adhesion via galectin binding. *Mol Immunol.* (2015) 65:1–16. doi: 10.1016/j.molimm.2014.12.010
88. Nieminen J, St-Pierre C, Bhaumik P, Poirier F, Sato S. Role of galectin-3 in leukocyte recruitment in a murine model of lung infection by *Streptococcus pneumoniae*. *J Immunol.* (2008) 180:2466–73. doi: 10.4049/jimmunol.180.4.2466
89. Farnworth SL, Henderson NC, Mackinnon AC, Atkinson KM, Wilkinson T, Dhaliwal K, et al. Galectin-3 reduces the severity of pneumococcal pneumonia by augmenting neutrophil function. *Am J Pathol.* (2008) 172:395–405. doi: 10.2353/ajpath.2008.070870

90. Elmwall J, Kwiecinski J, Na M, Ali AA, Osla V, Shaw LN, et al. Galectin-3 is a target for proteases involved in the virulence of *Staphylococcus aureus. Infect Immun.* (2017) 85:e00177–17. doi: 10.1128/IAI.00177-17
91. Ferraz LC, Bernardes ES, Oliveira AF, Ruas LP, Fermino ML, Soares SG, et al. Lack of galectin-3 alters the balance of innate immune cytokines and confers resistance to *Rhodococcus equi* infection. *Eur J Immunol.* (2008) 38:2762–75. doi: 10.1002/eji.200737986
92. Steichen AL, Simonson TJ, Salmon SL, Metzger DW, Mishra BB, Sharma J. Alarmin function of galectin-9 in murine respiratory tularemia. *PLoS ONE* (2015) 10:e0123573. doi: 10.1371/journal.pone.0123573
93. Vega-Carrascal I, Bergin DA, McElvaney OJ, McCarthy C, Banville N, Pohl K, et al. Galectin-9 signaling through TIM-3 is involved in neutrophil-mediated Gram-negative bacterial killing: an effect abrogated within the cystic fibrosis lung. *J Immunol.* (2014) 192:2418–31. doi: 10.4049/jimmunol.1300711
94. Jayaraman P, Sada-Ovalle I, Beladi S, Anderson AC, Dardalhon V, Hotta C, et al. Tim3 binding to galectin-9 stimulates antimicrobial immunity. *J Exp Med.* (2010) 207:2343–54. doi: 10.1084/jem.20100687
95. Sada-Ovalle I, Chavez-Galan L, Torre-Bouscoulet L, Nava-Gamino L, Barrera L, Jayaraman P, et al. The Tim3-galectin 9 pathway induces antibacterial activity in human macrophages infected with *Mycobacterium tuberculosis. J Immunol.* (2012) 189:5896–902. doi: 10.4049/jimmunol.1200990
96. Jayaraman P, Sada-Ovalle I, Nishimura T, Anderson AC, Kuchroo VK, Remold HG, et al. IL-1beta promotes antimicrobial immunity in macrophages by regulating TNFR signaling and caspase-3 activation. *J Immunol.* (2013) 190:4196–204. doi: 10.4049/jimmunol.1202688
97. Wang F, Xu J, Liao Y, Wang Y, Liu C, Zhu X, et al. Tim-3 ligand galectin-9 reduces IL-17 level and accelerates *Klebsiella pneumoniae* infection. *Cell Immunol.* (2011) 269:22–8. doi: 10.1016/j.cellimm.2011.03.005
98. Sharma S, Sundararajan A, Suryawanshi A, Kumar N, Veiga-Parga T, Kuchroo VK, et al. T cell immunoglobulin and mucin protein-3 (Tim-3)/Galectin-9 interaction regulates influenza A virus-specific humoral and CD8 T-cell responses. *Proc Natl Acad Sci USA.* (2011) 108:19001–6. doi: 10.1073/pnas.1107087108
99. Lu X, McCoy KS, Xu J, Hu W, Chen H, Jiang K, et al. Galectin-9 ameliorates respiratory syncytial virus-induced pulmonary immunopathology through regulating the balance between Th17 and regulatory T cells. *Virus Res.* (2015) 195:162–71. doi: 10.1016/j.virusres.2014.10.011
100. Shim JA, Park S, Lee ES, Niki T, Hirashima M, Sohn S. Galectin-9 ameliorates herpes simplex virus-induced inflammation through apoptosis. *Immunobiology* (2012) 217:657–66. doi: 10.1016/j.imbio.2011.11.002
101. Sehrawat S, Reddy PB, Rajasagi N, Suryawanshi A, Hirashima M, Rouse BT. Galectin-9/TIM-3 interaction regulates virus-specific primary and memory CD8 T cell response. *PLoS Pathog.* (2010) 6:e1000882. doi: 10.1371/journal.ppat.1000882
102. Rodrigues LC, Secatto A, Sorgi CA, Dejani NN, Medeiros AI, Prado MK, et al. Protective Effect of galectin-1 during *Histoplasma capsulatum* infection is associated with prostaglandin E2 and nitric oxide modulation. *Mediators Inflamm.* (2016) 2016:5813794. doi: 10.1155/2016/5813794
103. Wu SY, Yu JS, Liu FT, Miaw SC, Wu-Hsieh BA. Galectin-3 negatively regulates dendritic cell production of IL-23/IL-17-axis cytokines in infection by *Histoplasma capsulatum. J Immunol.* (2013) 190:3427–37. doi: 10.4049/jimmunol.1202122
104. Ruas LP, Bernardes ES, Fermino ML, de Oliveira LL, Hsu DK, Liu FT, et al. Lack of galectin-3 drives response to *Paracoccidioides brasiliensis* toward a Th2-biased immunity. *PLoS ONE* (2009) 4:e4519. doi: 10.1371/journal.pone.0004519
105. Paz I, Sachse M, Dupont N, Mounier J, Cederfur C, Enninga J, et al. Galectin-3, a marker for vacuole lysis by invasive pathogens. *Cell Microbiol.* (2010) 12:530–44. doi: 10.1111/j.1462-5822.2009.01415.x
106. Thurston TL, Wandel MP, von Muhlinen N, Foeglein A, Randow F. Galectin 8 targets damaged vesicles for autophagy to defend cells against bacterial invasion. *Nature* (2012) 482:414–8. doi: 10.1038/nature10744
107. Cheng YL, Wu YW, Kuo CF, Lu SL, Liu FT, Anderson R, et al. Galectin-3 inhibits galectin-8/parkin-mediated ubiquitination of group A *Streptococcus. MBio* (2017) 8:e00899-17. doi: 10.1128/mBio.00899-17
108. Staring J, von Castelmur E, Blomen VA, van den Hengel LG, Brockmann M, Baggen J, et al. PLA2G16 represents a switch between entry and clearance of *Picornaviridae. Nature* (2017) 541:412–6. doi: 10.1038/nature21032
109. Montespan C, Marvin SA, Austin S, Burrage AM, Roger B, Rayne F, et al. Multi-layered control of Galectin-8 mediated autophagy during adenovirus cell entry through a conserved PPxY motif in the viral capsid. *PLoS Pathog.* (2017) 13:e1006217. doi: 10.1371/journal.ppat.1006217
110. Mansilla Pareja ME, Bongiovanni A, Lafont F, Colombo MI. Alterations of the *Coxiella burnetii* replicative vacuole membrane integrity and interplay with the autophagy pathway. *Front Cell Infect Microbiol.* (2017) 7:112. doi: 10.3389/fcimb.2017.00112
111. Truchan HK, Christman HD, White RC, Rutledge NS, Cianciotto NP. Type II secretion substrates of *Legionella pneumophila* translocate out of the pathogen-occupied vacuole via a semipermeable membrane. *MBio* (2017) 8:e00870-17. doi: 10.1128/mBio.00870-17
112. Feeley EM, Pilla-Moffett DM, Zwack EE, Piro AS, Finethy R, Kolb JP, et al. Galectin-3 directs antimicrobial guanylate binding proteins to vacuoles furnished with bacterial secretion systems. *Proc Natl Acad Sci USA.* (2017) 114:E1698–706. doi: 10.1073/pnas.1615771114
113. Chauhan S, Kumar S, Jain A, Ponpuak M, Mudd MH, Kimura T, et al. TRIMs and galectins globally cooperate and TRIM16 and galectin-3 co-direct autophagy in endomembrane damage homeostasis. *Dev Cell* (2016) 39:13–27. doi: 10.1016/j.devcel.2016.08.003
114. Kumar S, Chauhan S, Jain A, Ponpuak M, Choi SW, Mudd M, et al. Galectins and TRIMs directly interact and orchestrate autophagic response to endomembrane damage. *Autophagy* (2017) 13:1086–7. doi: 10.1080/15548627.2017.1307487

15

Combination of Antibodies and Antibiotics as a Promising Strategy Against Multidrug-Resistant Pathogens of the Respiratory Tract

Mirian Domenech[1,2], Julio Sempere[1,2], Sara de Miguel[1,2] and Jose Yuste[1,2]*

[1] Centro Nacional de Microbiología, Instituto de Salud Carlos III, Madrid, Spain, [2] Centro de Investigación Biomédica en Red de Enfermedades Respiratorias, Madrid, Spain

***Correspondence:**
Jose Yuste
jyuste@isciii.es

The emergence of clinical isolates associated to multidrug resistance is a serious threat worldwide in terms of public health since complicates the success of the antibiotic treatment and the resolution of the infectious process. This is of great concern in pathogens affecting the lower respiratory tract as these infections are one of the major causes of mortality in children and adults. In most cases where the respiratory pathogen is associated to multidrug-resistance, antimicrobial concentrations both in serum and at the site of infection may be insufficient and the resolution of the infection depends on the interaction of the invading pathogen with the host immune response. The outcome of these infections largely depends on the susceptibility of the pathogen to the antibiotic treatment, although the humoral and cellular immune responses also play an important role in this process. Hence, prophylactic measures or even immunotherapy are alternatives against these multi-resistant pathogens. In this sense, specific antibodies and antibiotics may act concomitantly against the respiratory pathogen. Alteration of cell surface structures by antimicrobial drugs even at sub-inhibitory concentrations might result in greater exposure of microbial ligands that are normally hidden or hardly exposed. This alteration of the bacterial envelope may stimulate opsonization by natural and/or specific antibodies or even by host defense components, increasing the recognition of the microbial pathogen by circulating phagocytes. In this review we will explain the most relevant studies, where vaccination or the use of monoclonal antibodies in combination with antimicrobial treatment has demonstrated to be an alternative strategy to overcome the impact of multidrug resistance in respiratory pathogens.

Keywords: antibodies, antibiotics, resistance, respiratory infections, immune response

INTRODUCTION

One third of the annual deaths occurring in the world are estimated to be due to infectious diseases and notably, infections affecting the respiratory tract are responsible of 4 million deaths worldwide (1). According to estimates of the World Health Organization, pneumonia kills more children worldwide than any other disease, even more than acquired immune deficiency syndrome (AIDS), malaria and measles combined (2–4). In adults, the impact of community acquired pneumonia (CAP) or nosocomial pneumonia (including hospital-acquired pneumonia and ventilator-acquired pneumonia) is also very worrisome as they are associated with remarkably high morbidity and mortality rates worldwide (5). One the major causes of these pathologies is *Streptococcus pneumoniae* (pneumococcus) that has greater incidence in children under 5 years old and adults over 60 years old, although the mortality is much higher in elderly population worldwide (4, 5). Pneumococcus is indeed, the main etiologic agent of CAP, as well as, non-epidemic bacterial meningitis and acute otitis media (AOM), but is also one of the major causes of bacterial sepsis (6). Other frequent causes of CAP include *Haemophilus influenzae, Pseudomonas aeruginosa, Staphylococcus aureus,* and also other pathogens grouped as atypical bacteria (including *Mycoplasma* spp, *Chlamydia* spp, and *Legionella* spp) (7).

The search of effective treatments to fight against infectious diseases has been, since many years, among the main challenges of medicine. Before the discovery of antibiotics, there were very few choices against bacterial infections. In the last decade of XX century, therapies based in antibodies to treat these infections were commonly used (8) and, in the 20's of last century, serum therapy was used against many bacterial diseases including infections affecting the respiratory tract, such as those caused by *S. pneumoniae* (9). These treatments reduced in a 50%, the mortality caused by this pathogen (10). However, when antibiotic chemotherapy emerged in the 30's decade of last century, serum therapy was abandoned and it was substituted by antibiotic treatment due to its higher effectivity and lower toxicity. Interestingly, the appearance of resistant strains appeared promptly after the general use of antibiotics. Resistance to several antibiotics is a common phenotype in the majority of these pathogens including multidrug resistant (MDR) strains of pneumococcus. In some cases, such as extended spectrum β-lactamase producing enterobacteriaceae and methicillin-resistant *S. aureus* (MRSA) dissemination of resistance has become a serious threat worldwide (7). In the last years, the use of monoclonal antibodies has been proposed as an alternative for the treatment of MDR pathogens, due to their marked specificity against the bacterial pathogen, their limited possibility of creating resistance and their ability to act synergistically with antibiotics (11). A different approach to reduce the burden of disease caused by MDR pathogens and also limit the dissemination of resistance genes is based in the implementation of effective vaccines with high coverage rates among the pediatric and adult population (12, 13).

IMPACT OF VACCINATION AGAINST ANTIBIOTIC RESISTANCE IN RESPIRATORY PATHOGENS

To control antibiotic resistance, vaccines have been proposed as promising intervention measures to control the spread and dissemination of MDR strains. Indeed, existing vaccines against important pathogens, such as *S. pneumoniae* or *H. influenzae* type b may contribute to reduce the burden of antimicrobial resistance (14–17). One of the best examples is the reduction of MDR serotypes after the introduction of pneumococcal conjugate vaccines. Hence, preventive and therapeutic measures against infection produced by *S. pneumoniae* have modified the resistance pattern of this pathogen. PCV7 and later PCV10 and PCV13, are pneumococcal vaccines containing the capsular polysaccharides of the main serotypes causing invasive pneumococcal disease (IPD) protecting against the most common serotypes that are resistant to antibiotics. These vaccines were commercialized at the beginning of this century to promote immunization against pediatric population, although PCV13 is also indicated for adults. The general use of these vaccines induced a drastic decrease of the incidence of IPD caused by serotypes included in the vaccines and also reduced the prevalence of non-susceptible serotypes to antibiotics (18–20). As a consequence, PCV7 and later PCV13 have had a clear impact in the epidemiology of clinical isolates obtained from adults, who have been indirectly beneficiated from pediatric vaccination (18–22). Another example is vaccination against *H. influenzae* type b that has reduced the overall morbidity and mortality by this microorganism showing an impact on antibiotic resistance by declining ampicillin resistant strains (23). Additional evidence is the influenza virus vaccine and how can diminish the impact of antibiotic resistance in bacterial pathogens affecting the respiratory tract. Although, the best studied interaction of influenza virus with a bacterial specimen is with *S. pneumoniae* (24–26), there are many studies demonstrating possible associations between influenza and other respiratory bacterial pathogens, such as *S. aureus, H. influenzae, Streptococcus pyogenes,* and *Neisseria meningitidis* (27–29). Preventing infection by influenza virus due to vaccine strategies, may decrease the subsequent infection by some of the bacterial pathogens mentioned above, which in some cases may harbor high levels of antibiotic resistance.

IMMUNOMODULATORY EFFECTS OF ANTIBIOTICS

The emergence of strains with high levels of antibiotic resistance might jeopardize the success of the antibiotic therapy (30). Antibiotics play their role against bacteria in a more complex mechanism when they exert its activity *in vivo* in comparison to the *in vitro* conditions due to the presence of serum proteins and components of the host immune response (31). Immunomodulation mediated by antimicrobial drugs can be explained as an induction of immunity to pathogens triggered by the chemotherapy compound. In this sense, immunoglobulins and complement components can improve the activity of β-lactam antibiotics (32, 33) whereas the presence of albumin and globulins limit free-drug plasma concentrations affecting the expected antibacterial *in vitro* effect (34–38). This effect is only relevant if the binding to plasma proteins is high (more common in cephalosporins than in penicillins) (37, 38). However, other authors using a pharmacodynamic simulation at physiological conditions including binding proteins levels similar to those found in humans, demonstrated that the presence of binding proteins did not impair the anti-pneumococcal activity of cefditoren (CDN), which is a high binding protein cephalosporin (39). β-lactam antibiotics display its antibacterial activity by a direct action against the microorganism. However,

IPD is associated to high levels of morbidity and mortality despite an appropriate antibiotic therapy (40). The lack of antibiotic efficacy is very common being especially evident in immunocompromised patients, suggesting that the recovery of these patients depends on the joint action of antibiotics and the host defense mechanisms.

Alteration of bacterial surface structures caused by certain antibiotics might contribute to a major exposition of antigenic epitopes that are deeply or hardly exposed. This greater exposure might promote the opsonization by different components of the host immune response, such as acute phase proteins, enhancing the recognition of the respiratory pathogens by professional phagocytes. Pentraxins, such as C-reactive protein (CRP) and serum amyloid P component (SAP) are the main acute phase proteins in human and mice, respectively (41). CRP levels increase during different respiratory infections, demonstrating the importance of this protein as a sentinel molecule (42). One of the most important functions by CRP and SAP in host defense against invading pathogens is the opsonization of microorganisms and later the activation of the phagocytosis process by Fcγ receptors (41, 43–45). In this sense, it has been demonstrated that the recognition by CRP and SAP of different clinical isolates of *S. pneumoniae* is enhanced when the bacteria is opsonized with serum containing sub-inhibitory concentrations of β-lactams, suggesting that these antibiotics allow these pentraxins to recognize *S. pneumoniae* in a more efficient manner increasing the phagocytosis (32, 33). A different acute phase protein termed pentraxin 3 also has demonstrated to be very effective in combination with antimycotic drugs against infections produced by *Aspergillus fumigatus*, stimulating the antifungal activity of phagocytes (46). Moreover, the use of cephalosporins has been associated to an increased in the serum bactericidal activity against important pathogens, such as *Escherichia coli* and *P. aeruginosa* (47, 48), whereas the treatment with erythromycin (ERY) seems to produce small rupture points (breakpoints) in the cell wall, causing the breakage of the envelope of *Legionella pneumophila* (49, 50). In addition, it has been demonstrated that the macrolide azithromycin (AZM), in concentrations lower than the minimum inhibitory concentration (MIC), destabilizes the outer membrane increasing the permeability and producing the death of *P. aeruginosa* (51).

As an alternative, antibiotics might reduce the expression of certain virulence factors involved in the inhibition of complement activation and phagocytosis. Indeed, a recent study has confirmed that certain antibiotics in sub-inhibitory concentrations modify the expression of virulent genes of *S. aureus* (52). An additional explanation for the enhanced activation of the host immune response by macrolides could be related to its mechanism of action as these antibiotics interact with the ribosomal 50s subunit inhibiting the protein biosynthesis (31). This is an important aspect in terms of pathogenesis as sub-inhibitory concentrations of macrolides inhibit the production of pneumolysin (Ply) which is an important virulence factor involved in C3 evasion (53, 54). Furthermore, certain macrolides, such as ERY, AZM, or clarithromycin, inhibit negatively the synthesis of Ply and pneumococcal surface protein A (PspA) (55–57). This is relevant from the antimicrobial and immunological perspectives because the combination of both proteins has an additive effect and is very effective inhibiting the activation of complement immunity (54). Additional evidence demonstrate that macrolides exhibit immunomodulatory effects by inhibiting neutrophil inflammation and macrophage activation, reducing the levels of Th2 cytokines which might be important for the treatment of chronic inflammatory diseases using this antibiotic (58).

Overall, antimicrobial drugs can trigger the humoral and cellular response using a broader range of mechanisms including the recognition by acute phase proteins and complement-mediated immunity, inhibition of bacterial virulence factors involved in immune evasion and reduction of the inflammatory response.

THE HOST IMMUNE RESPONSE AGAINST RESPIRATORY PATHOGENS IS BOOSTED BY THE COOPERATION OF ANTIBIOTICS AND ANTIBODIES

One of the major risks of respiratory infections is that are frequently associated to high morbidity and mortality rates despite appropriate antibiotic therapy with poor prognosis when the infective pathogen is highly resistant to the antibiotic prescribed (40). In the absence of antibiotic treatment, the outcome of the infection depends on the balance of the interaction between bacterial virulence factors and host defense mechanisms. Antibiotics normally display their antibacterial activity by a direct action against the microorganism. Clearance of respiratory pathogens from the systemic circulation depends on the opsonization by the complement system and the phagocytosis process (59, 60). In this sense, it has been observed that antibodies bound to *Cryptococcus neoformans* modify the genetic expression and the metabolism of certain genes, increasing the susceptibility of the pathogen to different antifungal drugs (61). Vaccination against respiratory pathogens including *S. pneumoniae*, induces the generation of specific antibodies that can interfere with the growth and metabolism of different microorganisms, suggesting a novel mechanism for antibodies mediated immunity (62). The damage produced on the surface of the pathogen by antimicrobial drugs might allow certain components of the cellular envelope to be more accessible and therefore, improve the recognition by complement components and specific antibodies. For example, exposure of MDR strains of *Klebsiella pneumoniae* to serum and β-lactam antibiotics increased the C3 levels on the bacterial surface (63).

Considering *S. pneumoniae*, the classical pathway of the complement system is the most important pathway for complement activation (64, 65). Activation of this pathway *in S. pneumoniae* was significantly increased in the presence of β-lactam antibiotics confirming that alterations caused by these antibiotics, even at sub-inhibitory concentrations, improve the complement mediated immunity by a mechanism that is dependent on the activation of the classical pathway (33). Once the complement cascade is activated and after numerous enzymatic reactions, the key component C3 is formed. In the presence of serum containing antibodies to pneumococcus and sub-inhibitory concentrations of β-lactam antibiotics or macrolides, C3 deposition on the surface of different MDR strains was markedly increased (33, 66). Overall, activation of the recognition by acute phase proteins and complement proteins by certain antibiotics, such as β-lactams and macrolides in the presence of specific antibodies has functional consequences increasing the phagocytosis process and the clearance of the microorganism (**Figure 1**) (32, 33, 66). Previous studies using a sepsis model of infection in mice, have demonstrated that protective doses of amoxicillin and cefotaxime were, approximately, eight times lower in the presence of antibodies than in their absence (67, 68). It is important to mention that whatsoever, the possible benefit of the synergistic effect mediated by antibodies will not be based in a reduction of the antibiotic doses. The benefit would be to obtain a higher efficacy from the therapeutic perspective after the administration of the common doses used against IPD cases produced by clinical isolates with high MIC levels (32, 33, 66, 67). Hence, vaccination reduces the magnitude of the pharmacodynamics indices (i.e., drug exposure defined from pharmacokinetic/pharmacodynamic ratio, ft > MIC, fCmax/MIC or fAUC/MIC), needed to reach a certain effect. Consequently, in the presence of antibodies, usual doses of the antibacterial agent would necessarily cover clinical isolates with higher levels of resistance (32, 67).

The early onset of antibiotic treatment is essential to prevent the spread of the bacterial pathogens through the respiratory tract and the dissemination to the systemic circulation because any delay initiating the treatment may lead to the high fatality rates associated to respiratory infections (69). This problem gets worse when the bacterial pathogens harbor high levels of antibiotic resistance. In this case, treatment with β-lactams or macrolides may suppose a new strategy to reduce the possibility of treatment failure in those individuals who have been previously vaccinated against *S. pneumoniae*. This assertion is based in the enhanced efficiency of the host immune response to clear the bacterial pathogen in the presence of specific antibodies and these antibiotics (32, 33, 66–68, 70). This cooperative effect between antibodies and antibiotics it seems to be limited to

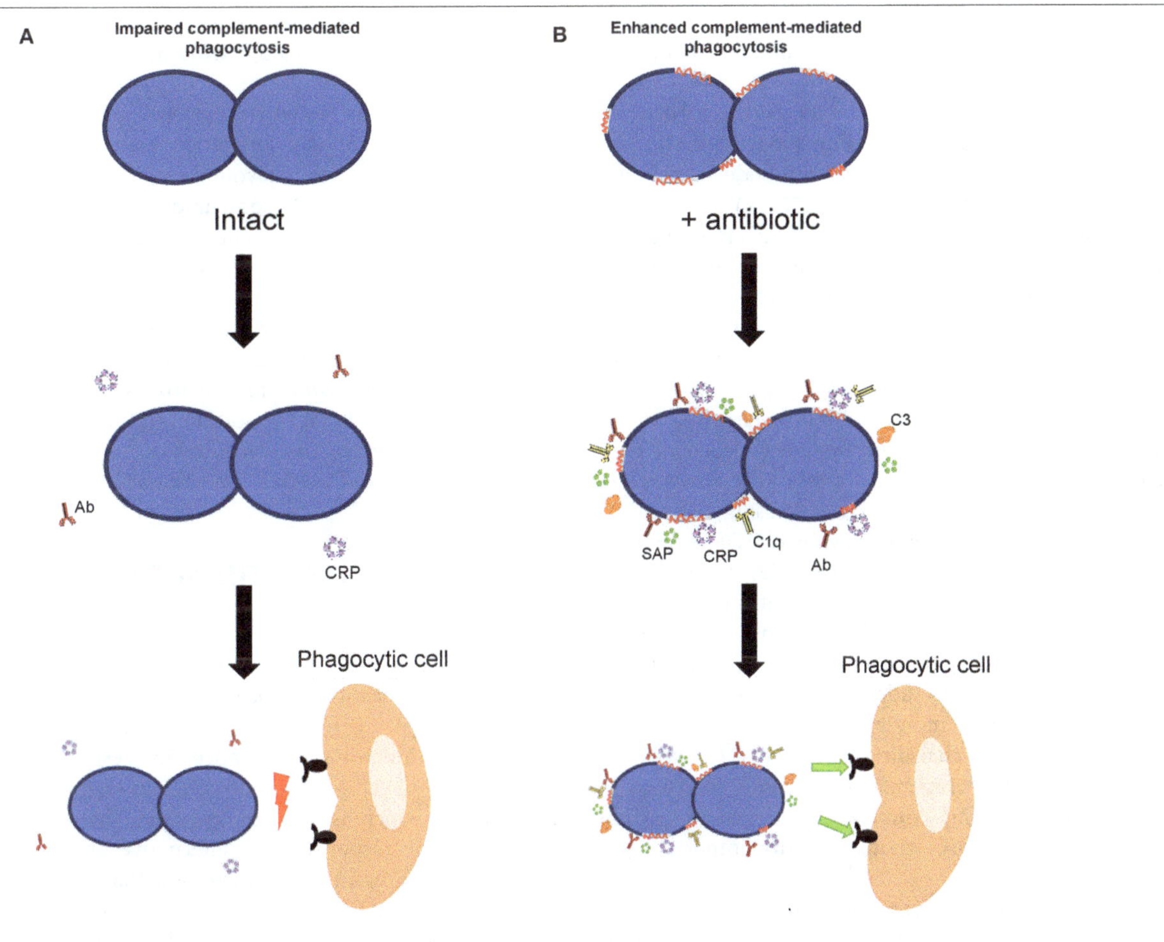

FIGURE 1 | Effect of host immune components on bacterial opsonization and phagocytosis. **(A)** Interaction of the host immune response with a bacterial pathogen in the absence of antibiotics. **(B)** Interaction of different components of the host immune response in the presence of antibiotics. In the presence of antibodies, acute phase proteins (CRP and SAP) and complement components (C1q and C3), the recognition of the bacterial pathogen is greatly enhanced when antibiotics are present (right panel).

β-lactams and macrolides because the presence of sub-inhibitory concentrations of levofloxacin and specific antibodies did not affect the opsonization by C3 against *S. pneumoniae* (66). These results explain why the treatment with sub-inhibitory concentrations of levofloxacin in mice previously immunized against *S. pneumoniae* did not increase the survival rate (71). Boosting effects on the host immune response by macrolides have been studied in other bacterial pathogens including Gram-positive and Gram-negative bacteria (31). Antimicrobial activity of macrolides is increased against resistant strains of *E. coli* and *S. aureus* when clinical isolates are exposed to sub-inhibitory concentrations of ERY and AZM in the presence of human serum. In the case of *S. pneumoniae*, exposure of resistant strains to sub-inhibitory concentrations of different macrolides increased C3 activation on the bacterial surface (66). Moreover, in the absence of the main autolytic pneumococcal enzyme, the amidase LytA, C3 deposition remained altered regardless the presence of opsonic antibodies and antibiotics demonstrating that LytA play a key role in the recognition by the complement system (66).

The rise of drug resistance to the majority of all antibiotic classes is particularly critical from the therapeutic perspective within the designated ESKAPE pathogens (*Enterococcus faecium*, *S. aureus*, *K. pneumoniae*, *A. baumannii*, *P. aeruginosa*, and *Enterobact*er spp.) (72). To fight these infections, the use of monoclonal or polyclonal antibodies has been proposed as antimicrobial alternatives against MDR strains including ESKAPE pathogens, with several antibodies being tested in different phase I-IV clinical trials (11, 73, 74). The possibility that these antibodies might confer boosting effects with antibiotics is a promising field to explore. In this sense, polyclonal antibodies to efflux pump proteins of *Stenotrophomonas maltophilia* have demonstrated additive or synergistic effects with a variety of antibiotics including cotrimoxazole, ticarcillin–clavulanate, and ciprofloxacin (75).

In *P. aeruginosa*, bispecific antibodies targeting the serotype-independent type III secretion system (injectisome) virulence factor PcrV and persistence factor Psl exopolysaccharide have shown to be very effective increasing the antimicrobial activity of different antibiotics against MDR strains (76, 77). Synergistic activity of these antibodies with ciprofloxacin, meropenem, ceftazidime, and tobramycin was observed, demonstrating enhanced effect against lung injury and prevented bacterial dissemination from the lung to the systemic circulation (76, 77). In addition, the use of panobacumab which is an IgM/κ monoclonal antibody directed against the LPS O-polysaccharide moiety of *P. aeruginosa* in combination with meropenem significantly increased bacterial clearance in the lung confirming the benefits of the joint therapy against MDR strains of this important pathogen (78).

In the case of *S. aureus*, monoclonal antibodies targeting different toxins and virulence factors have demonstrated synergistic effects in combination with several antibiotics. Therapeutic administration of a monoclonal antibody against the pore-forming toxin, alpha toxin in combination with vancomycin or linezolid resulted in improved survival against induced pneumonia by reducing inflammation and lung damage (79, 80). This combination results in a more robust immune response leading to reduced disease severity and accelerated healing relative to those with linezolid or vancomycin monotherapy. As a consequence, addition of antibodies to alpha toxin to antibiotic monotherapy may provide a benefit over antibiotics alone through its complementary mechanism of action (79, 80). Similar results were observed by other authors using monoclonal antibodies against different staphylococcal cytotoxins including alpha hemolysin and leukocidins demonstrating synergistic effects in the combination with linezolid that allowed a significant increment in survival rates (81). Among the numerous staphylococcal toxins, enterotoxin B has been classified as a class B biological warfare agent. Monoclonal antibodies to this toxin in combination with vancomycin increased survival rates and altered cytokine responses, compared with monotherapy with either monoclonal antibody or vancomycin alone (82).

Another warfare pathogen for which joint therapy using antibodies and antibiotics has been proposed is *Bacillus anthracis*. The most lethal route of exposure is via inhalation, and the disease is characterized by extensive bacteremia and toxemia which, without aggressive prophylaxis or intervention, results in a high mortality rate mainly due to anthrax exotoxin-driven pathogenesis. Monoclonal antibodies to the anthrax toxin protective antigen in combination with levofloxacin or doxycycline resulted in increased survival compared to the antibiotic alone and would provide an effective therapeutic strategy against symptomatic anthrax, even late in the course of the disease (83, 84).

Finally, a randomized, double-blind, placebo-controlled study of two neutralizing, fully human monoclonal antibodies against *Clostridium difficile* toxins A (CDA1) and B (CDB1) demonstrated that the addition of these antibodies to antibiotics metronidazole or vancomycin, significantly reduced the recurrence of *C. difficile* infection (85).

CONCLUDING REMARKS

The use of prophylactic measures including vaccination or even the use of monoclonal antibodies to treat or prevent severe infections caused by MDR pathogens is a realistic approach to fight these infections and reduce the impact of antimicrobial resistance in respiratory pathogens. The ability of certain antibiotics of showing an immunomodulatory effect which is strongly enhanced by the action of the host immune response is an alternative and promising strategy to eradicate or at least ameliorate the impact of MDR bacterial isolates in clinical practice. Further research in this field will contribute to identify and characterize novel prophylactic and therapeutic measures that in combination with current antimicrobial drugs may be effective solutions against the emergence of MDR pathogens, limiting their impact in public health.

AUTHOR CONTRIBUTIONS

MD, JS, SdM, and JY prepared the text. JS and JY produced the included figure. All authors assisted in the conception of this review, interpretation of the relevant literature and editing the manuscript. All authors gave approval of the final version submitted.

REFERENCES

1. Schluger NW, Koppaka R. Lung disease in a global context. A call for public health action. *Ann Am Thorac Soc.* (2014) 11:407–16. doi: 10.1513/AnnalsATS.201312-420PS
2. Wardlaw T, Salama P, Johansson EW, Mason E. Pneumonia: the leading killer of children. *Lancet* (2006) 368:1048–50. doi: 10.1016/S0140-6736(06)69334-3
3. O'Brien KL, Wolfson LJ, Watt JP, Henkle E, Deloria-Knoll M, McCall N, et al. Burden of disease caused by *Streptococcus pneumoniae* in children younger than 5 years: global estimates. *Lancet* (2009) 374:893–902. doi: 10.1016/S0140-6736(09)61204-6
4. Liu L, Oza S, Hogan D, Chu Y, Perin J, Zhu J, et al. Global, regional, and national causes of under-5 mortality in 2000-15: an updated systematic analysis with implications for the sustainable development goals. *Lancet* (2016) 388:3027–35. doi: 10.1016/S0140-6736(16)31593-8
5. Collaborators GBDLRI. Estimates of the global, regional, and national morbidity, mortality, and aetiologies of lower respiratory infections in 195 countries, 1990-2016: a systematic analysis for the Global Burden of Disease Study 2016. *Lancet Infect Dis.* (2018) 18: 1191–210. doi: 10.1016/S1473-3099(18)30310-4
6. Backhaus E, Berg S, Andersson R, Ockborn G, Malmstrom P, Dahl M, et al. Epidemiology of invasive pneumococcal infections: manifestations, incidence and case fatality rate correlated to age, gender and risk factors. *BMC Infect Dis.* (2016) 16:367. doi: 10.1186/s12879-016-1648-2
7. Prina E, Ranzani OT, Torres A. Community-acquired pneumonia. *Lancet* (2015) 386:1097–108. doi: 10.1016/S0140-6736(15)60733-4
8. Casadevall A. Crisis in infectious diseases: time for a new paradigm? *Clin Infect Dis.* (1996) 23:790–4.
9. Casadevall A, Scharff MD. Return to the past: the case for antibody-based therapies in infectious diseases. *Clin Infect Dis.* (1995) 21:150–61.
10. Casadevall A, Scharff MD. Serum therapy revisited: animal models of infection and development of passive antibody therapy. *Antimicrob Agents Chemother.* (1994) 38:1695–702.
11. Motley MP, Fries BC. A new take on an old remedy: generating antibodies against multidrug-resistant gram-negative bacteria in a postantibiotic world. *mSphere* (2017) 2:e00397-17. doi: 10.1128/mSphere.00397-17
12. Jansen KU, Knirsch C, Anderson AS. The role of vaccines in preventing bacterial antimicrobial resistance. *Nat Med* (2018) 24:10–9. doi: 10.1038/nm.4465
13. Esposito S, Principi N, European Society of Clinical Microbiology Infectious Diseases Vaccine Study G. Influenza vaccination and prevention of antimicrobial resistance. *Expert Rev Vaccines* (2018) 17:881–8. doi: 10.1080/14760584.2018.1525298
14. Atkins KE, Flasche S. Vaccination to reduce antimicrobial resistance. *Lancet Glob Health* (2018) 6:e252. doi: 10.1016/S2214-109X(18)30043-3
15. Atkins KE, Lafferty EI, Deeny SR, Davies NG, Robotham JV, Jit M. Use of mathematical modelling to assess the impact of vaccines on antibiotic resistance. *Lancet Infect Dis.* (2018) 18:e204–13. doi: 10.1016/S1473-3099(17)30478-4
16. Ginsburg AS, Klugman KP. Vaccination to reduce antimicrobial resistance. *Lancet Glob Health* (2017) 5:e1176–7. doi: 10.1016/S2214-109X(17)30364-9
17. Lipsitch M, Siber GR. How can vaccines contribute to solving the antimicrobial resistance problem? *mBio* (2016) 7:e00428–16. doi: 10.1128/mBio.00428-16
18. Fenoll A, Granizo JJ, Aguilar L, Giménez MJ, Aragoneses-Fenoll L, Hanquet G, et al. Temporal trends of invasive *Streptococcus pneumoniae* serotypes and antimicrobial resistance patterns in Spain from 1979 to 2007. *J Clinical Microbiol.* (2009) 47:1012–20. doi: 10.1128/JCM.01454-08
19. Pilishvili T, Lexau C, Farley MM, Hadler J, Harrison LH, Bennett NM, et al. Sustained reductions in invasive pneumococcal disease in the era of conjugate vaccine. *J Infect Dis.* (2010) 201:32–41. doi: 10.1086/648593
20. Fenoll A, Granizo JJ, Giménez MJ, Yuste J, Aguilar L. Secular trends (1990-2013) in serotypes and associated non-susceptibility of *S. pneumoniae* isolates causing invasive disease in the pre-/post-era of pneumococcal conjugate vaccines in Spanish regions without universal paediatric pneumococcal vaccination. *Vaccine* (2015) 33:5691–9. doi: 10.1016/j.vaccine.2015.08.009
21. Ladhani SN, Collins S, Djennad A, Sheppard CL, Borrow R, Fry NK, et al. Rapid increase in non-vaccine serotypes causing invasive pneumococcal disease in England and Wales, 2000-17: a prospective national observational cohort study. *Lancet Infect Dis.* (2018) 18:441–51. doi: 10.1016/S1473-3099(18)30052-5
22. Tomczyk S, Lynfield R, Schaffner W, Reingold A, Miller L, Petit S, et al. Prevention of antibiotic-nonsusceptible invasive pneumococcal disease with the 13-valent pneumococcal conjugate vaccine. *Clin Infect Dis.* (2016) 62:1119–25. doi: 10.1093/cid/ciw067
23. Giufre M, Cardines R, Caporali MG, Accogli M, D'Ancona F, Cerquetti M. Ten years of Hib vaccination in Italy: prevalence of non-encapsulated *Haemophilus influenzae* among invasive isolates and the possible impact on antibiotic resistance. *Vaccine* (2011) 29:3857–62. doi: 10.1016/j.vaccine.2011.03.059
24. Bosch AA, Biesbroek G, Trzcinski K, Sanders EA, Bogaert D. Viral and bacterial interactions in the upper respiratory tract. *PLoS Pathog.* (2013) 9:e1003057. doi: 10.1371/journal.ppat.1003057
25. Nakamura S, Davis KM, Weiser JN. Synergistic stimulation of type I interferons during influenza virus coinfection promotes *Streptococcus pneumoniae* colonization in mice. *J Clin Invest.* (2011) 121:3657–65. doi: 10.1172/JCI57762
26. Walters KA, D'Agnillo F, Sheng ZM, Kindrachuk J, Schwartzman LM, Kuestner RE, et al. 1918 pandemic influenza virus and *Streptococcus pneumoniae* co-infection results in activation of coagulation and widespread pulmonary thrombosis in mice and humans. *J Pathol.* (2016) 238:85–97. doi: 10.1002/path.4638
27. Morens DM, Taubenberger JK, Fauci AS. Predominant role of bacterial pneumonia as a cause of death in pandemic influenza: implications for pandemic influenza preparedness. *J Infect Dis.* (2008) 198:962–70. doi: 10.1086/591708
28. Rameix-Welti MA, Zarantonelli ML, Giorgini D, Ruckly C, Marasescu M, van der Werf S, et al. Influenza A virus neuraminidase enhances meningococcal adhesion to epithelial cells through interaction with sialic acid-containing meningococcal capsules. *Infect Immun.* (2009) 77:3588–95. doi: 10.1128/IAI.00155-09
29. Opatowski L, Baguelin M, Eggo RM. Influenza interaction with cocirculating pathogens and its impact on surveillance, pathogenesis, and epidemic profile: a key role for mathematical modelling. *PLoS Pathog.* (2018) 14:e1006770. doi: 10.1371/journal.ppat.1006770
30. Aguinagalde L, Corsini B, Domenech A, Domenech M, Cámara J, Ardanuy C, et al. Emergence of amoxicillin-resistant variants of Spain9V-ST156 pneumococci expressing serotype 11A correlates with their ability to evade the host immune response. *PLoS ONE* (2015) 10:e0137565. doi: 10.1371/journal.pone.0137565

31. Labro MT. Interference of antibacterial agents with phagocyte functions: immunomodulation or "immuno-fairy tales"? *Clin Microbiol Rev.* (2000) 13:615–50. doi: 10.1128/CMR.13.4.615
32. Cafini F, Yuste J, Giménez MJ, Sevillano D, Aguilar L, Alou L, et al. Enhanced *in vivo* activity of cefditoren in pre-immunized mice against penicillin-resistant *S. pneumoniae* (serotypes 6B, 19F and 23F) in a sepsis model. *PLoS ONE* (2010) 5:e12041. doi: 10.1371/journal.pone.0012041
33. Ramos-Sevillano E, Rodríguez-Sosa C, Cafini F, Giménez MJ, Navarro A, Sevillano D, et al. Cefditoren and ceftriaxone enhance complement-mediated immunity in the presence of specific antibodies against antibiotic-resistant pneumococcal strains. *PLoS ONE* (2012) 7:e44135. doi: 10.1371/journal.pone.0044135
34. Schmidt S, Rock K, Sahre M, Burkhardt O, Brunner M, Lobmeyer MT, et al. Effect of protein binding on the pharmacological activity of highly bound antibiotics. *Antimicrob Agents Chemother.* (2008) 52:3994–4000. doi: 10.1128/AAC.00427-08
35. Beer J, Wagner CC, Zeitlinger M. Protein binding of antimicrobials: methods for quantification and for investigation of its impact on bacterial killing. *AAPS J.* (2009) 11:1–12. doi: 10.1208/s12248-008-9072-1
36. Burian A, Wagner C, Stanek J, Manafi M, Bohmdorfer M, Jager W, et al. Plasma protein binding may reduce antimicrobial activity by preventing intra-bacterial uptake of antibiotics, for example clindamycin. *J Antimicrob Chemother.* (2011) 66:134–7. doi: 10.1093/jac/dkq400
37. Cafini F, Aguilar L, González N, Giménez MJ, Torrico M, Alou L, et al. *In vitro* effect of the presence of human albumin or human serum on the bactericidal activity of daptomycin against strains with the main resistance phenotypes in Gram-positives. *J Antimicrob Chemother.* (2007) 59:1185–9. doi: 10.1093/jac/dkm078
38. Sevillano D, Giménez MJ, Alou L, Aguilar L, Cafini F, Torrico M, et al. Effects of human albumin and serum on the *in vitro* bactericidal activity of cefditoren against penicillin-resistant *Streptococcus pneumoniae*. *J Antimicrob Chemother.* (2007) 60:156–8. doi: 10.1093/jac/dkm115
39. Sevillano D, Aguilar L, Alou L, Giménez MJ, González N, Torrico M, et al. High protein binding and cidal activity against penicillin-resistant *S. pneumoniae*: a cefditoren *in vitro* pharmacodynamic simulation. *PLoS ONE* (2008) 3:e2717. doi: 10.1371/journal.pone.0002717
40. Collaborators GL. Estimates of the global, regional, and national morbidity, mortality, and aetiologies of lower respiratory tract infections in 195 countries: a systematic analysis for the Global Burden of Disease Study 2015. *Lancet Infect Dis.* (2017) 17:1133–61. doi: 10.1016/S1473-3099(17)30396-1
41. Yuste J, Botto M, Bottoms SE, Brown JS. Serum amyloid P aids complement-mediated immunity to *Streptococcus pneumoniae*. *PLoS Pathog.* (2007) 3:1208–19. doi: 10.1371/journal.ppat.0030120
42. Almirall J, Bolibar I, Toran P, Pera G, Boquet X, Balanzo X, et al. Contribution of C-reactive protein to the diagnosis and assessment of severity of community-acquired pneumonia. *Chest* (2004) 125:1335–42. doi: 10.1378/chest.125.4.1335
43. Bharadwaj D, Mold C, Markham E, Du Clos TW. Serum amyloid P component binds to Fcγ receptors and opsonizes particles for phagocytosis. *J Immunol.* (2001) 166:6735–41. doi: 10.4049/jimmunol.166.11.6735
44. Mold C, Gresham HD, Du Clos TW. Serum amyloid P component and C-reactive protein mediate phagocytosis through murine Fc gamma Rs. *J Immunol.* (2001) 166:1200–5. doi: 10.4049/jimmunol.166.2.1200
45. Thomas-Rudolph D, Du Clos TW, Snapper CM, Mold C. C-reactive protein enhances immunity to *Streptococcus pneumoniae* by targeting uptake to FcγR on dendritic cells. *J Immunol.* (2007) 178:7283–91. doi: 10.4049/jimmunol.178.11.7283
46. Gaziano R, Bozza S, Bellocchio S, Perruccio K, Montagnoli C, Pitzurra L, et al. Anti-*Aspergillus fumigatus* efficacy of pentraxin 3 alone and in combination with antifungals. *Antimicrob Agents Chemother.* (2004) 48:4414–21. doi: 10.1128/AAC.48.11.4414-4421.2004
47. Darveau RP, Cunningham MD. Influence of subinhibitory concentrations of cephalosporins on the serum sensitivity of *Pseudomonas aeruginosa*. *J Infect Dis.* (1990) 162:914–21.
48. Jung E, Feldhoff RC, Walz BM, Drehs MM, Buchheit JQ, Lassiter HA. Complement component C9 enhances the capacity of beta-lactam antibiotics to kill *Escherichia coli in vitro* and *in vivo*. *Am J Med Sci* (1998) 315:307–13.
49. Verbrugh HA, Lee DA, Elliott GR, Keane WF, Hoidal JR, Peterson PK. Opsonization of *Legionella pneumophila* in human serum: key roles for specific antibodies and the classical complement pathway. *Immunology* (1985) 54:643–53.
50. Rodgers FG, Tzianabos AO, Elliott TS. The effect of antibiotics that inhibit cell-wall, protein, and DNA synthesis on the growth and morphology of *Legionella pneumophila*. *J Med Microbiol.* (1990) 31:37–44. doi: 10.1099/00222615-31-1-37
51. Imamura Y, Higashiyama Y, Tomono K, Izumikawa K, Yanagihara K, Ohno H, et al. Azithromycin exhibits bactericidal effects on *Pseudomonas aeruginosa* through interaction with the outer membrane. *Antimicrob Agents Chemother.* (2005) 49:1377–80. doi: 10.1128/AAC.49.4.1377-1380.2005
52. Subrt N, Mesak LR, Davies J. Modulation of virulence gene expression by cell wall active antibiotics in *Staphylococcus aureus*. *J Antimicrob Chemother.* (2011) 66:979–84. doi: 10.1093/jac/dkr043
53. Ramos-Sevillano E, Urzainqui A, Campuzano S, Moscoso M, González-Camacho F, Domenech M, et al. Pleiotropic effects of cell wall amidase LytA on *Streptococcus pneumoniae* sensitivity to the host immune response. *Infect Immun.* (2015) 83:591–603. doi: 10.1128/IAI.02811-14
54. Yuste J, Botto M, Paton JC, Holden DW, Brown JS. Additive inhibition of complement deposition by pneumolysin and PspA facilitates *Streptococcus pneumoniae* septicemia. *J Immunol.* (2005) 175:1813–9. doi: 10.4049/jimmunol.175.3.1813
55. Fukuda Y, Yanagihara K, Higashiyama Y, Miyazaki Y, Hirakata Y, Mukae H, et al. Effects of macrolides on pneumolysin of macrolide-resistant *Streptococcus pneumoniae*. *Eur Resp J.* (2006) 27:1020–5. doi: 10.1183/09031936.06.00116805
56. Anderson R, Steel HC, Cockeran R, von Gottberg A, de Gouveia L, Klugman KP, et al. Comparison of the effects of macrolides, amoxicillin, ceftriaxone, doxycycline, tobramycin and fluoroquinolones, on the production of pneumolysin by *Streptococcus pneumoniae in vitro*. *J Antimicrob Chemother.* (2007) 60:1155–8. doi: 10.1093/jac/dkm338
57. Yasuda Y, Kasahara K, Mizuno F, Nishi K, Mikasa K, Kita E. Roxithromycin favorably modifies the initial phase of resistance against infection with macrolide-resistant *Streptococcus pneumoniae* in a murine pneumonia model. *Antimicrob Agents Chemother.* (2007) 51:1741–52. doi: 10.1128/AAC.01459-06
58. Zimmermann P, Ziesenitz VC, Curtis N, Ritz N. The immunomodulatory effects of macrolides-A systematic review of the underlying mechanisms. *Front Immunol.* (2018) 9:302. doi: 10.3389/fimmu.2018.00302
59. Bogaert D, De Groot R, Hermans PW. *Streptococcus pneumoniae* colonisation: the key to pneumococcal disease. *Lancet Infect Dis.* (2004) 4:144–54. doi: 10.1016/S1473-3099(04)00938-7
60. van der Poll T, Opal SM. Pathogenesis, treatment, and prevention of pneumococcal pneumonia. *Lancet* (2009) 374:1543–56. doi: 10.1016/S0140-6736(09)61114-4
61. McClelland EE, Nicola AM, Prados-Rosales R, Casadevall A. Ab binding alters gene expression in *Cryptococcus neoformans* and directly modulates fungal metabolism. *J Clin Invest.* (2010) 120:1355–61. doi: 10.1172/JCI38322
62. Casadevall A, Pirofski LA. New concepts in antibody-mediated immunity. *Infect Immun.* (2004) 72:6191–6. doi: 10.1128/IAI.72.11.6191-6196.2004
63. Williams P. Sub-MICs of cefuroxime and ciprofloxacin influence interaction of complement and immunoglobulins with *Klebsiella pneumoniae*. *Antimicrob Agents Chemother.* (1987) 31:758–62.
64. Brown JS, Hussell T, Gilliland SM, Holden DW, Paton JC, Ehrenstein MR, et al. The classical pathway is the dominant complement pathway required for innate immunity to *Streptococcus pneumoniae* infection in mice. *Proc Natl Acad Sci USA.* (2002) 99:16969–74. doi: 10.1073/pnas.012669199
65. Yuste J, Sen A, Truedsson L, Jönsson G, Tay LS, Hyams C, et al. Impaired opsonization with C3b and phagocytosis of *Streptococcus pneumoniae* in sera from subjects with defects in the classical complement pathway. *Infect Immun.* (2008) 76:3761–70. doi: 10.1128/IAI.00291-08
66. Ramos-Sevillano E, Rodríguez-Sosa C, Díez-Martínez R, Giménez MJ, Olmedillas E, García P, et al. Macrolides and beta-lactam antibiotics enhance C3b deposition on the surface of multidrug-resistant *Streptococcus pneumoniae* strains by a LytA autolysin-dependent mechanism. *Antimicrob Agents Chemother.* (2012) 56:5534–40. doi: 10.1128/AAC.01470-12

67. Casal J, Aguilar L, Jado I, Yuste J, Giménez MJ, Prieto J, et al. Effects of specific antibodies against *Streptococcus pneumoniae* on pharmacodynamic parameters of beta-lactams in a mouse sepsis model. *Antimicrob Agents Chemother.* (2002) 46:1340–4. doi: 10.1128/AAC.46.5.1340-1344.2002
68. Yuste J, Fenoll A, Casal J, Giménez MJ, Aguilar L. Combined effect of specific antibodies (as serotherapy or preimmunization) and amoxicillin doses in treatment of *Streptococcus pneumoniae* sepsis in a mouse model. *Antimicrob Agents Chemother.* (2002) 46:4043–4. doi: 10.1128/AAC.46.12.4043-4044.2002
69. Woodhead M, Blasi F, Ewig S, Garau J, Huchon G, Ieven M, et al. Guidelines for the management of adult lower respiratory tract infections–full version. *Clin Microbiol Infect.* (2011) 17(Suppl. 6):E1–59. doi: 10.1111/j.1469-0691.2011.03672.x
70. Yuste J, Giménez MJ, Jado I, Fenoll A, Aguilar L, Casal J. Enhanced decrease of blood colony counts by specific anti-pneumococcal antibodies in the presence of sub-inhibitory concentrations of amoxicillin. *J Antimicrob Chemother.* (2001) 48:594–5. doi: 10.1093/jac/48.4.594
71. Tarragó D, Lara N, Fenoll A, Casal J, Giménez MJ, Aguilar L, et al. Specific antibodies, levofloxacin, and modulation of capsule-associated virulence in *Streptococcus pneumoniae. Antimicrob Agents Chemother.* (2005) 49:3095–6. doi: 10.1128/AAC.49.7.3095-3096.2005
72. Pendleton JN, Gorman SP, Gilmore BF. Clinical relevance of the ESKAPE pathogens. *Expert Rev Anti Infect Ther.* (2013) 11:297–308. doi: 10.1586/eri.13.12
73. DiGiandomenico A, Sellman BR. Antibacterial monoclonal antibodies: the next generation? *Curr Opin Microbiol.* (2015) 27:78–85. doi: 10.1016/j.mib.2015.07.014
74. Sparrow E, Friede M, Sheikh M, Torvaldsen S. Therapeutic antibodies for infectious diseases. *Bull World Health Organ.* (2017) 95:235–7. doi: 10.2471/BLT.16.178061
75. Al-Hamad A, Burnie J, Upton M. Enhancement of antibiotic susceptibility of *Stenotrophomonas maltophilia* using a polyclonal antibody developed against an ABC multidrug efflux pump. *Can J Microbiol.* (2011) 57:820–8. doi: 10.1139/w11-076
76. DiGiandomenico A, Keller AE, Gao C, Rainey GJ, Warrener P, Camara MM, et al. A multifunctional bispecific antibody protects against *Pseudomonas aeruginosa. Sci Transl Med.* (2014) 6:262ra155. doi: 10.1126/scitranslmed.3009655
77. Song Y, Baer M, Srinivasan R, Lima J, Yarranton G, Bebbington C, et al. PcrV antibody-antibiotic combination improves survival in *Pseudomonas aeruginosa*-infected mice. *Eur J Clin Microbiol Infect Dis.* (2012) 31:1837–45. doi: 10.1007/s10096-011-1509-2
78. Secher T, Fas S, Fauconnier L, Mathieu M, Rutschi O, Ryffel B, et al. The anti-*Pseudomonas aeruginosa* antibody Panobacumab is efficacious on acute pneumonia in neutropenic mice and has additive effects with meropenem. *PLoS ONE* (2013) 8:e73396. doi: 10.1371/journal.pone.0073396
79. Hua L, Hilliard JJ, Shi Y, Tkaczyk C, Cheng LI, Yu X, et al. Assessment of an anti-alpha-toxin monoclonal antibody for prevention and treatment of *Staphylococcus aureus*-induced pneumonia. *Antimicrob Agents Chemother.* (2014) 58:1108–17. doi: 10.1128/AAC.02190-13
80. Hilliard JJ, Datta V, Tkaczyk C, Hamilton M, Sadowska A, Jones-Nelson O, et al. Anti-alpha-toxin monoclonal antibody and antibiotic combination therapy improves disease outcome and accelerates healing in a *Staphylococcus aureus* dermonecrosis model. *Antimicrob Agents Chemother.* (2015) 59:299–309. doi: 10.1128/AAC.03918-14
81. Rouha H, Badarau A, Visram ZC, Battles MB, Prinz B, Magyarics Z, et al. Five birds, one stone: neutralization of alpha-hemolysin and 4 bi-component leukocidins of *Staphylococcus aureus* with a single human monoclonal antibody. *MAbs* (2015) 7:243–54. doi: 10.4161/19420862.2014.985132
82. Varshney AK, Wang X, MacIntyre J, Zollner RS, Kelleher K, Kovalenko OV, et al. Humanized staphylococcal enterotoxin B (SEB)-specific monoclonal antibodies protect from SEB intoxication and *Staphylococcus aureus* infections alone or as adjunctive therapy with vancomycin. *J Infect Dis.* (2014) 210:973–81. doi: 10.1093/infdis/jiu198
83. Migone TS, Bolmer S, Zhong J, Corey A, Vasconcelos D, Buccellato M, et al. Added benefit of raxibacumab to antibiotic treatment of inhalational anthrax. *Antimicrob Agents Chemother.* (2015) 59:1145–51. doi: 10.1128/AAC.04606-14
84. Biron B, Beck K, Dyer D, Mattix M, Twenhafel N, Nalca A. Efficacy of ETI-204 monoclonal antibody as an adjunct therapy in a New Zealand white rabbit partial survival model for inhalational anthrax. *Antimicrob Agents Chemother.* (2015) 59:2206–14. doi: 10.1128/AAC.04593-14
85. Lowy I, Molrine DC, Leav BA, Blair BM, Baxter R, Gerding DN, et al. Treatment with monoclonal antibodies against *Clostridium difficile* toxins. *N Engl J Med.* (2010) 362:197–205. doi: 10.1056/NEJMoa0907635

16

A Beneficial Effect of Low-Dose Aspirin in a Murine Model of Active Tuberculosis

*Vera Marie Kroesen[1,2], Paula Rodríguez-Martínez[3], Eric García[1], Yaiza Rosales[1], Jorge Díaz[1], Montse Martín-Céspedes[3], Gustavo Tapia[3], Maria Rosa Sarrias[4,5], Pere-Joan Cardona[1,6] and Cristina Vilaplana[1,6]**

[1]Experimental Tuberculosis Unit (UTE), Fundació Institut Germans Trias i Pujol (IGTP), Universitat Autònoma de Barcelona (UAB), Badalona, Spain, [2]Carl-von-Ossietzky University Oldenburg, Oldenburg, Germany, [3]Pathology Department, Hospital Universitari Germans Trias i Pujol (HUGTIP), Universitat Autònoma de Barcelona (UAB), Badalona, Spain, [4]Innate Immunity Group, Fundació Institut Germans Trias i Pujol (IGTP), Badalona, Spain, [5]Centro de Investigación Biomédica en Red de Enfermedades Hepáticas y Digestivas (CIBEREhD), Madrid, Spain, [6]Centro de Investigación Biomédica en Red de Enfermedades Respiratorias (CIBERES), Madrid, Spain

***Correspondence:**
Cristina Vilaplana
cvilaplana@gmail.com,
cvilaplana@igtp.cat

An excessive, non-productive host-immune response is detrimental in active, chronic tuberculosis (TB) disease as it typically leads to tissue damage. Given their anti-inflammatory effect, non-steroidal anti-inflammatory drugs can potentially attenuate excessive inflammation in active TB disease. As such, we investigated the prophylactic and therapeutic effect of low-dose aspirin (LDA) (3 mg/kg/day), either alone or in combination with common anti-TB treatment or BCG vaccination, on disease outcome in an experimental murine model of active TB. Survival rate, bacillary load (BL) in lungs, and lung pathology were measured. The possible mechanism of action of LDA on the host's immune response was also evaluated by measuring levels of CD5L/AIM, selected cytokines/chemokines and other inflammatory markers in serum and lung tissue. LDA increased survival, had anti-inflammatory effects, reduced lung pathology, and decreased bacillary load in late-stage TB disease. Moreover, in combination with common anti-TB treatment, LDA enhanced survival and reduced lung pathology. Results from the immunological studies suggest the anti-inflammatory action of LDA at both a local and a systemic level. Our results showed a systemic decrease in neutrophilic recruitment, decreased levels of acute-phase reaction cytokines (IL-6, IL-1β, and TNF-α) at late stage and a delay in the decrease in T cell response (in terms of IFN-γ, IL-2, and IL-10 serum levels) that occurs during the course of *Mycobacterium tuberculosis* infection. An anti-inflammatory milieu was detected in the lung, with less neutrophil recruitment and lower levels of tissue factor. In conclusion, LDA may be beneficial as an adjunct to standard anti-TB treatment in the later stage of active TB by reducing excess, non-productive inflammation, while enhancing Th1-cell responses for elimination of the bacilli.

Keywords: aspirin, host-directed therapies, non-steroidal anti-inflammatory drugs, tuberculosis, *Mycobacterium tuberculosis*, mouse model

INTRODUCTION

Tuberculosis (TB), which is a chronic infectious disease caused by *Mycobacterium tuberculosis*, ranks among the top 10 causes of death worldwide (1). In a clinical context, human TB presents with a wide spectrum of disease, ranging from asymptomatic infection to active TB disease (2).

Patients can usually be divided into having latent TB infection or suffering from active TB disease, depending on whether they show clinical signs of the disease or not (2). Patients with co-morbidities that induce a pro-inflammatory milieu, such as diabetes mellitus and tobacco smoking, an impaired immune response, such as the elderly, children, people relying on immunosuppressive therapy, such as anti-TNFs (3) or with immunodeficiencies, such as those co-infected with HIV (1), are particularly at risk of developing active TB disease once infected with *M. tuberculosis*.

The current approach to treating TB entails antimicrobial drugs that target the mycobacteria (4). Thus, the standard 6-month treatment for TB patients consists of a four-drug regimen containing rifampicin, isoniazid, pyrazinamide, and ethambutol (4). Multi-drug resistant tuberculosis (MDR-TB), defined as resistance to at least two first-line drugs isoniazid and rifampicin, and extensively-drug resistant tuberculosis, where additional resistance to any fluoroquinolone or any of the injectable second-line aminoglycosides occurs, is an emerging challenge in the treatment of TB (1, 5). In 2015, the WHO reported an incidence of 450,000 new cases of MDR-TB worldwide, and it has been reported in virtually every country (1). One strategy that has been suggested to more effectively fight against TB, MDR-TB, and TB/HIV involves drugs that target host immune functions as adjuvants to classic antimicrobial treatment rather than focusing on the bacteria themselves (6). By not targeting the infecting microorganisms, these drugs have the potential advantage of not selecting TB drug resistance. The majority of these so-called host-directed therapies (HDTs) (7), which include non-steroidal anti-inflammatory drugs (NSAIDS) (8, 9), aim to balance host immune responses in order to decrease damage and are potentially able to achieve clinical improvement and decreased morbidity and mortality. Pathological immune reactions in the host, such as an insufficient or excessive inflammatory response, the latter of which leads to severe tissue damage, are considered to be a major cause of failure of current TB treatments (7).

Upon infection, *M. tuberculosis* is phagocytosed by alveolar macrophages, where it prevents phagosome–lysosome fusion and elimination by the lysosome (10). Infected antigen-presenting cells secrete various cytokines and chemokines to activate the innate immune response and influx of neutrophils (11, 12). Neutrophils usually represent a protective immune response during early infection by secreting oxidizing and hydrolytic agents that target the bacteria (11). However, although this neutrophil-dominated inflammation is beneficial in acute infections, where a fast and strong immune response can potentially lead to control or even clearance of the bacilli, it can be detrimental when non-productive and excessive, as described above, in the context of HIV co-infection (13), or simply in chronic infection (11). In active, chronic TB disease, an early and strong immune response has been reported to destroy delicate neighboring host tissues, thus leading to necrosis and resulting in cavitation, which facilitates spread of the bacilli, rather than containing *M. tuberculosis* replication and the continuous, excessively aggressive immune response (14). Attenuating the excessive host inflammatory response in active TB disease might thus be vital for treatment and disease outcome (11). Given their anti-inflammatory effect, NSAIDS can potentially attenuate neutrophil-mediated inflammation in TB (9, 8). Similarly, cyclooxygenase (COX) inhibitors have also been suggested to have potential therapeutic applications in other infections, such as in the control of parasite replication and dissemination in Chagas disease (15–17), in *Leishmania major* infection (18) and in pneumonia and pneumococcal-influenza co-infection (19).

In this study, we aimed to investigate the effect of low-dose aspirin (AAS) (LDA), administered alone or as an adjunct to common anti-TB treatment with the standard antibiotic treatment-regimen for human patients or with preventative BCG vaccination, in a murine model of active TB. Disease outcome was quantified in terms of survival rate, bacillary load (BL) in lungs, and lung pathology. LDA has previously been shown to prolong survival and enhance control of BL in the late stages of TB (12) and was, therefore, to confirm this finding. AAS is a salicylate that inhibits the two isoforms of COX in an irreversible manner, while leaving LOX activity unaffected (20, 21). The LOX pathway results in the synthesis of lipoxins (LX), which are known to be immunoresolvents with a potent anti-inflammatory effect and potential antimicrobial properties (22). The resulting synthesis of LX promotes the switching from a pro-inflammatory to anti-inflammatory milieu, with a decrease in pro-inflammatory cytokines and less neutrophil recruitment. Inhibition of the COX pathway also has an impact on vascularization and is widely used in the prevention of cardiovascular disease and stroke (21).

In light of the above, we decided to explore whether the described beneficial effects of LDA on survival rate, pathology, and BL in lungs in active TB are mediated by an anti-inflammatory effect, as previously found with ibuprofen (23). To assess the potential anti-inflammatory effect of LDA, we measured immunological profiles in serum and lungs in a murine model of active TB. Our specific objectives were: (1) to provide further evidence for the described beneficial effects of LDA on disease outcome in a murine model of active TB, when given prophylactically or therapeutically, by assessing survival rate, pulmonary BL, and lung pathology; (2) to investigate whether the potential beneficial effects are mediated by an anti-inflammatory mechanism of action; (3) to draw conclusions regarding the general immune responses in TB (as possible target for HDTs) by comparing immunological profiles in infected animals and non-infected negative control mice.

MATERIALS AND METHODS

Experimental Design

A murine model of active TB based on a single intravenous (i.v.) infection [4×10^4–2×10^5/mL colony forming units (CFU)/mL per mouse] with *M. tuberculosis* H37Rv Pasteur strain in C3HeB/FeJ mice was used, as described previously (15). Animals (n = 164) were divided into five experiments (see **Table 1**):

(a) To evaluate the prophylactic effect of LDA: Experiments 1 and 2. AAS was given from 1 week before infection and

TABLE 1 | Experimental design of the five experiments included in the study.

Experimental design							
Experiment 1: prophylaxis, survival experiment	Group	W-1	W1	W3→			
	Control	–	Day 0: infection	–			
	AAS	AAS 3 mg/kg/ day	Day 0: infection. AAS 3mg/kg/ day	AAS 3 mg/kg/day continued until death			
Experiment 2: prophylaxis, scheduled timepoints	Group	W-1	W1	W2	W3	W4	
	Control	–	Day 0: infection	Day 14: euthanasia of 6 mice; serum collection	Day 21: euthanasia of 6 mice; serum collection	Day 28: euthanasia of 6 mice; serum collection	
	AAS	AAS 3 mg/kg/ day	Day 0: infection. AAS 3 mg/kg/ day	Day 14: euthanasia of 6 mice; serum collection. AAS 3 mg/ kg/day	Day 21: euthanasia of 6 mice; serum collection. AAS 3 mg/kg/day	Day 28: euthanasia of 6 mice; serum collection. AAS 3 mg/kg/day	
Experiment 3: therapeutics, survival experiment	Group	W-1	W1	W2–W4	W5	W6	W7→
	Control		Infection	–	–	–	–
	AAS		Infection	–	AAS 3 mg/kg/day	AAS 3 mg/kg/day	–
Experiment 4: therapeutics, synergy with BCG	Group	W-1	W1	W2–6	W7	W8	W9→
	Sham		Vacc.		Infection		
	BCG		Vacc.		Infection		
	BCG + AAS		Vacc.		Infection		AAS 3 mg/kg/ day continued until death
Experiment 5: therapeutics, synergy with Rimstar	Group	W-1	W1	W2–4	W5	W6	W7→
	RIMSTAR		Infection		RIMSTAR	RIMSTAR	RIMSTAR continued until death
	RIMSTAR + AAS		Infection		RIMSTAR + AAS 3 mg/ kg/day	RIMSTAR + AAS 3 mg/kg/day	RIMSTAR continued until death

AAS, aspirin; BCG, bacille Calmette–Guerin vaccine; Vacc., vaccination; RIMSTAR, rifampicin 150 mg + isoniazid 75 mg + pyrazinamid 400 mg + ethambutol 275 mg, adjusted to mouse weight; W, week; W-1, one week before challenge; W2, 3, 4, 5, 6, etc., means weeks after challenge.

disease outcome compared in aspirin-treated and non-treated animals.

(b) To evaluate the therapeutic effect of LDA: Experiments 3 to 5. In Experiment 3 ($n = 24$), disease outcome was compared in LDA-treated and non-treated animals. In Experiment 4, LDA was evaluated as a coadjuvant with BCG vaccination ($n = 36$). Mice were subcutaneously vaccinated with sham (SF) or BCG 10^6 CFU/animal [ImmunoCyst® BCG, Sanofi Pasteur (batch E-5-C4042A)] alone or in combination with therapeutical LDA (administered 2 weeks post-challenge). The results for the BCG- and BCG + AAS-treated groups were compared with those obtained for the sham group. The endpoint was established at week 18 after the start of the experiment as these BCG-vaccinated or BCG-vaccinated and AAS-treated mice did not die. Experiment 5 ($n = 24$) was designed to assess the therapeutic effect of LDA in combination with RIMSTAR, the standard antibiotic combination used in human TB treatment.

The Murine Model of Acute Active TB (C3HeB/FeJ Mice)

The C3HeB/FeJ murine model of acute active TB disease in humans was selected due to its suitability for investigating the effect of therapeutical strategies on disease outcome and immune mechanisms during active TB disease with excess inflammation and granuloma formation (12).

Endpoints to Assess the Impact of LDA on Disease Outcome

The effect of LDA on disease outcome was measured in terms of survival rate (all experiments except number 2; $n = 108$), BL in lungs at different timepoints (days 14, 21, and 28 post-infection; $n = 48$) and lung pathology analysis (histometry; $n = 138$) (**Table 2**). For the BL assessment, samples of lung lobes from animals from experiment 2 were collected, homogenized, and several dilutions plated on nutrient Middlebrook 7H11 agar (BD Diagnostics, Spark, USA). The number of CFU was counted after incubation for 28 days at 37°C and the results expressed as CFU/mL.

For the assessment of lung pathology, histological lung sections from C3HeB/FeJ mice from all experimental groups were analyzed by histometry. Lungs were fixed in 10% buffered formalin, embedded in paraffin and 5-μm sections stained with hematoxylin-eosin (HE) stain for histometric analysis. All slides were scanned at a resolution of 300 dpi (dots per inch), and scanned images analyzed using NIS-Elements Documentation 3.0 Software (by Nikon Instruments; Shinjuku, Tokio, Japan). The percentage of affected area in relation to total lung area was measured.

Methods to Assess the Impact of LDA on Immunological Profiles in Serum and Lung Tissue

The immunological profiles in sera from the experimental groups were assessed in Experiment 2 (**Table 2**). Ten selected cytokines and chemokines (G-CSF, KC, MIP-2, IL-1α, IL-1β, IL-6, TNFα, IL-2, IFNγ, and IL-17) were measured in serum samples obtained at days 14 (week 2), 21 (week 3), and 28 (week 4) post-infection, using the Luminex MILLIPLEX® MAP Kit, Mouse Cytokine/Chemokine Magnetic Bead Panel, 96-Well Plate Assay (EMD Millipore). Six non-infected mice were used as negative control in the Luminex assay. Circulating CD5L/AIM protein was assessed using the CircuLex Mouse AIM/CD5L/Spα ELISA Kit (MBL International Corporation, Woburn, USA) and the same sera samples. Both kits were used in accordance with their manufacturer's instructions.

Immunohistochemical stains on paraffined sections were performed using the ultraView DAB (Ventana Medical Systems) in accordance with the manufacturer's protocol. Monoclonal antibodies against TNF-α (rabbit polyclonal ab6671; Abcam, dilution 1:100), STAT1 (phospho S727) (rabbit monoclonal EPR3146; Abcam, dilution 1:500), myeloperoxidase (MPO) (rabbit polyclonal ab45977, Abcam, dilution 1:500), arginase 1 (rabbit polyclonal ab91279, Abcam, dilution 1:200), iNOS (rabbit polyclonal ab15323, Abcam, dilution 1:100), CD5L (dilution 1:50), tissue factor (TF) (rabbit monoclonal ab151748, Abcam, dilution 1:200) were used. Granulomas were imaged with a camera and NIS-Elements Documentation 3.0 Software connected to a microscope (Nikon Instruments; Shinjuku, Tokyo, Japan). As individual tissue sections from different animals with active TB contain multiple granulomas, we decided to image regions from five different granulomas with representative features, and to use them to analyze the IHC staining (5 per experimental group and timepoint). Images were acquired as TIFF-format images and analyzed with ImageJ (available at https://imagej.nih.gov/ij/). The median stained area for each antibody was graphically represented as square pixels.

Graphics and Statistics

Data are shown as median ± SEM. A non-parametric comparison (Mann–Whitney test) was used for comparisons between LDA and control groups (GraphPad Software v6.0). Statistically significant differences are designated as follows: $^{*}p < 0.05$; $^{**}p < 0.01$; $^{***}p < 0.001$.

RESULTS

Survival Rate

Low-dose aspirin increased the survival rate when compared to controls in all experiments in which survival was assessed

TABLE 2 | Overview of the experiments and methods employed.

Experiment	Experimental group	Treatment	No. of mice	Survival assessed	BL assessed	No. of slides for histometry	Serum samples for Luminex and ELISA
1	Positive control	–	12	Yes	No	12	No
	AAS	LDA	12			11	No
2	Positive control	–	24	No	Yes	18	Yes
	AAS	LDA	24			13	Yes
3	Positive control	–	12	Yes	No	12	No
	AAS	LDA	12			12	No
4	sham	sham	12			12	No
	BCG	BCG	12			12	No
	BCG + AAS	BCG + LDA	12			12	No
5	Rimstar	Rimstar	12	Yes	No	12	No
	Rimstar + AAS	Rimstar + LDA	12			12	No
Negative ct	Negative ct	–	6	No	No	No	Yes, only Luminex

AAS, aspirin; LDA, low-dose aspirin 3 mg/kg/day; BCG, bacille Calmette–Guerin vaccine; RIMSTAR, rifampicin 150 mg + isoniazid 75 mg + pyrazinamid 400 mg + ethambutol 275 mg, adjusted to mouse weight; Negative ct, negative control, healthy animals.

(experiments 1, 3, 4, and 5) (**Figure 1**). Both prophylactic and therapeutic treatment with LDA (experiments 1 and 3) increased survival compared to non-treated controls in a statistically significant manner ($p < 0.001$ and $p = 0.0032$, respectively). Both BCG vaccination alone and in combination with LDA (experiment 4) showed a statistically significant increase in survival compared to the control group ($p < 0.001$), although no additional effect of LDA was found, at least until termination of the experiment. Two weeks of LDA in addition to antibiotic treatment (experiment 5) increased survival compared to RIMSTAR-only treated animals, although the differences between the survival curves were not statistically significant, at least not with the number of animals included in each treatment group ($n = 12$).

BL in Lungs

Prophylactic treatment with LDA (experiment 2) showed a statistically significant increase in BL on day 14 post-infection ($p = 0.0022$), but a statistically significant decrease at later stages (day 21, $p = 0.0050$; day 28, $p = 0.0152$) when compared to controls (**Figure 2A**).

Lung Pathology (Histometry)

Histological lung sections obtained from mice from all experiments were stained with HE-stain and analyzed in terms of granulomatous area in lungs (%). A statistically significant increase in lung pathology in both treatment groups over the course of infection was seen in those animals used to evaluate the BL at different timepoints (experiment 2). This increase was statistically significantly delayed and mitigated by preventive treatment with LDA only. As shown in **Figure 2B**, the % affected area was significantly reduced in LDA-treated mice compared to controls in late-stage infection (day 21, $p = 0.0286$; day 28, $p = 0.0286$).

BCG vaccination was found to prevent excess lung pathology compared to sham ($p = 0.0169$) (**Figure 2C**), keeping lung pathology very low at least until the end of the experiment at 4 months post-infection [mean of 39.78%; SD 24.5% (BCG group) and 72.07%; SD 9.335% (sham group)]. Adjunctive LDA treatment had an additional beneficial impact on this effect, although this was not statistically significant when compared to BCG alone.

Immunological Studies

Figure 3 shows the results of the Luminex assay in serum for the cytokines. All median serum concentrations (pg/mL, plus 25–75% confidence intervals) for all cytokines/chemokines and CD5L measured by Luminex and ELISA at weeks 2 (day 14), 3 (day 21), and 4 (day 28) post-challenge are shown in Table S1 in Supplementary Material. The IHC values in lungs are shown in **Figure 4**, and the results of CD5L measurements in serum (measured by ELISA, **Figure 5A**) and lungs (assessed by IHC, **Figure 5B**) are shown in **Figure 5**.

Neutrophil Recruitment (G-CSF, KC, and MIP-2)

Our findings in serum (**Figure 3**) underline a general increase in the recruitment of granulocytes during TB, as the G-CSF and KC (CXCL-1) values for infected groups differed from the negative control in a statistically significant manner. As regards G-CSF

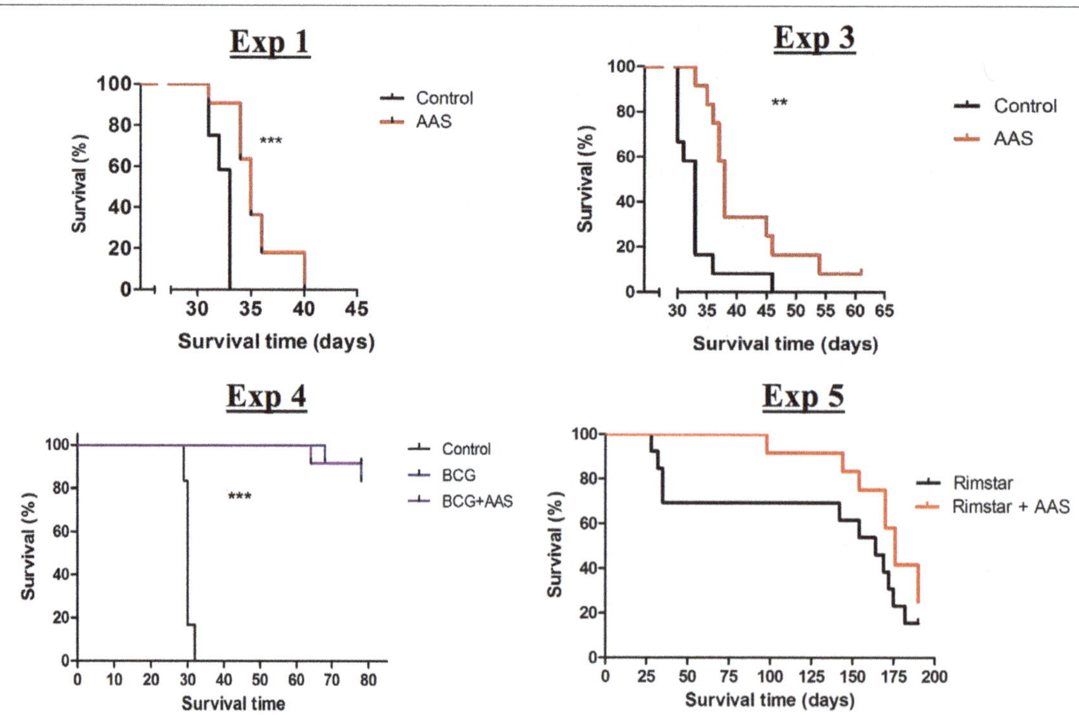

FIGURE 1 | Survival assessment. Curves for the experimental groups achieved in the four experiments in which the impact of treatment on survival was assessed. Abbreviations: AAS, aspirin; BCG, bacille Calmette–Guerin vaccine; Vacc., vaccination; RIMSTAR, rifampicin 150 mg + isoniazid 75 mg + pyrazinamid 400 mg + ethambutol 275 mg, adjusted to mouse weight.

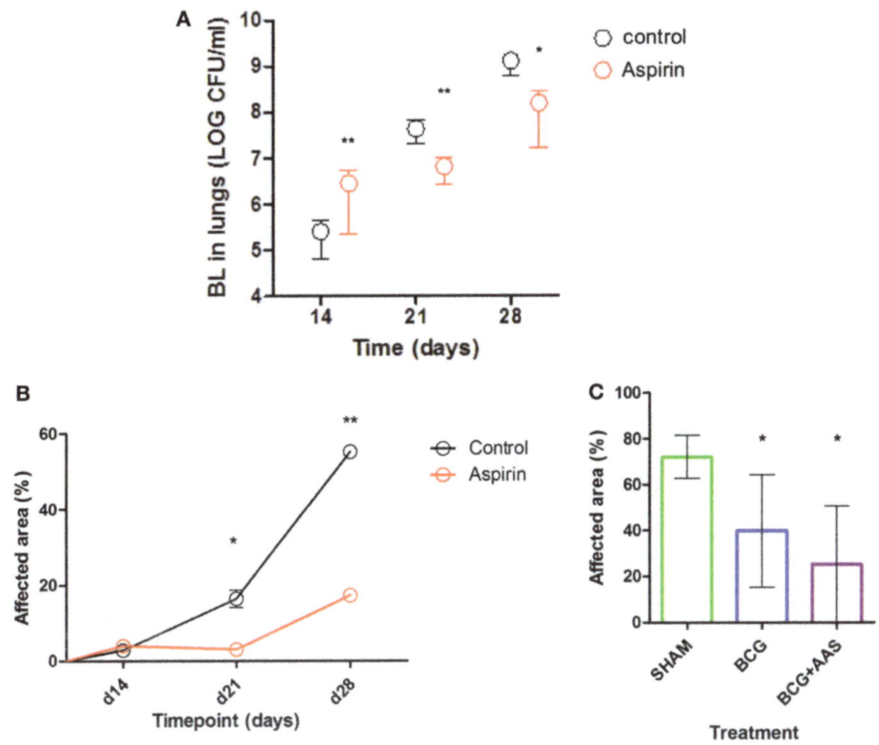

FIGURE 2 | Impact of AAS on the BL and histometry. AAS, aspirin; BCG, bacille Calmette–Guerin vaccine; BL, bacillary load. Panel **(A)** shows the impact of AAS on the BL with time post-challenge. Panels **(B,C)** show the impact of AAS on the histometry in terms of affected lung area, both alone [**(B)**: experiment 2] and in combination with BCG vaccine [**(C)**: experiment 4].

serum levels, there were no statistically significant differences between treatment groups, although LDA reduced serum levels in late-stage disease. For KC, serum levels seemed to reach a plateau in week 3 in LDA-treated mice, while in the untreated infected animals (positive control) they appeared to keep rising through week 4, although the difference was not statistically significant. MIP-2 (CXCL2) levels in infected groups remained similar to those in healthy mice, except for week 4 (day 28), when the levels in the positive control animals increased (difference not statistically significant).

Acute-Phase Reaction: IL-1α, IL-1β, IL-6, and TNFα

Our results (**Figure 3**) suggest an expected systemic (acute-phase) inflammatory reaction in TB. Thus, IL-1α values in infected groups were below the range in healthy animals (not statistically significant), and levels in the LDA group were lower than those obtained from the positive control group on days 14 and 28 post-infection. IL-1β levels in both infected groups increased over time, showing the greatest differences at week 4 (day 28) when compared to healthy animals. This rise seemed to be less pronounced in the LDA group, although no changes were found to be statistically significant. IL-6 and TNFα values in infected groups differed with respect to the negative control at all timepoints in a statistically significant manner. Indeed, there was a statistically significant increase in serum IL-6 levels over the course of infection, with this being mitigated in the AAS group in later stages. TNFα levels in the LDA group peaked at week 3 (day 21) post-infection in a statistically significant manner, but returned to day 14 levels by week 4 (day 28).

T-Cell Response: IL-2, IFNγ, and IL-17

Animals from both infected groups showed increased IFNγ values at weeks 2 and 3 (days 14 and 21) when compared to negative controls, with these levels decreasing to those of healthy animals by day 28 (week 4). AAS significantly delayed this decrease. Thus, on day 28 post-infection, the IL-17 values for infected groups were statistically significantly higher than those for the negative control. No differences were encountered between the control and AAS groups. Although serum IL-2 levels were generally low, they were elevated in the infected groups with respect to levels in healthy mice, dropping back over the course of infection. This effect was less evident in the AAS group (not statistically significant).

The Anti-Inflammatory Cytokine: IL-10

IL-10 levels in infected groups were higher at week 2 (day 14) post-challenge when compared to the negative control, subsequently decreasing to the level found in healthy animals by day 28. The drop in the AAS group in week 3 (day 21) was less pronounced ($p = 0.01$).

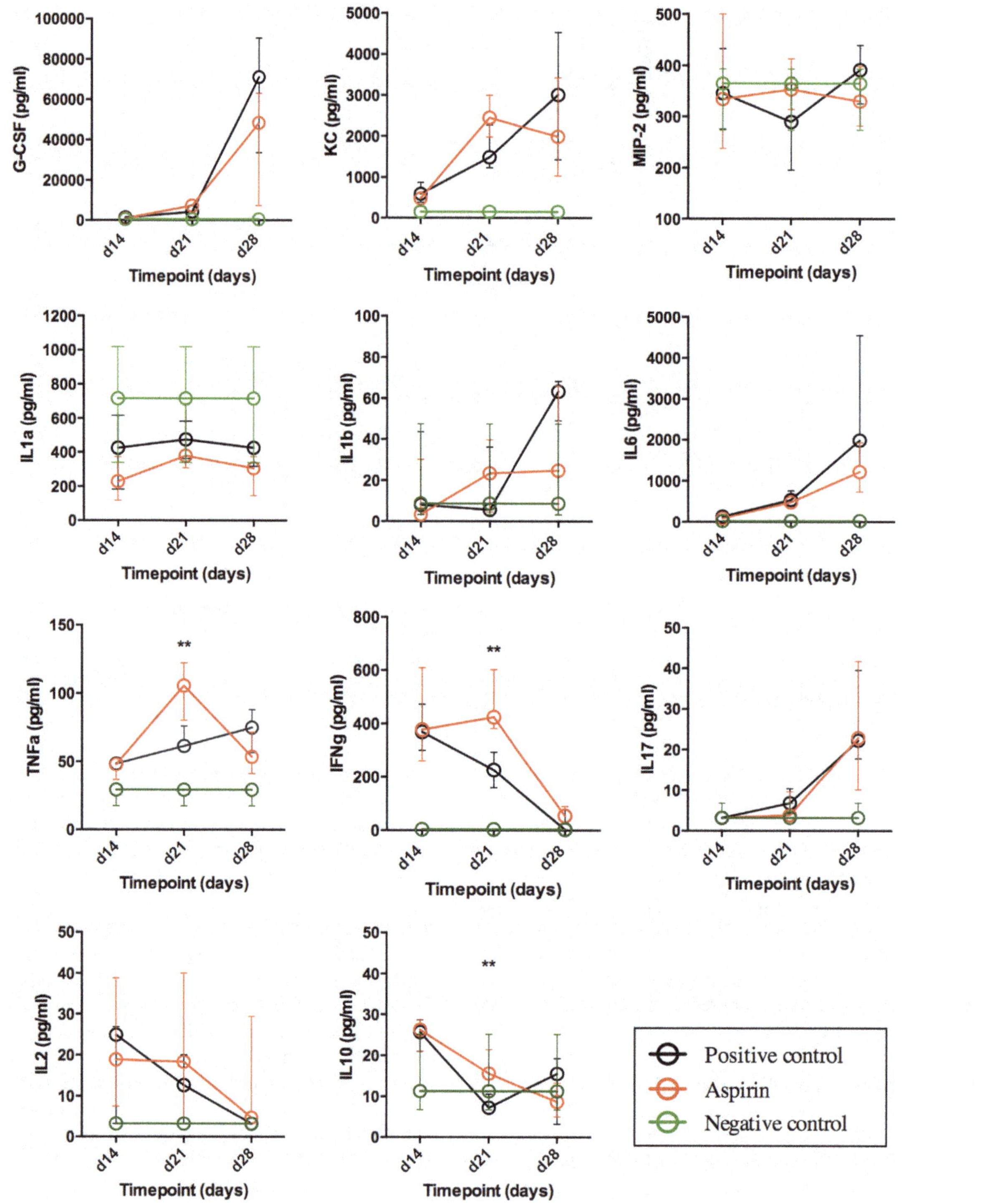

FIGURE 3 | Impact of AAS on serum cytokine/chemokine levels. All data are presented in pg/mL. Abbreviations: AAS, aspirin; G-CSF, granulocyte-colony stimulating factor; KC, chemokine (C-X-C motif) ligand 1 (CXCL-1); MIP-2, macrophage inflammatory protein 2-alpha [also named chemokine (C-X-C motif) ligand 2 (CXCL2)]; IL, interleukin; TNFa, tumor necrosis α; IFNg, interferon γ.

IHC Results

The IHC results (**Figure 4**) showed differences in terms of stained area in pixels when using anti-TNF and anti-STAT1 antibodies. These differences were observed at a tissue level both over time and when comparing the two experimental groups. The presence of TNF was slightly lower in the AAS group, especially at week 3 post-infection (difference not statistically significant). In contrast, STAT1 was found to be elevated at week 3 and decreased at week

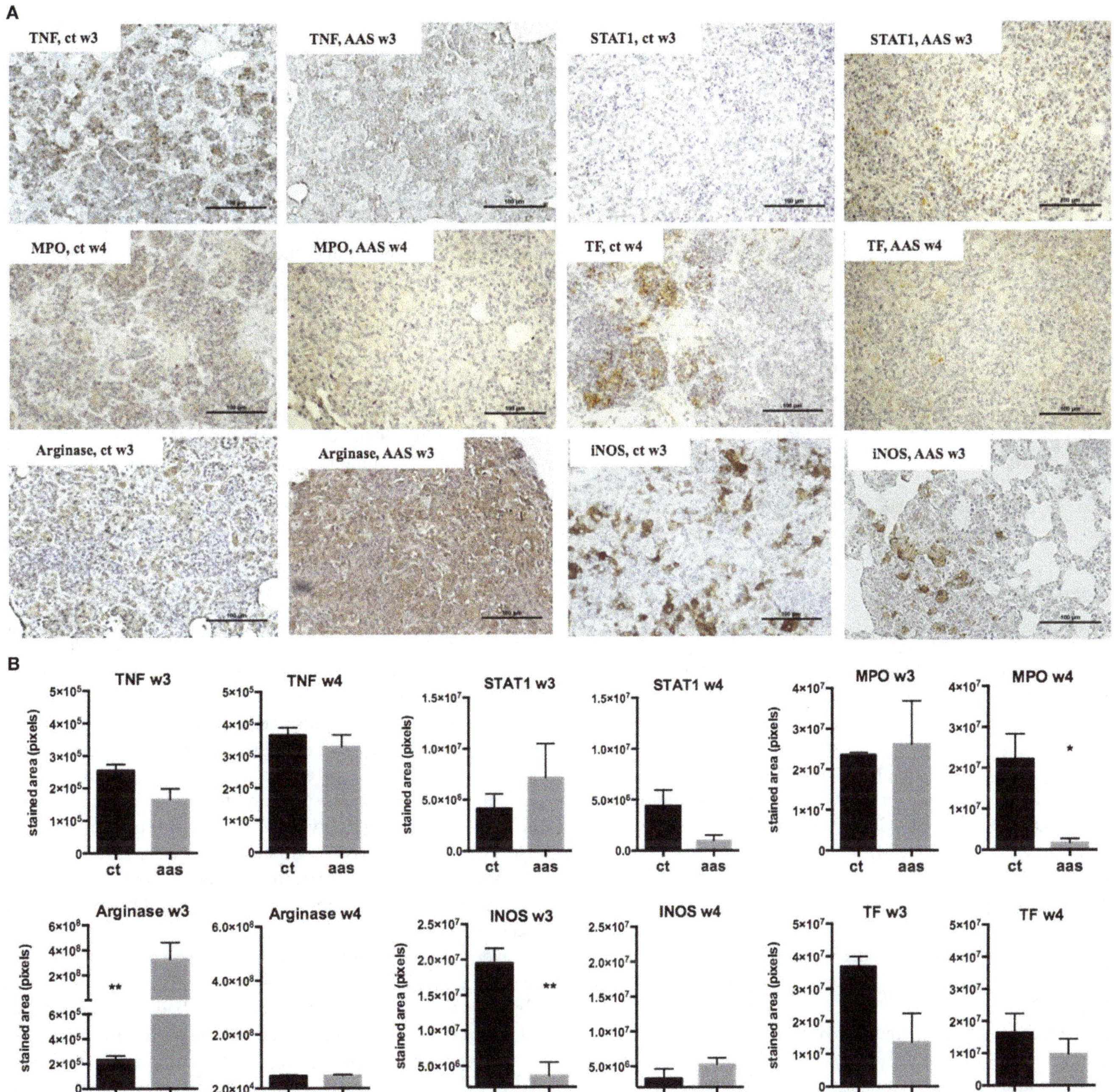

FIGURE 4 | Impact of AAS in lung measured by IHQ. Panel **(A)** shows some pictures of the staining. The bar represents 100 μm. Panel **(B)** shows the results of the staining quantification by experimental group and timepoint. Abbreviations: AAS, aspirin; TNF, tumor necrosis α; STAT1, signal transducer and activator of transcription 1; MPO, myeloperoxidase; INOS, inducible nitric oxide synthase; TF, tissue factor.

4 in the AAS group with respect to the control group. MPO+ cells were statistically significantly decreased in the AAS group in late-stage disease (week 4). Differences were encountered for both arginase and INOS detection at week 3. Thus, while arginase staining increased, INOS staining decreased in the AAS group, with the differences being statistically significant in both cases. Tissue factor was found to be decreased in the AAS group at both weeks 3 and 4 post-infection, although this decrease was more important at week 3 and was not statistically significant at either timepoint.

CD5L/AIM

Significant changes in serum CD5L/AIM levels were observed in both experimental groups over the course of the infection, dominated by a pronounced peak in week 3 post-infection (day 21), followed by a decrease. Serum CD5L/AIM levels were lower for

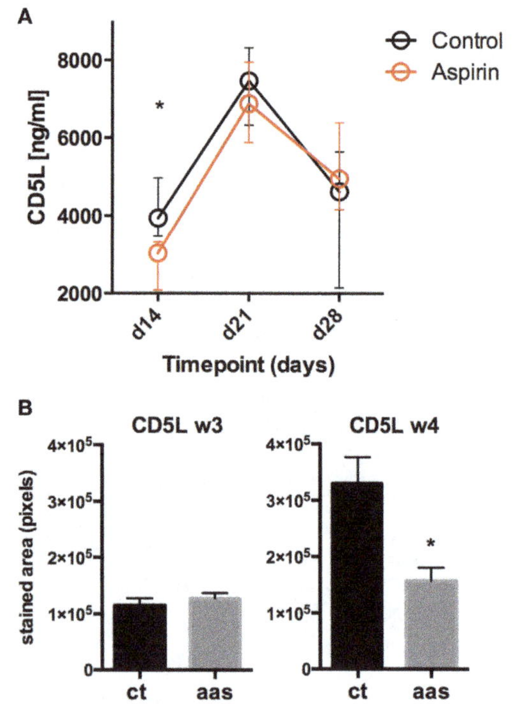

FIGURE 5 | Impact of AAS on CD5L at a systemic and local level. Panel **(A)** shows serum levels (in pg/mL) for CD5L over time. Panel **(B)** shows CD5L in lung tissue on days 21 (week 3) and 28 (week 4) after challenge. Abbreviations: Ct, control; AAS, aspirin; d, day; w, week.

the LDA group at weeks 2 and 3, although the difference was only statistically significant in week 2 (p = 0.0159) (**Figure 5A**). The IHC study revealed less CD5L/AIM in lung sections from the AAS-treated group at week 4 (p = 0.031).

DISCUSSION

The present study provides information on different LDA administration regimens (3 mg/kg) and their effect in a murine model of active TB.

The effect of AAS obtained *in vivo* has been classically considered to depend on the doses used. Thus, while low doses are commonly known to have an antithrombotic effect, only intermediate doses (500 mg to 3 g) were classically considered to be anti-inflammatory (24). However, the literature on preclinical and clinical studies in sepsis (25) shows that LDA triggers lipoxin synthesis, thus mediating anti-inflammatory and inflammation-resolving effects (26). Our results proved that maintained LDA also had an anti-inflammatory effect in the active TB model.

In our hands, when given preventatively or therapeutically in the absence of any other treatment, LDA statistically significantly increased survival in C3HeB/FeJ mice infected with TB, even enhancing the effect of RIMSTAR treatment. This is important as it stands in contrast with other findings, where AAS was described to antagonize the action of isoniazid (27) (which might raise the fear of the drug interfering with the standard treatment), and thus supporting the feasibility of AAS as an adjunct to TB drug therapy. Our findings, therefore, support the feasibility of AAS as an adjunct to TB drug therapy and provide evidence for the beneficial effects of LDA being mediated by an anti-inflammatory and an anti-mycobacterial mechanism, thereby reducing lung pathology over the course of the infection and BL in lungs, at least in late-stage TB.

As regards lung pathology, preventive treatment with LDA alone statistically significantly mitigated and delayed excess pulmonary damage in C3HeB/FeJ mice when compared to controls. Our results suggest that BCG vaccination can indeed prevent or delay terminal pathology due to *M. tuberculosis* infection in C3HeB/FeJ mice, and that treatment with LDA given therapeutically in addition to BCG vaccination does not provide any additional benefit, at least in the 4 months of this study. To determine whether LDA, administered therapeutically either alone or in combination with RIMSTAR or BCG vaccination, can statistically significantly mitigate and delay pulmonary damage during the course of infection, further experiments should be carried out using the same model, but with an experimental design considering several scheduled timepoints.

Analysis of serum levels for selected cytokines/chemokines showed that, as expected, TB itself generates a systemic inflammatory reaction with elevated levels of major neutrophil recruitment factors. Indeed, our results showed a significant increase in serum G-CSF, KC, IL-6, TNFα, and IL-17 levels when compared to negative controls. In contrast, the infection alone showed an inadequate drop in IFNγ, IL-2, and IL-10 levels over the course of infection. We observed a pronounced increase in serum IL-17 levels in late-stage disease, with this increase correlating with a decrease in IL-10 and CD5L. CD5L usually limits IL-17 production in Th17 and enhances IL-10 production in Th17 (28), and IL-10 has been suggested to play a role in controlling the anti-microbial activity and subsequent pulmonary tissue caseation (29). The observed late-stage rise in IL-17, therefore, probably reflects an increase in pathogenic Th17, thus leading to an increase in PMN infiltration and possibly explaining the excess late-stage lung pathology.

Overall, and although not reaching statistical significance for all measurements, our results suggest a systemic anti-inflammatory effect due to AAS treatment, as also described by Marzo et al. and Vilaplana et al. for ibuprofen in the same mouse model (12, 23). First, our findings point toward a systemic modulating effect of LDA on systemic neutrophil recruitment, thus resulting in a reduction in serum G-CSF and KC levels in late-stage disease. The IHC results confirmed the presence of fewer neutrophils in lungs, with a statistically significant decrease in MPO+ staining being observed at day 28 (week 4). With regards to the effects on neutrophil recruitment, it has been suggested that the anti-inflammatory mechanism of action of LDA is mitigated by both the reduced number (recruitment) of neutrophils and by reduced prostaglandin production in monocytes, lymphocytes, and neutrophils, which is implicated in the origin and development of granulomas (8, 14). These cells possess COX-2 activity and produce the prostaglandins (PG) implicated in the inflammation and lung damage associated with active TB, although in the short-term PGE2 might be beneficial (8). Moreover, the results for the AAS group showed less acute phase reaction cytokines

(IL-6, IL-1β, and TNF-α) in the later stages. It has been observed that increased IL-6 levels directly correlate with increased BL (30) and X-ray severity in active TB in humans, therefore, this could be a valuable marker for predicting response to anti-TB treatment, with a pronounced reduction of serum levels being observed following treatment (31). Serum IL-1β levels in infected mice rose above the levels for healthy mice in late-stage disease. It has been described that increased IL-1β levels directly correlate with X-ray severity in active pulmonary TB in humans (31), and increased lung pathology was also observed in our study over the course of infection. Consequently, the lower levels achieved with LDA could be a reflection of the reduced lung pathology found in late-stage TB in the animals in this group.

Eisen et al. previously suggested that the beneficial anti-inflammatory effect of AAS might be mediated by a balancing effect on TNFα and that this could only be achieved at high dose, commonly known as the anti-inflammatory dose (32). Our results suggest that LDA does indeed balance TNF-α in TB in C3HeB/FeJ mice, significantly increasing serum levels in earlier stages (week 3) and reducing serum levels in the later stages of infection compared to non-treated positive controls. However, this increase could also be a consequence of the increase in BL at week 3 observed in the AAS group. Indeed, according to our IHQ results, TNF-α was slightly decreased in lung tissue (especially at week 3). However, the TNF-α increase observed at a serum level was not associated with worsened lung damage at that precise timepoint or subsequently according to the pathology results (33). The increase detected in serum levels at week 3 in the AAS group might enhance the Th1 response, the macrophage response and, consequently, clearance of the mycobacteria, acting synergistically with IL-2 and IFNγ. Increased levels of IFNγ and IL-2 have been found to be associated with moderate cases of human TB rather than more severe cases (34). Indeed, with LDA treatment we see a delay in the decrease in T cell response at a serum level (IFN-γ, IL-2, and IL-10) observed over the course of the infection, which reaches statistical significance at week 3. This delay at this precise timepoint might be responsible for controlling the tissue damage and BL by week 4, when infected animals are usually critically ill because of TB.

Signal transducer and activator of transcription 1 (STAT-1) was found to be elevated in lung tissue from LDA-treated animals compared to controls at week 3 and decreased at week 4, thus mirroring the results obtained in serum. The decrease in serum IL-10 levels over the course of the infection was also delayed in LDA-treated mice, and although the AAS group showed the lowest values in late-stage disease, the anti-inflammatory effect observed, as represented by higher IL-10 levels at week 3, could be considered a problem. It has been found that high serum IL-10 levels in patients with pulmonary TB lead to a slower response to treatment and a lack of bacterial control, thereby underlining the importance of a strong pro-inflammatory response when lung tissues are still intact (30, 35). In addition, reduced IL-10 (and IL-4) levels are associated with more moderate cases of human TB (34). In our study, the impact of the anti-inflammatory effect achieved by LDA seems to be beneficial rather than detrimental as, overall, AAS manages to decrease the inflammation in late-stage disease without impairing the T cell response in the short term. At a tissue level, we were able to demonstrate an increase in arginase-1 and a decrease in INOS at a lung level by week 3 in animals treated with LDA compared to controls. Arginase and INOS have been reported to be markers for characterizing and differentiating different macrophage functions as pro-healing/anti-inflammatory (Arginase) or pro-inflammatory (INOS) in the context of TB (36). As such, LDA treatment may be temporarily switching the phenotype of lung macrophages toward a more pro-healing/anti-inflammatory mode at week 3, which could have an important impact on disease outcome.

As regards CD5L measurements, mice from the AAS group had lower values than those from the control group at early timepoints (weeks 2 and 3) in serum and at later stages (week 4) at a lung level. CD5L/AIM is an innate protein that has been previously described to peak in plasma at week 3 post-infection, which may reflect a strong early innate immune response aimed at controlling *M. tuberculosis* growth. This enhances autophagy for elimination of the bacilli and acts in an anti-inflammatory (regulatory) manner on macrophages and Th1 (28, 37, 38). According to our results, the observations at a serum level may not be mirrored at the lung level as we see increased CD5L in lungs by IHC in week 4 (less pronounced in AAS-treated animals). This could suggest that this protein may play a role both during early infection and also in late stages of the disease, a point that should be studied in further experiments.

Finally, the measurement of TF by IHQ showed high levels at week 3, which was diminished by AAS treatment. TF is the principal initiator of the coagulation cascade, which plays a role in inflammation (39) and innate immunity and is expressed in response to different stimuli, such as infections and inflammation (40). The role of TF in TB is controversial. Thus, while some authors have stated that although this factor is increased, TF-mediated coagulation does not contribute to the host's defense (41), others have suggested a protective role for TF during *M. tuberculosis* infection by demonstrating, in a mouse model of TB, that TF deficiency is associated with increased *M. tuberculosis* replication in lungs (42). LXA4 was found to be able to promote a proinflammatory and prothrombotic profile *in vitro* by inducing TF expression (43). However, a tendency toward hypercoagulation is a known problem in TB patients, especially in severe cases, therefore, the modulation of this state has been proposed as a target for AAS treatment in TB meningitis (9, 44). Indeed, our results point in this direction.

Our results are in contrast to some previous *in vitro* and *in vivo* studies in the literature, which suggest that inhibition of prostaglandin pathways involving a decrease in PGE2 and production of LXA4 is detrimental in terms of immunity to TB and might impair T cell immunity (45–47). In our opinion, the coexistence of contradictory results in the literature in this sense is probably due to the important matter of timing in HDT administration during TB, as a strong inflammatory response is needed at the beginning of the infection for possible control or even clearance of the mycobacteria. Our study was performed using a murine model based on intravenous infection of C3HeB/FeJ mice, which consistently develop lesions with liquefactive necrosis after infection with *M. tuberculosis* and die after

30 days in the absence of treatment. The characteristics of these lesions well mimic active TB in humans at diagnosis (when the disease is exacerbated, with an important inflammatory component and subsequent host tissue destruction), but not human latent infection or disease without a predominant inflammatory response. For this reason, we consider that results from studies in C3HeB/FeJ mice are not applicable to immune-competent humans chronically infected with *M. tuberculosis* or suffering from mild forms of TB. In light of the above, and as a conclusion to our work, we propose that LDA should only be considered as an adjunct to antibiotic treatment and/or vaccination in patients who present with clinical signs of disease (wasting, cough, etc.). On the other hand, the finding that preventative treatment with LDA increases survival, delays excess granuloma formation in lungs, and reduces BL in late-stage TB disease in our model suggests LDA could be given to patients at high risk for TB as a preventive measure, although further studies should be performed to confirm this point.

AUTHOR CONTRIBUTIONS

CV headed the project. CV, MS, and P-JC conceived and planned the experiments. VK, PR-M, MM-C, GT, EG, and JD carried out the experiments. VK, GT, MS, P-JC, and CV contributed to the interpretation of the results. VK and CV took the lead in writing the manuscript. All authors provided critical feedback and helped to shape the research, analysis, and manuscript.

REFERENCES

1. World Health Organization (WHO). *Global TB Report 2017* (2017). Available from: http://www.who.int/tb/publications/global_report/en/ (Accessed: April 8, 2018).
2. Pai M, Behr MA, Dowdy D, Dheda K, Divangahi M, Boehme CC, et al. Tuberculosis. *Nat Rev Dis* (2016) 2:16076. doi:10.1038/nrdp.2016.76
3. Bourigault M-L, Segueni N, Rose S, Court N, Vacher R, Vasseur V, et al. Relative contribution of IL-1α, IL-1β and TNF to the host response to *Mycobacterium tuberculosis* and attenuated *M. bovis* BCG. *Immun Inflamm Dis* (2013) 1(1):47–62. doi:10.1002/iid3.9
4. World Health Organization (WHO). *Treatment of Tuberculosis: Guidelines*. 4th ed. Geneva: World Health Organization (2010). 160 p. Available from: https://www.ncbi.nlm.nih.gov/books/NBK138741/
5. World Health Organization (WHO). *Treatment Guidelines for Drug-Resistant Tuberculosis*. Geneva: World Health Organization (2016). 61 p. Available from: http://www.who.int/tb/areas-of-work/drug-resistant-tb/MDRTBguidelines2016.pdf%0Ahttp://www.who.int/kms/handbook_2nd_ed.pdf (Accessed: April 8, 2018).
6. Zumla A, Maeurer M, Chakaya J, Hoelscher M, Ntoumi F, Rustomjee R, et al. Host-directed therapies for tackling multi-drug resistant TB – learning from the Pasteur-Bechamp debates, and the Host-Directed Therapies Network (HDT-NET). *Clin Infect Dis* (2015) 61(9):1432–8. doi:10.1093/cid/civ631
7. Zumla A, Maeurer M, Chakaya J, Hoelscher M, Ntoumi F, Rustomjee R, et al. Towards host-directed therapies for tuberculosis. *Nat Rev Drug Discov* (2015) 14:511–2. doi:10.1038/nrd4696
8. Ivanyi J, Zumla A. Nonsteroidal antiinflammatory drugs for adjunctive tuberculosis treatment. *J Infect Dis* (2013) 208(2):185–8. doi:10.1093/infdis/jit153
9. Kroesen VM, Gröschel MI, Martinson N, Zumla A, Maeurer M, van der Werf TS, et al. Non-steroidal anti-inflammatory drugs as host-directed therapy for tuberculosis: a systematic review. *Front Immunol* (2017) 8:772. doi:10.3389/fimmu.2017.00772
10. Kimmey JM, Huynh JP, Weiss LA, Park S, Kambal A, Debnath J, et al. Unique role for ATG5 in neutrophil-mediated immunopathology during *M. tuberculosis* infection. *Nature* (2015) 528(7583):565–9. doi:10.1038/nature16451
11. Hawn TR, Matheson AI, Maley SN, Vandal O. Host-directed therapeutics for tuberculosis: can we harness the host? *Microbiol Mol Biol Rev* (2013) 77(4):608–627. doi:10.1128/MMBR.00032-13
12. Marzo E, Vilaplana C, Tapia G, Diaz J, Garcia V, Cardona P-J. Damaging role of neutrophilic infiltration in a mouse model of progressive tuberculosis. *Tuberculosis* (2014) 94(1):55–64. doi:10.1016/j.tube.2013.09.004
13. Nusbaum RJ, Calderon VE, Huante MB, Sutjita P, Vijayakumar S, Lancaster KL, et al. Pulmonary tuberculosis in humanized mice infected with HIV-1. *Sci Rep* (2016) 6:21522. doi:10.1038/srep21522
14. Kiran D, Podell BK, Chambers M, Basaraba RJ. Host-directed therapy targeting the *Mycobacterium tuberculosis* granuloma: a review. *Semin Immunopathol* (2016) 38(2):167–83. doi:10.1007/s00281-015-0537-x
15. Freire-De-Lima CG, Nascimento DO, Soares MBP, Bozza PT, Castro-Faria-Neto HC, De Mello FG, et al. Uptake of apoptotic cells drives the growth of a pathogenic trypanosome in macrophages. *Nature* (2000) 403(6766):199–203. doi:10.1038/35003208
16. Lonien SCH, Malvezi AD, Suzukawa HT, Yamauchi LM, Yamada-Ogatta SF, Rizzo LV, et al. Response to *Trypanosoma cruzi* by human blood cells enriched with dentritic cells is controlled by cyclooxygenase-2 pathway. *Front Microbiol* (2017) 8:2020. doi:10.3389/fmicb.2017.02020
17. Luna-Gomes T, Filardy AA, Rocha JDB, Decote-Ricardo D, LaRocque-de-Freitas IF, Morrot A, et al. Neutrophils increase or reduce parasite burden in *Trypanosoma cruzi*-infected macrophages, depending on host strain: role of neutrophil elastase. *PLoS One* (2014) 9(3):e90582. doi:10.1371/journal.pone.0090582
18. Arcanjo AF, LaRocque-de-Freitas IF, Rocha JDB, Zamith D, Costa-da-Silva AC, Nunes MP, et al. The PGE2/IL-10 axis determines susceptibility of B-1 cell-derived phagocytes (B-1CDP) to *Leishmania* major infection. *PLoS One* (2015) 10(5):e0124888. doi:10.1371/journal.pone.0124888
19. Wang H, Anthony D, Yatmaz S, Wijburg O, Satzke C, Levy B, et al. Aspirin-triggered resolvin D1 reduces pneumococcal lung infection and inflammation in a viral and bacterial coinfection pneumonia model. *Clin Sci* (2017) 131(18):2347–62. doi:10.1042/CS20171006
20. *Aspirin Monograph for Professionals*. Available from: https://www.Drugs.com
21. Dennis EA, Norris PC. Eicosanoid storm in infection and inflammation. *Nat Rev Immunol* (2015) 15(8):511–23. doi:10.1038/nri3859
22. Romano M, Cianci E, Simiele F, Recchiuti A. Lipoxins and aspirin-triggered lipoxins in resolution of inflammation. *Eur J Pharmacol* (2015;) 760:49–63. doi:10.1016/j.ejphar.2015.03.083
23. Vilaplana C, Marzo E, Tapia G, Diaz J, Garcia V, Cardona P-J. Ibuprofen therapy resulted in significantly decreased tissue bacillary loads and increased survival in a new murine experimental model of active tuberculosis. *J Infect Dis* (2013) 208(2):199–202. doi:10.1093/infdis/jit152
24. Hankey GJ, Eikelboom JW. Antithrombotic drugs for patients with ischaemic stroke and transient ischaemic attack to prevent recurrent major vascular events. *Lancet Neurol* (2010) 9:273–84. doi:10.1016/S1474-4422(10)70038-7
25. Sossdorf M, Otto GP, Boettel J, Winning J, Lösche W. Benefit of low-dose aspirin and non-steroidal anti-inflammatory drugs in septic patients. *Crit Care* (2012) 17(1):1–2. doi:10.1186/cc11886
26. Eisen DP. Manifold beneficial effects of acetyl salicylic acid and nonsteroidal anti-inflammatory drugs on sepsis. *Intensive Care Med* (2012) 38:1249–57. doi:10.1007/s00134-012-2570-8
27. Byrne ST, Denkin SM, Zhang Y. Aspirin antagonism in isoniazid treatment of tuberculosis in mice. *Antimicrob Agents Chemother* (2007) 51(2):794–5. doi:10.1128/AAC.01145-06
28. Wang C, Yosef N, Gaublomme J, Wu C, Lee Y, Clish CB, et al. CD5L/AIM regulates lipid biosynthesis and restrains Th17 cell pathogenicity. *Cell* (2015) 163(6):1413–27. doi:10.1016/j.cell.2015.10.068

29. Marakalala MJ, Raju RM, Sharma K, Zhang YJ, Eugenin EA, Prideaux B, et al. Inflammatory signaling in human tuberculosis granulomas is spatially organized. *Nat Med* (2016) 22(5):531–8. doi:10.1038/nm.4073
30. Mesquita EDD, Gil-Santana L, Ramalho D, Tonomura E, Silva EC, Oliveira MM, et al. Associations between systemic inflammation, mycobacterial loads in sputum and radiological improvement after treatment initiation in pulmonary TB patients from Brazil: a prospective cohort study. *BMC Infect Dis* (2016) 16:368. doi:10.1186/s12879-016-1736-3
31. Chowdhury IH, Ahmed AM, Choudhuri S, Sen A, Hazra A, Pal NK, et al. Alteration of serum inflammatory cytokines in active pulmonary tuberculosis following anti-tuberculosis drug therapy. *Mol Immunol* (2014) 62(1):159–68. doi:10.1016/j.molimm.2014.06.002
32. Eisen DP, McBryde ES, Walduck A. Low-dose aspirin and ibuprofen's sterilizing effects on *Mycobacterium tuberculosis* suggest safe newadjuvant therapies for tuberculosis. *J Infect Dis* (2013) 208(11):1925–7. doi:10.1093/infdis/jit476
33. Kaufmann SHE, Dorhoi A, Hotchkiss RS, Bartenschlager R. Host-directed therapies for bacterial and viral infections. *Nat Rev Drug Discov* (2018) 17:35–56. doi:10.1038/nrd.2017.162
34. Dlugovitzky D, Torres-Morales A, Rateni L, Farroni MA, Largacha C, Molteni O, et al. Circulating profile of Th1 and Th2 cytokines in tuberculosis patients with different degrees of pulmonary involvement. *FEMS Immunol Med Microbiol* (1997) 18(3):203–7. doi:10.1111/j.1574-695X.1997.tb01046.x
35. Djoba Siawaya JF, Beyers N, Van Helden P, Walzl G. Differential cytokine secretion and early treatment response in patients with pulmonary tuberculosis. *Clin Exp Immunol* (2009) 156(1):69–77. doi:10.1111/j.1365-2249.2009.03875.x
36. Mattila JT, Ojo OO, Kepka-Lenhart D, Marino S, Kim JH, Eum SY, et al. Microenvironments in tuberculous granulomas are delineated by distinct populations of macrophage subsets and expression of nitric oxide synthase and arginase isoforms. *J Immunol* (2013) 191(2):773–84. doi:10.4049/jimmunol.1300113
37. Sanjurjo L, Amézaga N, Vilaplana C, Cáceres N, Marzo E, Valeri M, et al. The scavenger protein apoptosis inhibitor of macrophages (AIM) potentiates the antimicrobial response against *Mycobacterium tuberculosis* by enhancing autophagy. *PLoS One* (2013) 8(11):e79670. doi:10.1371/journal.pone.0079670
38. Sanjurjo L, Aran G, Roher N, Valledor AF, Sarrias M-R. AIM/CD5L: a key protein in the control of immune homeostasis and inflammatory disease. *J Leukoc Biol* (2015) 98(2):173–84. doi:10.1189/jlb.3RU0215-074R
39. Schuliga M. The inflammatory actions of coagulant and fibrinolytic proteases in disease. *Mediators Inflamm* (2015) 2015:437695. doi:10.1155/2015/437695
40. Caccamo N, Dieli F. Inflammation and the coagulation system in tuberculosis: tissue factor leads the dance. *Eur J Immunol* (2016) 46:303–6. doi:10.1002/eji.201546225
41. Kothari H, Keshava S, Vatsyayan R, Mackman N, Rao LVM, Pendurthi UR. Role of tissue factor in *Mycobacterium tuberculosis*-induced inflammation and disease pathogenesis. *PLoS One* (2014) 9(12):e114141. doi:10.1371/journal.pone.0114141
42. Venkatasubramanian S, Tripathi D, Tucker T, Paidipally P, Cheekatla S, Welch E, et al. Tissue factor expression by myeloid cells contributes to protective immune response against *Mycobacterium tuberculosis* infection. *Eur J Immunol* (2016) 46(2):464–79. doi:10.1002/eji.201545817
43. Maderna P, Godson C, Hannify G, Murphy M, Brady HR. Influence of lipoxin A4 and other lipoxygenase-derived eicosanoids on tissue factor expression. *Am J Physiol Cell Physiol* (2000) 279(4):C945–53. doi:10.1152/ajpcell.2000.279.4.C945
44. Schoeman J, Mansvelt E, Springer P, Van Rensburg AJ, Carlini S, Fourie E. Coagulant and fibrinolytic status in tuberculous meningitis. *Pediatr Infect Dis J* (2007) 26(5):428–31. doi:10.1097/01.inf.0000261126.60283.cf
45. Mayer-Barber KD, Andrade BB, Oland SD, Amaral EP, Barber DL, Gonzales J, et al. Host-directed therapy of tuberculosis based on interleukin-1 and type I interferon crosstalk. *Nature* (2014) 511(7507):99–103. doi:10.1038/nature13489
46. Divangahi M, Desjardins D, Nunes-Alves C, Remold HG, Behar SM. Eicosanoid pathways regulate adaptive immunity to *Mycobacterium tuberculosis*. *Nat Immunol* (2010) 11(8):751–8. doi:10.1038/ni.1904
47. Chen M, Divangahi M, Gan H, Shin DSJ, Hong S, Lee DM, et al. Lipid mediators in innate immunity against tuberculosis: opposing roles of PGE2 and LXA4 in the induction of macrophage death. *J Exp Med* (2008) 205(12):2791–801. doi:10.1084/jem.20080767

17

Neutrophil Elastase Subverts the Immune Response by Cleaving Toll-Like Receptors and Cytokines in Pneumococcal Pneumonia

*Hisanori Domon[1,2], Kosuke Nagai[1], Tomoki Maekawa[1,2,3], Masataka Oda[4], Daisuke Yonezawa[1,2,5], Wataru Takeda[6], Takumi Hiyoshi[1,3], Hikaru Tamura[1,2,3], Masaya Yamaguchi[7], Shigetada Kawabata[7] and Yutaka Terao[1,2]**

[1] Division of Microbiology and Infectious Diseases, Niigata University Graduate School of Medical and Dental Sciences, Niigata, Japan, [2] Research Center for Advanced Oral Science, Niigata University Graduate School of Medical and Dental Sciences, Niigata, Japan, [3] Division of Periodontology, Niigata University Graduate School of Medical and Dental Sciences, Niigata, Japan, [4] Department of Microbiology and Infection Control Sciences, Kyoto Pharmaceutical University, Kyoto, Japan, [5] Division of Oral Science for Health Promotion, Niigata University Graduate School of Medical and Dental Sciences, Niigata, Japan, [6] Faculty of Dentistry, Niigata University, Niigata, Japan, [7] Department of Oral and Molecular Microbiology, Osaka University, Graduate School of Dentistry, Osaka, Japan

***Correspondence:**
Yutaka Terao
terao@dent.niigata-u.ac.jp

Excessive activation of neutrophils results in the release of neutrophil elastase (NE), which leads to lung injury in severe pneumonia. Previously, we demonstrated a novel immune subversion mechanism involving microbial exploitation of this NE ability, which eventually promotes disruption of the pulmonary epithelial barrier. In the present study, we investigated the effect of NE on host innate immune response. THP-1-derived macrophages were stimulated with heat-killed *Streptococcus pneumoniae* or lipopolysaccharide in the presence or absence of NE followed by analysis of toll-like receptor (TLR) and cytokine expression. Additionally, the biological significance of NE was confirmed in an *in vivo* mouse intratracheal infection model. NE downregulated the gene transcription of multiple cytokines in THP-1-derived macrophages through the cleavage of TLRs and myeloid differentiation factor 2. Additionally, NE cleaved inflammatory cytokines and chemokines. In a mouse model of intratracheal pneumococcal challenge, administration of an NE inhibitor significantly increased proinflammatory cytokine levels in bronchoalveolar lavage fluid, enhanced bacterial clearance, and improved survival rates. Our work indicates that NE subverts the innate immune response and that inhibition of this enzyme may constitute a novel therapeutic option for the treatment of pneumococcal pneumonia.

Keywords: neutrophil elastase, pneumonia, innate immune response, toll-like receptor, *Streptococcus pneumoniae*, cytokines

INTRODUCTION

Bacterial pneumonia constitutes a leading cause of morbidity and mortality worldwide, being responsible for approximately 3.5 million deaths annually (1). Among all bacteria, *Streptococcus pneumoniae* represents the most common cause of pneumonia in all age groups. Although antibiotics comprise the primary treatment of choice for pneumonia, antimicrobial resistance among *S. pneumoniae*

Abbreviations: BALF, bronchoalveolar lavage fluid; CFU, colony forming units; ELISA, enzyme-linked immunosorbent assay; HK-Spn, heat-killed *S. pneumoniae*; IL, interleukin; LPS, lipopolysaccharide; MD2, myeloid differentiation factor 2; hNE, human neutrophil elastase; PBS, phosphate buffered saline; rh, recombinant human; SSH, sivelestat sodium hydrate; TLR, toll-like receptor; TNF, tumor necrosis factor.

has increased significantly in past decades. Additionally, the total costs of pneumococcal pneumonia reach $2.5 billion per year and are predicted to increase with the growth in the aging population in the United States (2). Therefore, basic research is essential to provide novel therapeutic targets for pneumococcal pneumonia.

Neutrophil elastase (NE) is a serine protease that degrades outer membrane proteins localized on the surface of Gram-negative bacteria and exerts antimicrobial activity (3). Although NE is required for host defense against a wide variety of bacteria, NE also degrades host extracellular-matrix proteins as well as epithelial cadherin, which is a cell–cell adhesion molecule with pivotal roles in epithelial cell behavior and tissue formation, and causes lung epithelial disruption (4, 5). Additionally, NE cleaves various host proteins, such as lung-surfactant proteins (6), vascular endothelial growth factor (7), C1 inhibitor (8), and C5a receptor (9), modulates inflammation, and promotes tissue remodeling. Generally, the proteolytic activity of NE is regulated by α1-antitrypsin, an endogenous NE inhibitor. However, during an acute inflammatory response, macrophages and neutrophils release a variety of proteases, including NE, proteinase 3, matrix metalloproteinases (MMPs), and cathepsins (10). Among these, MMPs, particularly MMP-12, degrade and inactivate α1-antitrypsin, thereby enhancing the activity of NE and causing tissue injury (11). In this regard, it has been reported that NE level is increased in bronchoalveolar lavage fluid (BALF) from patients with severe pneumonia (12). In animal models, intratracheal *S. pneumoniae* infection causes acute lung injury characterized by an increase in neutrophil accumulation and NE activity in BALF (13, 14). Together, these findings indicate that excessive release of NE from neutrophils can damage surrounding tissues and contribute to the lung dysfunction associated with pneumonia.

In order to reduce the excess inflammatory response and lung injury, various inhibitors of NE have been tested in various lung diseases, including severe pneumonia (15). Studies evaluating the effect of NE in the animal model of *Pseudomonas aeruginosa*-induced pneumonia have reported conflicting results. Cantin and Woods reported that the NE inhibitor significantly decreased NE activity and enhanced clearance of bacteria in the lungs (16), whereas Honoré et al. did not obtain positive results (17). In the animal model of pneumococcal pneumonia, NE inhibitor enhanced bacterial clearance and delayed mortality (13, 14). Although there are few descriptive studies of NE inhibitors in humans with bacterial pneumonia, a previous study suggested that early administration of NE inhibitor may improve acute lung injury and survival rate in severe pneumonia (18). Taken together, these findings suggest that not only bacterial pathogens but also NE contribute, at least in part, to the pathological progression of bacterial pneumonia.

We have previously reported that pneumolysin, a pneumococcal pore-forming toxin, induced cell lysis in human neutrophils, leading to the release of NE (19). Subsequently, NE induced the detachment of alveolar epithelial cells, leading to the disruption of pulmonary defenses. NE also impaired phagocytic activity in macrophages *in vitro*. We have also suggested the possibility that NE decreases interleukin (IL)-8 level in the culture supernatant from human alveolar epithelial cells (19). These data suggest that *S. pneumoniae* exploits NE leakage from neutrophils to subvert host innate immune responses. However, the effects of NE on innate immune responses are not fully understood. The main objective of this study was, therefore, to understand how NE inhibits cytokine production from innate immune cells and to determine its roles in a mouse model of pneumococcal pneumonia. Our data presented here demonstrate the immune subversion mechanism of NE, which caused development of pneumococcal bacteremia in experimental pneumonia. Our study thus provides a novel host modulation therapy for pneumonia utilizing an NE-specific inhibitor.

MATERIALS AND METHODS

Mice and Bacteria

Male 10- to 12-week-old BALB/c mice were obtained from Nihon CLEA (Tokyo, Japan). Mice were maintained under standard conditions in accordance with our institutional guidelines. All animal experiments were approved by the Institutional Animal Care and Use Committee of Niigata University (SA00002). *S. pneumoniae* D39 (NCTC 7466) was grown in tryptic soy broth (Becton Dickinson, Franklin Lakes, NJ, USA). For *in vitro* cytokine assays, *S. pneumoniae* D39 was inactivated by heating at 60°C for 1 h.

Cell Line

The monocytic cell line THP-1 was maintained in 25 mM HEPES-buffered RPMI 1640, supplemented with 10% fetal bovine serum, 100 U/mL penicillin, and 100 μg/mL streptomycin (Wako Pure Chemical Industries, Osaka, Japan) at 37°C in 95% air and 5% CO_2. For the experiments, the cells were incubated in a 24-well culture plate at a concentration of 2×10^5 cells/mL in medium supplemented with 200 nM phorbol 12-myristate 13-acetate to induce differentiation into macrophage-like cells, hereafter referred to as macrophages. After 48 h incubation, the cells were washed with RPMI 1640 and cultured further in RPMI 1640 for 12 h. Then, cells were stimulated with heat-killed *S. pneumoniae* (HK-Spn) or *Escherichia coli* lipopolysaccharide (LPS) (100 ng/mL; Sigma-Aldrich, St. Louis, MO, USA) in the presence or absence of human neutrophil elastase (hNE; Innovative Research, Novi, MI, USA) and the NE inhibitor sivelestat (100 μg/mL; ONO Pharmaceutical Co., Osaka, Japan) for 3 h under serum-free conditions.

Quantitative Real-Time PCR

Gene transcription in THP-1-derived macrophages was quantified using quantitative real-time PCR. Briefly, RNA was extracted from cell lysates using TRI Reagent (Molecular Research Center, Inc., Cincinnati, OH, USA) and quantified by spectrometry at 260 and 280 nm. The RNA was reverse transcribed using SuperScript VILO Master Mix (Thermo Fisher Scientific, Waltham, MA, USA), and quantitative real-time PCR with cDNA was performed with the StepOnePlus real-time PCR system (Thermo Fisher Scientific) according to manufacturer protocol. TaqMan probes, sense primers, and antisense primers for expression of *GAPDH*, *TNF*, *IL6*, and *IL8* were purchased from Thermo Fisher Scientific.

Immunofluorescence Analysis

Human neutrophil elastase-treated macrophages stimulated with HK-Spn or LPS were fixed and permeabilized using a cell fixation and permeabilization kit (Thermo Fisher Scientific) according to manufacturer instructions, followed by incubation of the cells in a blocking solution (Thermo Fisher Scientific) for 30 min. Samples were stained with rabbit anti-NF-κB p65 antibody (Santa Cruz Biotechnology, Dallas, TX, USA), anti-toll-like receptor (TLR) 2 antibody (clone TL2.1; Thermo Fisher Scientific), or anti-TLR4 antibody (clone HTA125; Thermo Fisher Scientific) in blocking solution. After overnight incubation at 4°C, secondary AlexaFluor 594-conjugated goat anti-rabbit IgG antibody or AlexaFluor 488-conjugated goat anti-mouse IgG antibody (Thermo Fisher Scientific) in blocking buffer was added, followed by a 2-h incubation in the dark. Then, samples were observed using a confocal laser-scanning microscope (Carl Zeiss, Jena, Germany). In addition, samples were observed with fluorescence microscopy using Hybrid cell-count software (Keyence, Osaka, Japan) to calculate fluorescence intensity per cell.

Western Blot Analysis

Whole cell lysates were prepared in 100 μL of lysis reagent (Thermo Fisher Scientific). For recombinant proteins cleavage assay, 100 ng of recombinant human (rh) TLR2 (R&D Systems, Minneapolis, MN, USA), rhTLR4 (R&D Systems), rh-myeloid differentiation factor 2 (MD2) (Abcam, Cambridge, UK), rh-tumor necrosis factor (TNF) (R&D Systems), rhIL-6 (PeproTech, Rocky Hill, NJ, USA), or rhIL-8 (R&D Systems) was treated with various concentrations of hNE (125–500 mU/mL) in the presence or absence of the NE inhibitor sivelestat (100 μg/mL) at 37°C for 3 h and mixed with 2% SDS-sample buffer. All samples were separated by SDS-PAGE and transferred to polyvinylidene difluoride membranes (Merck Millipore, Billerica, MA, USA) followed by incubation with blocking reagent (Nacalai Tesque, Kyoto, Japan). The membrane was probed with an anti-TLR2 antibody (Rockland Immunochemicals, Limerick, PA, USA), anti-TLR4 antibody (Novus Biologicals, Littleton, CO, USA), anti-MD2 antibody (Abcam), anti-NF-κB antibody (Santa Cruz Biotechnology), anti-GAPDH antibody (Abcam), anti-TNF antibody (Cell Signaling Technology, Beverly, MA, USA), anti-IL-6-antibody (Abcam), or anti-IL-8 antibody (R&D Systems) and then incubated with a HRP-conjugated secondary antibody (Cell Signaling Technology) in Tris-buffered saline containing 0.05% tween 20. The membrane was treated with HRP substrates (GE Healthcare, Chicago, IL, USA) and analyzed using a chemiluminescence detector (Fujifilm, Tokyo, Japan).

Cytokine Assay

The levels of TNF, IL-6, and IL-8 in the cell culture supernatants were determined by using enzyme-linked immunosorbent assay (ELISA) kits (BioLegend, San Diego, CA, USA).

Bead-Based Multiplex Assay for Cytokines

Comprehensive hNE-induced cytokine cleavage assays were performed using the MILLIPLEX MAP human cytokine/chemokine magnetic bead panel (Merck Millipore) by determining 18 cytokine concentrations (G-CSF, GM-CSF, IFNα2, IFN-γ, IL-10, IL12p40, IL-12p70, IL-17, IL-1β, IL-2, IL-3, IL-4, IL-6, IL-8, MCP-1, MIP1α, MIP1β, and TNF). Human cytokine/chemokine cocktail (Merck Millipore) was treated with various concentrations of hNE (125–500 mU/mL) in the presence or absence of the NE inhibitor sivelestat (100 μg/mL) at 37°C for 3 h followed by addition of sivelestat (100 μg/mL; final concentration) to inactivate hNE. These samples were assayed according to the manufacturer's instructions. Briefly, standards, controls, and samples were loaded into 96-well plates, followed by addition of antibody-immobilized beads. Plates were incubated for 2 h on a plate shaker and then washed twice with wash buffer. Detection antibodies were then added to the wells and incubated for 1 h. Finally, streptavidin-phycoerythrin was added to the wells and incubated for 30 min. Plates were gently washed twice with wash buffer before resuspending the beads in sheath fluid followed by analysis on a Luminex 200 (Merck Millipore). Using xPONENT software version 3.1 (Luminex Corporation, Austin, TX, USA), a standard curve was generated using a 5-parameter logistic curve for each mediator ranging from 10,000 to 3.2 pg/mL, and then cytokine concentrations were calculated.

Intratracheal Infection of Pneumococcus *In Vivo*

Following mouse anesthesia with isoflurane using an inhalational anesthesia system (Natsume Seisakusho, Tokyo, Japan), the trachea was aseptically exposed and an *S. pneumoniae* inoculum [2×10^8 colony forming units (CFUs) in 50 μL phosphate buffered saline (PBS)] was administered *via* a 26-gauge needle (20). Unchallenged naïve mice were administered PBS only. NE inhibitor (40 mg/kg) or PBS was administered intraperitoneally to the infected mice every 6 h. Groups of animals were sacrificed at 18 h postinfection. To obtain BALF, 1.0 mL PBS was instilled into mouse lungs and then slowly aspirated. BALF samples were then plated onto blood-agar plates and cultured aerobically for enumerating recovered CFU. To determine NE activity, cytokine levels, and recruitment of inflammatory cells, BALF was centrifuged at 500 *g*, and the supernatant was used for subsequent NE activity assay and cytokine analysis. The cell pellet was analyzed for total leukocyte count using Turk's solution (Nacalai Tesque). NE activity in BALF was determined by a method using the NE-specific substrate *N*-methoxysuccinyl-Ala-Ala-Pro-Val *p*-nitroanilide (Merck Millipore) as described elsewhere (14). Briefly, samples were incubated in 0.1 M Tris-HCl buffer (PH 8.0) containing 0.5 M NaCl and 1 mM substrate at 37°C for 24 h, and then absorbance at 405 nm was measured. The levels of TNF and IL-6 in BALF and serum were determined by using ELISA kits (BioLegend). To determine the concentration of pneumococcal DNA, DNA was isolated from 50 μL of serum from the infected mice using QIAamp Spin Columns (QIAGEN, Hilden, Germany). Then, absolute quantification by real-time PCR was performed using the StepOnePlus real-time PCR system *via* the SYBR Green detection protocol. The primers used for real-time PCR were based on published sequence (21). The forward primer oligonucleotide sequence was

5′-AGCGATAGCTTTCTCCAAGTGG-3′ and the reverse primer sequence was 5′-CTTAGCCAACAAATCGTTTACCG-3′.

To determine the effect of the NE inhibitor on the mouse pneumococcal pneumonia model, mice were intratracheally infected with *S. pneumoniae* (5×10^8 CFU in 50 μL PBS), and then the NE inhibitor (40 mg/kg) or PBS was administered intraperitoneally to these mice every 6 h. Survival was monitored following the treatments.

Statistical Analysis

Data were analyzed statistically by analysis of variance with Tukey's multiple-comparison test. Where appropriate (comparison of two groups only), unpaired *t* tests were conducted. The Kaplan–Meier survival curve was analyzed using the log-rank test equivalent to the Mantel–Haenszel test. All statistical analyses were performed using Graph Pad Prism Software version 6.05 (GraphPad Software, Inc., La Jolla, CA, USA). Values of $P < 0.05$ were considered significant.

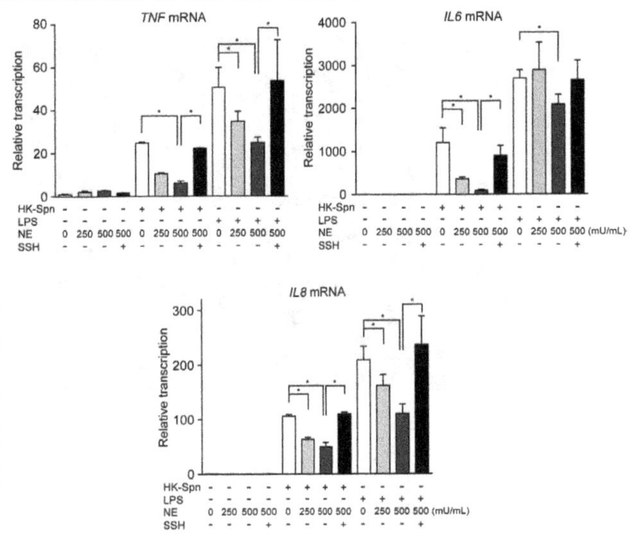

FIGURE 1 | Neutrophil elastase (NE) downregulates cytokine gene transcription in macrophages stimulated with TLR agonists. THP-1-derived macrophages were stimulated with HK-Spn D39 or *Escherichia coli* LPS (100 ng/mL) in the presence or absence of hNE (250–500 mU/mL) and/or SSH (100 μg/mL) for 4 h under serum-free conditions. Real-time PCR was performed to quantify *TNF*, *IL6*, and *IL8* mRNA in the macrophages exposed to these stimuli. The relative quantity of these cytokine mRNAs was normalized to the relative quantity of *GAPDH* mRNA. Data represent the mean ± SD of quadruplicate experiments and were evaluated using one-way analysis of variance with Tukey's multiple-comparisons test. *Significantly different within the same activation status at $P < 0.05$. HK-Spn, heat-killed *S. pneumoniae*; LPS, lipopolysaccharide; hNE, human neutrophil elastase; SSH, sivelestat sodium hydrate; TLR, toll-like receptor; TNF, tumor necrosis factor.

RESULTS

NE Downregulates Cytokine Gene Transcription in Macrophages by Inhibiting NF-κB Nuclear Translocation

We first investigated whether hNE affects cytokine gene transcription in macrophages. Accordingly, macrophages were stimulated with HK-Spn and LPS, which are recognized by TLR2 (22) and TLR4 (23), respectively, in the presence or absence of hNE. Strikingly, hNE significantly and dose-dependently reduced HK-Spn- and LPS-induced *TNF*, *IL6*, and *IL8* gene transcription in the macrophages, with the exception of *TNF* and *IL6* in the cells treated with 250 mU/mL hNE (**Figure 1**). Furthermore, downregulation of these cytokines in hNE-treated macrophages was counteracted by the administration of sivelestat. hNE did not show cytotoxicity toward macrophages up to 500 mU/mL (Figure S1 in Supplementary Material). As hNE downregulated the transcription of various cytokine genes, we hypothesized that hNE inhibits TLR signaling in the macrophages. Therefore, we next examined whether hNE could inhibit NF-κB nuclear translocation in the macrophages stimulated with HK-Spn or LPS. Although HK-Spn and LPS-induced NF-κB activation and subsequent nuclear translocation, 500 mU/mL hNE significantly inhibited the latter (**Figures 2A,B**), suggesting that hNE-induced inhibition of TLR signaling can downregulate cytokine gene transcription.

NE Cleaves TLRs and MD2 on Macrophages

It has been reported that NE mediates intracellular signaling through proteinase-activated receptor (PAR)-1 or PAR-2 (24, 25). These findings prompted us to further examine whether NE-dependent activation of these receptors is involved in the downregulation of cytokine gene transcription. However, neither a PAR-1 antagonist (SCH79797) nor PAR-2 antagonist (FSLLRY-NE2) could counteract the downregulation of *TNF* gene transcription in the hNE-treated macrophages (Figure S2 in Supplementary Material), indicating that the effect of hNE is not mediated by PARs. Given that NE can cleave some cell-surface receptors, such as urokinase receptor and C5a receptor (9, 26), we investigated whether hNE cleaves TLRs. Indeed, hNE decreased the protein expression of TLR2, TLR4, and MD2 in hNE-treated macrophages (**Figures 3A,B**). Moreover, we observed that rhTLR2, rhTLR4, and rhMD2 were cleaved by hNE after 3 h of coincubation (**Figure 3C**). Taken together, our findings indicate that hNE inhibits TLR signaling by cleaving TLRs and MD2.

NE Also Cleaves Various Proinflammatory Cytokines *In Vitro*

To confirm hNE-induced inhibition of TLR signaling, we measured *in vitro* cytokine levels (TNF, IL-6, and IL-8) in culture supernatants of HK-Spn- or LPS-stimulated macrophages in the presence of absence of hNE. Consistent with the repression of cytokine gene transcription, treatment of the macrophages with hNE resulted in marked reduction of these cytokine levels in the supernatant (**Figure 4A**). Among these, IL-6 levels were almost completely abolished in the supernatant of hNE-treated macrophages stimulated with HK-Spn. We thus speculated that hNE cleaves not only TLRs but also proinflammatory cytokines. To test this, rhTNF, rhIL-6, and rhIL-8 were treated

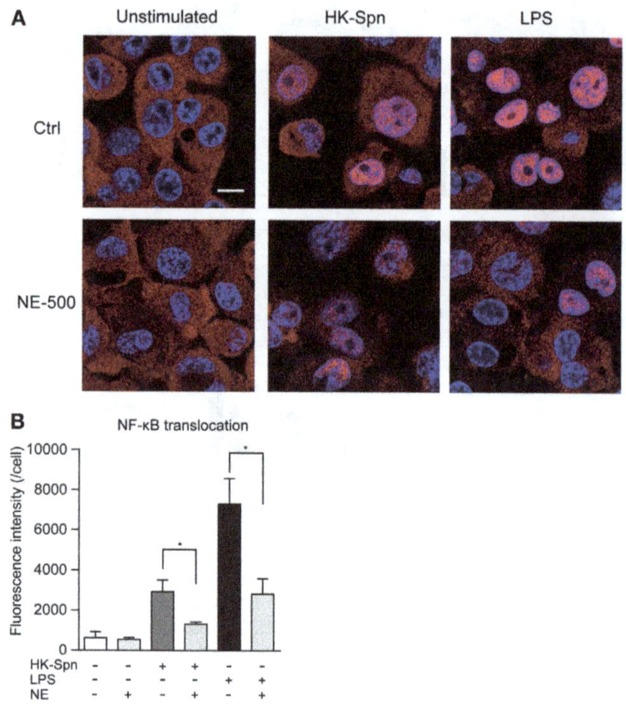

FIGURE 2 | Neutrophil elastase (NE) inhibits NF-κB translocation to the nucleus in macrophages. THP-1-derived macrophages were exposed to hNE (500 mU/mL) in the presence or absence of HK-Spn or LPS (100 ng/mL) for 30 min. **(A)** Representative fluorescence microscopy images of macrophages stained for DNA (DAPI; blue) and NF-κB p65 (red). Scale bar: 10 μm. **(B)** The fluorescence intensity of NF-κB p65 in the nucleus per cell was calculated. Data represent the mean ± SD of quadruplicate experiments and were evaluated using one-way analysis of variance with Tukey's multiple-comparisons test. *Significantly different within the same activation status at $P < 0.05$. HK-Spn, heat-killed *S. pneumoniae*; LPS, lipopolysaccharide; hNE, human neutrophil elastase.

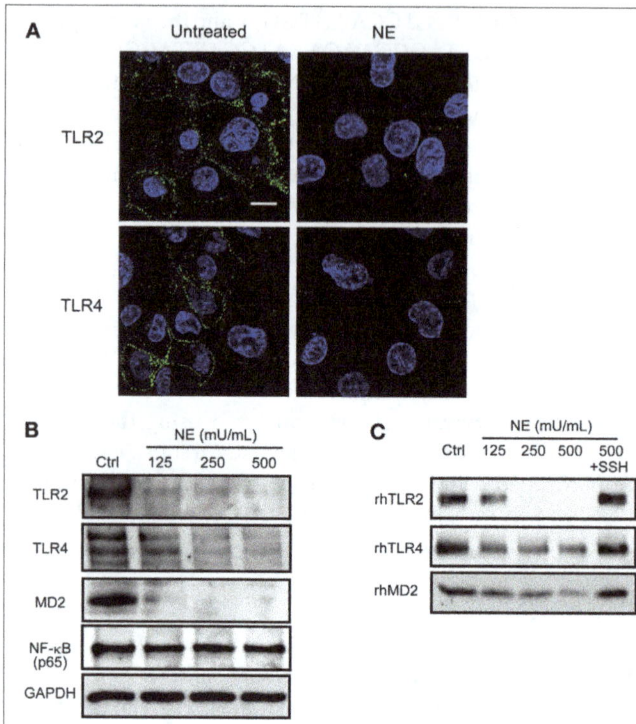

FIGURE 3 | Neutrophil elastase (NE) cleaves TLRs and MD2 on macrophages. **(A,B)** THP-1-derived macrophages were cultured in serum free RPMI 1640 and exposed to hNE (125–500 mU/mL) for 4 h. **(A)** Representative fluorescence microscopy images of untreated and hNE-treated (500 mU/mL) macrophages stained for DNA (DAPI; blue) and TLRs (green). **(B)** TLR2, TLR4, and TLR-related molecules were determined by western blot analysis. **(C)** Recombinant human (rh) TLR2, rhTLR4, and rhMD2 were exposed to hNE (125–500 mU/mL) in the presence or absence of SSH (100 μg/mL) for 3 h and determined by western blot analysis. MD2, myeloid differentiation factor 2; hNE, human neutrophil elastase; SSH, sivelestat sodium hydrate; TLR, toll-like receptor.

with varying concentrations of hNE in the presence or absence of sivelestat. **Figure 4B** shows that hNE cleaved these cytokines, whereas this effect was counteracted by sivelestat. Additionally, rhTNF and rhIL-6 that had been treated by hNE exhibited lower-molecular-mass fragments. We next evaluated the effect of hNE on the cytokine levels in the supernatant from mouse peritoneal macrophages infected with *S. pneumoniae*. Figure S3 in Supplementary Material shows that hNE treatment almost completely obliterated mouse IL-6 in the supernatant, which is consistent with the results shown in **Figure 4A**, whereas hNE treatment did not decrease mouse TNF levels. These findings suggest the possibility that mouse proteins show different sensitivity to hNE-induced proteolysis as compared with human proteins.

Although the role of cytokines in pneumonia is not fully understood, various cytokines may be involved in innate and acquired pulmonary defense (1). Therefore, we comprehensively investigated the cleavage activity of hNE on 18 cytokines. Of these, 17 cytokine levels were significantly decreased by hNE treatment but showed different susceptibility to hNE (**Figure 5**). For example, IL-17 level was decreased by 20% in 500 mU/mL hNE, whereas G-CSF, IL-12p70, MIP-1α, and MIP-1β levels were almost abolished by 125 mU/mL hNE. Conversely, IL-10 was not significantly affected by hNE. These findings suggest that hNE cleaves a variety of cytokines and may subvert host immune responses during lung infections.

In contrast to our findings, it has been reported that NE treatment itself induces *IL8* gene transcription and protein release in alveolar epithelial cells and bronchial epithelial cells in the culture medium containing 10% fetal bovine serum (27, 28); however, 125 mU/mL hNE treatment did not result in an increase in IL-8 protein levels in the supernatant of A549 alveolar epithelial cells under serum-free conditions (Figure S4A in Supplementary Material). Higher concentrations (>100 mU/mL) of hNE induced the detachment of A549 cells as described previously (19). The catalytic function of NE is blocked by serum α1-antitrypsin (29); therefore, we treated A549 cells with hNE under serum-containing conditions. Figure S4B in Supplementary Material shows that treatment with excessive concentrations (2,000–5,000 mU/mL) of hNE significantly increased IL-8 protein levels under serum-containing conditions, whereas treatment with 500–1,000 mU/mL hNE did not.

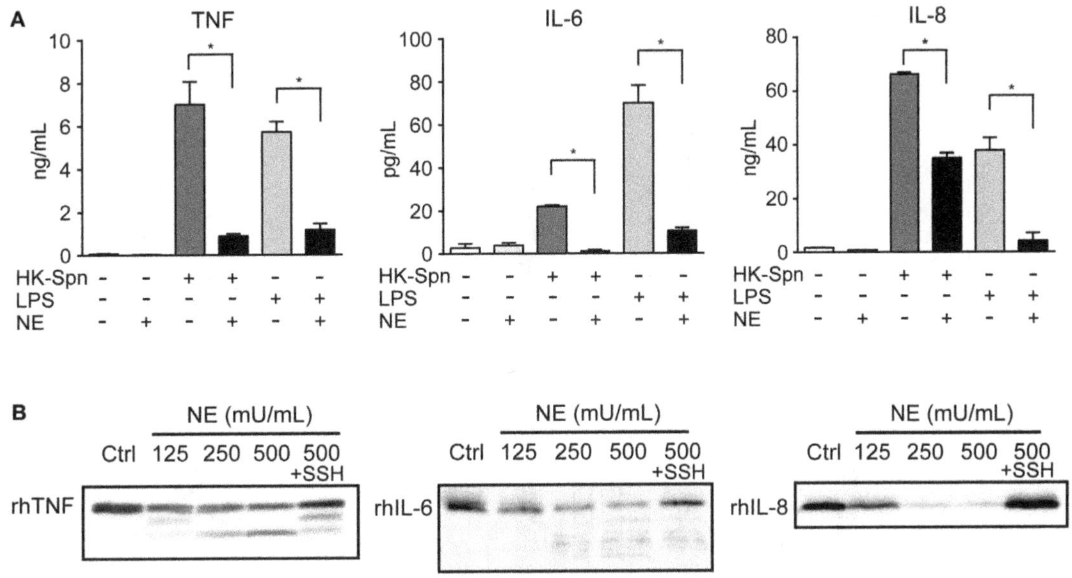

FIGURE 4 | Neutrophil elastase (NE) degrades TNF, IL-6, and IL-8 **(A)**. THP-1-derived macrophages were exposed to hNE (125–500 mU/mL) in the presence or absence of HK-Spn or LPS (100 ng/mL) for 4 h. TNF, IL-6, and IL-8 concentrations in the culture supernatants were determined by ELISA. Data represent the mean ± SD of quadruplicate experiments and were evaluated using one-way analysis of variance with Tukey's multiple-comparisons test. *Significantly different within the same activation status at $P < 0.05$. **(B)** rhTNF, rhIL-6, and rhIL-8 were exposed to hNE (125–500 mU/mL) in the presence or absence of SSH (100 μg/mL) for 3 h and determined by western blot analysis. ELISA, enzyme-linked immunosorbent assay; HK-Spn, heat-killed *S. pneumoniae*; LPS, lipopolysaccharide; hNE, human neutrophil elastase; rh, recombinant human; SSH, sivelestat sodium hydrate; IL, interleukin; TNF, tumor necrosis factor.

Administration of an NE Inhibitor Increased BALF Cytokine Level and Decreased Bacterial Load *In Vivo*

To confirm whether NE alters cytokine homeostasis and induces immune subversion *in vivo*, we investigated the effect of NE in mice after intratracheal infection with pneumococcus, in the presence or absence of sivelestat. First, we confirmed that sivelestat does not possess direct antimicrobial activity against *S. pneumoniae* (Figure S5 in Supplementary Material). Although pulmonary infection causes the infiltration of neutrophils and serum proteins, including α1-antitrypsin, into lungs (30), NE activity was significantly elevated in BALF from sivelestat-untreated mouse compared with uninfected mouse (sham) at 18 h postinfection (average: 431.6 vs. 2.6 mU/mL; Figure S6A in Supplementary Material). This data suggests that increased IL-8 protein levels in the supernatant due to ≥2,000 mU/mL hNE-treated cells under the serum-containing condition *in vitro* likely does not reflect the *in vivo* status. Figure S6A in Supplementary Material also shows that BALF from sivelestat-treated mice contained significantly lower NE activity compared to that of untreated control mice (>65% reduction). In addition, sivelestat treatment significantly decreased pneumococcal CFU in BALF (>65% reduction; **Figure 6A**). By contrast, IL-6 and TNF levels were significantly higher in sivelestat-treated BALF (**Figure 6B**). These data suggest that NE-dependent cleavage of these cytokines was inhibited following treatment with sivelestat, resulting in the apparent increase in the BALF cytokine level. Sivelestat treatment did not affect the number of leukocytes in BALF (Figure S6B in Supplementary Material). Although hNE reduced cytokine gene transcription in the macrophages *in vitro*, the *Il6* and *Tnf* gene transcription levels in whole lung samples appeared similar between untreated and sivelestat-treated mice (Figure S6C in Supplementary Material); this observation could be attributed to the higher bacterial loads in untreated control mice. These data indicate that decreased proinflammatory cytokine levels in sivelestat-untreated mice were mainly attributed to the NE-dependent cleavage of cytokines in this mouse model.

A recent human study demonstrated that serum IL-6 and TNF levels are associated with early mortality of patients with pneumonia (31). Therefore, we next investigated whether higher IL-6 and TNF levels in BALF from sivelestat-treated mice are correlated with these cytokine levels in serum samples. However, IL-6 and TNF levels were significantly lower in the serum from sivelestat-treated mice (**Figure 6C**). The significantly higher serum cytokine levels in untreated control mice, which contradicts the NE-induced lower cytokine levels in BALF, is partly explained by the α1-antitrypsin-mediated blockade of NE activity in serum. Additionally, the untreated control mice were found to be bacteremic for *S. pneumoniae* (pneumococcal DNA detection in four out of seven blood samples in this group), whereas lower prevalence of bacteremia (one out of seven blood samples) could be detected in the sivelestat-treated group. Serum pneumococcal DNA concentration correlated directly with serum IL-6 ($r = 0.82$, $P < 0.001$) and TNF ($r = 0.88$, $P < 0.001$) levels after inoculation with *S. pneumoniae* (Figure S6D in Supplementary Material). These data suggest that pneumococcal bacteremia induced increases in serum cytokine levels in untreated control mice. **Figure 6D** illustrates the cumulative survival of mice after intratracheal infection. The mortality of sivelestat-treated mice

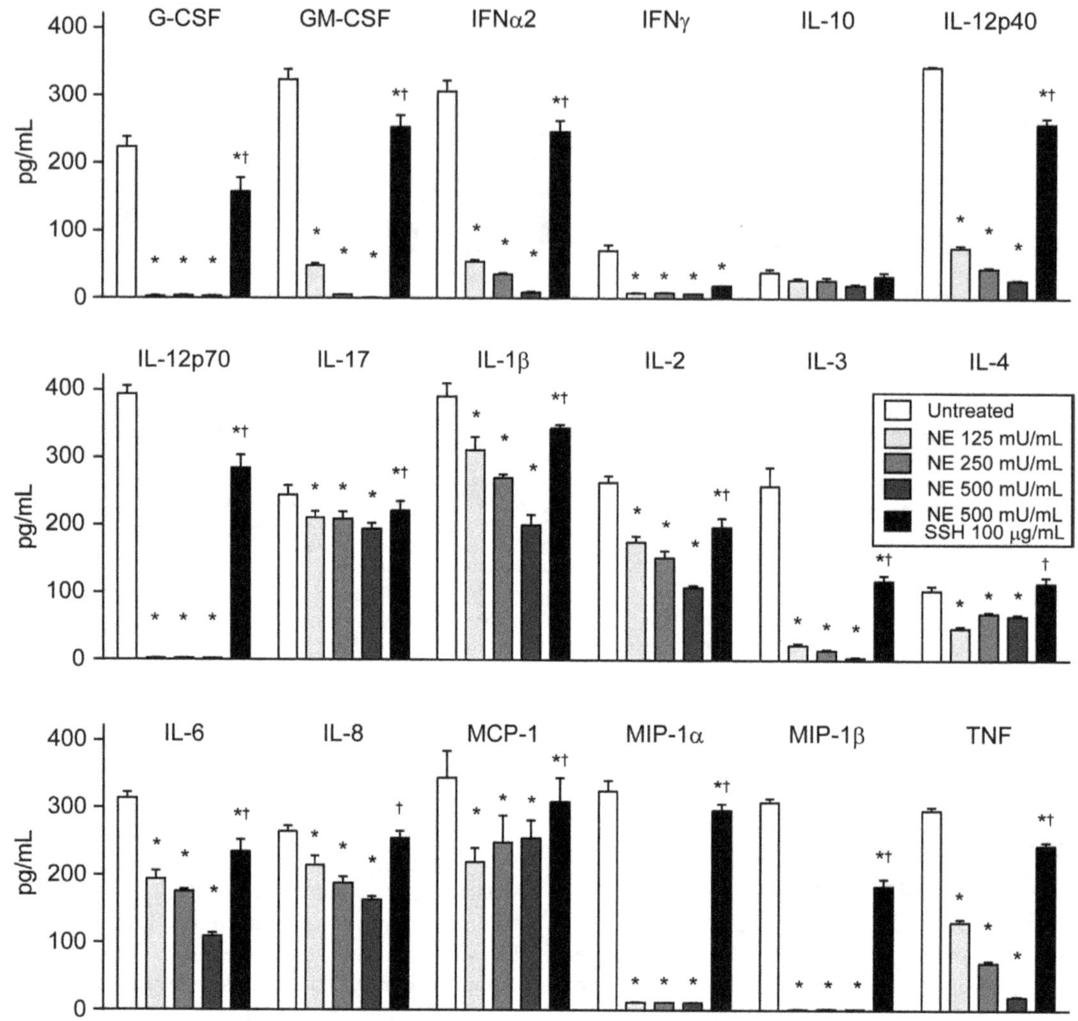

FIGURE 5 | Multiplex assay reveals that neutrophil elastase (NE) degrades various cytokines. Human cytokine/chemokine cocktail was exposed to hNE (125–500 mU/mL) in the presence or absence of SSH (100 μg/mL) for 3 h. Then, cytokines were detected using a multiplex assay. Data represent the mean ± SD of quadruplicate experiments and were evaluated using two-way ANOVA. *Significantly different from the hNE-untreated control at $P < 0.05$. †Significantly different from the hNE-treated (500 mU/mL) group in the absence of SSH at $P < 0.05$. hNE, human neutrophil elastase; SSH, sivelestat sodium hydrate.

inoculated with *S. pneumoniae* was significantly lower than that of untreated control mice ($P = 0.001$); in particular, 90% (18/20) of the untreated mice died by 4 days after infection, whereas 55% (11/20) of sivelestat-treated mice dead within 5 days of infection. These *in vivo* findings demonstrate that the subversion of host immune responses by NE causes bacterial invasion of the bloodstream followed by death.

DISCUSSION

Innate immune defenses are primarily responsible for the clearance of foreign particles deposited on the surface of airways and elimination of bacterial pathogens from the alveolus (32). The development of pneumonia indicates a defect in host defense, exposure to an overwhelming inoculum of virulent microorganism, or a combination of these factors (33). Here, we addressed the intriguing possibility that at least some of the innate immune receptors, such as TLR2 and TLR4, were cleaved by NE, which was originally identified as a powerful host defense component, leading to the inhibition of downstream signaling pathways followed by downregulation of cytokine gene transcription (**Figure 7**). Furthermore, NE also cleaves various cytokines secreted from macrophages in response to TLR agonists and leads to the impairment of host innate immune defenses and death. The pneumococcal intracellular toxin, pneumolysin, constitutes such an NE-inducing factor through its ability to promote pore formation in the neutrophilic plasma membrane (19). Together, these observations indicate that pneumococcus exploits NE as an etiological agent during pneumonia.

Toll-like receptors are key molecules that recognize pathogen-associated molecular patterns and induce an inflammatory response (23). Among these, TLR2 and TLR4 are thought to be critical in bacterial infections and have been studied in pneumococcal pneumonia. Although TLR2, which recognizes various pathogen-associated

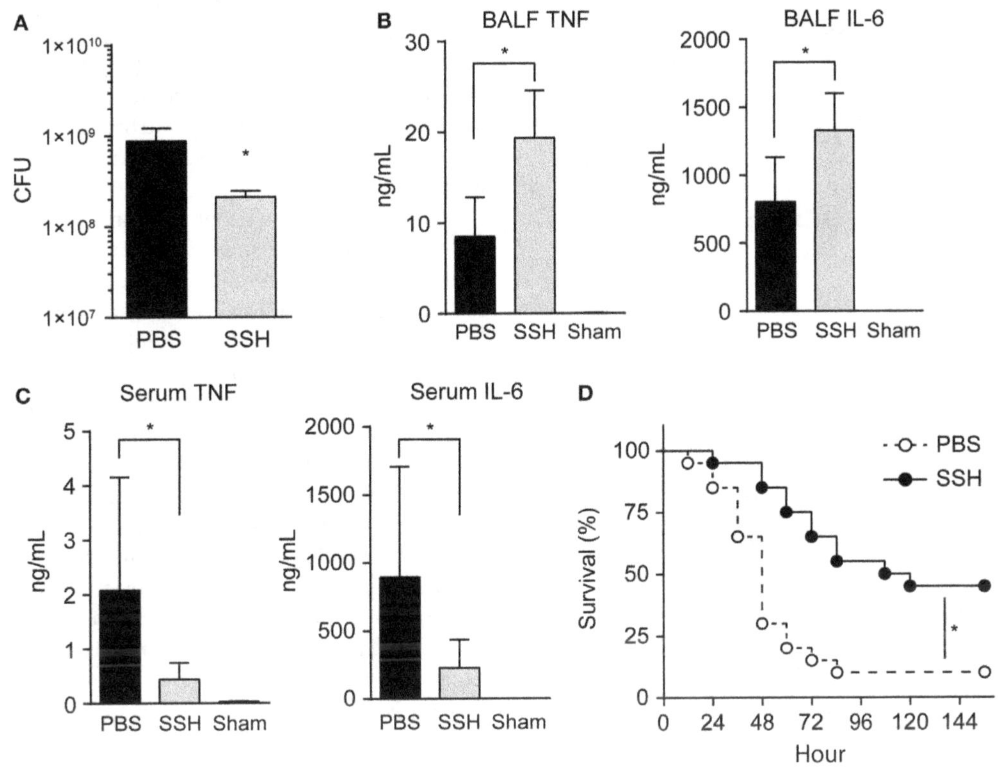

FIGURE 6 | Administration of NE inhibitor increases cytokine level and decreases bacterial load in BALF. BALB/c mice (seven mice each) were intratracheally infected with *Streptococcus pneumoniae* D39 (2 × 10^8 CFU in 50 µL PBS). Unchallenged naive mice (Sham group) were administered PBS only. NE inhibitor (SSH group; 50 mg/kg) or PBS (PBS group) was administrated intraperitoneally to the infected mice every 6 h. **(A–C)** Groups of animals were sacrificed at 18 h postinfection. **(A)** BALF samples were plated onto blood-agar plates and cultured aerobically for enumerating recovered CFU. Data represent the mean ± SD and were evaluated using unpaired *t* tests. *Significantly different from the infected control group at $P < 0.05$. **(B)** The levels of TNF and IL-6 in BALF were determined by using ELISA kits. **(C)** Serum TNF and IL-6 levels were determined. **(B,C)** Data represent the mean ± SD and were evaluated using one-way analysis of variance with Tukey's multiple-comparisons test. *Significantly different from the infected control group at $P < 0.05$. **(D)** Survival of BALB/c (twenty mice each) mice was monitored following the intratracheal infection with *S. pneumoniae* (5 × 10^8 CFU) in the presence or absence of intraperitoneal administration of an NE inhibitor. Statistical analysis was performed with log-rank test. *Significantly different from the SSH-untreated control at $P < 0.001$. BALF, bronchoalveolar lavage fluid; CFUs, colony forming units; ELISA, enzyme-linked immunosorbent assay; NE, neutrophil elastase; PBS, phosphate buffered saline; SSH, sivelestat sodium hydrate; IL, interleukin; TNF, tumor necrosis factor.

molecular patterns of Gram-positive microbes, plays a limited role in the survival of a mouse pneumococcal pneumoniae model, the responsiveness of alveolar macrophages against *S. pneumoniae* depends on the presence of TLR2 (34). In addition to LPS of Gram-negative bacteria, pneumococcal pneumolysin is also considered to be a TLR4 ligand (35). Accordingly, TLR4-deficient mice showed impaired antibacterial defense against *S. pneumoniae* and reduced survival (36). In a human study, genetic variability in the *TLR4* gene was associated with an increased risk of developing invasive disease in patients infected with *S. pneumoniae* (37). These findings indicate that TLR2, TLR4, or a combination of these receptors play an essential role in pneumococcal pneumonia; thus, it is consistent that cleavage of these receptors by NE results in impaired immune responses and decreased survival for pneumococcal infections.

Several studies have demonstrated the importance of proinflammatory cytokines in host defense during pneumonia and other infectious diseases. TNF activates phagocytosis, oxidative burst, and bacterial killing (38). Our previous findings of NE-induced impairment of phagocytosis in macrophages (19) suggest that the NE-dependent cleavage of TNF and other cytokines observed in the present study may mediate the reduction of phagocytic activity, which leads to the increment of bacterial load in the lungs of NE inhibitor-untreated mice. Consistent with this, it has been reported that treatment with neutralizing anti-TNF monoclonal antibody resulted in an enhanced outgrowth of *S. pneumoniae* in the lungs and blood, along with significantly earlier death in mice with pneumococcal pneumonia as compared with control mice (39). Moreover, IL-6 and IFN-γ knockout mice showed impaired defense against pneumococcal pneumonia and demonstrated higher mortality (40, 41). Chemokines, such as KC, MCP-1, and MIP-1α, contribute to pulmonary neutrophil recruitment and macrophage infiltration (42). G-CSF- and GM-CSF-treated mice showed improved lung clearance of pneumococci, suggesting the protective role of these cytokines in pneumonia (43, 44). Although cytokine and chemokine networks in pneumococcal pneumonia are highly complex and not fully understood, NE-induced dysregulation of these networks may cause the disruption of pulmonary homeostasis, which leads to bacterial growth in the lungs thereby potentially causing death.

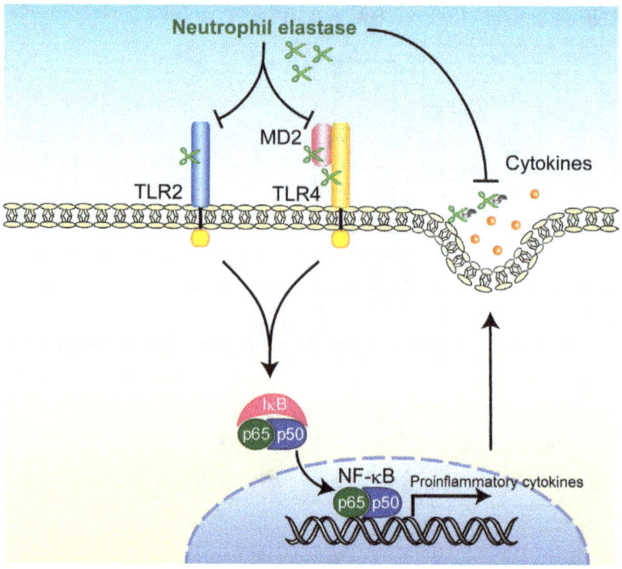

FIGURE 7 | Summary of neutrophil elastase-induced suppression of toll-like receptor (TLR) signaling. Human neutrophil elastase (hNE) degrades TLRs and myeloid differentiation factor 2 (MD2) followed by inhibition of downstream signaling pathways including NF-κB activation, which subsequently downregulates cytokine gene transcription. hNE also degrades secreted cytokines and eventually impairs the host innate immune response.

Neutrophil elastase has been recognized as a double-edged sword of innate immunity as it can act as both a host defensive and tissue destructive factor (13). Although NE plays an important role in intracellular pneumococcal killing by neutrophils (45), leakage of NE into the extracellular space promotes lung injury without killing the pneumococcal cells (19). In recent years, several experimental NE inhibitors, including sivelestat with low cellular permeability, have been tested in animal studies of pneumococcal pneumonia, with positive results (15). However, the mechanisms by which NE inhibitors improve survival rates in animal pneumonia models were not fully understood. One possible mechanism was that the NE inhibitor blocks NE-induced disruption of pulmonary epithelial cells and prevents bacterial invasion into bloodstream (14, 19). However, this alone cannot explain how an NE inhibitor enhanced clearance of pneumococci in the lung in this and previous studies (13). Our findings suggest that the NE inhibitor abolishes the effect of extracellular NE and subversion of the host innate immune response without impairing intracellular pneumococcal killing. Accordingly, we observed lower serum cytokine levels associated with decreased prevalence of bacteremia in sivelestat-treated mice as compared with untreated control mice.

In the present study, 40 mg/kg sivelestat were intraperitoneally administered to mice every 6 h, resulting in significantly decreased NE activity in BALF and markedly reduced mortality of mice inoculated with *S. pneumoniae* compared with untreated control mice. Yanagihara et al. demonstrated that administration of sivelestat (30 mg/mL per 12 h) resulted in moderately delayed mortality in pneumococcal pneumonia mouse model (14), whereas Mikumo et al. reported that administration of 150 mg/kg/day of sivelestat ameliorates pneumonitis and that there is significant improvement in the survival of mice administered naphthalene and gefinitib (46). Higher dose or increased frequency of administration could have effectively blocked NE activity in the present study. Further investigation is required to evaluate the optimal dose and frequency of administration of sivelestat.

Reportedly, NE-deficient mice in a model of *P. aeruginosa*-induced pneumonia showed that the absence of NE significantly increased bacterial CFU in BALF, which is caused by NE-mediated killing of Gram-negative bacteria by neutrophils in wild-type mice (47). Consistent with our findings, the same group also demonstrated the possibility of NE-dependent cleavage of TLR4 protein in wild-type mice (48). These data led us to predict the elevation of inflammatory cytokines in the BALF from the pneumonia model of NE-deficient mice. However, NE deficiency was associated with decreased levels of proinflammatory cytokines, such as TNF and IL-6, in BALF, which is inconsistent with our findings (48). This discrepancy may be caused by *P. aeruginosa*-induced proteolytic inactivation of these cytokines. *P. aeruginosa* possesses several proteases, including alkaline protease, elastase A, elastase B, and protease IV, that have been isolated and shown to be involved in pathogenesis. Additionally, *P. aeruginosa* produces two other proteases: modified elastase and *P. aeruginosa* small protease (49). Of these proteases, the cytokine degradation activities of alkaline protease and elastase B were reported (50). Although the *P. aeruginosa* strain 103, which was inoculated into NE-deficient mouse (47), is a low-protease-producing strain (51), it is possible that increased bacterial loads in the lungs of NE-deficient mice resulted in the elevation of local protease activity responsible for the degradation of host cytokines.

Although numerous studies have focused on the biological functions of hNE, little is known about how mouse NE acts *in vitro*. Although we demonstrated that hNE cleaved human TLRs and TNF, hNE did not significantly decrease mouse TNF levels *in vitro*. In an *in vivo* mouse intratracheal infection model, specific inhibition of NE by sivelestat significantly upregulated BALF TNF levels, suggesting that mouse NE cleaves mouse TNF. These results suggest that the peptide substrate specificities of human and mouse NE are different despite their conserved catalytic triad and close structural resemblance (52). In this regard, it has been reported that mouse and human NE may generate different peptide profiles from a common substrate (53). Therefore, there are limitations in the use of mouse models for studying NE pathogenesis for understanding human disease.

To our knowledge, this is the first study that has comprehensively examined the impact of NE on host innate immune receptors and cytokines. The NE inhibitor restored alveolar homeostasis and induced intrinsic innate immune responses during pneumococcal pneumonia. From a therapeutic viewpoint and in addition to antibiotic use, novel strategies for pneumonia treatment might include restraint of excessive neutrophil infiltration or NE-specific inhibition (13, 15, 54). Our findings further suggested that the evolutionary progression of pneumococcus has allowed the bacterium to exploit host molecules for developing severe pneumonia.

AUTHOR CONTRIBUTIONS

HD and YT designed the study. HD, TM, KN, TH, HT, and WT performed all of the experiments. HD, MO, DY, MY, and SK analyzed the data. MY and SK prepared the materials. HD and YT wrote the paper. All authors discussed the results and approved the manuscript.

ACKNOWLEDGMENTS

We thank Ms. Chisato Jimbo (Niigata University, Niigata, Japan) for providing technical assistance.

REFERENCES

1. Rendon A, Rendon-Ramirez EJ, Rosas-Taraco AG. Relevant cytokines in the management of community-acquired pneumonia. *Curr Infect Dis Rep* (2016) 18(3):10. doi:10.1007/s11908-016-0516-y
2. Wroe PC, Finkelstein JA, Ray GT, Linder JA, Johnson KM, Rifas-Shiman S, et al. Aging population and future burden of pneumococcal pneumonia in the United States. *J Infect Dis* (2012) 205(10):1589–92. doi:10.1093/infdis/jis240
3. Belaaouaj A, Kim KS, Shapiro SD. Degradation of outer membrane protein A in *Escherichia coli* killing by neutrophil elastase. *Science* (2000) 289(5482):1185–8. doi:10.1126/science.289.5482.1185
4. Chua F, Laurent GJ. Neutrophil elastase: mediator of extracellular matrix destruction and accumulation. *Proc Am Thorac Soc* (2006) 3(5):424–7. doi:10.1513/pats.200603-078AW
5. Boxio R, Wartelle J, Nawrocki-Raby B, Lagrange B, Malleret L, Hirche T, et al. Neutrophil elastase cleaves epithelial cadherin in acutely injured lung epithelium. *Respir Res* (2016) 17(1):129. doi:10.1186/s12931-016-0449-x
6. Hirche TO, Crouch EC, Espinola M, Brokelman TJ, Mecham RP, DeSilva N, et al. Neutrophil serine proteinases inactivate surfactant protein D by cleaving within a conserved subregion of the carbohydrate recognition domain. *J Biol Chem* (2004) 279(26):27688–98. doi:10.1074/jbc.M402936200
7. Kurtagic E, Jedrychowski MP, Nugent MA. Neutrophil elastase cleaves VEGF to generate a VEGF fragment with altered activity. *Am J Physiol Lung Cell Mol Physiol* (2009) 296(3):L534–46. doi:10.1152/ajplung.90505.2008
8. Pemberton PA, Harrison RA, Lachmann PJ, Carrell RW. The structural basis for neutrophil inactivation of C1 inhibitor. *Biochem J* (1989) 258(1):193–8. doi:10.1042/bj2580193
9. van den Berg CW, Tambourgi DV, Clark HW, Hoong SJ, Spiller OB, McGreal EP. Mechanism of neutrophil dysfunction: neutrophil serine proteases cleave and inactivate the C5a receptor. *J Immunol* (2014) 192(4):1787–95. doi:10.4049/jimmunol.1301920
10. Fischer BM, Pavlisko E, Voynow JA. Pathogenic triad in COPD: oxidative stress, protease-antiprotease imbalance, and inflammation. *Int J Chron Obstruct Pulmon Dis* (2011) 6:413–21. doi:10.2147/COPD.S10770
11. Shapiro SD. Proteinases in chronic obstructive pulmonary disease. *Biochem Soc Trans* (2002) 30(2):98–102. doi:10.1042/bst0300098
12. Wilkinson TS, Morris AC, Kefala K, O'Kane CM, Moore NR, Booth NA, et al. Ventilator-associated pneumonia is characterized by excessive release of neutrophil proteases in the lung. *Chest* (2012) 142(6):1425–32. doi:10.1378/chest.11-3273
13. Hagio T, Kishikawa K, Kawabata K, Tasaka S, Hashimoto S, Hasegawa N, et al. Inhibition of neutrophil elastase reduces lung injury and bacterial count in hamsters. *Pulm Pharmacol Ther* (2008) 21(6):884–91. doi:10.1016/j.pupt.2008.10.002
14. Yanagihara K, Fukuda Y, Seki M, Izumikawa K, Miyazaki Y, Hirakata Y, et al. Effects of specific neutrophil elastase inhibitor, sivelestat sodium hydrate, in murine model of severe pneumococcal pneumonia. *Exp Lung Res* (2007) 33(2):71–80. doi:10.1080/01902140701198500
15. Polverino E, Rosales-Mayor E, Dale GE, Dembowsky K, Torres A. The role of neutrophil elastase inhibitors in lung diseases. *Chest* (2017) 152(2):249–62. doi:10.1016/j.chest.2017.03.056
16. Cantin AM, Woods DE. Aerosolized prolastin suppresses bacterial proliferation in a model of chronic *Pseudomonas aeruginosa* lung infection. *Am J Respir Crit Care Med* (1999) 160(4):1130–5. doi:10.1164/ajrccm.160.4.9807166
17. Honoré S, Attalah HL, Azoulay E, Soussy CJ, Saudubray F, Harf A, et al. Beneficial effect of an inhibitor of leukocyte elastase (EPI-hNE-4) in presence of repeated lung injuries. *Shock* (2004) 22(2):131–6. doi:10.1097/01.shk.0000126861.77543.d0
18. Nakamura S, Yanagihara K, Izumikawa K, Seki M, Kakeya H, Yamamoto Y, et al. Efficacy of sivelestat for acute lung injury due to severe bacterial pneumonia with systemic inflammatory response syndrome. *Nihon Kokyuki Gakkai Zasshi* (2008) 46(10):793–7.
19. Domon H, Oda M, Maekawa T, Nagai K, Takeda W, Terao Y. *Streptococcus pneumoniae* disrupts pulmonary immune defence via elastase release following pneumolysin-dependent neutrophil lysis. *Sci Rep* (2016) 6:38013. doi:10.1038/srep38013
20. Hajishengallis G, Wang M, Bagby GJ, Nelson S. Importance of TLR2 in early innate immune response to acute pulmonary infection with *Porphyromonas gingivalis* in mice. *J Immunol* (2008) 181(6):4141–9. doi:10.4049/jimmunol.181.6.4141
21. Greiner O, Day PJ, Bosshard PP, Imeri F, Altwegg M, Nadal D. Quantitative detection of *Streptococcus pneumoniae* in nasopharyngeal secretions by real-time PCR. *J Clin Microbiol* (2001) 39(9):3129–34. doi:10.1128/JCM.39.9.3129-3134.2001
22. Tomlinson G, Chimalapati S, Pollard T, Lapp T, Cohen J, Camberlein E, et al. TLR-mediated inflammatory responses to *Streptococcus pneumoniae* are highly dependent on surface expression of bacterial lipoproteins. *J Immunol* (2014) 193(7):3736–45. doi:10.4049/jimmunol.1401413
23. Kawai T, Akira S. TLR signaling. *Cell Death Differ* (2006) 13(5):816–25. doi:10.1038/sj.cdd.4401850
24. Mihara K, Ramachandran R, Renaux B, Saifeddine M, Hollenberg MD. Neutrophil elastase and proteinase-3 trigger G protein-biased signaling through proteinase-activated receptor-1 (PAR1). *J Biol Chem* (2013) 288(46): 32979–90. doi:10.1074/jbc.M113.483123
25. Zhao P, Lieu T, Barlow N, Sostegni S, Haerteis S, Korbmacher C, et al. Neutrophil elastase activates protease-activated receptor-2 (PAR2) and transient receptor potential vanilloid 4 (TRPV4) to cause inflammation and pain. *J Biol Chem* (2015) 290(22):13875–87. doi:10.1074/jbc.M115.642736
26. Beaufort N, Leduc D, Rousselle JC, Magdolen V, Luther T, Namane A, et al. Proteolytic regulation of the urokinase receptor/CD87 on monocytic cells by neutrophil elastase and cathepsin G. *J Immunol* (2004) 172(1):540–9. doi:10.4049/jimmunol.172.1.540
27. Devaney JM, Greene CM, Taggart CC, Carroll TP, O'Neill SJ, McElvaney NG. Neutrophil elastase up-regulates interleukin-8 via toll-like receptor 4. *FEBS Lett* (2003) 544(1–3):129–32. doi:10.1016/S0014-5793(03)00482-4
28. Kuwahara I, Lillehoj EP, Lu W, Singh IS, Isohama Y, Miyata T, et al. Neutrophil elastase induces *IL-8* gene transcription and protein release through p38/NF-κB activation via EGFR transactivation in a lung epithelial cell line. *Am J Physiol Lung Cell Mol Physiol* (2006) 291(3):L407–16. doi:10.1152/ajplung.00471.2005
29. Mansuy-Aubert V, Zhou QL, Xie X, Gong Z, Huang JY, Khan AR, et al. Imbalance between neutrophil elastase and its inhibitor α1-antitrypsin in obesity alters insulin sensitivity, inflammation, and energy expenditure. *Cell Metab* (2013) 17(4):534–48. doi:10.1016/j.cmet.2013.03.005
30. Braun J, Dalhoff K, Schaaf B, Wood WG, Wiessmann KJ. Characterization of protein-antiproteinase imbalance in bronchoalveolar lavage from patients with pneumonia. *Eur Respir J* (1994) 7(1):127–33. doi:10.1183/09031936.94.07010127
31. Bacci MR, Leme RC, Zing NP, Murad N, Adami F, Hinnig PF, et al. IL-6 and TNF-alpha serum levels are associated with early death in community-acquired pneumonia patients. *Braz J Med Biol Res* (2015) 48(5):427–32. doi:10.1590/1414-431X20144402
32. Zhang P, Summer WR, Bagby GJ, Nelson S. Innate immunity and pulmonary host defense. *Immunol Rev* (2000) 173:39–51. doi:10.1034/j.1600-065X.2000.917306.x

33. Sligl WI, Marrie TJ. Severe community-acquired pneumonia. *Crit Care Clin* (2013) 29(3):563–601. doi:10.1016/j.ccc.2013.03.009
34. Knapp S, Schultz MJ, van der Poll T. Pneumonia models and innate immunity to respiratory bacterial pathogens. *Shock* (2005) 24(Suppl 1):12–8. doi:10.1097/01.shk.0000191385.41689.f3
35. Malley R, Henneke P, Morse SC, Cieslewicz MJ, Lipsitch M, Thompson CM, et al. Recognition of pneumolysin by toll-like receptor 4 confers resistance to pneumococcal infection. *Proc Natl Acad Sci U S A* (2003) 100(4):1966–71. doi:10.1073/pnas.0435928100
36. Branger J, Knapp S, Weijer S, Leemans JC, Pater JM, Speelman P, et al. Role of toll-like receptor 4 in Gram-positive and Gram-negative pneumonia in mice. *Infect Immun* (2004) 72(2):788–94. doi:10.1128/IAI.72.2.788-794.2004
37. Yuan FF, Marks K, Wong M, Watson S, de Leon E, McIntyre PB, et al. Clinical relevance of TLR2, TLR4, CD14 and FcγRIIA gene polymorphisms in *Streptococcus pneumoniae* infection. *Immunol Cell Biol* (2008) 86(3):268–70. doi:10.1038/sj.icb.7100155
38. Beutler B. TNF, immunity and inflammatory disease: lessons of the past decade. *J Investig Med* (1995) 43(3):227–35.
39. Takashima K, Tateda K, Matsumoto T, Iizawa Y, Nakao M, Yamaguchi K. Role of tumor necrosis factor alpha in pathogenesis of pneumococcal pneumonia in mice. *Infect Immun* (1997) 65(1):257–60.
40. Rubins JB, Pomeroy C. Role of gamma interferon in the pathogenesis of bacteremic pneumococcal pneumonia. *Infect Immun* (1997) 65(7):2975–7.
41. van der Poll T, Keogh CV, Guirao X, Buurman WA, Kopf M, Lowry SF. Interleukin-6 gene-deficient mice show impaired defense against pneumococcal pneumonia. *J Infect Dis* (1997) 176(2):439–44. doi:10.1086/514062
42. Fillion I, Ouellet N, Simard M, Bergeron Y, Sato S, Bergeron MG. Role of chemokines and formyl peptides in pneumococcal pneumonia-induced monocyte/macrophage recruitment. *J Immunol* (2001) 166(12):7353–61. doi:10.4049/jimmunol.166.12.7353
43. Hebert JC, O'Reilly M, Gamelli RL. Protective effect of recombinant human granulocyte colony-stimulating factor against pneumococcal infections in splenectomized mice. *Arch Surg* (1990) 125(8):1075–8. doi:10.1001/archsurg.1990.01410200141022
44. Hebert JC, O'Reilly M. Granulocyte-macrophage colony-stimulating factor (GM-CSF) enhances pulmonary defenses against pneumococcal infections after splenectomy. *J Trauma* (1996) 41(4):663–6. doi:10.1097/00005373-199610000-00011
45. Standish AJ, Weiser JN. Human neutrophils kill *Streptococcus pneumoniae* via serine proteases. *J Immunol* (2009) 183(4):2602–9. doi:10.4049/jimmunol.0900688
46. Mikumo H, Yanagihara T, Hamada N, Harada E, Ogata-Suetsugu S, Ikeda-Harada C, et al. Neutrophil elastase inhibitor sivelestat ameliorates gefitinib-naphthalene-induced acute pneumonitis in mice. *Biochem Biophys Res Commun* (2017) 486(1):205–9. doi:10.1016/j.bbrc.2017.03.031
47. Hirche TO, Benabid R, Deslee G, Gangloff S, Achilefu S, Guenounou M, et al. Neutrophil elastase mediates innate host protection against *Pseudomonas aeruginosa*. *J Immunol* (2008) 181(7):4945–54. doi:10.4049/jimmunol.181.7.4945
48. Benabid R, Wartelle J, Malleret L, Guyot N, Gangloff S, Lebargy F, et al. Neutrophil elastase modulates cytokine expression: contribution to host defense against *Pseudomonas aeruginosa*-induced pneumonia. *J Biol Chem* (2012) 287(42):34883–94. doi:10.1074/jbc.M112.361352
49. Tang A, Marquart ME, Fratkin JD, McCormick CC, Caballero AR, Gatlin HP, et al. Properties of PASP: a *Pseudomonas* protease capable of mediating corneal erosions. *Invest Ophthalmol Vis Sci* (2009) 50(8):3794–801. doi:10.1167/iovs.08-3107
50. Parmely M, Gale A, Clabaugh M, Horvat R, Zhou WW. Proteolytic inactivation of cytokines by *Pseudomonas aeruginosa*. *Infect Immun* (1990) 58(9):3009–14.
51. Sokol PA, Ohman DE, Iglewski BH. A more sensitive plate assay for detection of protease production by *Pseudomanas aeruginosa*. *J Clin Microbiol* (1979) 9(4):538–40.
52. Belaaouaj A, Walsh BC, Jenkins NA, Copeland NG, Shapiro SD. Characterization of the mouse neutrophil elastase gene and localization to chromosome 10. *Mamm Genome* (1997) 8(1):5–8. doi:10.1007/s003359900337
53. Kalupov T, Brillard-Bourdet M, Dadé S, Serrano H, Wartelle J, Guyot N, et al. Structural characterization of mouse neutrophil serine proteases and identification of their substrate specificities: relevance to mouse models of human inflammatory diseases. *J Biol Chem* (2009) 284(49):34084–91. doi:10.1074/jbc.M109.042903
54. Maekawa T, Hosur K, Abe T, Kantarci A, Ziogas A, Wang B, et al. Antagonistic effects of IL-17 and D-resolvins on endothelial Del-1 expression through a GSK-3β-C/EBPβ pathway. *Nat Commun* (2015) 6:8272. doi:10.1038/ncomms9272

18

Stabilization of Hypoxia-Inducible Factor-1 Alpha Augments the Therapeutic Capacity of Bone Marrow-Derived Mesenchymal Stem Cells in Experimental Pneumonia

Naveen Gupta[1,2] and Victor Nizet[3,4]*

[1] *Division of Pulmonary and Critical Care, Department of Medicine, School of Medicine, University of California, San Diego, La Jolla, CA, United States,* [2] *Department of Molecular Medicine, The Scripps Research Institute, La Jolla, CA, United States,* [3] *Division of Host-Microbe Systems and Therapeutics, Department of Pediatrics, School of Medicine, University of California, San Diego, La Jolla, CA, United States,* [4] *Skaggs School of Pharmacy and Pharmaceutical Sciences, School of Medicine, University of California, San Diego, La Jolla, CA, United States*

***Correspondence:**
Naveen Gupta
n6gupta@ucsd.edu,
ngupta@scripps.edu

Bone marrow-derived mesenchymal stem cells (MSCs) have therapeutic effects in experimental models of lung injury. Hypoxia-inducible factor-1 alpha (HIF-1α) is a transcriptional regulator that influences cellular metabolism, energetics, and survival under hypoxic conditions. The current study investigated the effects of stabilizing HIF-1α on the therapeutic capacity of MSCs in an experimental mouse model of bacterial pneumonia. HIF-1α stabilization was achieved by the small molecule prolyl-hydroxlase inhibitor, AKB-4924 (Aerpio Therapeutics, Inc.), which blocks the pathway for HIF-1α degradation in the proteosome. *In vitro*, pre-treatment with AKB-4924 increased HIF-1α levels in MSCs, reduced the kinetics of their cell death when exposed to cytotoxic stimuli, and increased their antibacterial capacity. *In vivo*, AKB-4924 enhanced MSC therapeutic capacity in experimental pneumonia as quantified by a sustainable survival benefit, greater bacterial clearance from the lung, decreased lung injury, and reduced inflammatory indices. These results suggest that HIF-1α stabilization in MSCs, achieved *ex vivo*, may represent a promising approach to augment the therapeutic benefit of these cells in severe pneumonia complicated by acute lung injury.

Keywords: mesenchymal stem cells, hypoxia-inducible factor-1 alpha, lung injury, pneumonia, sepsis

INTRODUCTION

Severe pneumonia is the most common cause of sepsis and respiratory failure among critically ill patients. The mortality in the most severe cases can approach 50%, and treatment options have become increasingly limited due to the rapid emergence of multi-drug resistant bacterial strains, particularly among enteric Gram-negative bacteria (1–3). New treatment options that can harness the potential of the innate immune system are needed to more effectively manage this complex condition.

Bone marrow-derived mesenchymal stem cells (MSCs) have been studied as a potential source for cell-based therapy for a wide range of experimental organ injury models. In particular, there has been a considerable amount of focus on using MSCs as a therapy for severe lung injury and sepsis as there are no proven pharmacological therapies in this field (4–9). MSCs have a number of biological properties that lend them to producing a favorable outcome in lung injury and sepsis including immunomodulation, secretion of epithelial and endothelial growth factors, and augmentation of host defense to infection (6, 10, 11). However, the clinical benefits of MSCs in trials have been modest, which may be due to a lack of sustained benefit given MSC death and clearance under inflammatory conditions *in vivo*. It has previously been shown that non-viable MSCs exert no therapeutic benefit (5). Thus, methods to enhance MSC survival and augment their therapeutic capacity should improve their efficacy in clinical lung injury and sepsis.

Hypoxia-inducible factor-1 alpha (HIF-1α) is an important transcriptional regulator that controls many cellular processes under hypoxic conditions, and the injured lung represents a low-oxygen tension environment that presents a metabolic stress to cells introduced into that space. Prior efforts suggested that stabilization of cellular HIF-1α levels could increase the therapeutic function of MSCs in cardiac and vascular injury models (12–14). Consequently, we hypothesized that HIF-1α stabilization in MSCs would enhance their therapeutic efficacy in experimental lung injury and pneumonia, potentially by improving cell survival in the face of inflammatory, cytotoxic stimuli. To that end, we pharmacologically stabilized HIF-1α in MSCs using AKB-4924 (Aerpio Therapeutics, Blue Ash, OH, USA) given our previous experience with the selective potency of this compound (15–17).

METHODS

Isolation, Characterization, and Culturing of MSCs

Mouse MSCs were isolated from 8- to 10-week old male C57BL/6J mice and characterized as published before (8). MSCs were then cultured using MEM-alpha media (Gibco, catalog #12561) with 15% FBS (Gibco, catalog #12662-029) and 1% Pen/Strep/L-Glutamine and used for *in vitro* and *in vivo* experiments from passages 5 to 10.

HIF-1α Stabilization in MSCs and Western Blotting

Mesenchymal stem cells were incubated in the presence of AKB-4924 in a 12-well plates for 4 and 24 h to determine the optimal time and concentration for HIF-1α stabilization in MSCs. AKB-4924 was used at 10 and 100 μM in MEM-alpha supplemented with 5% FBS. MSCs were then lysed and the protein fraction isolated, quantified, and analyzed for HIF-1α expression by Western blotting (see Supplementary Material for details). Based on the data, AKB-4924 was used at 100 μM for 4 h on MSCs to stabilize HIF-1α in most *in vitro* and *in vivo* studies.

In Vitro Bacterial Killing Studies

To determine if AKB-4924 enhances MSC killing of bacteria, separate assays were done with live MSCs and MSC-derived conditioned media in the presence of *Escherichia coli* (see Supplementary Material). Mouse cathelicidin-related antimicrobial protein (CRAMP ELISA, MyBioSource, catalog #MBS280706) was specifically measured to determine if it accounted for the antimicrobial effects induced by AKB-4924. Gene expression for CRAMP was quantified using qPCR as outlined below.

In Vitro Cell Death and Caspase 3/7 Activity

To measure the effect of AKB-4924 on MSC death when exposed to cytotoxic, inflammatory stimuli, studies were done to measure caspase 3/7 activity in a plate-based assay (Promega, catalog #G7790). TNF-α and cycloheximide were chosen as the stimuli since this combination resulted in the most reproducible quantity of cell death for MSCs, and it has been published as an *in vitro* method to model cell death in an inflammatory environment (18, 19) (see Supplementary Material).

RNA Isolation and qPCR

In vitro studies were done to determine if AKB-4924 regulated expression of selected genes (CRAMP, Oct4, TWIST) in MSCs that could account for the observed *in vitro* and *in vivo* effects. RNA was isolated and qPCR was carried out using standard procedures (see Supplementary Material).

In Vivo E. coli Pneumonia Model and Experimental Design

All mice used for these experiments were male C57BL/6J (Jackson Labs) between the ages of 10 and 15 weeks of age. All experiments were approved by the University of California, San Diego (UCSD) Institutional Animal Care and Use Committee, and mice were housed in a UCSD facility approved by the Association for Assessment and Accreditation of Laboratory Animal Care. The general experimental design that we followed is as previously published (5, 8) (see Supplementary Material).

Assessment of Lung Injury, Inflammation, and Bacterial Burden

Lung injury was assessed by histological methods and scored using a previously published method (20). Markers of inflammation and permeability were measured in the bronchoalveolar lavage (BAL) fluid (5, 8), and bacterial burden was calculated from whole lung homogenate (see Supplementary Material).

Statistical Analysis

The majority of the data is presented as mean ± SD for each group analyzed. An unpaired, two-sided Student's t-test was used for comparisons between sets of data. For sets of data with a small sample size (total $n < 20$), a Mann–Whitney U test was used. If multiple groups of data were compared simultaneously, an ANOVA was used. Survival data were analyzed using a log-rank test. A p-value <0.05 was used for statistical significance for all analyses.

RESULTS

AKB-4924 Stabilizes HIF-1α in MSCs and Reduces MSC Death Under Cytotoxic Conditions

AKB-4924 stabilization of HIF-1α protein levels in MSCs occurred at a concentration of 10 or 100 μM and was readily apparent after 4 h incubation (**Figure 1A**). MSCs treated with AKB-4924 exhibited significantly reduced cell death, as measured by caspase 3/7 activity, when exposed to TNF-α and cycloheximide (**Figure 1B**).

AKB-4924 Enhances the Antibacterial Capacity of MSCs

In vitro, AKB-4924 was able to significantly improve MSC-based reduction of viable *E. coli*. The effect of AKB-4924 occurred under both basal and TNF-α stimulated conditions (**Figure 1C**). Conditioned media from AKB-4924 stimulated and TNF-α + LPS stimulated MSCs demonstrated an approximate 20% reduction in viable *E. coli* compared with conditioned media from unstimulated MSCs (**Figure 1D**). This suggests that release of an antimicrobial factor into the conditioned media may account for part of the increased bacterial killing by MSCs that is induced by AKB-4924. We hypothesized that this factor may be mouse CRAMP given previous literature demonstrating that the human cathelicidin antimicrobial protein LL-37 is a potential transcriptional target of HIF-1α, and that human MSCs exert antibacterial effects *via* LL-37 secretion (10, 21). However, under the conditions utilized in this study, we did not detect a significant increase in CRAMP protein secretion in HIF-1α stabilized MSCs (**Figure 1E**).

AKB-4924 Improves MSC-Derived Therapeutic Capacity *In Vivo*

To determine if the *in vitro* benefits with AKB-4924 described above translated into greater MSC-derived therapeutic capacity *in vivo*, the experimental design using an *E. coli* pneumonia model outlined in **Figure 2A** was utilized. While both unstimulated and AKB-4924 stimulated MSCs exerted significant survival benefits at 72 h (**Figure 2B**), only MSCs incubated with AKB-4924 conferred sustained protection against mortality over the course of 7 days (**Figure 2C**). Bacterial clearance from the lung at 24 h post-infection was significantly improved with MSCs incubated with AKB-4924 as well (**Figure 2D**). In addition, HIF-1α stabilized MSCs led to a significant reduction in inflammatory indices such as BAL myeloperoxidase (MPO) and macrophage inflammatory protein-2 (MIP-2) levels 24 h after infection (**Figures 2F,G**, respectively), though there was not a significant reduction in the total BAL cell count (**Figure 2E**) or BAL albumin concentration

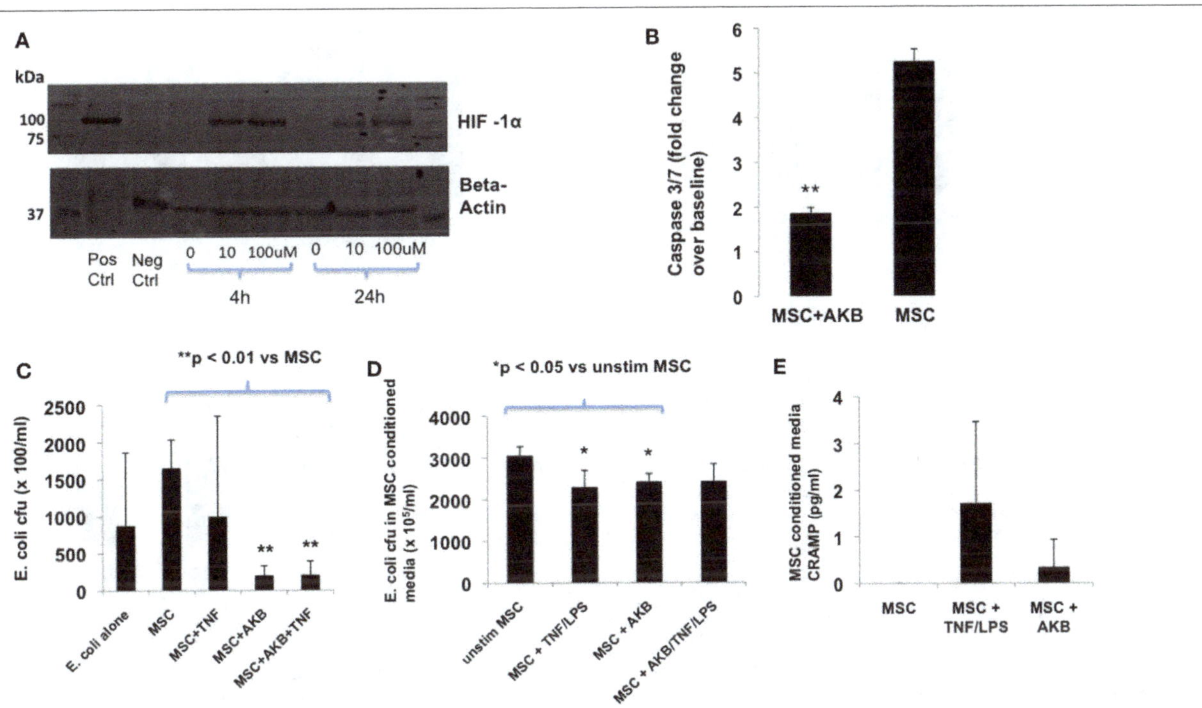

FIGURE 1 | AKB-4924 stabilizes hypoxia-inducible factor 1α (HIF-1α) in mesenchymal stem cells (MSCs) and improves MSC survival and bacterial clearance under *in vitro* conditions. Use of AKB-4924 at both 10 and 100 μM resulted in detectable amounts of HIF-1α protein in MSCs after 4 and 24 h of incubation **(A)**. AKB-4924 significantly reduced caspase 3/7 activity in MSCs exposed to TNF-α and cycloheximide for 5 h [**(B)**, $^{**}p < 0.01$ for MSC + AKB vs MSC, $n = 6$ per group]. MSCs pre-stimulated with AKB-4924 exhibited enhanced bacterial clearance at 6 h [**(C)**, $^{**}p < 0.01$ when compared with MSC group, $n = 4$ per group] that may be partially due to a soluble antimicrobial factor [**(D)**, $^{*}p < 0.05$ compared with unstim group, $n = 4$ per group]. Cathelicidin-related antimicrobial protein (CRAMP) was not significantly increased in the conditioned media of MSCs pre-treated with AKB-4924 when compared with unstimulated MSCs [**(E)**, $n = 3$ per group].

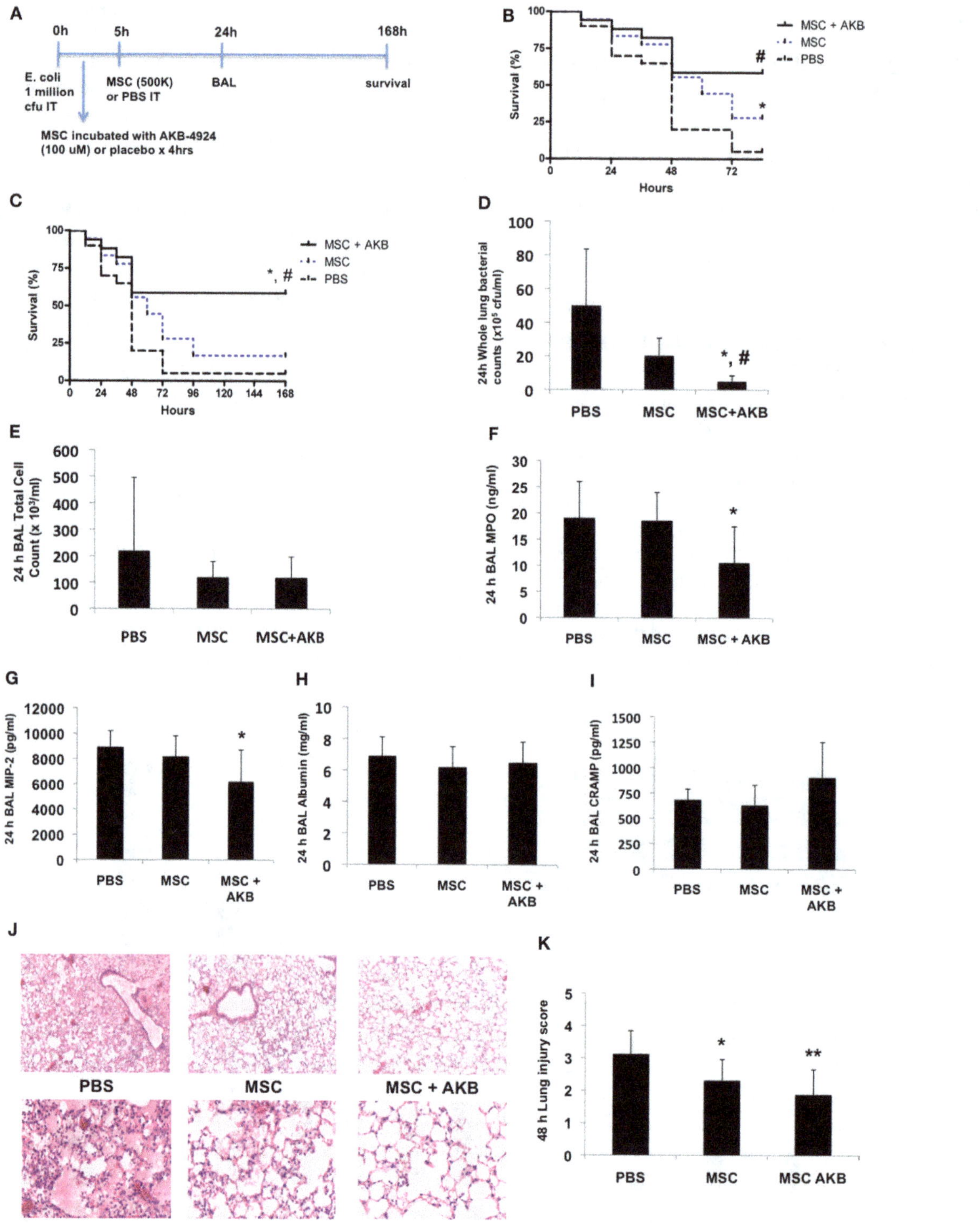

FIGURE 2 | AKB-4924 augments the therapeutic capacity of mesenchymal stem cells (MSCs) in an *Escherichia coli* pneumonia model. Following the experimental design outlined in panel **(A)**, both unstimulated MSCs and MSCs pre-incubated with AKB-4924 (100 µM × 4 h) significantly improved the survival of mice at 72 h [**(B)**, $^{\#}p < 0.05$ for MSC + AKB vs PBS, $^{*}p < 0.05$ for MSC vs PBS, $n = 17$–20 per group], while only AKB-4924 stimulated MSCs increased survival over 7 days [**(C)**, $^{*,\#}p < 0.05$ for MSC + AKB vs MSC and PBS treated groups, respectively, $n = 17$–20 per group]. AKB-4924 also significantly improved the ability of MSCs to reduce whole lung bacterial burden [**(D)**, $^{*,\#}p < 0.05$ for MSC + AKB vs MSC and PBS treated groups, respectively, $n = 5$–6 per group], alveolar neutrophil influx as measured by bronchoalveolar lavage (BAL) MPO levels [**(F)**, $^{*}p < 0.05$ for MSC + AKB vs PBS treated group, $n = 6$–12 per group], and inflammation as measured by BAL MIP-2 levels [**(G)**, $^{*}p < 0.05$ for MSC + AKB vs PBS treated group, $n = 6$ per group]. Total BAL cell counts [**(E)**, $n = 5$ per group], albumin concentration [**(H)**, $n = 5$ per group], and cathelicidin-related antimicrobial protein (CRAMP) levels [**(I)**, $n = 5$ per group] were not significantly changed in the BAL of mice treated with AKB-4924 stimulated MSCs. Lung injury was significantly reduced in both MSC and MSC + AKB treated groups, though the magnitude of improvement was greater in mice treated with AKB-4924 stimulated MSCs [**(J,K)**, $^{*}p < 0.05$ for MSC vs PBS treated group, $^{**}p < 0.01$ for MSC + AKB vs PBS treated group, $n = 8$–12 per group; images taken at 2.5 and 20x magnification].

(**Figure 2H**). BAL CRAMP was measured to see if it correlated with the reduction in bacterial burden seen in **Figure 2D**, but the increase in CRAMP observed with HIF-1α stabilized MSCs did not reach statistical significance (**Figure 2I**). The improvements in bacterial clearance and inflammation were associated with a reduction in lung injury at 48 h post-infection, as assessed by histological methods, that was more pronounced in mice treated with HIF-1α stabilized MSCs (**Figures 2J,K**).

DISCUSSION

Mesenchymal stem cells have been extensively studied as a potential therapy for severe lung injury and sepsis and have shown promise in several pre-clinical models (4–11). However, strategies to improve the survival of MSCs in inflammatory environments and thus augment their therapeutic potential are needed. This proof-of-principle study sought to enhance the therapeutic potential of MSCs in experimental lung injury due to pneumonia by stabilizing the transcription factor HIF-1α with the pharmacological agent AKB-4924. Results from this study substantiated our hypothesis by demonstrating that AKB-4924 improved: (a) MSC survival under *in vitro* cytotoxic conditions; (b) MSC antibacterial activity *in vitro*; and (c) MSC-derived therapeutic capacity *in vivo* with reduced mortality, bacterial burden, inflammation, and lung injury. Though, it is interesting to note that while BAL MPO levels were reduced, total BAL cell counts were not in this study. This discordance may due to a greater effect on neutrophil degranulation as opposed to absolute neutrophil recruitment to the alveolar space. Also, the lack of reduction in BAL albumin at 24 h is not concordant with the other parameters measured, which may be because it represents a summation of permeability over the entire time period and is not sensitive enough to detect changes that develop later in the timeframe being studied. Nevertheless, the overall findings suggest that methods to stabilize HIF-1α in MSCs could be implemented in order to boost the therapeutic effect achieved in critically ill patients with lung injury, and are consistent with recent promising results in cardiac and vascular disease models (12–14).

Mesenchymal stem cells have been tested in several hundred clinical trials to date targeting a wide range of clinical diseases, but their clinical efficacy has not been reproducibly robust to date (22, 23). One of the potential explanations that has been suggested is the relatively short half-life of MSCs *in vivo* (24, 25). HIF-1α represents an intuitive target to augment survival of MSCs in lung injury applications since the injured lung is a hypoxic environment requiring metabolic adaptations. Recent studies in experimental models of ischemia-reperfusion and radiation-induced lung injury have shown that hypoxic preconditioning of MSCs enhances their therapeutic efficacy (26, 27). The mechanisms demonstrated include improved MSC survival and antioxidant ability.

In this study, HIF-1α stabilization in MSCs with the use of AKB-4924 resulted in significantly improved MSC survival under cytotoxic conditions and MSC-derived therapeutic capacity *in vivo*. While improving MSC survival is likely an important contributor to the augmented biological effect achieved with HIF-1α stabilized MSCs, there are other possible mechanisms to consider. We provide some preliminary data that HIF-1α stabilization augments the antibacterial property of MSCs, and it is possible that HIF-1α stabilization in MSCs may be boosting other biological effects of MSCs such as growth factor secretion and immunomodulation. We also tested the possibility that HIF-1α stabilization could keep MSCs in an undifferentiated, "stem-like" state that permits them to retain their reparative properties for a longer duration (28). However, screening qPCR analyses to determine if HIF-1α stabilization upregulated-specific genes involved in maintaining an undifferentiated MSC phenotype (Oct4, TWIST) were unable to detect a significant difference compared with unstimulated MSCs (Figure S1 in Supplementary Material). Finally, HIF-1α stabilized MSCs may be modulating the survival and function of other cell types that are known to be present in the injured lung such as alveolar epithelial cells, endothelial cells, neutrophils, and macrophages. These other potential mechanisms remain the focus of ongoing and future investigations.

While we used a small molecule, AKB-4924, to stabilize HIF-1α in MSCs there are other potential methods that could be used to achieve this goal. Previous studies have used hypoxic preconditioning (i.e., growing MSCs under hypoxic conditions) to augment HIF-1α expression. In addition, genetic editing could be applied to MSCs in order to inactivate the prolyl hydroxylase enzymes responsible for HIF-1α degradation under normoxic conditions. However, genetic editing may carry an increased risk of malignant transformation of MSCs due to sustained dysregulation of HIF-1α expression, particularly since HIF-1α has been implicated in tumor development and invasiveness (29–31). In this regard, the use of AKB-4924 affords the advantage of stabilizing HIF-1α for a defined time period that is determined by its own half-life. For acute inflammatory processes, such as lung injury due to bacterial pneumonia, even transient stabilization of HIF-1α can lead to significant beneficial outcomes as we observed.

In summary, stabilization of HIF-1α in MSCs, with the use of AKB-4924, significantly boosts MSC-derived therapeutic capacity in an *E. coli* model of bacterial pneumonia. Mechanistically, this may be due, in part, to improved MSC survival under cytotoxic conditions. This study and other recent publications suggest that strategies to stabilize HIF-1α should be incorporated into MSC-based clinical trials for critically ill patients with lung injury.

AUTHOR CONTRIBUTIONS

NG and VN planned the experiments, wrote the manuscript, and funded the studies. NG carried out the experiments.

ACKNOWLEDGMENTS

The authors thank Aerpio Therapeutics for supplying AKB-4924 to be utilized in this study. The study was supported by funding by the University of California, San Diego Department of Medicine (NG), and the National Institutes of Health/National Heart, Lung, and Blood Institute (HL125352, VN).

REFERENCES

1. Angus DC, Linde-Zwirble WT, Lidicker J, Clermont G, Carcillo J, Pinsky MR. Epidemiology of severe sepsis in the United States: analysis of incidence, outcome, and associated costs of care. *Crit Care Med* (2001) 29:1303–10. doi:10.1097/00003246-200107000-00002
2. World Health Organization. *Antimicrobial Resistance: Global Report on Surveillance*. Geneva (2014).
3. Bellani G, Laffey JG, Pham T, Fan E, Brochard L, Esteban A, et al. Epidemiology, patterns of care, and mortality for patients with acute respiratory distress syndrome in intensive care units in 50 countries. *JAMA* (2016) 315:788–800. doi:10.1001/jama.2016.0291
4. Xu J, Woods CR, Mora AL, Joodi R, Brigham KL, Iyer S, et al. Prevention of endotoxin-induced systemic response by bone marrow-derived mesenchymal stem cells in mice. *Am J Physiol Lung Cell Mol Physiol* (2007) 293:L131–41. doi:10.1152/ajplung.00431.2006
5. Gupta N, Su X, Popov B, Lee JW, Serikov V, Matthay MA. Intrapulmonary delivery of bone marrow-derived mesenchymal stem cells improves survival and attenuates endotoxin-induced acute lung injury in mice. *J Immunol* (2007) 179:1855–63. doi:10.4049/jimmunol.179.3.1855
6. Lee JW, Fang X, Gupta N, Serikov V, Matthay MA. Allogeneic human mesenchymal stem cells for treatment of E. coli endotoxin-induced acute lung injury in the ex vivo perfused human lung. *Proc Natl Acad Sci U S A* (2009) 106:16357–62. doi:10.1073/pnas.0907996106
7. Mei SH, Haitsma JJ, Dos Santos CC, Deng Y, Lai PF, Slutsky AS, et al. Mesenchymal stem cells reduce inflammation while enhancing bacterial clearance and improving survival in sepsis. *Am J Respir Crit Care Med* (2010) 182:1047–57. doi:10.1164/rccm.201001-0010OC
8. Gupta N, Sinha R, Krasnodembskaya A, Xu X, Nizet V, Matthay MA, et al. The TLR4-PAR1 axis regulates bone marrow mesenchymal stromal cell survival and therapeutic capacity in experimental bacterial pneumonia. *Stem Cells* (2018). doi:10.1002/stem.2796
9. McIntyre LA, Moher D, Fergusson DA, Sullivan KJ, Mei SH, Lalu M, et al. Efficacy of mesenchymal stromal cell therapy for acute lung injury in preclinical animal models: a systematic review. *PLoS One* (2016) 11:e0147170. doi:10.1371/journal.pone.0147170
10. Krasnodembskaya A, Song Y, Fang X, Gupta N, Serikov V, Lee JW, et al. Antibacterial effect of human mesenchymal stem cells is mediated in part from secretion of the antimicrobial peptide LL-37. *Stem Cells* (2010) 28:2229–38. doi:10.1002/stem.544
11. Nemeth K, Leelahavanichkul A, Yuen PS, Mayer B, Parmelee A, Doi K, et al. Bone marrow stromal cells attenuate sepsis via prostaglandin E2-dependent reprogramming of host macrophages to increase their interleukin-10 production. *Nat Med* (2009) 15:42–9. doi:10.1038/nm0409-462b
12. Cerrada I, Ruiz-Sauri A, Carrero R, Trigueros C, Dorronsoro A, Sanchez-Puelles JM, et al. Hypoxia-inducible factor 1 alpha contributes to cardiac healing in mesenchymal stem cells-mediated cardiac repair. *Stem Cells Dev* (2013) 22:501–11. doi:10.1089/scd.2012.0340
13. Liu XB, Wang JA, Ji XY, Yu SP, Wei L. Preconditioning of bone marrow mesenchymal stem cells by prolyl hydroxylase inhibition enhances cell survival and angiogenesis in vitro and after transplantation into the ischemic heart of rats. *Stem Cell Res Ther* (2014) 5:111. doi:10.1186/scrt499
14. HoWangYin KY, Loinard C, Bakker W, Guerin CL, Vilar J, d'Audigier C, et al. HIF-prolyl hydroxylase 2 inhibition enhances the efficiency of mesenchymal stem cell-based therapies for the treatment of critical limb ischemia. *Stem Cells* (2014) 32:231–43. doi:10.1002/stem.1540
15. Okumura CY, Holands A, Tran DN, Olson J, Dahesh S, von Kockritz-Blickwede M, et al. A new pharamacological agent (AKB-4924) stabiliizes hypoxia inducible factor-1 (HIF-1) and increases skin innate defenses against bacterial infection. *J Mol Med* (2012) 90:1079–89. doi:10.1007/s00109-012-0882-3
16. Leire E, Olson J, Isaacs H, Nizet V, Hollands A. Role of hypoxia inducible factor-1 in keratinocyte inflammatory response and neutrophil recruitment. *J Inflamm* (2013) 10:28. doi:10.1186/1476-9255-10-28
17. Lin AE, Beasley FC, Olson J, Keller N, Shalwitz RA, Hannan TJ, et al. Role of hypoxia inducible factor-1α in innate defense against uropathogenic *Escherichia coli* Infection. *PLoS Pathog* (2015) 11:e1004818. doi:10.1371/journal.ppat.1004818
18. Polunovsky VA, Wendt CH, Ingbar DH, Peterson MS, Bitterman PB. Induction of endothelial cell apoptosis by TNF alpha: modulation by inhibitors of protein synthesis. *Exp Cell Res* (1994) 214:584–94. doi:10.1006/excr.1994.1296
19. Tsuchida H, Takeda Y, Takei H, Shinzawa H, Takahashi T, Sendo F. In vivo regulation of rat neutrophil apoptosis occurring spontaneously or induced with TNF-alpha or cycloheximide. *J Immunol* (1995) 154:2403–12.
20. Mrozek JD, Smith KM, Bing DR, Meyers PA, Simonton SC, Connett JE, et al. Exogenous surfactant and partial liquid ventilation: physiologic and pathologic effects. *Am J Respir Crit Care Med* (1997) 156:1058–65. doi:10.1164/ajrccm.156.4.9610104
21. Peyssonnaux C, Datta V, Cramer T, Doedens A, Theodorakis EA, Gallo RL, et al. HIF-1 alpha expression regulates the bactericidal capacity of phagocytes. *J Clin Invest* (2005) 115:1806–15. doi:10.1172/JCI23865
22. Squillaro T, Peluso G, Galderisi U. Clinical trials with mesenchymal stem cells: an update. *Cell Transplant* (2016) 25:829–48. doi:10.3727/096368915X689622
23. Trounson A, McDonald C. Stem cell therapies in clinical trials: progress and challenges. *Cell Stem Cell* (2015) 17:11–22. doi:10.1016/j.stem.2015.06.007
24. Eggenhofer E, Luk F, Dahlke MH, Hoogduijn MJ. The life and fate of mesenchymal stem cells. *Front Immunol* (2014) 5:148. doi:10.3389/fimmu.2014.00148
25. Li L, Chen X, Wang WE, Zeng C. How to improve the survival of transplanted mesenchymal stem cell in ischemic heart? *Stem Cells Int* (2016) 2016:9682757. doi:10.1155/2016/9682757.
26. Liu Y-Y, Chiang C-H, Hung S-C, Chian C-F, Tsai C-L, Chen W-C, et al. Hypoxia-preconditioned mesenchymal stem cells ameliorate ischemia/reperfusion-induced lung injury. *PLoS One* (2017) 12:e0187637. doi:10.1371/journal.pone.0187637
27. Li B, Li C, Zhu M, Zhang Y, Du J, Xu Y, et al. Hypoxia-induced mesenchymal stromal cells exhibit an enhanced therapeutic effect on radiation-induced lung injury in mice due to an increased proliferation potential and enhanced antioxidant ability. *Cell Physiol Biochem* (2017) 44:1295–310. doi:10.1159/000485490
28. Tsai C-C, Chen Y-J, Yew T-L, Chen L-L, Wang J-Y, Chiu C-H, et al. Hypoxia inhibits senescence and maintains mesenchymal stem cell properties through down-regulation of E2A-p21 by HIF-TWIST. *Blood* (2011) 117:459–69. doi:10.1182/blood-2010-05-287508
29. Lu X, Kang Y. Hypoxia and hypoxia-inducible factors: master regulators of metastasis. *Clin Cancer Res* (2010) 16:5928–35. doi:10.1158/1078-0432.CCR-10-1360
30. Soni S, Padwad YS. HIF-1 in cancer therapy: two decade long story of a transcription factor. *Acta Oncol* (2017) 56:503–15. doi:10.1080/0284186X.2017.1301680
31. Qiu GZ, Jin MZ, Dai JX, Sun W, Feng JH, Jin WL. Reprogramming of the tumor in the hypoxic niche: the emerging concept and associated therapeutic strategies. *Trends Pharmacol Sci* (2017) 38:669–86. doi:10.1016/j.tips.2017.05.002

19

Lung Surfactant Lipids Provide Immune Protection Against *Haemophilus influenzae* Respiratory Infection

Belén García-Fojeda[1,2], Zoe González-Carnicero[1], Alba de Lorenzo[1], Carlos M. Minutti[1,2†], Lidia de Tapia[1], Begoña Euba[2,3], Alba Iglesias-Ceacero[1], Sonia Castillo-Lluva[1], Junkal Garmendia[2,3] and Cristina Casals[1,2]*

[1] Department of Biochemistry and Molecular Biology I, Complutense University of Madrid, Madrid, Spain, [2] Centro de Investigación Biomédica en Red de Enfermedades Respiratorias (CIBERES), Instituto de Salud Carlos III, Madrid, Spain, [3] Instituto de Agrobiotecnología, Mutilva, Spain

***Correspondence:**
Cristina Casals
ccasalsc@ucm.es

Non-typeable *Haemophilus influenzae* (NTHi) causes persistent respiratory infections in patients with chronic obstructive pulmonary disease (COPD), probably linked to its capacity to invade and reside within pneumocytes. In the alveolar fluid, NTHi is in contact with pulmonary surfactant, a lipoprotein complex that protects the lung against alveolar collapse and constitutes the front line of defense against inhaled pathogens and toxins. Decreased levels of surfactant phospholipids have been reported in smokers and patients with COPD. The objective of this study was to investigate the effect of surfactant phospholipids on the host-pathogen interaction between NTHi and pneumocytes. For this purpose, we used two types of surfactant lipid vesicles present in the alveolar fluid: (i) multilamellar vesicles (MLVs, $> 1\ \mu m$ diameter), which constitute the tensioactive material of surfactant, and (ii) small unilamellar vesicles (SUVs, $0.1\ \mu m$ diameter), which are generated after inspiration/expiration cycles, and are endocytosed by pneumocytes for their degradation and/or recycling. Results indicated that extracellular pulmonary surfactant binds to NTHi, preventing NTHi self-aggregation and inhibiting adhesion of NTHi to pneumocytes and, consequently, inhibiting NTHi invasion. In contrast, endocytosed surfactant lipids, mainly via the scavenger receptor SR-BI, did not affect NTHi adhesion but inhibited NTHi invasion by blocking bacterial uptake in pneumocytes. This blockade was made possible by inhibiting Akt phosphorylation and Rac1 GTPase activation, which are signaling pathways involved in NTHi internalization. Administration of the hydrophobic fraction of lung surfactant *in vivo* accelerated bacterial clearance in a mouse model of NTHi pulmonary infection, supporting the notion that the lipid component of lung surfactant protects against NTHi infection. These results suggest that alterations in surfactant lipid levels in COPD patients may increase susceptibility to infection by this pathogen.

Keywords: nontypeable *Haemophilus influenzae*, pulmonary surfactant, phospholipids, alveolar epithelial cells, host-pathogen interaction, bacterial invasion, RAC-1, PI3K/Akt

INTRODUCTION

Non-typeable *Haemophilus influenzae* (NTHi) is a non-capsulated Gram-negative bacterium that has been recognized as a major causative pathogen of mucosal infections such as otitis media in children and exacerbations of chronic obstructive pulmonary disease (COPD) in adults (1–5). NTHi is a common commensal of the human nasopharynx that induces a polymicrobial disease, typically due to concurrent or predisposing respiratory viral infection (3). In the upper respiratory tract, the main pathological condition caused by NTHi is acute otitis media, with almost 60% of the cases attributable to this bacterium (1). In the lower airways, NTHi infections are highly prevalent in individuals suffering from COPD, bronchiectasis, cystic fibrosis, and pneumonia (1, 2). In particular, NTHi is a very common bacterial colonizer in the airways of COPD patients, and is the most frequently isolated bacterium in exacerbations of COPD, contributing to inflammation and disease progression (2, 5).

One of the mechanisms likely to be involved in the persistence of respiratory infections by NTHi is its capacity to invade airway epithelial cells (2, 5–7). Intracellular NTHi has been detected in epithelial cells from bronchial biopsies of patients suffering chronic bronchitis (8) and COPD (9). Intracellular invasion of lung epithelial cells enables NTHi to escape from the host immune system and to reside inside cells with high access to essential nutrients (10). Moreover, intracellular NTHi is protected from high concentrations of antibiotics, hampering clinical treatment (11). Therefore, we put forward the notion that preventing NTHi from invading lung epithelial cells is crucially important for the prophylaxis and treatment of respiratory NTHi infections.

To penetrate into airway epithelial cells, adherence of NTHi to such cells is essential, and several adhesion molecules on NTHi have been identified (12–15). They can bind either integrin receptors on the epithelial cell surface (6) or extracellular matrix proteins that interact with the epithelium (13, 15). In healthy individuals, the alveolar epithelium is exceptionally well-defended from bacterial infection through multiple mechanisms of bacterial clearance, including expression of antimicrobial peptides, lung collectins (SP-A and SP-D), and active surveillance of airway macrophages (16–18). In this study, we wondered whether the complicated network of extracellular membranes, called pulmonary surfactant, could also protect the host from NTHi adhesion and invasion.

Pulmonary surfactant is a complex lipoprotein system, exquisitely conserved across species. Surfactant is composed of 90 wt % lipids and 10 wt % proteins. Phospholipids are the major lipid component of surfactant, especially dipalmitoylphosphatidylcholine (DPPC) (19, 20). Phosphatidylglycerol (PG) represents a major unsaturated anionic component (19, 20). Four surfactant proteins form part of this material: the hydrophobic proteins SP-B and SP-C, which are inserted in surfactant membranes and are essential for surfactant biophysical function, and the soluble collectins SP-A and SP-D, which are involved in innate immune host defense (18–24). Lung surfactant is synthesized and secreted by type II pneumocytes. After secretion to the alveolar space, SP-B/SP-C and phospholipids form a multilayered surface film at the air-liquid interface that decreases alveolar surface tension on expiration, and thus prevents lung collapse and respiratory failure (19, 20). Airway instillation of surfactant is in general use for treatment of respiratory distress syndrome in preterm babies (25, 26). Replacement surfactants consist of lipid extract preparations obtained from animal bronchoalveolar fluids, containing phospholipids, mainly DPPC, and the hydrophobic proteins SP-B and SP-C (26). Interestingly, replacement surfactants also improve recovery of animal models of otitis media (27, 28). Lipoprotein structures similar to lung surfactant seems to be present in other mucosal surfaces exposed to the external environment, suggesting the importance of these lipoprotein structures.

In healthy individuals, the amount of surfactant phospholipids (particularly saturated phosphatidylcholine) is tightly regulated and does not significantly change through life (29). However, in pathological conditions, such as COPD, pulmonary fibrosis, or pneumonia, the concentration of surfactant phospholipids decreases (30–33). Whether the decrease of surfactant lipids increases susceptibility to infection by inhaled pathogens in these respiratory diseases remains mostly unaddressed.

In the present study, we tested the hypothesis that surfactant lipids may protect against NTHi infection in the lung. We found that extracellular large surfactant aggregates bind to NTHi and act as a physical barrier that inhibits adhesion of NTHi to pneumocytes and, consequently, invasion. In addition, endocytosed small lipid vesicles interfere with cytoskeletal reorganization required for bacterial entry in pneumocytes, inhibiting NTHi invasion. The protective effect of the hydrophobic fraction of pulmonary surfactant was assessed in a mouse model of NTHi infection.

MATERIALS AND METHODS

Isolation of Lung Surfactant and Preparation of the Surfactant Hydrophobic Fraction

Pulmonary surfactant was obtained from bronchoalveolar lavages (BAL) of male Sprague Dawley rats (Envigo). Rats (~350 g) were euthanized with carbon dioxide and the cardiopulmonary block was extracted to perform BALs with 40 ml of PBS (0.2 mM EDTA). The isolation of lung surfactant experiment was reviewed and approved by the local ethics committee (both Complutense University of Madrid and Autonomous Community of Madrid), according to Directive 2010/63/EU of the European Parliament and the Spanish law RD53/2013 on protection of animals used for experimentation. The mouse lung infection assays were conducted with the approval of Animal Experimentation Committee from the Universidad Pública de Navarra and the authorization of the local government, under the same regulation as above, and following the FELASA and ARRIVE guidelines.

Large surfactant aggregates (heavy subtype surfactant) were obtained as previously described (34, 35). Briefly, BAL was centrifuged at 100,000 g for 1 h at 4°C to obtain large surfactant aggregates in the resulting pellet, which largely contains surfactant lipids and the apolipoproteins SP-A, SP-B, and SP-C. In contrast, about 80% of the total SP-D from BAL does not sediment and remains in the supernatant. The hydrophobic fraction of lung surfactant (composed of surfactant lipids, SP-B, and SP-C) was obtained by chloroform/methanol extraction as previously reported (34, 35). The organic solvent was then evaporated to dryness under a stream of nitrogen, and traces of solvent were subsequently removed by evacuation under reduced pressure overnight. Total phospholipid was determined from aliquots of the surfactant hydrophobic fraction by phosphorus analysis (36).

Multilamellar vesicles (MLVs) of the surfactant hydrophobic fraction were prepared by hydrating the dry proteolipid film in 10 mM phosphate buffered saline (138 mM NaCl, 2.7 mM KCl), pH 7.4, (PBS) and allowing them to swell for 1 h at 55° C. After vortexing, the resulting multilamellar vesicles were used for *in vitro* and *in vivo* assays. This surfactant preparation was used to test the effect of surfactant in a mouse model of NTHi infection.

Surfactant Lipid Vesicles Preparation

Experiments were done using a synthetic mixture of surfactant phospholipids (PL), in the form of either MLVs or small unilamellar vesicles (SUVs). Surfactant vesicles were composed of dipalmitoylphosphatidylcholine (DPPC), 1-palmitoyl-2-oleoyl-phosphatidylglycerol (POPG), and palmitic acid (PA) (Avanti Polar Lipids) at weight ratios of 23:10:1.6 as previously reported (37–39). The lipid composition of these vesicles was chosen according to the following criteria: (i) a high DPPC content, which is the main phospholipid constituent of pulmonary surfactant (~50 wt.% of the total surfactant PL); (ii) the presence of an unsaturated anionic phospholipid (POPG), which forms part of lung surfactant (~8–15 wt.%); and (iii) the presence of small amounts of palmitic acid in surfactant (19, 20).

Preparation of MLVs and SUVs from surfactant lipids was carried out as described in Sáenz et al. (37, 38), and Cañadas et al. (40). The required amounts of DPPC, POPG, and PA were dissolved in chloroform/methanol (2:1 v/v). The solvent was then evaporated to dryness under a gentle stream of nitrogen. Traces of solvent were subsequently removed in a vacuum centrifuge for 2 h. In cases where the lipofilic fluorescent tracer 1,1′-Dioctadecyl-3,3,3′,3′-tetramethylindocarbocyanine perchlorate [DiIC$_{18}$(3)] (Thermofisher Scientific) was incorporated in the lipid mixture, the lipofilic probe was dissolved in methanol and added to the lipid mixture at a DiIC$_{18}$/surfactant phospholipid molar ratio of 1:200, before solvent removal. MLVs were prepared by hydrating the dry lipid film with PBS, allowing them to swell for 1 h at 45°C, a temperature above the gel to liquid phase transition temperature (Tm) of these membranes (37, 38). To prepare SUVs, the resulting MLVs were sonicated at the same temperature (45°C) during 8 min at 390 W/cm^2 (burst of 0.6 s, with 0.4 s between bursts) in a UP 200S sonifier with a 2 mm microtip (Hielscher Ultrasonics).

The size of lipid vesicles was measured at 25°C in a Zetasizer Nano S (Malvern Instruments, Malvern, UK) equipped with a 633-nm HeNe laser, as previously reported (18, 22). Three scans were performed for each sample. Zeta potential measurements were performed with a Zetasizer Nano S (Malvern Instruments), applying an electric field across the dispersion. Measurements were performed in PBS in the presence and absence of 0.4 mM Ca^{2+}.

Bacterial Strains, Media, and Growth Conditions

The two NTHi strains used in this study are clinical isolates from patients with otitis media (NTHi375) (6) and COPD (NTHi398) (14). Frozen stocks of NTHi strains were thawed and then grown on chocolate agar plates (bioMérieux) or on brain heart infusion broth (BHI) supplemented with haemin 10 µg/ml and β-NAD 10 µg/ml (Sigma-Aldrich) (sBHI). Bacteria were grown overnight at 37°C in a humidified 5% CO_2 atmosphere.

Epithelial Cell Cultures and Bacterial Infection

Experiments were performed using the mouse lung epithelial cell line MLE-12 (ATTC® CRL-2110™, Manassas, VA, USA) and the human alveolar basal epithelial cell line A549 (ATTC® CCL-185™). Cells were maintained in RPMI 1640 supplemented with 10% (v/v) heat-inactivated fetal bovine serum (FBS), antibiotics (100 U/ml penicillin and 100 µg/ml streptomycin), and 2 mM L-glutamine (BioWhittacker). Lung epithelial cells were incubated at 37°C in a humidified 5% CO_2 atmosphere.

Bacterial adhesion and invasion assays were performed as described previously (6, 7) in the presence and absence of surfactant phospholipid vesicles (MLVs or SUVs). MLE-12 or A549 cells were seeded to a density of 50,000 cells per well in 24-well tissue culture plates for 24 h. Cells were grown in complete medium with 5% FBS [RPMI 1640 tissue culture medium supplemented with antibiotics (100 U/ml penicillin and 100 µg/ml streptomycin), 2 mM L-glutamine, and 5% FBS]. A confluence of 90% was reached at the time of the bacterial infection. The following day, cells were incubated with NTHi in the presence or absence of MLVs. For SUVs, cells were (i) pre-incubated with SUVs during 24 h to allow PL endocytosis before NTHi infection, (ii) co-incubated with SUVs at the onset of NTHi infection, or (iii) post-incubated with SUVs after NTHi infection.

For NTHi infection, bacteria were recovered with 1 ml PBS from a chocolate agar plate grown overnight. Bacterial suspensions were adjusted to $OD_{600} = 1$, $\sim 10^9$ colony forming units (C.F.U.)/ml. Cells were infected with 50 µl (10^8 C.F.U./ml) of the adjusted bacterial suspension in 1 ml of Hank's balanced buffered saline (HBBS) (137 mM NaCl, 5.4 mM KCl, 0.25 mM Na_2HPO_4, 0.44 mM KH_2PO_4, 1.3 mM $CaCl_2$, 1 mM $MgSO_4$, 4.2 mM $NaHCO_3$).

For adhesion experiments, cells were infected for 30 min, washed three times with PBS, and lysed with 300 µl of 0.025% (w/v) saponin in PBS for 10 min at room temperature. The resulting lysates were diluted serially 1/10 in PBS, and serial dilutions were plated on sBHI agar (6, 7).

Colonies were counted and the results were expressed as the percentage (%) of C.F.U. related to the control (not incubated with lipids).

For invasion assays, cells were infected for 2 h and washed three times with PBS. Cells were then incubated for an additional 1 h with RPMI 1640 containing 10% FBS and 200 μg/ml gentamicin to kill extracellular bacteria. Then, cells were washed three times with PBS and lysed as described above. Serial dilutions were plated on sBHI agar (6, 7). Colonies were counted and the results were expressed as % C.F.U. related to the control (not incubated with lipids).

In some experiments, cells were pre-incubated in the presence of anti-SR-BI blocking antibody for 30 min. Rabbit IgG anti-SR-BI [NB400-113 (Novus, Biologicals)] or its corresponding normal Rabbit IgG control (R&D Systems) were used at a working concentration of 1:100 in culture medium. Then, SUVs (250 μg/ml) were added to the medium for an additional 2 h. Afterwards, the NTHi infection assay was carried out as described above.

Bacterial Killing Assay

NTHi strains were grown on chocolate agar. Bacteria were harvested in PBS, NaCl 100 mM, 1% (w/v) trypticasein soy broth to a final concentration of 10^8 C.F.U./ml. Then, 100 μl of bacterial suspension (10^7 C.F.U.) were incubated with either 250 μg/ml of PL (present as MLVs) or 20 μg/ml of polymyxin B (PMB) for 2 h at 37°C in a humidified 5% CO_2 atmosphere. Bacteria were then stained with 5 μM 5-(and-6)-carboxyfluorescein diacetate, succinimidyl ester (CFSE) (ThermoFisher Scientific), which stains active and inactive bacteria (41). Bacteria were centrifuged, washed with PBS, and resuspended in 100 μl PBS with 7.5 μM propidium iodide, to stain dead bacteria. Bacteria were incubated for 5 min at 37°C in a humidified 5% CO_2 atmosphere, and then centrifuged, resuspended in 10 μl PBS, and placed on a microscope slide to be immediately analyzed. Micrographs were taken with a 40x objective in a fluorescence microscope Nikon ECLIPSE TE2000-U. Dead and live bacteria were counted in six micrographs of each experimental condition using Image J software. Data are shown as % of dead bacteria to total bacteria.

Bacterial Aggregation Assay

Otitis NTHi was grown on chocolate agar for 16 h and diluted in HBSS without $CaCl_2$ to $OD_{600} = 1$. Bacterial aggregation was assessed by measuring changes in light absorbance at 600 nm during 3 h without shaking, in a spectrophotometer DU-800 (Beckman Coulter, Fullerton, USA). Readings were taken every 3 min. Aggregation is observed as a decrease in absorbance as bacterial aggregates precipitate out of solution. To test the effect of surfactant phospholipids (MLVs or SUVs) on this process, a suspension of NTHi was carefully mixed with and without surfactant lipids (MLVs or SUVs) at room temperature, and bacterial aggregation was measured. Control experiments with phospholipid vesicles alone, without bacteria, were performed.

Confocal Microscopy

Endocytosis of lipid vesicles (either MLVs or SUVs) were analyzed by confocal microscopy. Cells were seeded to a density of 50,000 cells per well in 24-well tissue culture plates for 24 h. Each well-contained a plastic coverslip previously sterilized under UV light for 10 min. Cells were grown in complete medium with 5% FBS. The following day, cells were incubated for 5, 10, 30 min, 1, 4, or 24 h with MLVs or SUVs (250 μg PL/ml), fluorescently labeled with $DiIC_{18}(3)$ ($\lambda_{exc} = 549$ nm; $\lambda_{em} = 565$ nm).

To determine whether the internalization of PL was mediated by the scavenger receptors SR-BI or CD36, confocal microscopy experiments were performed in the presence of either blocking antibodies [mouse IgAκ anti-CD36 (Abcam) and rabbit IgG anti-SR-BI] or their isotype controls [mouse IgAκ isotype control (Abcam) and normal rabbit IgG control], at a working concentration of 1:100, for 30 min. Then, cells were incubated for 1 h with lipid vesicles (250 μg PL/ml) stained with $DiIC_{18}(3)$.

After incubation with vesicles, cells were washed three times with PBS and fixed with 4% paraformaldehyde (PFA) in PBS for 30 min at room temperature. Staining of plasma membrane and organelles was performed with 5 μg/ml wheat germ agglutinin (WGA) conjugated with Alexa Fluor 488 for 10 min at room temperature. Nuclei were stained with 1 μg/ml 4′, 6-diamino-2-phenylindol (DAPI) for 5 min. Coverslips were mounted onto glass slides using ProLong Diamond (Thermo Fisher Scientific), and micrographs were taken under an Olympus FV1200 confocal system.

NTHi invasion of alveolar epithelial cells was also analyzed by confocal microscopy as in Morey et al. (6) and López-Gómez

TABLE 1 | The average size distribution and zeta potential of MLVs and SUVs used in this study, determined in PBS in the absence and presence of physiological concentrations Ca^{2+}.

Vesicle type	Composition	$[Ca^{2+}]$ (mM)	Z-average (nm)	Z-potential (mV)
MLVs	PL/SP-B/SP-C (Native surfactant)	0.0	2,651 ± 45	−43.8 ± 0.1
		0.4	2,380 ± 28	−30.4 ± 0.3
Downsizing MLVs (sonication) **(a)**	PL/SP-B/SP-C (Native surfactant)	0.0	283 ± 2	−39.0 ± 0.2
		0.4	648 ± 15	−24.0 ± 0.2
MLVs	DPPC/POPC/PA (Surfactant lipid mixture)	0.0	1,057 ± 17	−39.5 ± 0.6
		0.4	3,100 ± 27	−27.5 ± 0.3
Downsizing MLVs (sonication) **(b)** SUVs	DPPC/POPC/PA (Surfactant lipid mixture)	0.0	98 ± 5	−36.0 ± 0.3
		0.4	110 ± 8	−26.0 ± 0.4

Phospholipid (PL) concentration: 0.25 mg/mL.

[a]Small vesicles from the hydrophobic fraction of native surfactant were not used in this study due to their instability and rapid aggregation induced by the presence of surfactant hydrophobic proteins SP-B and SP-C. They aggregated in the presence of calcium and tend to rapidly aggregate over time.

[b]This sample showed a polydispersed size-distribution, with two major peaks centered at 60 ±7 nm and 31 ± 2 nm, and a minor peak at 677 ± 5. The average size is ≤ 100 nm (SUVs).

et al. (7). Once invasion experiments were performed and cells were treated with gentamicin, as described above, cells were washed three times with PBS and fixed with 4% PFA in PBS for 30 min at room temperature. Then cells were permeabilized with 0.1% saponin in PBS, and staining was performed in 10% FBS and 0.1% saponin in PBS. NTHi was stained with rabbit anti-NTHi antibody at a working concentration of 1:800 (6), followed by a secondary antibody conjugated with Alexa Fluor 488 (1:100). Late endosomes were stained with anti-LAMP-1 antibody conjugated with phycoerythrin at a working concentration of 1:300 (eBioscience). Nuclei were stained with 1 μg/ml DAPI for 5 min. Coverslips were mounted onto glass slides using ProLong Diamond, and images were taken with an Olympus FV1200 confocal system. Quantification of internalized NTHi bacteria (colocalized with late endosomes) per cell number was performed using Image J software on each of 12 micrographs per treatment and experiment.

Flow Cytometry

Alveolar epithelial cells were seeded to a density of 80,000 cells per well in 24-well tissue culture plates and were grown overnight in complete medium with 5% FBS. For analysis of endocytosis of SUVs, cells were incubated for 30 min with or without either blocking antibodies for scavenger receptors

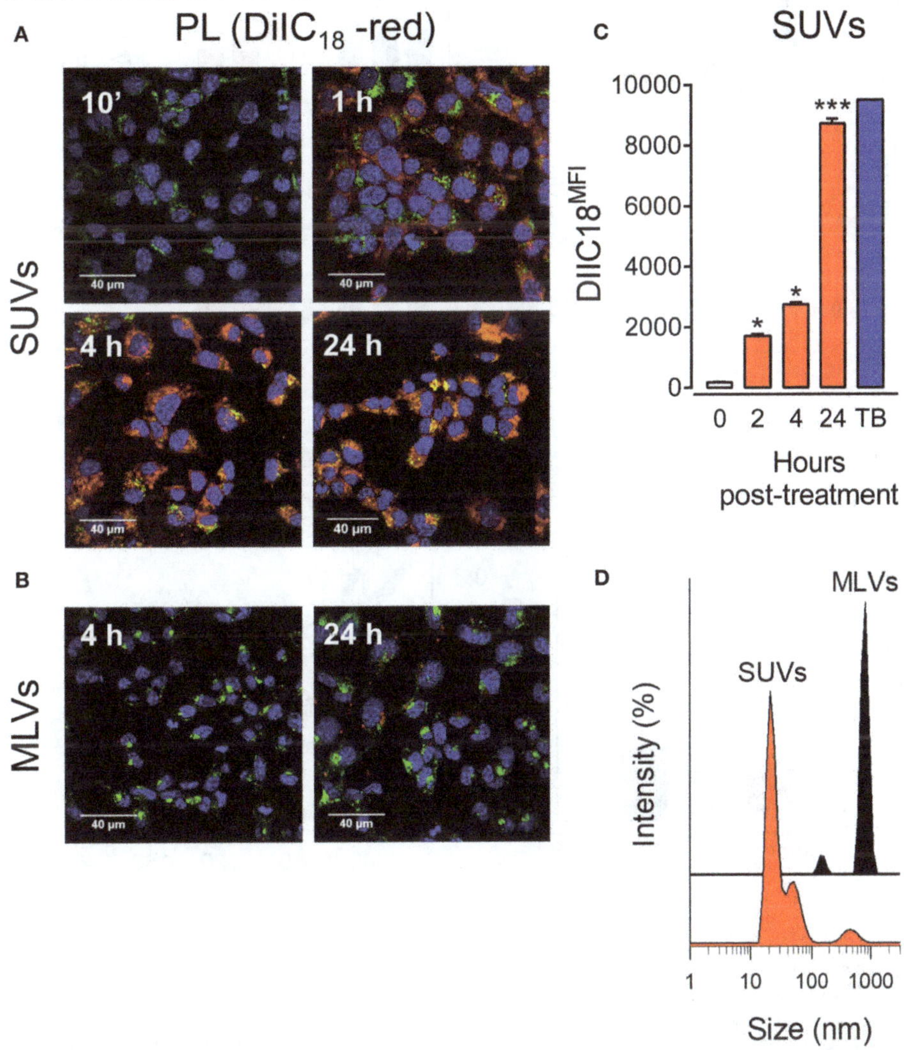

FIGURE 1 | Small vesicles, but not multilamellar vesicles, of pulmonary surfactant are internalized by pneumocytes. **(A)** MLE-12 pneumocytes were incubated with $DiIC_{18}(3)$-labeled SUVs composed of a mixture of surfactant lipids (250 μg PL/ml) for 10 min, 1, 4, or 24 h. Cells were fixed and stained with Alexa Fluor 488-conjugated WGA. Nuclei were stained with DAPI. Endocytosis of lipid vesicles was analyzed by confocal microscopy. **(B)** As in **(A)**, but cells were incubated with $DiIC_{18}(3)$-labeled MLVs (250 μg PL/ml) for 4 and 24 h. **(C)** Cells were incubated with $DiIC_{18}(3)$-labeled SUVs for the indicated times and analyzed by flow cytometry. ANOVA followed by Bonferroni multiple comparison test was used. $^{*}p < 0.05$ and $^{***}p < 0.001$ when compared to control cells in the absence of lipids. Trypan blue (TB) was used to quench extracellular vesicles attached to the cell membrane after 24 h incubation. **(D)** Hydrodynamic diameter of surfactant vesicles (SUVs and MLVs) determined by dynamic light scattering. The y-axis represents the relative intensity of the scattered light; the x-axis denotes the hydrodynamic diameter of the particles present in the solution. One representative experiment of three is shown.

(mouse IgAκ anti-CD36 and rabbit IgG anti-SR-BI) or their appropriate isotype controls, all used at a working concentration of 1:100 in medium. Then, SUVs fluorescently labeled with $DiIC_{18}(3)$ were added to the cells at a concentration of 100 μg PL/ml, and cells were incubated with lipid vesicles for the indicated times. Next, cells were trypsinized and collected in tubes for centrifugation. After two washes with PBS, cells were resuspended in 200 μl PBS and analyzed by flow cytometry using Becton-Dickinson FACSCan and Cell Quest software.

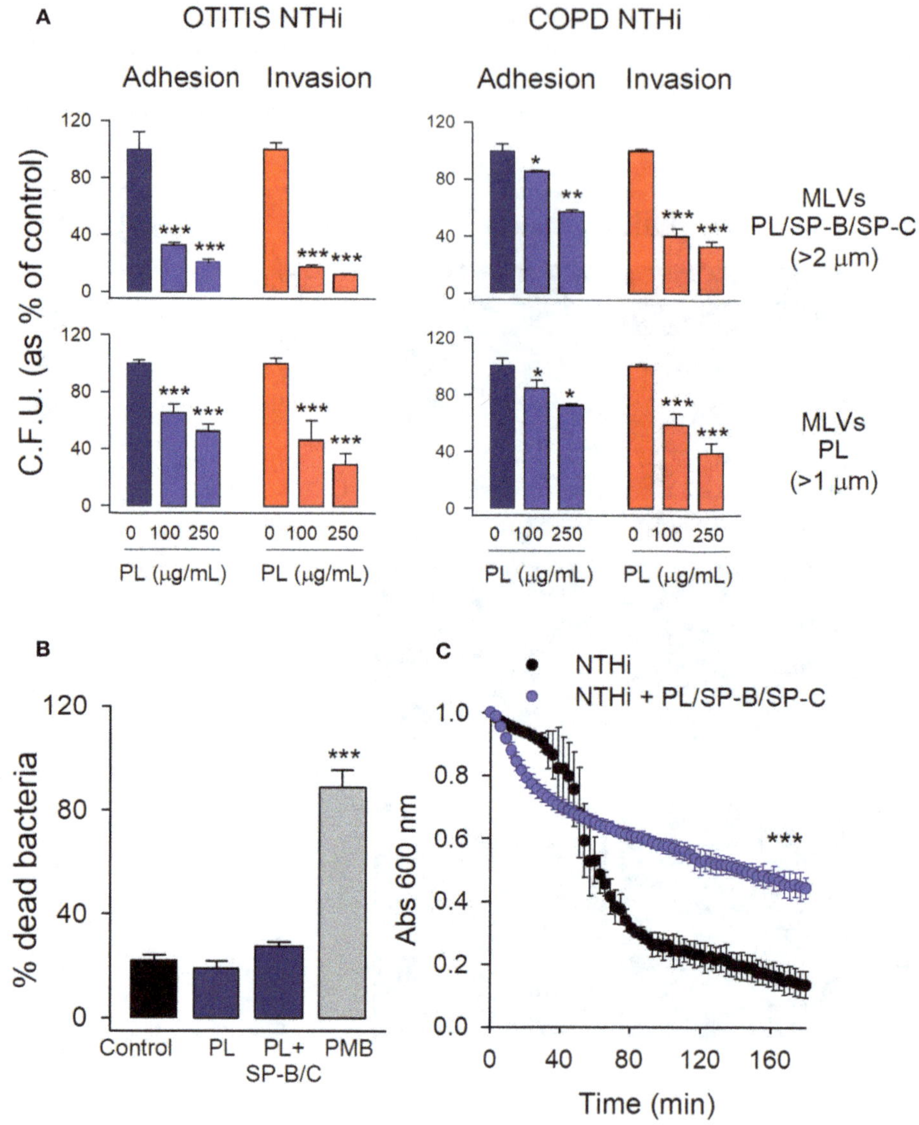

FIGURE 2 | Extracellular multilamellar vesicles of pulmonary surfactant inhibit adhesion of NTHi to pneumocytes and decrease NTHi self-aggregation. **(A)** MLE-12 cells were infected with NTHi clinical strains from patients with otitis media and COPD, in the presence or absence of MLVs (100 or 250 μg PL/ml) prepared from either the hydrophobic fraction of native surfactant (PL/SP-B/SP-C) or a mixture of surfactant lipids (PL). For adhesion experiments, cells were infected for 30 min, washed, and lysed. For invasion assays, cells were infected for 2 h, washed, and incubated for an additional 1 h with gentamicin to kill extracellular bacteria. The resulting lysates were plated on sBHI agar. Colonies were counted and the results were expressed as percentages of C.F.U. relative to infected cells in the absence of lipids. Results are mean ± SEM of three independent experiments run in triplicate. ANOVA followed by Bonferroni multiple comparison test was used. $^{*}p < 0.05$, $^{**}p < 0.01$, and $^{***}p < 0.001$ when compared with NTHi-infected pneumocytes in the absence of lipids. **(B)** NTHi (otitis strain) were incubated in the presence or absence of MLVs (250 μg/ml) composed of either a mixture of surfactant lipids (PL), or the hydrophobic fraction of native surfactant (PL/SP-B/C) for 30 min. Bacteria were then stained with carboxyfluorescein diacetate succinimidyl ester (green), and bacterial viability was assessed by propidium iodide exclusion. Polymixin B (PMB) (20 μg/ml) was used as a positive control of bacterial killing. Data were expressed as % of dead bacteria. Results are mean ± SEM. ANOVA followed by the Bonferroni multiple-comparison test was used. $^{***}p < 0.001$ vs. untreated bacteria. **(C)** Effect of surfactant vesicles on NTHi self-aggregation. NTHi (otitis strain) was incubated in the presence or absence of MLVs (250 μg PL/ml) prepared from the hydrophobic fraction of native surfactant. Bacterial aggregation was monitored by measuring the decrease of absorbance at 600 nm every 3 min. Four independent experiments were performed. Results are mean ± SEM. Student's *t*-test was used. $^{***}p < 0.001$.

To test the effect of phospholipid uptake on the expression of SR-BI or CD36 receptors on the cell surface, cells were incubated in the presence or absence of SUVs (250 μg PL/ml) for 2 h. Then cells were harvested with cold PBS 10 mM EDTA and incubated with 10% FBS-supplemented medium, followed by incubation with either anti-SR-BI, anti-CD36, or isotype controls and appropriate secondary Alexa Fluor 488-conjugated antibodies. Following surface staining, samples were analyzed by flow cytometry using Becton-Dickinson FACScalibur and Cell Quest Pro software.

Western Blot Analysis of Akt Phosphorylation

Cells were seeded to a density of 50,000 cells per well in 24-well tissue culture plates and were grown overnight in complete medium with 5% FBS. The following day, cells were pre-incubated for 24 h with different concentrations of surfactant PL (present in solution as SUVs) to allow their endocytosis by alveolar epithelial cells. Then, cells were infected with NTHi following the same conditions previously explained for invasion experiments. After 45 min of cell-pathogen contact, cells were washed three times with PBS and lysed with 120 μl lysis buffer composed of 10 mM HEPES, 1.5 mM $MgCl_2$, 10 mM KCl, 0.5 mM EDTA, 0.2% Triton X-100, 1 mM benzamidine, 20 μg/ml aprotinin, 20 μg/ml leupeptin, 20 mM β-glycerophosphate, 10 mM NaF, 10 mM sodium pyrophosphate, and 2 mM orthovanadate (Sigma-Aldrich). Samples were resolved by SDS-PAGE under reducing conditions and transferred to polyvinylidene fluoride (PVDF) membranes (Bio-Rad). Membranes were blocked with 5 % (w/v) skimmed milk in PBS and were incubated with the anti-phospho-Akt (Ser473) antibody (1:5000), or Akt antibody (Cell Signaling) (1:1000), overnight at 4°C. After a washing step in PBS, membranes were incubated for 1 h at room temperature with the appropriate secondary antibody conjugated with horseradish peroxidase (Cell Signaling). Membranes were washed in PBS and exposed to ECL reagents (Millipore). Immunoreactive bands were quantified using Quantity One Software (Bio-Rad). Results are shown as p-Akt normalized to total Akt, and expressed as % of pAkt/Akt induced by NTHi in cells in the absence of surfactant PL. Data were presented as the p-Akt intensity of each band normalized for the intensity of the corresponding total Akt band (same sample) and referred as the correspondent percentage in relation to cells infected with NTHi but not treated with phospholipids.

Rac1-GTP Pull Down

Pull down assays were performed as described in Castillo-Lluva et al. (42) and Woodcock et al. (43). Cells were seeded to a density of 500,000 cells per plate in 60 cm diameter tissue culture plates and were grown in complete medium with 5% FBS. The following day, SUVs (250 μg PL/ml) were added to the cells for 24 h to allow PL endocytosis. Then cells were infected with NTHi for 2 h as described above for bacterial invasion experiments.

To measure endogenous Rac GTPase activity, cells were lysed on ice in glutathione-S-transferase-fish buffer (50 mM TrisHCl, pH 7.5, 100 mM NaCl, 2 mM MgCl2, 1% (v/v) Nonidet P-40, 10% (v/v) glycerol, and protease inhibitors [0.5 mM benzamidine, 10 μg/ml aprotinin, 10 μg/ml leupeptin] (Sigma-Aldrich) containing 1.5 μg of a biotinylated p21-activated kinase (PAK) derived CRIB (Cdc42/Rac interacting binding) peptide per assay. Cleared cell lysates were incubated at 4°C for 30 min. Active Rac/CRIB complexes were precipitated using streptavidin-conjugated magnetic sepharose beads (GE Healthcare) for a further 15 min at 4°C. Following washes in glutathione-S-transferase-fish buffer, protein samples were retrieved with 1× SDS-PAGE sample buffer and processed for Western blotting with anti-Rac antibody (Becton Dickinson).

NTHi Mouse Lung Infection

CD1® IGS (Caesarian-derived 1 from Charles River Laboratories, Massachusetts, U.S.A.) mice were used to establish a model of NTHi lung infection, as previously described (44, 45). CD1 female mice (18–20 g) aged 4–5 weeks were purchased from Charles River Laboratories (France), housed under pathogen-free conditions at the Institute of Agrobiotechnology facility (registration number ES/31-2016-000002-CR-SU-US), and used at 22–25 g. Before NTHi infection, the surfactant hydrophobic fraction (or the same volume of PBS in the untreated group) was intratracheally instilled into the lung at 37°C at a dose of 25 mg PL/kg body weight (40 μl of surfactant at a PL concentration of 13.75 mg/ml). Subsequently, 10 μl of PBS (uninfected group) or a NTHi375 suspension containing 4×10^9 C.F.U./ml (4×10^7 C.F.U./mouse) (NTHi infected group) were intratracheally administered. Mice were randomly divided into 6 infected ($n = 5$) groups and 2 non-infected ($n = 3$) control groups. The NTHi-infected groups are: (i) animals treated with surfactant, euthanized at 6 h post-infection; (ii) treated with surfactant, euthanized at 12 h post-infection; (iii) treated with surfactant, euthanized at 24 h post-infection; and untreated groups instilled with PBS, (iv) euthanized at 6 h, (v) 12 h, and (vi) 24 h post-infection. The uninfected control groups are: (1) animals treated with surfactant; and (2) animals instilled with PBS.

In all animals, lungs were aseptically removed and weighed. The left lung was clamped and separated to obtain lung homogenates in 1:10 (w/v) sterile PBS. The right lung was lavaged five times with sterile PBS to obtain the bronchoalveolar lavage (BAL). BAL fluid was centrifuged at 2000 × g for 10 min, and the pellet was resuspended in 1 ml RPMI 10% FBS as described previously (18). A 50-μl aliquot was stained with an equal volume of 0.4% trypan blue (Sigma-Aldrich) for total cell count on a hemocytometer. Differential cell counts were made on cytospin preparations stained with May–Grünwald–Giemsa (Sigma-Aldrich). For bacterial count in cell-free BAL and lung homogenate, dilutions of BAL and lung homogenates were plated in triplicate on BHI-agar plates, and the number of CFUs was determined after an overnight incubation at 37°C. Data were expressed as $\log_{10}$ CFU ± SEM/mouse.

Statistical Methods

Data are presented as means ± SEM. Differences in means between groups were evaluated by one-way ANOVA, followed by the Bonferroni multiple comparison test. Student's t-test was used when comparing two groups. An α level $\leq 5\%$ ($p \leq 0.05$)

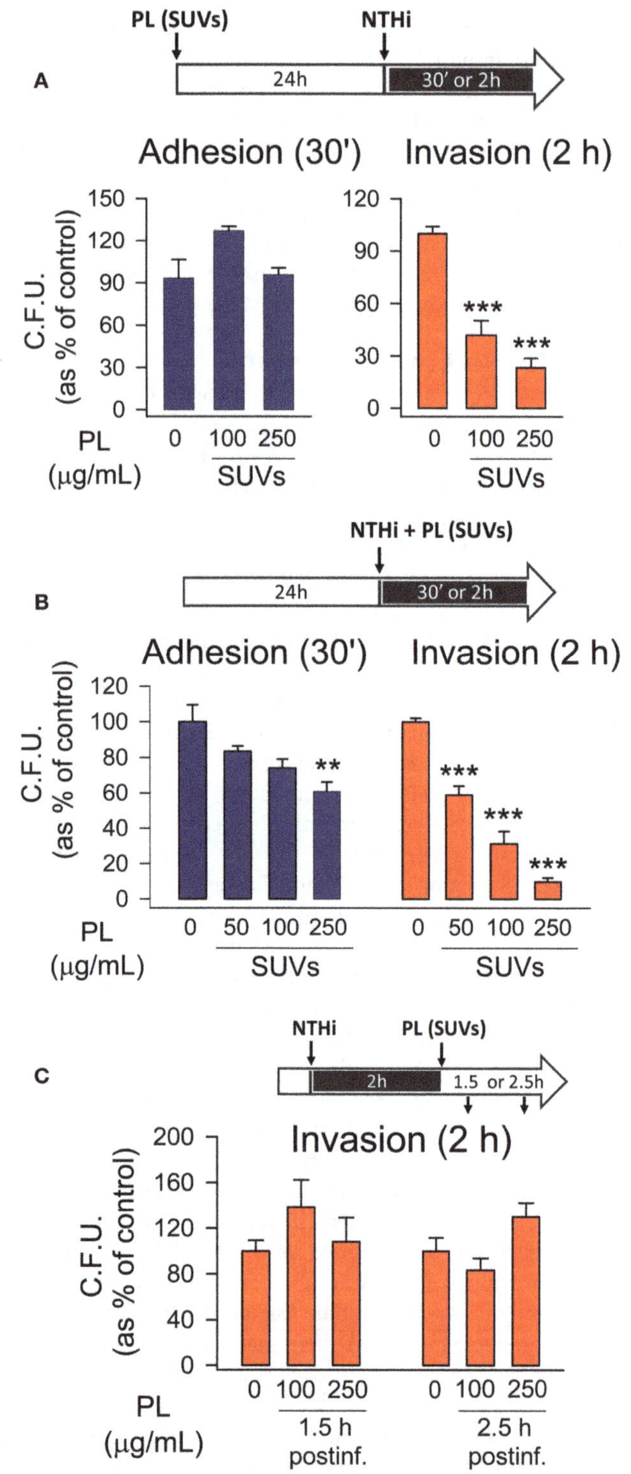

FIGURE 3 | Endocytosed surfactant vesicles inhibit NTHi invasion of pneumocytes. MLE-12 pneumocytes were incubated with SUVs composed of a mixture of surfactant lipids. Cells were either pre-incubated with SUVs for 24 h prior to infection **(A)**, co-incubated with SUVs and NTHi **(B)**, or post-incubated with SUVs for 1.5 or 2.5 h after infection with NTHi **(C)**. For bacterial adhesion experiments, cells were infected for 30 min. For invasion assays, cells were infected for 2 h, washed, and incubated with gentamicin *(Continued)*

FIGURE 3 | to kill extracellular bacteria. Cells were lysed and plated on sBHI agar. Data are shown as percentage of C.F.U. relative to infected cells in the absence of lipid vesicles. Results are mean ± SEM of three independent experiments performed in triplicate. ANOVA followed by the Bonferroni multiple-comparison test was used. $^{**}p < 0.01$, and $^{***}p < 0.001$ when compared with infected pneumocytes in the absence of lipids.

was considered significant. SigmaPlot version 11.0 was used for statistical tests.

RESULTS

Two different surfactant subtypes are present in the alveolar fluid: (i) a heavy subtype or large surfactant aggregates, rich in SP-B and SP-C, that form MLVs in solution and constitute the freshly secreted surfactant tensioactive material; and (ii) a light subtype characterized by the presence of small vesicles devoid of SP-B and SP-C and by poor surface activity. These small vesicles are generated after inspiration/expiration cycles (19).

In this study, we used two types of lipid vesicles with different sizes, composed of either the hydrophobic fraction of surfactant (PL/SP-B/SP-C) or a mixture of surfactant lipids (DPPC/POPG/PA). **Table 1** shows the average size distribution and zeta potential of MLVs and SUVs used in this study, determined in PBS in the absence and presence of physiological concentrations Ca^{2+}. Zeta potential measurements of lipid vesicles used in this study confirm that they are negatively charged due to the presence of anionic phospholipids. The Zeta potential value for lipid vesicles composed of a surfactant lipid mixture was -39.5 ± 0.6 mV, similar to that obtained for the hydrophobic fraction of native surfactant: -43.8 ± 0.1 mV (**Table 1**). The presence of calcium decreased Zeta potential values to -27.5 ± 0.3 and -30.4 ± 0.3 mV, respectively.

MLVs used in this study mimic the lung surfactant multilayers present in the hypophase of the air-liquid interface in the alveolus, whereas SUVs resemble the small lipid vesicles produced as a consequence of breathing compression-expansion cycles.

Lipid Vesicle Uptake by Alveolar Epithelial Cells Depends on Vesicle Size

Alveolar epithelial cells are always in contact with surfactant lipid vesicles and ingest abundant amounts of this material to maintain surfactant homeostasis. However, the process of lipid uptake by alveolar epithelial cells and the receptors involved are incompletely understood.

To directly assess the effect of vesicle size on lipid uptake by alveolar epithelial cells, we incubated lung epithelial cell lines (mouse MLE-12 and human A549 cells) stained with Alexa Fluor 488-conjugated wheat germ agglutinin and DAPI in the presence and absence of fluorescent lipid vesicles of different sizes (MLVs or SUVs) composed of surfactant lipids (DPPC/POPG/PA). Lipid uptake was analyzed by confocal microscopy. We observed a time-dependent increase in the engulfment of SUVs, but not MLVs, by mouse MLE-12 (**Figures 1A,B**) and human A549 (**Supplementary Figure 1**) cells. Fluorescent small lipid vesicles were observed inside pneumocytes after 1 h of incubation, and the greatest uptake of SUVs seems to occur at 24h (**Figure 1A**). MLVs were not internalized by mouse and human pneumocytes after 24 h (**Figure 1B** and **Supplementary Figure 1**). Flow cytometry analysis of the time-dependent entry of fluorescent small lipid vesicles in mouse pneumocytes indicated that maximal cell fluorescence was observed at 24 h (**Figure 1C**). At this time, no extracellular vesicles attached to the cell membrane are quenched by trypan blue. **Figure 1D** show the different hydrodynamic sizes of the vesicles (MLVs and SUVs) used in this study, determined by dynamic light scattering.

According to these results, MLVs, which cannot be internalized by pneumocytes, were used in this study to determine the extracellular effect of lung surfactant on NTHi infection *in vitro*, whereas SUVs, which can be internalized, can be used to analyze the intracellular effect of endocytosed surfactant lipids.

Extracellular Large Surfactant Aggregates Bind to NTHi and Inhibit Bacterial Adhesion to Pneumocytes

The analysis of the extracellular effect of surfactant lipids on the adhesion and invasion of NTHi to pneumocytes was performed with MLVs prepared from either the hydrophobic fraction of native surfactant (PL/SP-B/SP-C) or a mixture of surfactant lipids (PL). For adhesion experiments, cells were infected for 30 min, washed, and lysed. For invasion assays, cells were infected for 2 h, washed, and incubated for an additional 1 h with gentamicin to kill extracellular bacteria (6, 7). We used two NTHi clinical strains, isolated from patients with otitis media and COPD. **Figure 2A** shows that co-incubation of mouse MLE-12 cells with MLVs and NTHi strains results in reducing the number of bacteria adhered and internalized in the cells. For both NTHi strains, inhibition of bacterial adhesion and invasion was dose-dependent. For each concentration of PL, similar inhibition values were reached for adhesion and invasion of NTHi. These results suggest that the observed reduction in bacterial internalization relates to the inhibition of bacterial adhesion to the cell membrane.

To test the possibility that surfactant MLVs would have a direct bactericidal effect on NTHi that would lead to the observed decreased C.F.U. in infection experiments, we analyzed bacterial viability in the presence and absence of MLVs at the greatest PL concentration assayed. Polymyxin B was used as a positive control of bacterial killing. Bacterial viability was determined by propidium iodide exclusion. **Figure 2B** shows that MLVs from native or synthetic surfactant preparations did not have bactericidal action against NTHi.

To test whether NTHi can stick to MLVs, so that surfactant lipids might serve as a sink absorbing the bacteria, we analyzed NTHi aggregation in the presence and absence of MLVs prepared from the surfactant hydrophobic fraction (PL/SP-B/SP-C). **Figure 2C** shows that MLVs significantly decreased bacterial aggregation over time. These results indicate that surfactant MLVs bind to bacteria, impairing bacterial self-aggregation and bacterial attachment to epithelial cells.

Altogether, our results indicate that extracellular surfactant membranes would function as biological barriers that bind to bacteria and prevent bacterial adhesion to the epithelium.

Endocytosed Surfactant Lipids Inhibited NTHi Invasion by Blocking Bacterial Uptake in Pneumocytes

With the aim of analyzing intracellular effect of endocytosed surfactant vesicles on NTHi adhesion and invasion, mouse

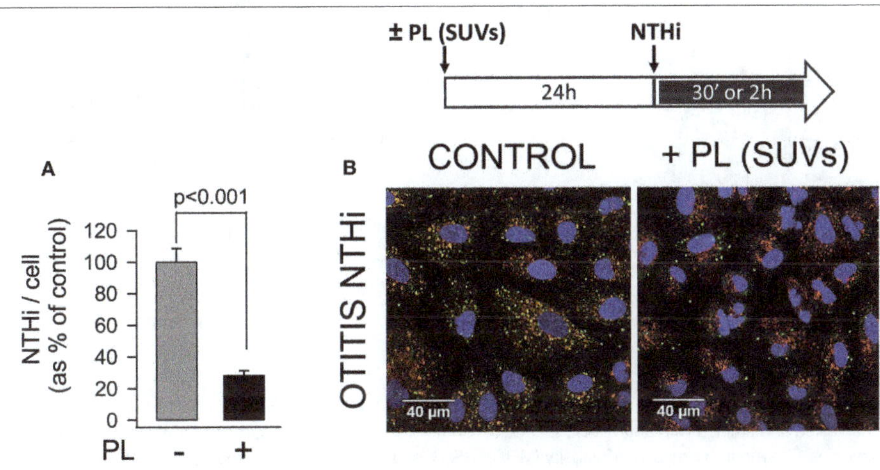

FIGURE 4 | Endocytosis of surfactant lipids attenuates NTHi entry in pneumocytes. MLE-12 cells were incubated with or without SUVs composed of surfactant lipids (250 µg PL/ml) for 24 h. Then cells were infected with otitis NTHi, and bacterial invasion assays were performed. Cells were then washed, fixed, and permeabilized with 0.1% saponin. For confocal microscopy analysis, internalized bacteria were stained with an anti-NTHi antibody and Alexa Fluor 488-conjugated secondary antibody. Late endosomes were stained with anti-LAMP1 antibody conjugated with phycoerytrin, and nuclei were stained with DAPI. **(A)** The graph shows the percentage of internalized bacteria relative to cell associated individual bacteria. Mean ± SEM of two independent experiments are shown. Student's *t*-test was used. **(B)** Representative micrographs are shown.

pneumocytes were preincubated with SUVs 24 h before infection. Then, cells were washed, independently infected with the two NTHi clinical strains, and both adhesion and invasion experiments were performed. Results indicated that endocytosed surfactant vesicles significantly inhibited otitis-NTHi invasion but not bacterial adhesion to mouse MLE-12 (**Figure 3A**) and human A549 (**Supplementary Figure 2A**) pneumocytes. Higher concentrations of PL are needed to inhibit COPD NTHi strain (**Supplementary Figure 2B**). This strain had a greater invasion capacity, as long as the number of C.F.U. recovered in invasion experiments was one order of magnitude greater than that of the otitis NTHi strain (data not shown). These experiments suggest that pneumocytes that endocytose small surfactant vesicles, as part of the surfactant recycling cycle, show reduced NTHi invasion.

When mouse pneumocytes were co-incubated with NTHi and SUVs for just 30 min, small PL vesicles also reduced bacterial adhesion to the epithelium (**Figure 3B**), but the PL concentration required for bacterial adhesion inhibition was greater for SUVs than for MLVs (**Figure 3A**). Small PL vesicles bound to NTHi decreasing NTHi self-aggregation at the highest concentration tested (**Supplementary Figure 2C**). Importantly, co-incubation of mouse pneumocytes with NTHi and SUVs for 2 h resulted in a robust inhibition of bacterial invasion at very low PL concentrations, likely due to SUV's endocytosis (**Figure 3B**). However, the effect of SUVs on NTHi invasion in coincubation

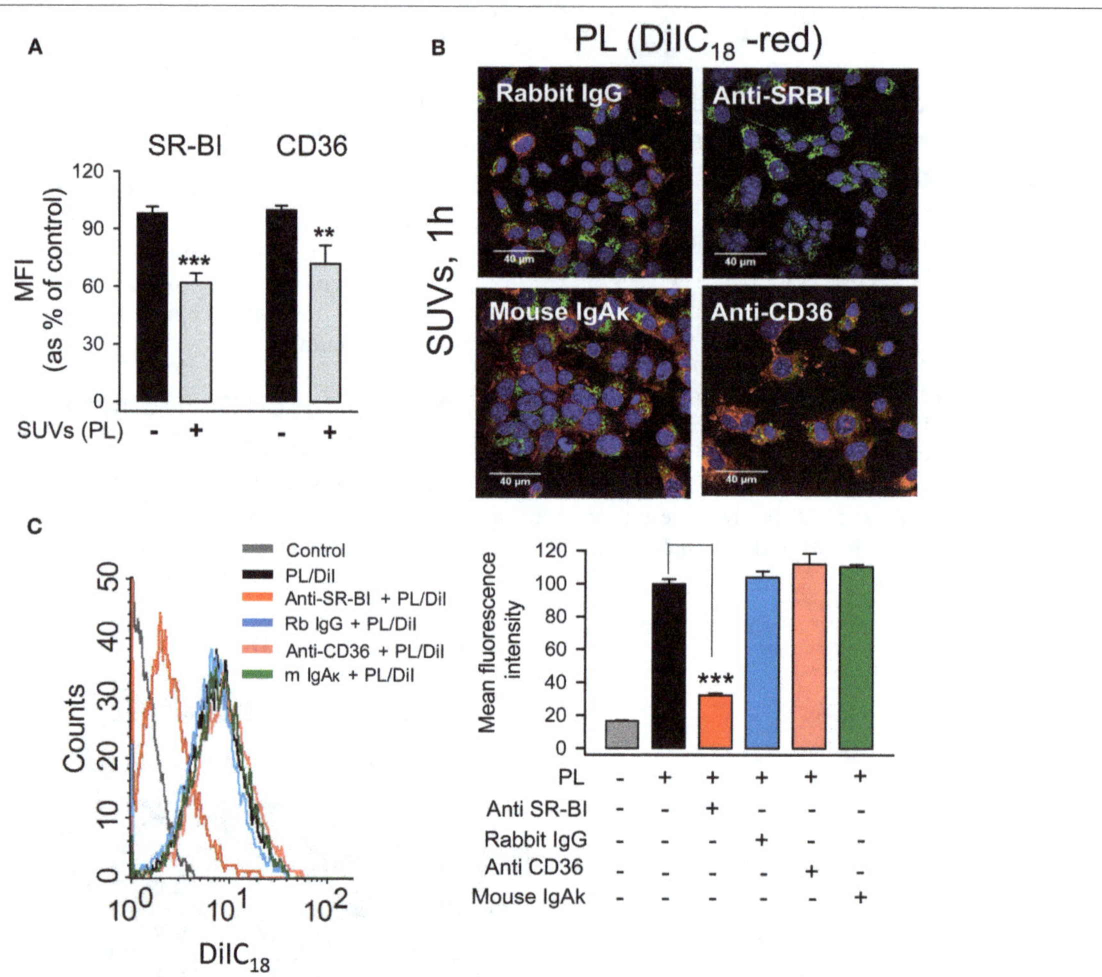

FIGURE 5 | SR-BI mediates endocytosis of small surfactant vesicles by pneumocytes. **(A)** MLE-12 cells were incubated in the presence or absence of SUVs (250 μg PL/ml) for 2 h, then cells were harvested and stained with anti-SR-BI, anti-CD36 or their respective controls, rabbit IgG or mouse IgAκ, and appropriate Alexa Fluor 488-conjugated secondary antibodies. The mean fluorescence intensity (MFI) of SR-BI and CD36 was measured by flow cytometry, and background fluorescence from IgG and IgAκ controls was subtracted. Data are presented as mean ± SEM of two independent experiments run in triplicate. Student's *t*-test was used. $^{**}p < 0.01$, and $^{***}p < 0.001$ when compared with control cells in the absence of lipids. In **(B,C)**, anti-SR-BI and anti-CD36 blocking antibodies or their respective controls, rabbit IgG or mouse IgAκ, were added to MLE-12 cells for 30 min. Then cells were incubated with $DiIC_{18}$(3)-labeled SUVs (100 μg/ml) for an additional 60 min. **(B)** Cells were fixed, stained with Alexa Fluor 488-WGA (cell membranes) and DAPI (nuclei), and analyzed by confocal microscopy. **(C)** Cells were fixed and analyzed by flow cytometry. A representative histogram is shown. The mean fluorescence intensity is represented as percentage of positive control, which is cells incubated with $DiIC_{18}$(3)-labeled SUVs in the absence of antibodies. Data are presented as mean ± SEM of three independent experiments run in triplicate. ANOVA followed by the Bonferroni multiple-comparison test was used. $^{***}p < 0.001$ when compared with cells incubated with SUVs in the absence of antibodies.

experiments was greater than that observed when SUVs were previously endocytosed by epithelial cells (**Figure 3A**), suggesting that the effect of SUVs on reducing NTHi aggregation and bacterial adhesion might also influence bacterial invasion.

Once epithelial cells were infected by NTHi, post-infection treatment with SUVs had no effect on the number of CFU recovered in invasion experiments (**Figure 3C**). This suggests that uptake of SUVs post-infection did not affect survival of previously internalized bacteria.

To assess that endocytosed surfactant lipids inhibited NTHi invasion by blocking bacterial uptake in pneumocytes, we analyzed internalized fluorescent bacteria by confocal microscopy (**Figure 4**). To this end, bacteria were stained with an antibody against NTHi and Alexa-488-conjugated secondary antibody, late endosomes were stained with a PE-conjugated anti-LAMP1 antibody, and cell nuclei were stained with DAPI. In absence of lipids, fluorescent NTHi bacteria co-localized with late endosomes, as previously described (6). However, when cells were preincubated with small surfactant vesicles for 24 h prior to infection, a 70% reduction of fluorescent bacteria was observed inside the cells. These results indicate that endocytosed surfactant lipids inhibited NTHi entry in pneumocytes.

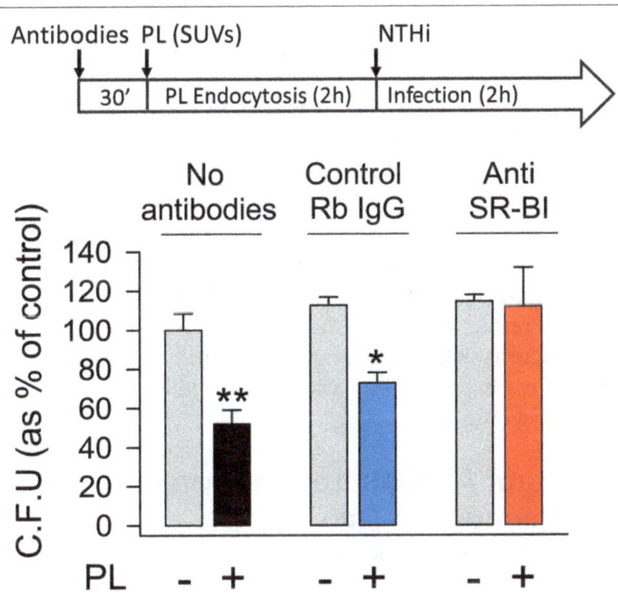

FIGURE 6 | Blocking scavenger receptor SR-BI abrogates surfactant lipid inhibition of NTHi invasion. Mouse pneumocytes were preincubated with or without anti-SR-BI or control rabbit IgG antibodies for 30 min, followed by 2 h incubation with SUVs composed of a mixture of surfactant lipids (100 µg PL/ml). Then, cells were infected with otitis NTHi, and invasion experiments were performed. Bacterial invasion was quantified by colony counting, and results were expressed as percentage of C.F.U. relative to cells infected in the absence of lipids and antibodies. The percentages of C.F.U. obtained in cells infected in the absence of lipids were not affected by the presence or absence of antibodies (control IgG or anti-SR-BI). Mean ± SEM of two independent experiments done in duplicate are shown. ANOVA followed by the Bonferroni multiple-comparison test was used. $^{*}p < 0.05$ and $^{**}p < 0.01$ when compared with infected pneumocytes in the absence of surfactant lipids and antibodies.

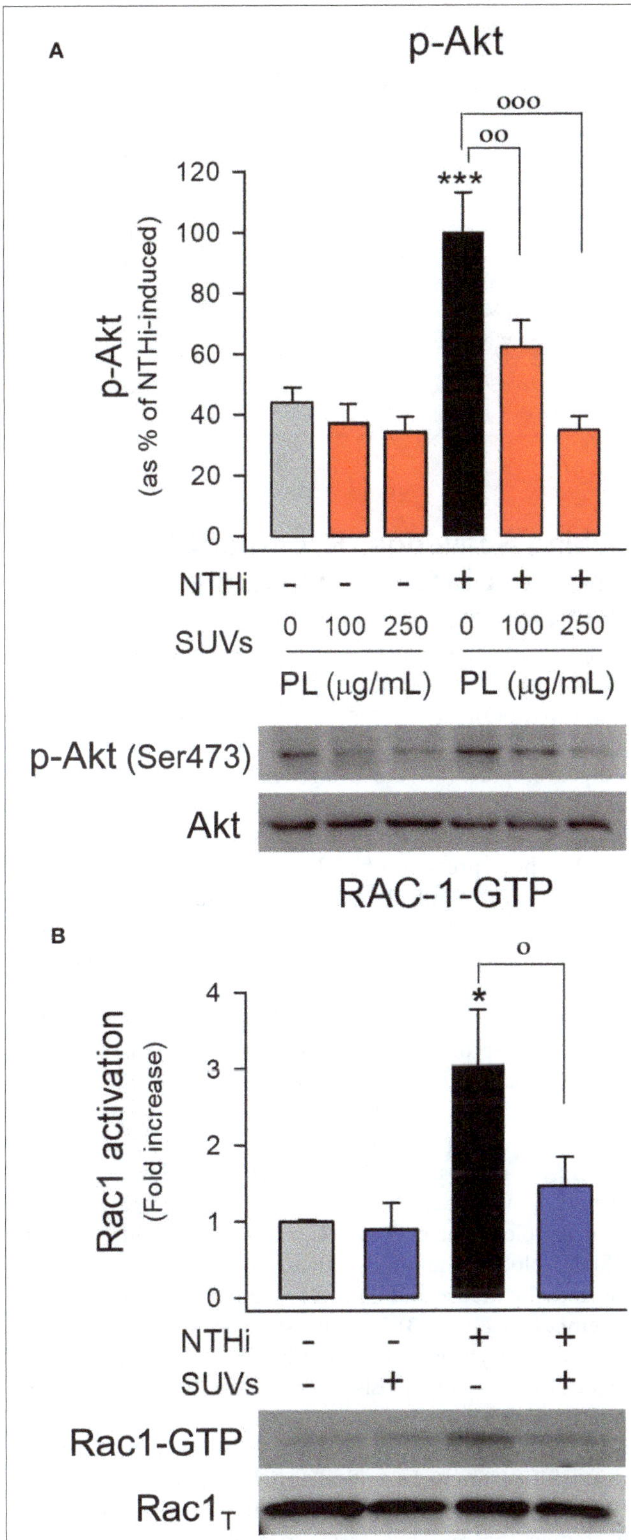

FIGURE 7 | Endocytosis of surfactant lipids inhibits signaling pathways involved in NTHi internalization. **(A)** Mouse pneumocytes were preincubated with SUVs of surfactant lipids (100 or 250 µg PL/ml) for 24 h. Then cells were washed and infected with otitis NTHi for 45 min. Cells were lysed, and p-Akt and total Akt were analyzed by western blot. p-Akt was normalized to total

(Continued)

FIGURE 7 | Akt, and data are shown as percentage of NTHi-induced Akt phosphorylation in the absence of lipids. Mean ± SEM of three independent experiments performed in triplicate are shown. ANOVA followed by Bonferroni multiple-comparison test was used. $^{***}p < 0.001$ when compared with untreated and uninfected cells. $^{\circ\circ}p < 0.01$ and $^{\circ\circ\circ}p < 0.001$ when compared with infected pneumocytes in the absence of surfactant lipid vesicles. **(B)** MLE-12 cells were preincubated with SUVs of surfactant lipids (250 μg PL /ml) for 24 h. Then cells were infected with otitis NTHi for 2 h and activation of the GTPase Rac1 was analyzed by pull-down and western blot. Rac1-GTP and total Rac1 were quantified, and data are shown as percentage of NTHi-induced Rac1 activation (fold increase) relative to uninfected cells in the absence of lipids. Mean ± SEM of four independent experiments performed in triplicate are shown. ANOVA followed by the Bonferroni multiple-comparison test was used. $^{*}p < 0.05$ when compared with untreated and uninfected cells. $^{\circ}p < 0.05$ when compared with infected pneumocytes in the absence of surfactant lipids.

Blocking Scavenger Receptor SR-BI Abrogates Surfactant Lipid Inhibition of NTHi Invasion

Although surfactant lipids may be endocytosed by type II pneumocytes via clathrin-dependent and -independent mechanisms (46), the receptors that mediate lipid vesicle endocytosis by pneumocytes have not been entirely identified. Scavenger receptors (SR) are involved in lipid uptake (47) and SR-BI and SR-BII (CD36) interact with anionic phospholipids (48). In addition, these receptors are expressed in airway epithelial cells (49). The expression of SR-BI and CD36 receptors on the surface of MLE-12 epithelial cells was examined in the presence and absence of surfactant PL. We observed that the expression of both SR-BI and CD36 was significantly reduced in response to lipid vesicle internalization (**Figure 5A**).

To determine the effect of blocking antibodies of SR-BI and CD36 receptors on the endocytosis of small surfactant vesicles, alveolar epithelial cells were preincubated with blocking antibodies or their respective immunoglobulin controls, and endocytosis of DiIC$_{18}$-fluorescent lipid vesicles was determined by confocal microscopy (**Figure 5B**) and flow cytometry (**Figure 5C**). We identified SR-BI as the receptor with a prominent role in the endocytosis of surfactant lipids, since the anti-SR-BI blocking antibody caused 70 % reduction of SUVs endocytosis by mouse and human pneumocytes (**Figure 5C** and **Supplementary Figure 3**). In contrast, anti-CD36 produced only 20 % PL endocytosis reduction by human cells, and it had no effect on PL endocytosis by mouse cells (**Figure 5C** and **Supplementary Figure 3**).

Next, we investigated whether the engulfment of surfactant lipids by SR-BI might be critical for the attenuation of NTHi invasion (**Figure 6**). To this end, MLE-12 cells were pre-incubated in the presence or absence of anti-SR-BI blocking antibody or its IgG control for 30 min before incubating with surfactant lipid vesicles for 2 h. After washing, cells were infected with NTHi and bacterial invasion experiments were performed. We found that, in the absence of lipids, anti-SR-BI antibody did not have any effect on NTHi invasion, because the number of bacteria internalized in the cells was similar to that of control experiments without blocking SR-BI antibody or in the presence of its IgG control (**Figure 6**). Importantly, in the presence of small lipid vesicles, the blockade of SR-BI impeded lipid-induced inhibition of NTHi invasion (**Figure 6**). Thus, blocking the endocytosis of lipid vesicles increased pneumocyte susceptibility to NTHi invasion. These results demonstrate that SR-BI-mediated internalization of surfactant lipids is required for lipid-dependent inhibition of NTHi invasion of alveolar epithelial cells.

Endocytosis of Surfactant Lipids Inhibits Signaling Pathways Involved in NTHi Internalization

NTHi was shown to enter bronchial epithelial cells through macropinocytosis (50). NTHi internalization seems to be mediated by either direct bacterium binding to integrins or indirect binding through extracellular matrix proteins (51, 52). Integrin signaling leads to phosphorylation of focal adhesion kinase (FAK), followed by activation of Rac1 GTPase and PI3K to induce actin polymerization and membrane protrusion (52). We previously showed that activation of both Rac1 and PI3K is essential for NTHi entry in A549 epithelial cells (7).

To determine whether endocytosed surfactant vesicles reduced bacterial entry into pneumocytes by blocking key signaling pathways required for NTHi internalization, the next step was to evaluate NTHi-induced PI3K-Akt and Rac1 activation in mouse and human pneumocytes preincubated with or without surfactant lipid vesicles (**Figure 7** and **Supplementary Figure 4**). We found that NTHi infection induced Akt phosphorylation (**Figure 7A**) and Rac1 GTPase activation (**Figure 7B**) in mouse pneumocytes, as previously described in human A549 cells (7). Endocytosed surfactant lipid vesicles inhibited NTHi-induced Akt phosphorylation in mouse (**Figure 7A**) and human (**Supplementary Figure 4**) pneumocytes. Furthermore, endocytosed surfactant lipids blocked NTHi-induced Rac1 activation (**Figure 7B**).

These results suggest that endocytosis of surfactant phospholipid vesicles interferes with cytoskeletal reorganization required for membrane protrusions that facilitate bacterial entry in pneumocytes.

Surfactant Administration Protects From NTHi Infection *in vivo*

Lastly, we wondered whether lung surfactant administration could protect from NTHi infection *in vivo*. To test this hypothesis, we infected CD1 mice intratracheally with a clinical NTHi strain from otitis patients, and simultaneously we instilled the hydrophobic fraction of native surfactant that contains surfactant lipids and the hydrophobic proteins SP-B and SP-C. Then, bacterial burden was assessed in whole lung tissue and BAL after 6, 12, and 24 h post infection. **Figure 8** shows that administration of exogenous lung surfactant significantly diminished bacterial load in lung tissue and BAL of NTHi infected mice 12–24 h after surfactant administration, supporting the notion that the lipid component of lung surfactant protects against NTHi infection. Analyses of cell types in BAL from infected mice treated with or without surfactant revealed that recruited cells consisted predominantly

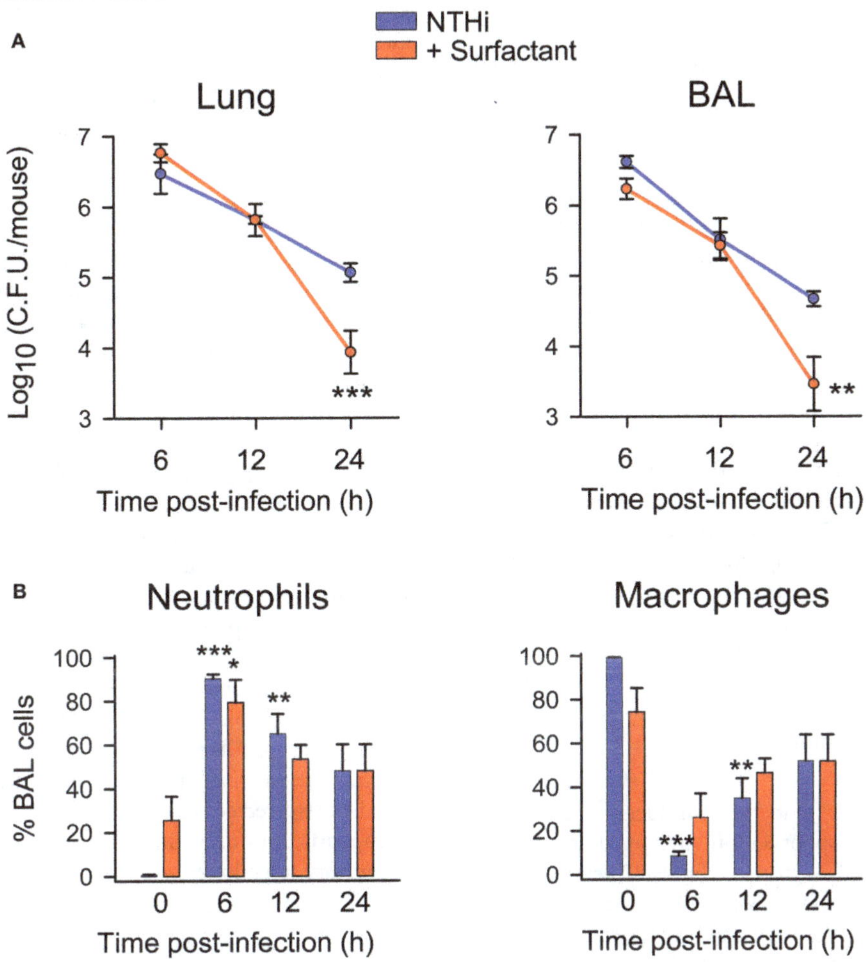

FIGURE 8 | Surfactant treatment accelerated bacterial clearance in lung tissue and BAL of NTHi infected mice. Mice were intratracheally infected with otitis NTHi strain (4×10^7 C.F.U./mouse), and the hydrophobic fraction of native pulmonary surfactant (25 mg PL/kg body weigh) was simultaneously instilled into the lungs (or the same volume of PBS in the untreated infected group). Mice were euthanized at 6, 12, or 24 h postinfection. Lungs were harvested, weighed, and homogenized (left lung) or used for BAL extraction (right lung) ($n = 5$ mice each infected group; $n = 3$ mice each uninfected group). **(A)** The numbers of viable bacteria in lung homogenates and BAL were assessed by colony counting and expressed as $\log_{10}$ (C.F.U./mouse). Results are mean ± SEM. ANOVA followed by Bonferroni multiple-comparison test was used. $^{**}p < 0.01$, and $^{***}p < 0.001$ when compared with untreated infected groups. **(B)** Percentage of alveolar macrophage and neutrophil counts in BAL. Results are mean ± SEM. ANOVA followed by the Bonferroni multiple-comparison test was used. $^{*}p < 0.05$, $^{**}p < 0.01$, and $^{***}p < 0.001$ when compared with the corresponding uninfected group.

of neutrophils (**Figure 8**). Neutrophil recruitment was similar in infected mice treated with surfactant compared with untreated infected animals. Control experiments indicate that neutrophil recruitment did not significantly increase in uninfected mice treated with surfactant compared with untreated uninfected mice (**Figure 8**). These results suggest that the accelerated clearance of NTHi in mice treated with surfactant was not associated with increased neutrophil infiltration at 6, 12, and 24 h post-infection in surfactant-treated mice compared with untreated mice.

DISCUSSION

Lung surfactant has two essential functions: keeping the alveolus open and host defense. These functions are inseparably coordinated and depend on the complexity of surfactant's components (19). Whereas surfactant proteins SP-A and SP-D have a clear role in lung defense, attention to surfactant lipids and hydrophobic surfactant proteins has been focused on surface tension properties. Whether surfactant lipids participate in the control of infection by inhaled pathogens remains mostly unaddressed.

In the present study, we demonstrated that the lipid component of pulmonary surfactant interferes with pathogen-host interaction between NTHi and pneumocytes through two different mechanisms. On the one hand, large extracellular surfactant vesicles bind to NTHi and function as biological barriers to reduce the number of bacteria adhered and internalized in alveolar epithelial cells. On the other hand, small surfactant vesicles were rapidly endocytosed by pneumocytes, mainly via the scavenger receptor SR-BI that mediates clathrin- and dynamin-independent endocytosis (53). The endocytosed surfactant lipids inhibited NTHi invasion by blocking bacterial uptake in pneumocytes.

Macropinocytosis is exploited by several intracellular pathogens as a means of entry into cells (54). This process is responsible for the uptake of large particles, >0.5 μm in diameter. The NTHi entry into pneumocytes requires direct or indirect bacterial binding to integrins, which initiate the activation of the Src/GEF Vav2/Rac1 GTPase/Pak1 signaling axis for polymerization of microtubules and cell ruffling (6, 7). These cytoskeletal remodeling proteins are bound to phosphatidylinositol (PtdIns)(4, 5)P2, which is enriched at the macropinocytic site in early stages of macropinosome development (54–56). Interestingly, PtdIns(4, 5)P2 disappearance is critical for macropinosome formation. At this stage, PtdIns(3,4,5)P3 is formed by PI3K activity. PtdIns(3,4,5)P3 is essential for cup closure (54–56). By recruiting adaptors, GEFs and GAPs that contain PtdIns(3,4,5)P3-interacting PH domains, the cell is able to dictate the activity of Rho family GTPases that direct the polymerization of actin required for macropinosome closure. Consistent with this, we previously found that inhibition of PI3K or Rac1 activation abrogates NTHi internalization (6, 7).

In this study, we show that NTHi-induced Rac1 GTPase activation and Akt phosphorylation by pneumocytes was inhibited by endocytosed surfactant lipids. Therefore, small surfactant lipid vesicles, once endocytosed, block intracellular signaling pathways that are required for NTHi entry into pneumocytes. The mechanism by which endocytosed lipid vesicles show such inhibitory effects is unknown. Given that clathrin-independent endocytosis of small particles also requires PtdIns(4,5)P2 for membrane curvature and invagination (55, 56) as well as Src, Rac1, or ARF signaling proteins that bind to PtdIns(4,5)P2, it is possible that endocytosis of lipid vesicles could shuttle PtdIns(4,5)P2 and associated proteins from the plasma membrane into internal membranes. The sequestration of PtdIns(4,5)P2 and Src, Rac1, or ARF could inhibit bacterial entry since depletion of PtdIns(4,5)P2 in the macropinocytic site reduces the macropinocytic or phagocytic efficiency (57).

To assess the beneficial role of lung surfactant lipids during NTHi infection, we performed *in vivo* experiments treating NTHi-infected mice with the hydrophobic fraction of native surfactant isolated from rat lungs. We found that this surfactant fraction, composed of PL, SP-B, and SP-C, was able to bind to NTHi, which led to a significant reduction of NTHi capability to self-aggregate. NTHi aggregation is responsible for microcolony formation on the epithelial surfaces, facilitating bacterial colonization of the airways (58). Administration of the hydrophobic fraction of native surfactant to NTHi infected mice significantly accelerated bacterial clearance in lung tissue and BAL. Surfactant treatment did not significantly affect early neutrophil recruitment in infected mice, suggesting that surfactant vesicles are directly involved in preventing bacterial adhesion to the epithelium and facilitating the actions of airway macrophages, neutrophils, antimicrobial proteins, and mucociliary clearance in promoting bacterial clearance.

Surfactant phospholipid concentration has been reported to decrease in COPD and idiopathic pulmonary fibrosis (30, 59). Smokers have reduced surfactant phospholipid levels, as well as impaired biophysical activity (30, 31). In asthma or pneumonia, reduced levels of phosphatidylcholine and changes in phospholipid composition have also been found (30). Surfactant lipids are also significantly altered in the aged lung in both mice and humans (60). In addition, pathological conditions, such as previous infection with rhinovirus, can reduce the inflammatory response and cause delay in NTHi clearance (61). Thus, in a context of immune dysregulation, the protective effect of pulmonary surfactant on NTHi respiratory infection may be more necessary. Therapeutic interventions with the hydrophobic fraction of surfactant might be of potential benefit in respiratory diseases with NTHi infection because exogenous surfactant protects against NTHi and improves lung biophysical function. In addition, the use of small surfactant-like vesicles as vehicles for inhaled drug administration may have further added value. This lipid-based host-directed strategy would offer novel prophylactic or therapeutic options against chronic, recurrent, or drug-resistant respiratory infections.

AUTHOR CONTRIBUTIONS

BG-F conceived, designed, and performed all the experiments, collected, analyzed, and interpreted all data, and wrote the manuscript. ZG-C, CM, AI-C, and LdT performed research. AdL, BE, and JG designed and performed *in vivo* experiments. SC-L contributed tools, and provided expertise. CC conceived the study, designed the experiments, interpreted and organized all data, and wrote the manuscript.

ACKNOWLEDGMENTS

We thank the animal facility of the Faculty of Biology and Confocal Microscopy Unit of Universidad Complutense de Madrid for excellent technical support. We acknowledge Dr. O. Cañadas's help in dynamic light scattering and zeta potential measurements, and Dr. I. Rodríguez-Arce's help with animal experiments.

REFERENCES

1. Duell BL, Su YC, Riesbeck K. Host-pathogen interactions of nontypeable *Haemophilus influenzae*: from commensal to pathogen. *FEBS Lett.* (2016) 590:3840–53. doi: 10.1002/1873-3468
2. King PT, Sharma R. The lung immune response to nontypeable *Haemophilus influenzae* (Lung immunity to NTHi). *J Immunol Res.* (2015) 2015:706376. doi: 10.1155/2015/706376
3. Bakaletz LO, Novotny LA. Nontypeable *Haemophilus influenzae* (NTHi). *Trends Microbiol.* (2018) 26:727–8. doi: 10.1016/j.tim.2018.05.001
4. Van Eldere J, Slack MPE, Ladhani S, Cripps AW. Non-typeable *Haemophilus influenzae*, an under-recognised pathogen. *Lancet Infect Dis.* (2014) 14:1281–92. doi: 10.1016/S1473-3099(14)70734-0
5. Ahearn CP, Gallo MC, Murphy TF. Insights on persistent airway infection by non-typeable *Haemophilus influenzae* in chronic obstructive pulmonary disease. *Pathog Dis.* (2017) 75:ftx042. doi: 10.1093/femspd/ftx042
6. Morey A, Cano V, Martí-Lliteras P, López-Gómez A, Regueiro V, Saus C, et al. Evidence for a non-replicative intracellular stage of nontypeable *Haemophilus influenzae* in epithelial cells. *Microbiology.* (2011) 157:234–50. doi: 10.1099/mic.0.040451-0
7. López-Gómez A, Cano V, Moranta D, Morey P, García del Portillo F, Bengoechea JA, et al. Host cell kinases, a5 and b1 integrins, and Rac1 signalling on the microtubule cytoskeleton are important for non-typable *Haemophilus influenzae* invasion of respiratory epithelial cells. *Microbiology.* (2012) 158:2384–98. doi: 10.1099/mic.0.059972-0
8. Bandi V, Apicella MA, Mason E, Murphy TF, Siddiqi A, Atmar RL, et al. Nontypeable *Haemophilus influenzae* in the lower respiratory tract of patients with chronic bronchitis. *Am J Respir Crit Care Med.* (2001) 164:2114–9. doi: 10.1164/ajrccm.164.11.2104093
9. Drömann D, Rupp J, Rohmann K, Osbahr S, Ulmer AJ, Marwitz S, et al. The TGF-beta-pseudoreceptor BAMBI is strongly expressed in COPD lungs and regulated by nontypeable *Haemophilus influenzae. Respir Res.* (2010) 11:67. doi: 10.1186/1465-9921-11-67
10. Raffel FK, Szelestey BR, Beatty WL, Mason KM. The *Haemophilus influenzae* Sap transporter mediates bacterium-epithelial cell homeostasis. *Infect Immun.* (2013) 81:43–54. doi: 10.1128/IAI.00942-12
11. Clementi CF, Murphy TF. Non-typeable *Haemophilus influenzae* invasion and persistence in the human respiratory tract. *Front Cell Infect Microbiol.* (2011) 1:1. doi: 10.3389/fcimb.2011.00001
12. van Schilfgaarde M, van Ulsen P, Eijk P, Brand M, Stam M, Kouame J, et al. Characterization of adherence of nontypeable *Haemophilus influenzae* to human epithelial cells. *Infect Immun.* (2000) 68:4658–65. doi: 10.1128/IAI.68.8.4658-4665.2000
13. Hallstrom T, Blom AM, Zipfel PF, Riesbeck K. Nontypeable *Haemophilus influenzae* protein E binds vitronectin and is important for serum resistance. *J Immunol.* (2009) 183:2593–60. doi: 10.4049/jimmunol.0803226
14. Marti-Lliteras P, Lopez-Gomez A, Mauro S, Hood DW, Viadas C, Calatayud L, et al. Nontypable *Haemophilus influenzae* displays a prevalent surface structure molecular pattern in clinical isolates. *PLoS ONE.* (2011) 6:e21133. doi: 10.1371/journal.pone.0021133
15. Eberhard T, Ullberg M. Interaction of vitronectin with *Haemophilus influenzae. FEMS Immunol Med Microbiol.* (2002) 34:215–9. doi: 10.1111/j.1574-695X.2002.tb00627.x
16. Iwasaki A, Foxman EF, Molony RD. Early local immune defences in the respiratory tract. *Nat Rev Immunol.* (2017) 17:7–20. doi: 10.1038/nri.2016.117
17. Zhang P, Summer WR, Bagby GJ, Nelson S. Innate immunity and pulmonary host defense. *Immunol Rev.* (2000) 173:39–51. doi: 10.1034/j.1600-065X.2000.917306.x
18. Coya JM, Akinbi HT, Sáenz A, Yang L, Weaver TE, Casals C. Natural anti-infective pulmonary proteins: *in vivo* cooperative action of surfactant protein SP-A and the lung antimicrobial peptide SP-BN. *J Immunol.* (2015) 195:1628–36. doi: 10.4049/jimmunol.1500778
19. Casals C, Cañadas O. Role of lipid ordered/disordered phase coexistence in pulmonary surfactant function. *Biochim Biophys Acta.* (2012) 1818:2550–62. doi: 10.1016/j.bbamem.2012.05.024
20. Olmeda B, Martínez-Calle M, Pérez-Gil J. Pulmonary surfactant metabolism in the alveolar airspace: biogenesis, extracellular conversions, recycling. *Ann Anat.* (2017) 209:78–92. doi: 10.1016/j.aanat.2016.09.008
21. Wright JR. Immunoregulatory functions of surfactant proteins. *Nat Rev Immunol.* (2005) 5:58–68. doi: 10.1038/nri1528
22. Minutti CM, García-Fojeda B, Sáenz A, de Las Casas-Engel M, Guillamat-Prats R, de Lorenzo A, et al. Surfactant protein A prevents IFN-γ/IFN-γ receptor interaction and attenuates classical activation of human alveolar macrophages. *J Immunol.* (2016) 197:590–8. doi: 10.4049/jimmunol.1501032
23. Minutti CM, Jackson-Jones LH, García-Fojeda B, Knipper JA, Sutherland TE, Logan N, et al. Local amplifiers of IL-4Rα-mediated macrophage activation promote repair in lung and liver. *Science.* (2017) 356:1076–80. doi: 10.1126/science.aaj2067
24. Sorensen GL. Surfactant protein D in respiratory and non-respiratory diseases. *Front Med.* (2018) 5:18. doi: 10.3389/fmed.2018.00018
25. Whitsett JA, Wert SE, Weaver TE. Diseases of pulmonary surfactant homeostasis. *Annu Rev Pathol.* (2015) 10:371–93. doi: 10.1146/annurev-pathol-012513-104644
26. Robertson B, Halliday HL. Principles of surfactant replacement. *Biochim Biophys Acta.* (1998) 1408:346–61. doi: 10.1016/S0925-4439(98)00080-5
27. Jang CH, Cho YB, Oh SE, Choi JU, Park H, Choi CH. Effect of nebulized bovine surfactant for experimental otitis media with effusion. *Clin Exp Otorhinolaryngol.* (2010) 3:13–7. doi: 10.3342/ceo.2010.3.1.13
28. Zhu ZH, Shan YJ, Han Y, Zhu LW, Ma ZX. Pathological study of otitis media with effusion after treatment with intranasal pulmonary surfactant. *Laryngoscope.* (2013) 123:3148–55. doi: 10.1002/lary.24166
29. Fessler MB, Summer RS. Surfactant Lipids at the Host-Environment Interface. Metabolic Sensors, Suppressors, and Effectors of Inflammatory Lung Disease. *Am J Respir Cell Mol Biol.* (2016) 54:624–35. doi: 10.1165/rcmb.2016-0011PS
30. Griese M. Pulmonary surfactant in health and human lung diseases: state of the art. *Eur Respir J.* (1999) 13:1455–76. doi: 10.1034/j.1399-3003.1999.13f36.x
31. Moré JM, Voelker DR, Silveira LJ, Edwards MG, Chan ED, Bowler RP. Smoking reduces surfactant protein D and phospholipids in patients with and without chronic obstructive pulmonary disease. *BMC Pulm Med.* (2010) 10:53. doi: 10.1186/1471-2466-10-53
32. Hite RD, Seeds MC, Bowton DL, Grier BL, Safta AM, Balkrishnan R, et al. Surfactant phospholipid changes after antigen challenge: a role for phosphatidylglycerol in dysfunction. *Am J Physiol Lung Cell Mol Physiol.* (2005) 288:L610–7. doi: 10.1152/ajplung.00273.2004
33. Wirtz HR, Schmidt M. Acute influence of cigarette smoke on secretion of pulmonary surfactant in rat alveolar type II cells in culture. *Eur Respir J.* (1996) 9:24–32. doi: 10.1183/09031936.96.09010024
34. Casals C, Herrera L, Miguel E, Garcia-Barreno P, Municio AM. Comparison between intra- and extracellular surfactant in respiratory distress induced by oleic acid. *Biochim Biophys Acta.* (1989) 1003:201–3. doi: 10.1016/0005-2760(89)90256-7
35. Casals C, Varela A, Ruano MLF, Valiño F, Pérez-Gil J, Torre N, et al. Increase of C-reactive protein and decrease of surfactant apolipoproteins SP-A and SP-B in surfactant after lung transplantation. *Am J Respir Crit Care Med.* (1998) 157:43–7. doi: 10.1164/ajrccm.157.1.9611106
36. Rouser G, Fleischer S, Yamamoto A. Two dimensional thin layer chromatographic separation of polar lipids and determination of phospholipids by phosphorus analysis of spots. *Lipids.* (1970) 5:494–6. doi: 10.1007/BF02531316
37. Sáenz A, Cañadas O, Bagatolli LA, Johnson ME, Casals C. Physical properties and surface activity of surfactant-like membranes containing the cationic and hydrophobic peptide KL4. *FEBS J.* (2006) 273:2515–27. doi: 10.1111/j.1742-4658.2006.05258.x
38. Sáenz A, Cañadas O, Bagatolli LA, Sánchez-Barbero F, Johnson ME, Casals C. Effect of surfactant protein A on the physical properties and surface activity of KL4-surfactant. *Biophys J.* (2007) 92:482–92. doi: 10.1529/biophysj.106.090217
39. Sáenz A, Alvarez L, Santos M, López-Sánchez A, Castillo-Olivares JL, Varela A, et al. Beneficial effects of synthetic KL4 surfactant in experimental lung transplantation. *Eur Respir J.* (2011) 37:925–32. doi: 10.1183/09031936.00020810
40. Cañadas O, Guerrero R, García-Cañero R, Orellana G, Menéndez M, Casals C. Characterization of liposomal FK506 in lung surfactant-like phospholipids and evaluation of its immunosuppressive activity. *Biochemistry.* (2004) 43:9926–38. doi: 10.1021/bi036227z

41. Hoefel D, Grooby WL, Monis PT, Andrews S, Saint CP. A comparative study of carboxyfluorescein diacetate and carboxyfluorescein diacetate succinimidyl ester as indicators of bacterial activity. *J Microbiol Methods.* (2003) 52:379–88. doi: 10.1016/S0167-7012(02)00207-5
42. Castillo-Lluva S, Tatham MH, Jones RC, Jaffray EG, Edmondson RD, Hay RT, et al. SUMOylation of the GTPase Rac1 is required for optimal cell migration. *Nat Cell Biol.* (2010) 12:1078–85. doi: 10.1038/ncb2112
43. Woodcock SA, Jones RC, Edmondson RD, Malliri A. A modified tandem affinity purification technique identifies that 14-3-3 proteins interact with Tiam1, an interaction which controls Tiam1 stability. *J Proteome Res.* (2009) 8:5629–41. doi: 10.1021/pr900716e
44. Rodríguez-Arce I, Martí S, Euba B, Fernández-Calvet A, Moleres J, López-López N, et al. Inactivation of the thymidylate synthase ThyA in non-typeable *Haemophilus influenzae* modulates antibiotic resistance and has a strong impact on its interplay with the host airways. *Front Cell Infect Microbiol.* (2017) 7:266. doi: 10.3389/fcimb.2017.00266
45. Euba B, López-López N, Rodríguez-Arce I, Fernández-Calvet A, Barberán M, Caturla N, et al. Resveratrol therapeutics combines both antimicrobial and immunomodulatory properties against respiratory infection by nontypeable *Haemophilus influenzae. Sci Rep.* (2017) 7:12860. doi: 10.1038/s41598-017-13034-7
46. Bates SR, Dodia C, Tao JQ, Fisher AB. Surfactant protein A plays an important role in lung surfactant clearance: evidence using the surfactant protein-A-gene-targeted mouse. *Am J Physiol Lung Cell Mol Physiol.* (2008) 294:L325–33. doi: 10.1152/ajplung.00341.2007
47. Martin C, Chevrot M, Poirier H, Passilly-Degrace P, Niot I, Besnard P. CD36 as a lipid sensor. *Physiol Behav.* (2011) 105:36–42. doi: 10.1016/j.physbeh.2011.02.029
48. Rigotti A, Acton SL, Krieger M. The class B scavenger receptors SR-BI and CD36 are receptors for anionic phospholipids. *J Biol Chem.* (1995) 270:16221–4. doi: 10.1074/jbc.270.27.16221
49. Dieudonné A, Torres D, Blanchard S, Taront S, Jeannin P, Delneste Y, et al. Scavenger receptors in human airway epithelial cells: role in response to double-stranded RNA. *PLoS ONE.* (2012) 7:e41952. doi: 10.1371/journal.pone.0041952
50. Ketterer MR, Shao JQ, Hornick DB, Buscher B, Bandi VK, Apicella MA. Infection of primary human bronchial epithelial cells by *Haemophilus influenzae*: macropinocytosis as a mechanism of airway epithelial cell entry. *Infect Immun.* (1999) 67:4161–70.
51. Singh B, Su YC, Riesbeck K. Vitronectin in bacterial pathogenesis: a host protein used in complement escape and cellular invasion. *Mol Microbiol.* (2010) 78:545–60. doi: 10.1111/j.1365-2958.2010.07373.x
52. Ikeda M, Enomoto N, Hashimoto D, Fujisawa T, Inui N, Nakamura Y, et al. Nontypeable *Haemophilus influenzae* exploits the interaction between protein-E and vitronectin for the adherence and invasion to bronchial epithelial cells. *BMC Microbiol.* (2015) 15:263. doi: 10.1186/s12866-015-0600-8
53. Sun B, Boyanovsky BB, Connelly MA, Shridas P, van der Westhuyzen DR, Webb NR. Distinct mechanisms for OxLDL uptake and cellular trafficking by class B scavenger receptors CD36 and SR-BI. *J Lipid Res.* (2007) 48:2560–70. doi: 10.1194/jlr.M700163-JLR200
54. Kumari S, Mg S, Mayor S. Endocytosis unplugged: multiple ways to enter the cell. *Cell Res.* (2010) 20:256–75. doi: 10.1038/cr.2010.19.56.2013
55. Bohdanowicz M, Grinstein S. Role of phospholipids in endocytosis, phagocytosis, and macropinocytosis. *Physiol Rev.* (2013) 93:69–106. doi: 10.1152/physrev.00002.2012
56. Ferreira APA, Boucrot E. Mechanisms of Carrier Formation during Clathrin-Independent Endocytosis. *Trends Cell Biol.* (2018) 28:188–200. doi: 10.1016/j.tcb.2017.11.004
57. Coppolino MG, Dierckman R, Loijens J, Collins RF, Pouladi M, Jongstra-Bilen J, et al. Inhibition of phosphatidylinositol-4-phosphate 5-kinase I alpha impairs localized actin remodeling and suppresses phagocytosis. *J Biol Chem.* (2002) 77:43849–57. doi: 10.1074/jbc.M2090 46200
58. Hendrixson DR, St Geme JW 3rd. The *Haemophilus influenzae* Hap serine protease promotes adherence and microcolony formation, potentiated by a soluble host protein. *Mol Cell.* (1998) 2:841–50.
59. Zhao CZ, Fang XC, Wang D, Tang FD, Wang XD. Involvement of type II pneumocytes in the pathogenesis of chronic obstructive pulmonary desease. *Respir Med.* (2010) 104:1391–5. doi: 10.1016/j.rmed.2010.06.018
60. Moliva JI, Rajaram MV, Sidiki S, Sasindran SJ, Guirado E, Pan XJ, et al. Molecular composition of the alveolar lining fluid in the aging lung. *Age.* (2014) 36:9633. doi: 10.1007/s11357-014-9633-4
61. Unger BL, Faris AN, Ganesan S, Comstock AT, Hershenson MB, Sajjan US. Rhinovirus attenuates non-typeable *Hemophilus influenzae*-stimulated IL-8 responses via TLR2-dependent degradation of IRAK-1. *PLoS Pathog.* (2012) 8:e1002969. doi: 10.1371/journal.ppat.10029

Permissions

All chapters in this book were first published by Frontiers; hereby published with permission under the Creative Commons Attribution License or equivalent. Every chapter published in this book has been scrutinized by our experts. Their significance has been extensively debated. The topics covered herein carry significant findings which will fuel the growth of the discipline. They may even be implemented as practical applications or may be referred to as a beginning point for another development.

The contributors of this book come from diverse backgrounds, making this book a truly international effort. This book will bring forth new frontiers with its revolutionizing research information and detailed analysis of the nascent developments around the world.

We would like to thank all the contributing authors for lending their expertise to make the book truly unique. They have played a crucial role in the development of this book. Without their invaluable contributions this book wouldn't have been possible. They have made vital efforts to compile up to date information on the varied aspects of this subject to make this book a valuable addition to the collection of many professionals and students.

This book was conceptualized with the vision of imparting up-to-date information and advanced data in this field. To ensure the same, a matchless editorial board was set up. Every individual on the board went through rigorous rounds of assessment to prove their worth. After which they invested a large part of their time researching and compiling the most relevant data for our readers.

The editorial board has been involved in producing this book since its inception. They have spent rigorous hours researching and exploring the diverse topics which have resulted in the successful publishing of this book. They have passed on their knowledge of decades through this book. To expedite this challenging task, the publisher supported the team at every step. A small team of assistant editors was also appointed to further simplify the editing procedure and attain best results for the readers.

Apart from the editorial board, the designing team has also invested a significant amount of their time in understanding the subject and creating the most relevant covers. They scrutinized every image to scout for the most suitable representation of the subject and create an appropriate cover for the book.

The publishing team has been an ardent support to the editorial, designing and production team. Their endless efforts to recruit the best for this project, has resulted in the accomplishment of this book. They are a veteran in the field of academics and their pool of knowledge is as vast as their experience in printing. Their expertise and guidance has proved useful at every step. Their uncompromising quality standards have made this book an exceptional effort. Their encouragement from time to time has been an inspiration for everyone.

The publisher and the editorial board hope that this book will prove to be a valuable piece of knowledge for researchers, students, practitioners and scholars across the globe.

List of Contributors

Neetika Jaisinghani, Stanzin Dawa, Kaurab Singh, Ananya Nandy, Dilip Menon, Purva Deepak Bhandari and Sheetal Gandotra
Chemical and Systems Biology Group, CSIR-Institute of Genomics and Integrative Biology, New Delhi, India Academy of Scientific and Innovative Research (AcSIR), New Delhi, India

Garima Khare
Department of Biochemistry, University of Delhi South Campus, New Delhi, India

Anil Tyagi
Department of Biochemistry, University of Delhi South Campus, New Delhi, India Guru Gobind Singh Indraprastha University, New Delhi, India

Jorge A. Soto, Nicolás M. S. Gálvez, Felipe M. Benavente, Magdalena S. Pizarro-Ortega, Susan M. Bueno and Pablo A. Gonzalez
Millennium Institute on Immunology and Immunotherapy, Departamento de Genética Molecular y Microbiología, Facultad de Ciencias Biológicas, Pontificia Universidad Católica de Chile, Santiago, Chile

Margarita K. Lay
Departamento de Biotecnología, Facultad de Ciencias del Mar y Recursos Biológicos, Universidad de Antofagasta, Antofagasta, Chile

Claudia Riedel
Departamento de Ciencias Biológicas, Facultad de Ciencias de la Vida, Universidad Andrés Bello, Santiago, Chile

Alexis M. Kalergis
Millennium Institute on Immunology and Immunotherapy, Departamento de Genética Molecular y Microbiología, Facultad de Ciencias Biológicas, Pontificia Universidad Católica de Chile, Santiago, Chile Departamento de Endocrinología, Facultad de Medicina, Pontificia Universidad Católica de Chile, Santiago, Chile

Roberto Vázquez, Ernesto García and Pedro García
Centro de Investigaciones Biológicas (CSIC), Madrid, Spain Centro de Investigación Biomédica en Red deEnfermedades Respiratorias (CIBERES), Madrid, Spain

Petr Konečný
Centre for Environmental and Occupational Health, School of Public Health and Family Medicine, University of Cape Town, Cape Town, South Africa Division of Immunology, Department of Pathology and Institute of Infectious Disease and Molecular Medicine, Faculty of Health Sciences, University of Cape Town, Cape Town, South Africa

Rodney Ehrlich
Centre for Environmental and Occupational Health, School of Public Health and Family Medicine, University of Cape Town, Cape Town, South Africa

Mary Gulumian
National Health Laboratory Service, Department of Toxicology and Biochemistry, National Institute for Occupational Health, Johannesburg, South Africa Division of Molecular Medicine and Haematology, University of the Witwatersrand, Johannesburg, South Africa National Health Laboratory Service, Johannesburg, South Africa

Muazzam Jacobs
Division of Immunology, Department of Pathology and Institute of Infectious Disease and Molecular Medicine, Faculty of Health Sciences, University of Cape Town, Cape Town, South Africa National Health Laboratory Service, Johannesburg, South Africa Immunology of Infectious Disease Research Unit, South African Medical Research Council, Cape Town, South Africa

Luis Solans and Camille Locht
Center of Infection and Immunity of Lille, Institut Pasteur de Lille, Lille, France Inserm U1019, Lille, France CNRS UMR8204, Lille, France Center for Infection and Immunity of Lille, Univ. Lille, Lille, France

Yu-Ching Su, John Thegerström and Kristian Riesbeck
Clinical Microbiology, Department of Translational Medicine, Faculty of Medicine, Lund University, Malmö, Sweden

Farshid Jalalvand
Clinical Microbiology, Department of Translational Medicine, Faculty of Medicine, Lund University, Malmö, Sweden, Department of Biology, Centre for Bacterial Stress Response and Persistence, University of Copenhagen, Copenhagen, Denmark

Jeroen D. Langereis and Marien I. de Jonge
Section Pediatric Infectious Diseases, Laboratory of Medical Immunology, Radboud Institute for Molecular Life Sciences, Nijmegen, Netherlands Radboud Center for Infectious Diseases, Nijmegen, Netherlands

Michiel van der Flier
Section Pediatric Infectious Diseases, Laboratory of Medical Immunology, Radboud Institute for Molecular Life Sciences, Nijmegen, Netherlands Radboud Center for Infectious Diseases, Nijmegen, Netherlands Pediatric Infectious Diseases and Immunology, Amalia Children's Hospital, Nijmegen, Netherlands Expertise Center for Immunodeficiency and Autoinflammation (REIA), Radboudumc, Nijmegen, Netherlands

Elisa Ramos-Sevillano, Giuseppe Ercoli and Jeremy S. Brown
Centre for Inflammation and Tissue Repair, UCL Respiratory, London, United Kingdom

Melinda E. Varney, Dylan T. Boehm, Katherine DeRoos, Evan S. Nowak, Ting Y. Wong, Emel Sen-Kilic, Shebly D. Bradford, Cody Elkins, Matthew S. Epperly, William T. Witt, Mariette Barbier and F. Heath Damron
Department of Microbiology, Immunology, and Cell Biology, West Virginia University School of Medicine, Morgantown, WV, United States Vaccine Development Center at West Virginia University Health Sciences Center, Morgantown, WV, United States

Manuel Alcalde-Rico, Jorge Olivares-Pacheco, Carolina Alvarez-Ortega and José Luis Martínez
Centro Nacional de Biotecnología, Consejo Superior de Investigaciones Científicas, Madrid, Spain

Miguel Cámara
Centre for Biomolecular Sciences, School of Life Sciences, University of Nottingham, Nottingham, United Kingdom

Oskar Thofte, Marta Brant, Nils Littorin, Benjamin Luke Duell, Vera Alvarado
Clinical Microbiology, Department of Translational Medicine, Faculty of Medicine, Lund University, Malmö, Sweden

Hongyi Liao, Yue Gao, Shenghui Yang, Xuexue Hu, Yibing Yin and Hong Wang
Key Laboratory of Diagnostic Medicine Designated by the Ministry of Education, Chongqing Medical University, Chongqing, China School of Laboratory Medicine, Chongqing Medical University, Chongqing, China

Xiaoqiong Peng
Department of Ultrasound, The First Affiliated Hospital of Chongqing Medical University, Chongqing, China

Lingling Gan and Jiafu Feng
Department of Clinical Laboratory, Mianyang Central Hospital, Mianyang, Sichuan, China

Liping Zhang and Xiuyu Xu
Department of Laboratory Medicine, The First Affiliated Hospital of Chongqing Medical University,

Chongqing, China
Alicia Lacoma, Raquel Villar-Hernandez, Jose Domínguez, Cristina Prat and Irene Latorre

Servei de Microbiologia, Hospital Universitari Germans Trias i Pujol, Institut d'Investigació Germans Trias Pujol, Universitat Autònoma de Barcelona, CIBER Enfermedades Respiratorias, Barcelona, Spain

Lourdes Mateo
Servei de Reumatologia, Hospital Universitari Germans Trias i Pujol, Institut d'Investigació Germans Trias I Pujol, Universitat Autònoma de Barcelona, Barcelona, Spain

Ignacio Blanco
Clinical Genetics and Genetic Counseling Program, Hospital Universitari Germans Trias i Pujol, Institut d'Investigació Germans Trias i Pujol, Barcelona, Spain

Maria J. Méndez
Servei de Pediatria, Hospital Universitari Germans Trias i Pujol, Institut d'Investigació GermansTrias I

Pujol, Universitat Autònoma de Barcelona, Barcelona, Spain

Carlos Rodrigo
Servei de Pediatria, Hospital Universitari Vall d'Hebron, Vall d'Hebron Institut de Recerca, Facultat de Medicina, Unitat Docent Germans Trias I Pujol, Universitat Autònoma de Barcelona, Barcelona, Spain

Cristina Casals and Belén García-Fojeda
Centro de Investigación Biomédica en Red de Enfermedades Respiratorias (CIBERES), Instituto de Salud Carlos III, Madrid, Spain Departamento de Bioquímica y Biología Molecular, Universidad Complutense de Madrid, Madrid, Spain

María A. Campanero-Rhodes and Dolores Solís
Centro de Investigación Biomédica en Red de Enfermedades Respiratorias (CIBERES), Instituto de Salud Carlos III, Madrid, Spain Instituto de Química Física Rocasolano, CSIC, Madrid, Spain

Mirian Domenech, Julio Sempere, Sara de Miguel and Jose Yuste
Centro Nacional de Microbiología, Instituto de Salud Carlos III, Madrid, Spain
Centro de Investigación Biomédica en Red de Enfermedades Respiratorias, Madrid, Spain

Vera Marie Kroesen
Experimental Tuberculosis Unit (UTE), Fundació Institut Germans Trias i Pujol (IGTP), Universitat Autònoma de Barcelona (UAB), Badalona, Spain Carl-von-Ossietzky University Oldenburg, Oldenburg, Germany

Paula Rodríguez-Martínez, Montse Martín-Céspedes and Gustavo Tapia
Pathology Department, Hospital Universitari Germans Trias i Pujol (HUGTIP), Universitat Autònoma de Barcelona (UAB), Badalona, Spain

Eric García, Yaiza Rosales and Jorge Díaz
Experimental Tuberculosis Unit (UTE), Fundació Institut Germans Trias i Pujol (IGTP), Universitat Autònoma de Barcelona (UAB), Badalona, Spain

Maria Rosa Sarrias
Innate Immunity Group, Fundació Institut Germans Trias i Pujol (IGTP), Badalona, Spain Centro de Investigación Biomédica en Red de Enfermedades Hepáticas y Digestivas (CIBEREhD), Madrid, Spain

Pere-Joan Cardona and Cristina Vilaplana
Experimental Tuberculosis Unit (UTE), Fundació Institut Germans Trias i Pujol (IGTP), Universitat Autònoma de Barcelona (UAB), Badalona, Spain Centro de Investigación Biomédica en Red de Enfermedades Respiratorias (CIBERES), Madrid, Spain

Hisanori Domon and Yutaka Terao
Division of Microbiology and Infectious Diseases, Niigata University Graduate School of Medical and Dental Sciences, Niigata, Japan Research Center for Advanced Oral Science, Niigata University Graduate School of Medical and Dental Sciences, Niigata, Japan

Kosuke Nagai
Division of Microbiology and Infectious Diseases, Niigata University Graduate School of Medical and Dental Sciences, Niigata, Japan

Tomoki Maekawa and Hikaru Tamura
Division of Microbiology and Infectious Diseases, Niigata University Graduate School of Medical and Dental Sciences, Niigata, Japan Research Center for Advanced Oral Science, Niigata University Graduate School of Medical and Dental Sciences, Niigata, Japan Division of Periodontology, Niigata University Graduate School of Medical and Dental Sciences, Niigata, Japan

Masataka Oda
Department of Microbiology and Infection Control Sciences, Kyoto Pharmaceutical University, Kyoto, Japan

Daisuke Yonezawa
Division of Microbiology and Infectious Diseases, Niigata University Graduate School of Medical and Dental Sciences, Niigata, Japan Research Center for Advanced Oral Science, Niigata University Graduate School of Medical and Dental Sciences, Niigata, Japan Division of Oral Science for Health Promotion, Niigata University Graduate School of Medical and Dental Sciences, Niigata, Japan

Wataru Takeda
Faculty of Dentistry, Niigata University, Niigata, Japan

Takumi Hiyoshi
Division of Microbiology and Infectious Diseases, Niigata University Graduate School of Medical and Dental Sciences, Niigata, Japan Division of Periodontology, Niigata University Graduate School of Medical and Dental Sciences, Niigata, Japan

Masaya Yamaguchi and Shigetada Kawabata
Department of Oral and Molecular Microbiology, Osaka University, Graduate School of Dentistry, Osaka, Japan

Naveen Gupta
Division of Pulmonary and Critical Care, Department of Medicine, School of Medicine, University of California, San Diego, La Jolla, CA, United States Department of Molecular Medicine, The Scripps Research Institute, La Jolla, CA, United States

Victor Nizet
Division of Host-Microbe Systems and Therapeutics, Department of Pediatrics, School of Medicine, University of California, San Diego, La Jolla, CA, United States Skaggs School of Pharmacy and Pharmaceutical Sciences, School of Medicine, University of California, San Diego, La Jolla, CA, United States

Zoe González-Carnicero, Alba de Lorenzo, Lidia de Tapia, Alba Iglesias-Ceacero and Sonia Castillo-Lluva
Department of Biochemistry and Molecular Biology I, Complutense University of Madrid, Madrid, Spain

Carlos M. Minutti
Department of Biochemistry and Molecular Biology I, Complutense University of Madrid, Madrid, Spain
Centro de Investigación Biomédica en Red de Enfermedades Respiratorias (CIBERES), Instituto de Salud Carlos III, Madrid, Spain

Begoña Euba and Junkal Garmendia
Centro de Investigación Biomédica en Red de Enfermedades Respiratorias (CIBERES), Instituto de Salud Carlos III, Madrid, Spain Instituto de Agrobiotecnología, Mutilva, Spain

Index

www.ingramcontent.com/pod-product-compliance
Lightning Source LLC
LaVergne TN
LVHW082140200926
848484LV00008B/2080